Equine Pathology

Equine Pathology

JAMES R. ROONEY, DVM
JOHN L. ROBERTSON, VMD, PhD

IOWA STATE UNIVERSITY PRESS / AMES

James R. Rooney received his AB degree from Dartmouth College and his DVM from Cornell University. Dr. Rooney also has an MS degree from Virginia Polytechnic Institute and State University and an MA degree from the University of Pennsylvania. His life's work has been devoted to the study of equine species, and he is recognized worldwide as an expert in equine pathology. Dr. Rooney is a Diplomate of the American College of Veterinary Pathologists, and is retired from the University of Kentucky.

John L. Robertson received his BS degree from the State University of New York at Stony Brook and his MS, VMD, and PhD degrees from the University of Pennsylvania. Dr. Rooney was his mentor while at the University of Pennsylvania. Dr. Robertson is presently Associate Professor of Anatomic Pathology in the Department of Biomedical Sciences and Pathobiology at Virginia–Maryland Regional College of Veterinary Medicine in Blacksburg, Virginia. He has had a lifelong interest in diseases of horses and other species. His current research is in the fields of oncology and immunology.

♾ Printed on acid-free paper in the United States of America

First edition, 1996

Library of Congress Cataloging-in-Publication Data

Rooney, James, R.
Equine pathology/James R. Rooney, John L. Robertson.—1st ed.
p. cm.
Includes bibliographical references and index.
ISBN 0-8138-2334-X (alk. paper)
1. Horses—Diseases. I. Robertson, John L. II. Title
SF951.R6835 1996
636.1'089607—dc20 96-4630

Contents

Illustrations

Cardiovascular System

Respiratory System

Gastrointestinal Tract

Endocrine System

Eyes and Ears

Locomotor System, General

Fore Leg

Rear Leg

Vertebral Column

Stability and Lameness

Female Reproductive System

Neonate

Male Reproductive System

Urinary Tract

Nervous System

Shock

Hemolymphatic System

Autopsy Method

Preface

THIS BOOK is not intended to replace other texts of general or special pathology. There is little to be gained in an era of many books and rapid change by repeating what is already available on the cutting edges of molecular pathology, immunopathology, and pathological physiology. Very little work on these frontiers is available specifically for the horse, in any case, and our task is to bring to the reader what has been done and what is known about that species without too much unwarranted speculation based on studies in other species.

Acknowledgments

OUR INDEBTEDNESS to others is so extensive that another book would be required to acknowledge them. First, of all, however, we thank the librarians—the keepers of our heritage—who have done all that they should and so much more to make this possible. We, also, owe an enormous debt to a select group of horse veterinarians who, over many years, have not only provided clinical background but intelligent and penetrating analyses of pathogenesis. Our special thanks go, as well, to the publisher and editor who have been patient with us and lived up to the distinguished name of their house.

Introduction

THIS BOOK is a collection and collation of experience and literature on the pathology of the horse. Pathogenesis is emphasized in the belief that lesions are to be interpreted in terms of the natural history of disease processes. In no case is the pathogenesis complete—a fully formed and documented theory of disease process. Pathogenesis is formulated insofar as the facts permit. The hypotheses are formulated with limited data and with the certain knowledge that they are ephemeral. A quotation from Dadd (1854) is not inappropriate: "The more a man knows of physiology, the less faith has he in medicine."

Normal anatomical and physiological information has been included since so much seems lost to those acquainted only with computer databases. While one may excuse the practitioner, how can one excuse the academic? Is not one of roles of the academy to preserve and transmit the wisdom of the past? However trite, Sanatayana's thought, in paraphrase, remains true: those who forget the lessons of history are doomed to repeat them. It would be a shame to lose the designation of horse thieves in Tudor and Stuart England as "priggers of prancers."

The literature in English, German, and French has been reviewed as completely as possible. Citations have been followed into other languages, but there are undoubtedly papers that have been missed, unobtainable, or beyond our language abilities. The older Italian literature would have been fruitful, but was hardly to be found in North American libraries, and the citations were usually incorrect if the journal was found. Readers aware of missed citations will, we hope, let us know of them. The translations, whether our own or by others, may be problematic in any given case, and we would appreciate kindly corrections and emendations. As has been truly said, translations are never really finished, they are abandoned. That is as true of citations from the English as other languages.

One cannot help the fascination of references to common, present-day problems of horses well known to the Greeks and earlier peoples long before the common era. Herbal prescriptions for horses existed as early as 1380 BCE, Gordon (1942). Where possible, entry citations have been made to that ancient, rich, and difficult to obtain, literature. We use the terms BCE, before the common era, instead of BC, before Christ, and CE for the common era rather than AD, anno Domini.

Although avoiding, whenever possible, citing what someone else has cited, obtaining original papers has sometimes been difficult or impossible. Hutyra and Marek (1920, 1926) and other old texts have been invaluable, but their references are usually incomplete and almost impossible to find. The older French literature is a gold mine of original case reports, Lyon after all being the first veterinary school in the world. Access to that literature has, however, been difficult, and we have been fortunate to have the remarkable series of texts by Cadeac, which cover French, German, Italian, English, and American literature.

Often, material from older editions of books has been used, newer not necessarily being better. Sometimes material in French or German texts has been extensively and carefully cited in an English text, for example, Colin (1886/88) in Smith (1917). Both texts were consulted and are cited.

Gross illustrations have been emphasized since it is in the gross lesion that the individuality of horse pathology is most apparent. As magnification increases species differences become less and less obvious, eventually to disappear altogether. More illustrations would obviously be desirable, but simply could not be done for this edition.

The lack of the biochemical, molecular, and ultrastructural aspects of pathogenesis is obvious, indicating the lack of such information in the literature and not lack of interest.

Insofar as possible we have followed the dictates of *Nomina Anatomica Veterinaria* (1983), at least indicating the preferred names even if continuing to use the names of our choice. It is usual to refer to joint movements as flexion and extension, but we find this incoherent with the digital joints and prefer to use the terms: *dorsiflexion* instead of extension and *palmarflexion* or *plantarflexion* instead of flexion. Similarly, we use dorsiflexion and ventroflexion for the movements of the vertebral column (Sisson and Grossman 1953).

It is unfortunate that medicine has taken a number of terms from mechanics and twisted them into tenuous new byways. We shall not do so: stress, strain, and displacement belong to mechanics and shall remain there. Tendons undergo strain and that is normal, the amount of elongation divided by the original length. When the strain is too great, tendons *tear*. Stress is the resistance to applied force. While Hans Selye brought much good to theoretical medicine, he did but harm with the word, *stress*. We shall usually use, *duress*. *Sprain* is a meaningless word and totally undefined in veterinary medicine. We shall use virtually no acronyms; if the word is appropriate, we shall use it. If an acronym seems necessary, we shall find another word. English is difficult enough without rendering it in code. Eponyms do not daunt us and will be used in the absence of more descriptive or etiological terms.

Breed designations, particularly in the older European literature, can be confusing. The *full blood* is certainly the Thoroughbred. Draft breeds may be given regional names or be referred to as *heavy* or *draft*. *Half bloods* are usually, but not invariably, crosses between Thoroughbred and draft animals. *Warm blood* seems to apply generally to animals of mixed breeding, often with the name of the region in which they originated or are indigenous. The Westphalian and Holsteiner, for example, are Warm bloods with regional names. Because of continued selection within a region, some "breeds" have become phenotypically distinct. Blood typing may eventually establish genotypic distinctiveness.

The Warm blood situation is not unlike the Standardbred, which was developed from the Thoroughbred with admixtures of many other breeds. With the closing of the stud book the Standardbred became, by definition, a distinct breed. The Warm blood has parallels with the American Quarter horse, as well, an animal of varying Thoroughbred and western horse admixtures. The western horse, in turn, is a mixture, though basically of Spanish origin. The phenotype is reasonably clear while the genotype awaits definition. Perhaps one might avoid the semantic difficulties and revert to the Latin of Albert the Great (1987): *dextrarii* = war horses, *palefridi* = palfrey, riding horse, *currili equi* = racehorse (chariot horse), *runcini* = work horse, plow horse.

Since this book is about the horse, a quotation from Smith (1917) is appropriate, albeit nonpathological, concerning the "psychical function" of the horse:

> As a rule the intelligence and affection of the horse only exist in books and the imagination of those who have the least to do with him; whatever region of the brain affection is located in, it does not occupy much space in the equine. ... If the horse possesses but little affection it is compensated for by cherishing no resentment; he will kick his friend as readily as a foe, or, in many cases, his groom with as much cheerfulness as a perfect stranger; to all his hard life and the abominable cruelties of domestication he shows no sign of resentment; water and feed him, and give him a place to lie in, and he forgets the past in his anxiety for the present. ... The horse is very conservative, he likes nothing new or any departure from his ordinary mode of life. ... His gregarious instincts are proverbial; he frets at the absence of his companions, and if used to work amongst a body of horses, as in cavalry, he will take any degree of punishment rather than leave them for five minutes. During the absence of his companions he neighs, sweats, paws with the fore-legs, and almost screams with delight on rejoining them, not because he loves them, but because he dislikes being alone.

The interacting role of genetics and environment, nature and nurture, in disease processes is well known, if often ignored. At any given point in this book we may appear inattentive to this interaction, but we are not. Only our lack of knowledge might make it appear so. Cantharidin requires no genetic assistance to damage the urinary tract, and the defective genes of Arabian combined immunodeficiency need no environmental assistance. Often the distinction is not so clear.

Cadeac (1909):

Assuredly, heredity does not transmit the lesion itself to the descendants; but it assures the transmission of the architectural terrain, physical and chemical, which assures its development.

Disease incidence

Only limited data is available on the frequency of disease in the modern horse. Case compilations usually emphasize medicine and surgery at the expense of data useful for the study of etiology and pathogenesis. Indeed, there is a singular lack of demographic data for horses, incidence of disease being expressed in terms of hospital or postmortem room populations, a parlous situation.

Bartke in *Bayer-Fröhner* (1900) provided a wealth of information on the frequency of disease in horses of the Prussian army. The number of horses in that population was not given, but probably averaged about 100,000, including cavalry and artillery horses, in any given year between 1886 and 1895, according to data in *Deutsche Reich* (1903). (We are indebted to Prof. James Albisetti, University of Kentucky, for this reference.) There were 278,323 sick horses during the 10-year period, or about 27,832 horses per year. Of that number 94.6% recovered, 1.3% were turned out or disposed of, 3.3% died, and 0.9% were killed (figures rounded). About 27% of the horses were on sick call in any given year.

Frequency by organ system [data from *Bayer-Fröhner* (1990)]:

locomotor	52.2%
skin	29.8
foot	12.7
eye	3.4
nervous system	0.5
cardiovascular	0.2
respiratory	0.2
urinary	0.2
ear	0.06
gastrointestinal	0.8 (11.0)

Gastrointestinal disease, at 0.8%, includes only cases considered surgically manageable by the methods of the time. Colics were not so considered, and a figure of 11% for the frequency of colic is undoubtedly more nearly correct and, so, included in parentheses (Dobberstein and Dinter 1942). These were working-age horses in heavy training, during peacetime, and with good care. Reproductive problems were irrelevant as were diseases of foals.

Jeffcott et al. (1982) provided similar data for 314 Thoroughbred horses in six racing stables in Newmarket, England, for 1 year. A one-to-one comparison cannot be made, but it was apparent that locomotor, skin, and gastrointestinal problems retained pride of place in the English horses. The one significant difference was a high rate of respiratory disease in the English as compared to the Prussian horses. The majority of the English horses were 2- and 3-year-olds while the Prussian horses were probably older, and it is well known that young horses experience more problems.

Equine Pathology

CHAPTER 1

Cardiovascular System

- Normal cardiovascular anatomy and physiology
  - Fenestration of valves
  - Ring-form lymphatic vessels
  - Asteroid bodies
- Incidence of cardiovascular pathology
  - Valvular lesions
  - Jet lesions
  - Myocardial lesions
  - Aortic lesions
- Sudden death
  - Cardiac rupture
  - Rupture of the aorta
  - Rupture of the pulmonary artery
- Inflammatory cardiovascular diseases
  - Viral diseases
  - Bacterial diseases
  - Fungal diseases
  - Parasitic diseases
  - Thrombosis of the jugular veins
  - Unknown
- Congenital and developmental cardiovascular disease
  - Aging changes
  - Endarteritis
  - Congenital defects
- Cardiovascular disease related to nutrition
- Rhythm abnormalities
  - Atrial fibrillation
  - Idioventricular tachycardia
  - Sinoatrial block
  - Second-degree atrioventricular block
  - Wandering pacemaker
  - Multiple atrial dysrhythmias
- Toxic cardiovascular disease
  - Phenylbutazone
  - Cantharidin
- Neoplasia
  - Lymphosarcoma
  - Lipoma
  - Mesothelioma
  - Hemangiosarcoma
- Cardiovascular diseases with unclassified etiology
  - Hypertension
  - Myocardial necrosis
  - Right atrial ossification

Cardiovascular disease seriously interferes with the ability to perform work and, so, is of great economic importance. Common signs of cardiovascular dysfunction include tiring, dyspnea, poor performance, organ dysfunction related to decreased perfusion, and sudden death (Bonagura 1985). Cardiovascular, respiratory, and musculoskeletal diseases are primary causes of poor performance. In a survey of 480 autopsies in Liverpool between 1958 and 1980, cardiovascular disease was fourth as cause of death, following diseases of the alimentary tract, locomotor, and nervous system (Baker and Ellis 1981).

Normal cardiovascular anatomy and physiology

There is a considerable literature on normal equine cardiovascular anatomy and physiology. Many early investigations of normal heart function and dysfunction were with horses. Aristotle described the *os cordis* (Peck 1979). Hales (1733) cited by Detweiler et al. (1972) measured arterial blood pressure in horses. German and French investigators in the 1800s used horses in determining the origin of heart sounds (Detweiler et al. 1972). In the early 1900s MacKenzie and Lewis used naturally occurring and induced atrial fibrillation in horses to clarify the nature of the disease in humans (Hoff et al. 1966). Roos (1928) cited by Hoff et al. (1966) studied atrial fibrillation in domestic animals, including horses and dogs. With primitive equipment, these early investigators determined the basic components of the equine electrocardiogram. They described the relative insensitivity of the atrioventricular node in rapid transmission of atrial depolarization and relationships between electrical activity and pulse pressure. Studies since that time have further defined equine cardiovascular function (Fregin 1982).

Physiological murmurs and cardiac arrhythmias are not uncommon in foals, yearlings, and adult horses and, often, do not have pathological significance (Hilwig 1977; Holmes 1977). Murmurs may occur in anemic horses and in otherwise normal animals during or shortly after exercise. Else and Holmes (1972) found murmurs in 27 horses without cardiac valvular lesions on postmortem examination. They found murmurs correlated with valvular lesions in 195 of 1557 horses. Reef (1985) found murmurs of patent ductus arteriosus through the first 4 days of life in many normal foals. She also noted the volatility of the heart rate in neonates.

Steel (1963) cited in Fregin (1982) made extensive observations on the normal electrocardiogram of Australian racehorses. Fregin (1982) reported that about 25% of horses have cardiac arrhythmias without signs of cardiac disease. Brown (1985), in a review of acquired cardiovascular disease based on the work of Else and Holmes (1972a,b,c,d), questioned the value of electrocardiography and auscultation in detecting and assessing murmurs and arrhythmias. Brown specifically questioned if electrocardiographic impulses on the body surface accurately represented cardiac electrical events.

Ventricular fibrillation is induced by, *inter alia*, electrical shock and cannot be reversed as it can in humans and smaller animals.

Gross evaluation of the status of the heart muscle, dilatation, and hypertrophy/hyperplasia, is fraught with the difficulties of antemortem and postmortem changes and *rigor mortis*. In general, heart muscle is in diastole immediately after death. Systolic contraction occurs rarely and only in special cases such as digitalis toxicity. Normal left ventricular firmness does not, alone, indicate systolic contraction.

The heart muscle usually enters rigor within 30 minutes to 1–2 hours after death and may disappear within 12–24 hours. Rigor disappears rapidly from the right ventricle, which invariably contains blood. Rigor disappears more slowly from the left ventricle, and blood will not be present unless there has been antemortem dilatation of cardiac disease or, more commonly, rigor has disappeared, allowing postmortem flow of bloody fluid into the ventricle. Putative hypertrophy/hyperplasia and/or dilatations of pathological significance must be supported by clinical and histological findings.

Fenestration of valves

Mahaffey (1958) described fenestration of the aortic and pulmonic valve cusps in 22 normal horses between 8 months of fetal life and 22 years. Delicate perforations and fenestrations occurred on the edges of one or more valve cusps (Fig. 1.1). Mahaffey speculated that these "lesions" did not cause valvular incompetence unless the fenestrae extended far into the leaflet or if the fenestrae of several valves overlapped, leaving a defect through which blood could regurgitate. These fenestrae are common and even more common as an artifact after even reasonably gentle handling. No clinical correlations have confirmed Mahaffey's speculations.

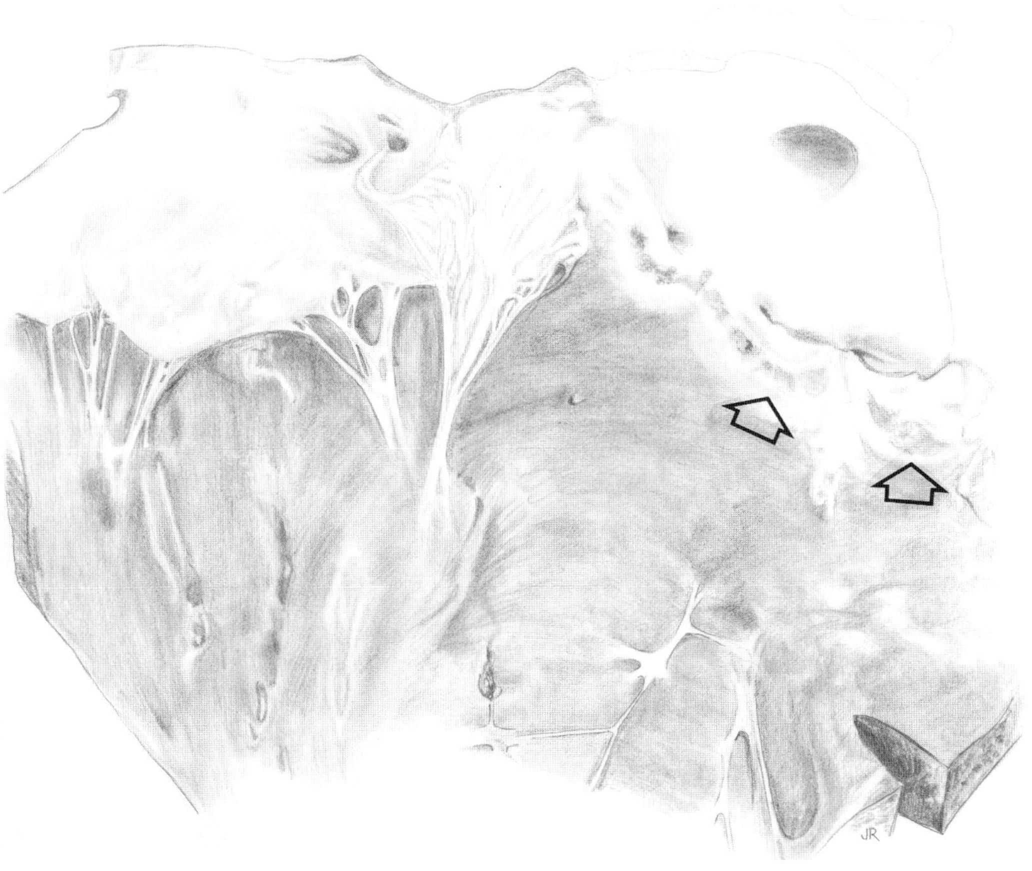

1.1. Fenestrations on valve cusps of semilunar valves (*arrows*).

Ring-form lymphatic vessels

Ring-form lymphatic vessels are not uncommon beneath the epicardium and have no pathological significance.

Asteroid bodies

Subendothelial deposits of partially mineralized material, asteroid or intimal bodies, are found in the blood vessels of horses of all ages (Fig. 1.2). Montali et al. (1970) studied the histochemical and electron microscopic appearance of these bodies in horses from 8 days to over 20 years of age. These bodies were common in the small arteries at all ages and more common in the gastrointestinal tract. We have not seen them in the fetus.

The cause of these bodies and their predilection for the horse is not known. Bollinger (1869) believed them to be related to *S. vulgaris* migrations while Montali et al. did not find evidence for such a cause. See also, Chapter 3, "Gastrointestinal Tract and Adnexa."

Incidence of cardiovascular pathology

Else and Holmes (1972a,b,c,d) surveyed cardiac lesions in 1557 English abattoir horses and reviewed the literature on equine cardiac pathology. They

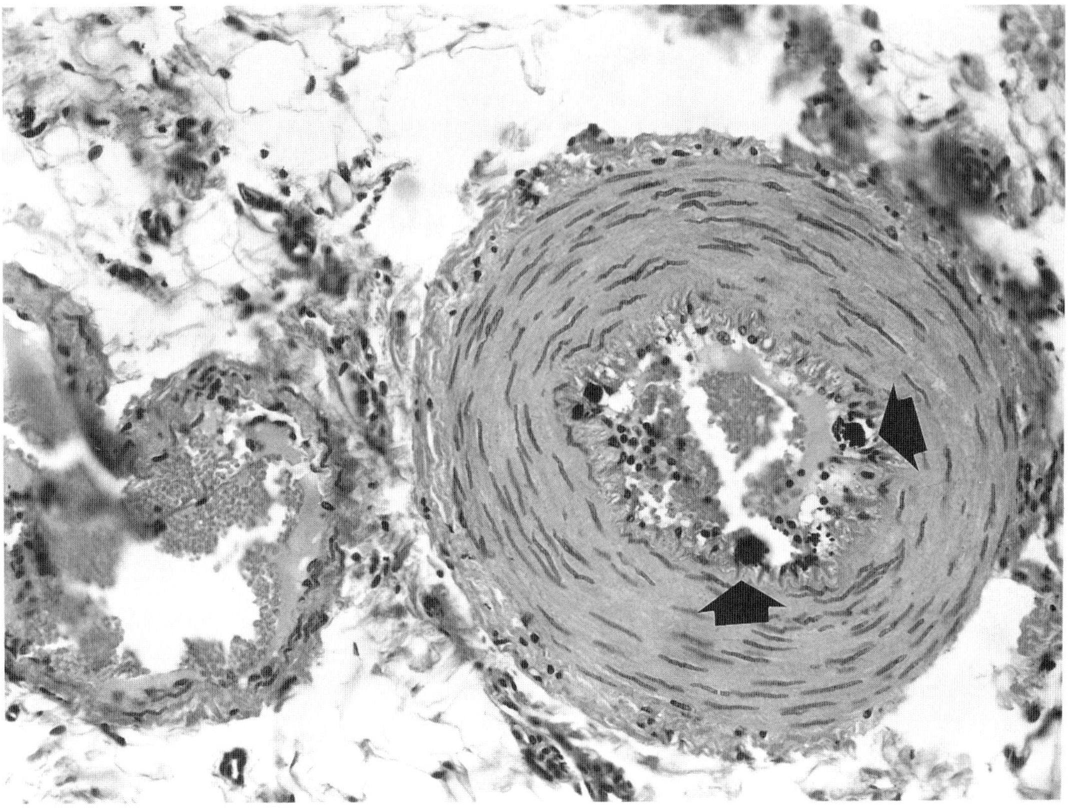

1.2. Several intimal bodies (*arrows*) in a small muscular artery in cecal submucosa.

attempted to correlate antemortem auscultation and postmortem lesions. No antemortem disease histories were available.

The animals ranged from a few months to over 20 years of age. There were Thoroughbreds, hunters, draft horses, and ponies. Gross cardiac and vascular lesions were present in 439 of 1557; valvular lesions were most frequent, occurring in 338 of 447; 91 horses had nonvalvular lesions; and 10 had both valvular and nonvalvular lesions. Lesions were more common and more severe on the left side.

Valvular lesions

Valvular lesions were commonest in the aortic valve, followed by the left atrioventricular, right atrioventricular, and pulmonary valves. The frequency of lesions increased with age. By 10 years, about 8% of the horses had lesions of the atrioventricular valves. Lesions in the semilunar valves were common in all age groups and a significant number were in horses 5 years old or less.

The incidence of **aortic valve lesions** [data from Else and Holmes (1972a)] was:

Horses with aortic valve lesions	311/1557
Cusps with lesions	641/933
Valve cusp nodules (of cusps with lesions)	59.7%
Valve cusp plaques	21.8%
Valve cusp fibrous bands	14.8%
Distortions of shape	3.6%

The nodules were simple, single thickenings of the valve cusps, large and eroded lesions, or mixtures. Fenestrations of valve cusps were as frequent as reported by Mahaffey (1958). There were few lesions (13/1557) of the **pulmonary valve** leaflets, most being fenestrations or nodules on cusps.

Lesions of the **left atrioventricular valve** were 2–3 times more common than of the right atrioventricular valve. Thickening of the free margin of valve cusps, minute fibrous nodules or "beads," thickened insertion points, and valve cusp nodules were the commonest lesions of both valves. Else and Holmes found only 2 cases of vegetative endocarditis in 1557 horses. The frequency of clinical and/or lethal endocarditis is very low.

The incidence of atrioventricular lesions [data from Else and Holmes (1972a)] was:

AV valve lesions	220/1557
Valve thickening	36.8%
(of horses with AV lesions)	
Valve beading	19.5%
Valve nodules	17.7%
Thick insertions	10.5%
Thick border	9.5%
Other lesions	6.0%

Many of the valvular lesions consisted of variable accumulations of fibroblasts and collagenous tissue, a mixture of inflammatory cells, and tissue tags such as villous papillary projections from the borders of valve leaflets. Diastolic and systolic murmurs were correlated with the presence of mitral, tricuspid, and aortic valve lesions or aortic stenosis in 74 horses. Some of these valvular lesions are aging changes of minor or no clinical significance.

Jet lesions

Jet lesions, discrete foci of endocardial fibrosis caused by continuous turbulent blood flow, were found in 27 of 1557 horses (Fig. 1.3).

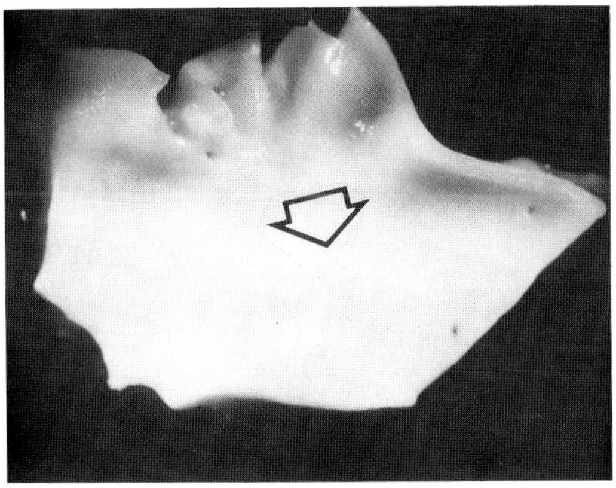

1.3. A jet lesion in an artery (*arrow*) consists of endothelial thickening due to turbulent blood flow.

Myocardial lesions

Myocardial lesions were found in 33 of 1557 hearts. Approximately 60% of horses over 20 years old had endocardial thickening and fibrosis at the left ventricular apex. In a few horses with presumed healed infarcts, myocardium was replaced with fibrous connective tissue.

Aortic lesions

Nodular or fibrotic aortic lesions were found in 83 of 1557 horses. Else and Holmes (1972a) attributed most of these lesions to migration of strongyle larvae. In many cases, the intima and collagenous matrix of the aortic wall was disrupted and infiltrated with eosinophils and lymphocytes with occasional foci of dystrophic mineralization.

Cadiot (1893) cited by Cadeac (1897a) reported strongyle thromboses in the coronary arteries. While coronary thrombosis certainly can cause myocardial infarction, this is extremely rare in the horse, whether caused by strongyle larvae or otherwise.

Baker and Ellis (1981a,b) found cardiovascular disease the fourth commonest cause of death: 8.5% of horses died of cardiovascular disease. The commonest lesions were verminous aneurysm of the mesenteric arteries (34.1% of total cardiovascular deaths), hemorrhage (31.7%), and cardiac arrest during anaesthesia or exercise (12.2%). They found lesions of the cardiovascular system not directly related to the cause of death in about 44% of horses. Most of these lesions were caused by *S. vulgaris* migration.

Sudden death

Cardiac rupture

For many years, unexpected deaths in foals and horses have been attributed to cardiovascular catastrophes. Leonhardt (1923) described cardiac rupture in Prussian army horses. Among 80,000–142,000 horses, he found 52 cases of cardiac rupture over a 19-year period. The location of the ruptures in 34 cases was: right ventricle, 15; left ventricle, 3; right atrium, 7; left atrium, 8; and rupture of the interventricular septum, 1.

Platt (1982) reviewed postmortem data of 69 foals and horses that died unexpectedly. All were autopsied soon after death. Twenty-four died suddenly, under observation, generally within a few minutes of exercise. Of these, 13 had lesions of the cardiovascular system considered the cause of death, including valvular lesions, ruptured blood vessels, or hemorrhage from unspecified sources. In 8 others, dying unexpectedly during or shortly after exercise, no significant lesions were found. A second group of horses and foals were found dead with no antemortem indication of illness. Seven died of cardiovascular lesions, including 4 brood mares that bled from the uterine artery. In a third group of horses, 6 of 17 other unexpected deaths were related to valvular endocarditis.

Cardiac lesions in sudden death in 10 racehorses was reported by Kiryu et al. (1987). Eight of 10 had no history of heart disease; 2 had either ventricular premature contractions or second-degree atrioventricular block. Eight of the 10 died immediately after or within hours of training; 2 died unobserved in their stalls at night. Seven of 8 died rapidly—collapsing, sweating, and in severe respiratory distress.

Gross lesions were found in the atria of 8 of 10 horses, primarily focal areas of myocardial ischemia and discoloration ranging from 0.5 cm to 4 cm diameter. Congestion of the viscera and massive subpleural ecchymotic hemorrhages were present in all 10 horses.

Microscopically, there was myocardial ischemia and fibrosis in the atria and in the atrioventricular junction. Foci of ischemia, necrosis, and fibrosis were found near the sinoatrial node, and sclerotic vascular changes were described in feeder arteries to the sinoatrial node. No lesions of strongyle migration were detected. No data were given for the frequency of any of these lesions in horses not dying suddenly, and the relevance of the lesions to the death of the animals is problematic. Indeed, sclerosis (endarteritis) is not uncommon in the coronary arteries and is unrelated to clinical disease.

Rupture of the aorta

There are two types of rupture of the aorta that usually, but not invariably, cause sudden death. The first is a rupture just distal to the aortic valves, causing death by cardiac tamponade (Cohrs 1961). Rupture of the aorta was apparently more common in middle-aged animals and particularly during prolonged transport. It is uncommon, in our experience, in the modern era.

The second type of rupture of the aorta was described by Rooney et al. (1967) as a cause of sudden death in stallions during or following breeding, particularly early in the breeding season. There is rupture of the aortic ring just at the junction of aorta and left ventricle. The tear is behind the aortic valve leaflet and easily overlooked (Fig. 1.4). Death, usually sudden, is related to massive bleeding into the region of the atrioventricular bundle. Some horses may survive for a time with signs of progressive right heart dilatation and failure. At postmortem there is a **cardioaortic fistula**, blood flowing from the rupture site through a fistula into the right ventricle. In a few animals, surviving for some weeks, vegetative endocarditis developed on the right atrioventricular valve, an otherwise unusual site.

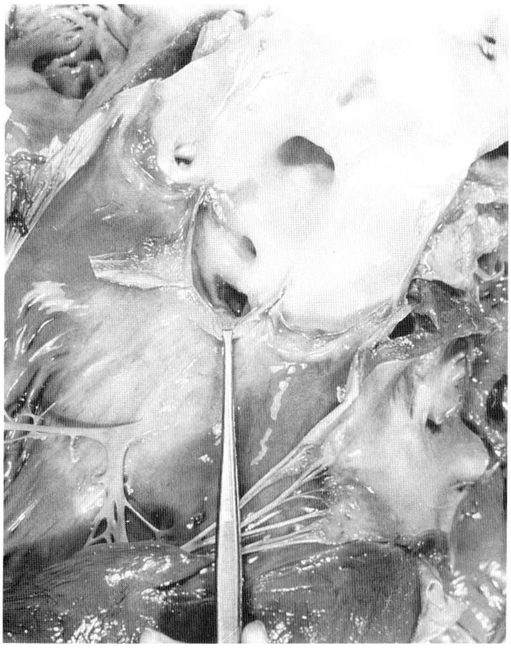

1.4. Rupture at the base of the aorta may be overlooked without meticulous examination of valve cusps; from a horse that died suddenly.

These ruptures were attributed to the force of recoil of the column of ejected blood at the end of systole with aortic valve closure, anatomic and mechanical demands on the aortic ring, age-related degenerative changes, and the increased blood pressure of breeding activities.

Rupture of the pulmonary artery

Rooney (1979a) described death in mares from rupture of the uterine, ovarian, or external iliac artery. See Chapter 11, "Female Reproductive System." An occasional rupture of the pulmonary artery has been seen in young foals, but rarely in older horses. The ruptures were so extensive that histological search for predisposing lesions was fruitless. Either **atrium** may be ruptured in dead, neonatal foals. Usually there is no hemorrhage in the torn edges, showing that the rupture was postmortem and the probable result of delivery of an already asphyxiated foal through an incompletely dilated cervical canal.

Inflammatory cardiovascular diseases

Viral diseases

Equine viral arteritis

Equine viral arteritis was reported in the United States in 1957 by Doll et al. The disease had been described in Europe since the 1800s under a variety of names, for example, pferdestaupe, grippe, influenza, typhoid fever, and pinkeye (Hutyra and Marek 1920). Zuill (1894) indicated that it may have been seen earlier than 1796. Clinical descriptions of epizootics among horses in Rome in 1301 and 1313 and even earlier suggest the disease.

Viral arteritis is spread by direct contact of infected and noninfected individuals, on fomites, by aerosols, and through coitus (Crawford and Henson 1972; Timoney and McCollum 1987a; Huntington et al. 1990). As early as 1885 it had been shown that recovered and apparently healthy stallions could infect mares by breeding. The disease was transmitted to mares by intravenous and subcutaneous injection of sperm from such stallions. Stallions were known to be infectious for 1–6 1/2 years after recovering from the disease (Hutyra and Marek 1920). The virus was first isolated by Doll et al. (1957a) from material collected in an epizootic abortion storm in Ohio. The virus is an RNA togavirus, the only member of the Arterivirus group of the Togaviradae. Related viruses in the togavirus group include hog cholera and bovine viral diarrhea (Mumford 1985). An effective modified live virus vaccine was developed by Doll and is available commercially (Timoney 1987b).

Viral arteritis is an epizootic disease with high morbidity and low mortality, the greatest danger being abortion of mares pregnant at the time of exposure and clinical disease. The epidemiology of the disease is still not completely clear, though it is apparent from the early studies, confirmed and extended by Timoney et al. (1987a,b,c), that the persistently infected carrier stallion plays a major role. Experimental studies have shown that almost 2 of 3 infected stallions become long-term carriers. No decrease in fertility has been observed in infected stallions, and a carrier state has not been demonstrated in mares (Timoney et al. 1987a).

There is serological evidence of the disease in many countries, but clinical disease is infrequent (McCollum et al. 1971; Huntington et al. 1990). Studies by McCollum et al. (1985) suggest that certain strains of the virus are more likely to cause clinical disease. Several investigators state that viral arteritis is more common in Standardbred and Thoroughbred horses, but outbreaks have been seen in other breeds and controlled epidemiological studies are needed (Godnik et al. 1981; Huntington et al. 1990).

The clinical signs and gross pathology have been known for many years (Hutyra and Marek 1920). Jones et al. (1957) added the histopathology, and Estes and Cheville (1970) elegantly described the ultrastructure of the vascular lesions.

Subclinical infections are common. McCollum and Bryans (1973) and Timoney et al. (1987b) estimated the ratio of clinical to subclinical cases at 1:4 to 1:6. In many animals, the disease is only detectable by seroconversion. The acute clinical picture is dominated by fever, inappetence, and depression 3–7 days after infection. The conjunctivae are characteristically reddened and edematous with multiple fine petechiae. Subcutaneous edema of the limbs and the ventral body wall is characteristic. Most animals recover uneventfully within a week to 2 weeks.

Pregnant mares abort during the course of the clinical illness as the result of arteritis and ischemia causing placental separation (Coignoul and Cheville 1984). Cole et al. (1986) reported a 71% rate of abortion in experimental infections. Higher and lower rates have been seen in natural outbreaks and in other experiments, depending upon the amount of viral inoculum.

The basic lesions are edema, hyperemia, and hemorrhage of various organs and tissues caused by necrotizing vasculitis of small muscular arteries and degeneration of endothelium of capillaries and venules (Jones et al. 1957; Crawford and Henson 1972). Studies in horses exposed by the respiratory route have shown that the virus first propagates in reticuloendothelial cells and endothelium in the lung for 1–5 days, after which there is generalized infection of endothelial cells throughout the body (Crawford and Henson 1972). Viral replication in regional lymph nodes occurred within 1–3 days of exposure. By day 4 viral replication was found in the epithelium of various organs. Edema surrounding thin-walled blood vessels was noted by day 5, and endothelial pyknosis, karyolysis, and proliferation was seen (Estes and Cheville 1970). Perivascular and perilymphatic neutrophil and lymphocyte infiltration appeared at this time.

Lesions of small muscular arteries became prominent 6–10 days following infection, several days after the appearance of endothelial damage and leakage from thin-walled vessels. Clinical disease is most evident while vascular lesions are widespread in venules and capillaries, 6–8 days following infection. Virus disappears from endothelial and epithelial cells after about 14 days. In one study vascular lesions were not detectable after 60 days (Crawford and Henson 1972).

Characteristic gross lesions are found in the gastrointestinal tract. There is intense segmental hyperemia and edema of the mucosa and submucosa of the small intestine. Submucosal edema is most apparent in the ventral colon and the apical portion of the cecum. There is marked edema of the neurovascular complexes of the large intestine and intense hyperemia and hemorrhage of the mucosa when there is diarrhea.

Hyperemia and multiple petechiae are present throughout the respiratory system. The lungs may be heavier than normal with edema of the subpleural and interlobular connective tissue interspersed with areas of emphysema. Petechiae and edema are present in the coronary grooves together with variably severe subendocardial hemorrhage.

The spleen is either normal or enlarged and congested. Small hemorrhagic infarcts occur, and there is depletion of lymphoid elements in germinal centers and in lymph nodes (Estes and Cheville 1970). The kidneys are pale with marked perirenal edema. Lymph nodes, particularly mediastinal and mesenteric, are edematous.

Specific histological changes variably reflect the gross changes in most organs and tissues. The changes are seen in arteries with a well-developed media, 0.5 mm in diameter or slightly larger, and in thin-walled vessels as noted. Lesions vary in size and shape and are distributed at irregular intervals along the arteries. They involve quadrants of the arteries, concentric outer media, or the entire media. There is necrosis of smooth muscle cells characterized by loss of nuclei and replacement of cytoplasm by homogeneous, eosinophilic, fibrinoid material. There is edema and infiltration of a few leukocytes in the early lesions, and the adventitia and media are infiltrated by lymphoid cells.

Crawford and Henson (1972) suggested that the vascular lesions were not directly caused by viral infection, but by the action of neutrophils and neutrophilic enzymes and inflammatory mediators. Estes and Cheville (1970) considered the arterial lesions anoxic, secondary to necrosis of endothelium and microthrombosis of the vasa vasorum. The role of viral-antibody immune complexes as mediators of the inflammatory response has not been addressed.

Edema, congestion, and hemorrhage accompany these changes in all tissues, together with necrosis of lymphocytes in the lymph nodes and spleen and focal infarction of the mucosa of the intestine and lung.

No specific gross or microscopic lesions are present in aborted fetuses despite the presence of large quantities of virus. Doll et al. (1957b) reported petechial hemorrhages on the pleural and peritoneal surfaces of aborted fetuses, and pulmonary and mediastinal edema. Cole et al. (1986) found few such lesions, and they are, in fact, nonspecific asphyxial changes. Johnson et al. (1991) found lymphoplasmacytic perivascular cuffing of vessels in the brain, foci of mixed inflammatory cells in the liver as well as foci of hepatic necrosis and arteritis, and necrosis of splenic lymphoid nodules in two freshly aborted fetuses. Necrotizing arteritis of the placenta was seen in one case. These findings are idiosyncratic and unconfirmed. In natural outbreaks, the fetus is usually decomposed, in contrast to the fresh condition of most herpesvirus (EHV)-1 abortions. Abortion may occur at any time and is directly related to clinical disease of the mare.

Equine infectious anemia

Cadeac (1897a) noted that there were a few nonspecific lesions seen in the hearts of horses with equine infectious anemia. In acute cases, there may be swelling and vacuolization of myocardial fibers, and round cell infiltration, particularly in the left ventricular myocardium. In chronic cases, round cell infiltration may be so extensive as to be visible grossly, especially in the left atrium.

Bacterial diseases

Myocarditis

Focal acute and chronic inflammatory lesions of the myocardium are not uncommon in horses. Cadeac (1897b) reported that acute interstitial myocarditis was associated with a variety of infectious diseases, including strangles. Focal lesions are found with strangles and influenza and incidentally at postmortem in the absence of relevant history. The lesions appear always to be secondary, there being no evidence for primary myocarditis in the horse. Rubarth (1943) reported sudden death of five horses with chronic pharyngitis and myocarditis associated with strangles infections.

The myocardium may be involved in metastatic septic processes, but this is not as common as in the kidney and in the liver. The association of myocardial inflammation and atrial fibrillation is discussed below.

Endocarditis

Endocarditis is uncommon in horses. There are single case reports of infection with *Streptococcus equi* (Detweiler et al. 1972), *Actinobacillus* (Shigella) *equuli* (Innes et al. 1949), and fungi (Peet et al. 1981). Winqvist (1945), in a seminal study, found *S. zooepidemicus* to be the commonest pathogen, according with our experience.

In the studies reviewed below, no consideration was given to aging changes of valves. The heart valves of horses do undergo gradual fibrosis and minor nodule formation together with some distortion with advancing age, and these are to be considered, or at least annotated, whenever valvular lesions are being evaluated.

Six cases reviewed by Buergelt et al. (1985) were in horses from 3 months to 14 years of age; 4 were 2 years old or less. Two of the 6 had signs of cardiac disease by auscultation and echocardiography. Endocarditis was found at postmortem in 4 others killed for noncardiac problems. Five horses had valvular vegetations and 1 had thrombi on the chordae tendinae. Vegetations were commonest on mitral valves. Valvular lesions consisted of roughened or disrupted endothelium, fibrovascular proliferations, fibrin strands, and infiltration with mixed populations of inflammatory cells. Gram-negative rods were seen in the vegetations of 2 horses, but were not cultured. In one case, the yeast, *Candida parapsilosis*, was identified by morphological characteristics of the pseudohyphae and growth in differential culture media.

Dobin (1968) found two types of endocarditis among 78 cases: ulcerating septic endocarditis and chronic fibrosing endocarditis. Lesions were found on the aortic valve in 22 cases of ulcerating septic endocarditis (Fig. 1.5). In 13 there was septicemia or pyemia. In 4 cases the horses had concurrent bronchopneumonia while others had purulent rhinitis or lymphangitis. Valve deformation and dysfunction were common. As in the cases reported by Buergelt et al. (1985), valvular lesions consisted of endothelial roughening, leukocytic infiltration, proliferation of fibrovascular aggregates, and foci of necrosis. Masses of bacteria were identified but not isolated. Dobin considered 47 cases of chronic fibrosing endocarditis to be caused by migration of strongyle larvae, a highly unlikely if not fantastic interpretation.

Collatos et al. (1990) described atrial myocardial enlargement, atrial fibrillation, and a mass in the wall of the left atrium of a 70-day-old Thoroughbred colt with septic arthropathy. Episodes of cardiac enlargement and fibrillation eventually resolved with aggressive medical therapy. *Rhodococcus equi* was cultured from an infected metatarsophalangeal joint.

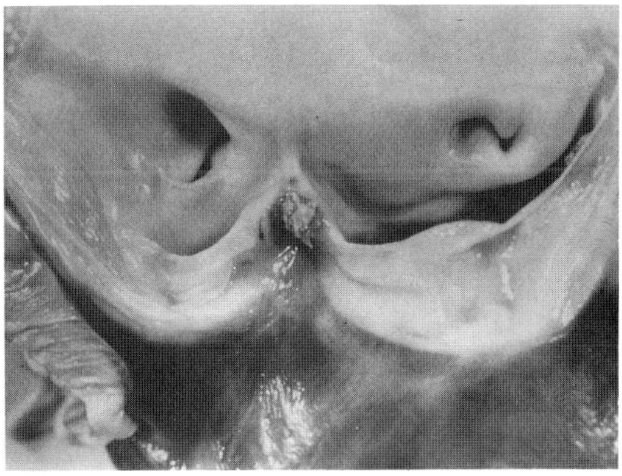

1.5. A focus of vegetative endocarditis between the cusps of the aortic valve.

Pericarditis

Fibrinous or eosinophilic pericarditis is uncommon. Reviews have been published (Dill et al. 1982; Freestone et al. 1987; Bernard et al. 1990; Robinson et al. 1992). An association of arthritis and pericarditis in Tasmanian horses was reported in the mid-1940s (Ryan and Ramey 1945). We have seen a case in an 18-month-old Percheron gelding (Robertson 1993).

There is a constellation of clinical signs including exercise intolerance, anorexia, dyspnea, congested or cyanotic mucous membranes, ascites, and subcutaneous edema. Several animals died of cardiac tamponade caused by pericardial and epicardial constriction. Animals with fibrinous pericarditis may have muffled heart sounds, nonspecific low amplitude complexes on electrocardiography, and jugular pulses. Conventional radiography and ultrasonography have shown enlargement of the cardiac shadow, dorsal tracheal displacement, and compression of the lung.

Gross pathological changes can be spectacular. After 1 week of increasing dyspnea, ascites, and pectoral edema, the Percheron gelding died suddenly. At autopsy 25 liters of ascitic fluid and 15 liters of pericardial fluid were collected. There was marked edema of the mesentery. Similar changes were reported by Dill et al. (1982) in four cases. The pericardial sac was enlarged and occupied half of the thoracic cavity and the pericardium was thickened and opaque. The epicardium was covered with a layer of fibrin 2-cm thick. There was pulmonary congestion and edema.

Fungal diseases

In a single case of **fungal myocarditis and nephritis** reported by Peet et al. (1981), a 4-year-old Thoroughbred had severe myocardial necrosis and inflammation with infiltration of fungal mycelia.

Although the fungus was not cultured, the morphological appearance was of *Mucor* or *Rhizopus* sp.

Parasitic diseases

Strongyle cardiopathy

Myocardial lesions caused by the migration of strongyle larvae have been described. Cranley and McCullagh (1981) examined the hearts and aortas of 2076 horses, ponies, and donkeys of various ages at an abattoir. Atrial and ventricular foci of fibrosis were found in 14.3%. Microthrombi and foci of acute infarction were more common in younger horses. Grossly, fibrotic and ischemic foci ranged from 0.5 to 3.0 cm in diameter and were evenly distributed in the right and left sides of the heart.

Microscopic examination revealed areas of acute and healed infarction with fibrosis of older lesions. There were arteriolar intimal hyperplasia and sclerosing arterial lesions adjacent to areas of infarction and fibrosis. Thrombi and nodular fibrotic plaques associated with migrating larvae of *Strongylus vulgaris* were found in the aortas of 9.4% of the horses. Thirty-five percent of the aortic plaques were in the proximal 10 cm of the aorta, in agreement with Poynter (1960). Statistical analysis showed a high degree of association between strongyle proximal aortic lesions and foci of myocardial ischemia and fibrosis (Poynter 1960).

Vascular lesions

Vascular lesions associated with infection by *Dirofilaria immitis* were reported in a 20-month-old Quarter horse dying of cantharidin toxicosis (Thurman et al. 1984). There were gross and microscopic lesions of pulmonary endarteritis obliterans. *D. immitis* infestation is extremely rare in horses.

Aortic-iliac thrombosis

One cause of rear leg lameness is aortic-iliac thrombosis, Hutyra and Marek (1920). The lameness may affect one or both rear legs with pulse deficit, coolness of the affected leg(s), failure to sweat when exercised, and remission of lameness when rested (Maxie and Physick-Sheard 1985). The condition appears to be progressive and irreversible.

In South Africa, Azzie found the condition in 1%–1.5% of racing horses. Maxie and Physick-Sheard (1985) reviewed the literature and incidence of the condition. While it is generally accepted that the lesion is caused by strongyle migration, other causes including infection with *Streptococcus equi*, equine influenza, embolization, or treatment with procoagulant drugs for pulmonary hemorrhage have been proposed (Adams 1966; Mayhew and Kryger 1975; Smith et al. 1983). There is, however, no hard evidence that the lesion is anything other than reaction to *S. vulgaris* larval migration.

Maxie and Physick-Sheard (1985) studied the pathogenesis of aortic-iliac thrombosis in 17 horses with rear limb lameness. Clinical signs were consistent with lesions at the aortic quadrification, and thrombosed vessels were palpated per rectum. The mean age was 5.2 years; there were more geldings than stallions or mares. There was no breed predisposition, although some consider this a disease of light, rather than draft, horses (Merillat 1917). Autopsies were done on 10 of the 17 horses and 6 normal controls. Thrombosed vessels were found from the aortic bifurcation to the level of medium-sized muscular arteries (internal pudendal, femoral, and tibial). In some cases the process appeared to be multicentric, with thrombi forming at several points in the arterial tree. Fresh, hemorrhagic thrombi were present cranial to the bifurcation while fibrotic, organized, and recanalized thrombi were present at and beyond the bifurcation. Foci of intimal thickening and fibrosis were found in control horses, but no thrombi, despite the presence of strongyle tracts in the vessels of most horses. The microscopic description of the thrombi included fibrosis, bony metaplasia, fatty infiltration, and minimal inflammation.

Thrombosis of the jugular veins

Thrombosis of the jugular veins is a common complication of venepuncture. Irritant solutions, repetitive disruption of the vascular wall and endothelium, catheterization, bacterial infection, and systemic disease are known risk factors. Signs of jugular thrombosis and thrombophlebitis include enlargement of the vein, firm thickening of the wall, localized heat, and pain on palpation (Gardner et al. 1991). Risk factors associated with jugular thrombosis and thrombophlebitis were studied in 46 horses by Gardner et al. There was no breed or sex predisposition. Nearly 90% of the horses had only one vein affected. Of these, 58.5% were in the left jugular, a common site of injection and catheterization; 37% of the thrombosed veins had been catheterized.

Resolution of the thrombosis may be prolonged. The vessel may be lost entirely, recanalization may occur, or, unusually, the thrombus is removed with restitution to normal.

The role of needle puncture in thrombus formation is readily demonstrated in the postmortem room. Blunt or slow insertion raises the intima in tentlike fashion on the tip of the needle until the intima splits into a rent of considerably greater size than the needle.

While bilateral thrombosis is uncommon, it can occur, with massive edema of the head and neck and asphyxia an immediate danger. In such instances, the horse does not have *internal jugular veins*. Indeed, most horses do not have them (Ellenberger and Scheunert 1910), and are at risk once one vein has been thrombosed and the other invaded.

Unknown

Acute necrotizing vasculitis

Vascular inflammation not associated with viral or other infectious agents is rare. Werner et al. (1984) reported acute necrotizing vasculitis and thrombocytopenia in a 2-year-old Quarter horse with limb edema and pain. The skin of the right rear leg was necrotic and ulcerated with exuberant granulation tissue. Transmural necrosis and inflammation of arterioles and venules was seen microscopically, associated with the deposition of immunoglobulins G, A, and M on the endothelium of dermal arterioles. There were also antinuclear antibodies. No antibodies for equine viral arteritis were found. Immune-mediated necrotizing vasculopathy was diagnosed and immunosuppressive therapy led to an apparently uneventful recovery.

Granulomatous enteritis and cutaneous arteritis

An association between granulomatous enteritis and cutaneous arteritis was found by Woods et al. (1993). A 5-year-old Quarter horse with progressive weight loss had foci of ulcerative alopecia on the nose, neck, and coronary band. Granulomatous enteritis was confirmed with rectal biopsies showing typical histological lesions and staining with antisera to immunoglobulins G, M, and A. Multiple skin biopsies revealed necrotizing, ulcerative dermatitis and vasculitis with immunoglobulin deposition on epidermal basement membranes together with vesicle formation.

Affected arteries had segmental fibrinoid necrosis with mixed inflammatory cell infiltration. When the horse was killed, there were severe granulomatous lesions in the gastrointestinal tract. An immune-mediated vasculitis of the Schwartzman-type was suspected.

Congenital and developmental cardiovascular disease

Aging changes

In the fetus the large elastic arteries, such as the aorta, pulmonary artery, carotids, vertebral, and femoral, are lined by a thin intima covered by endothelium. The intima consists of collagen fibers and fine elastic tissue fibers, which become denser as they approach the media. The internal elastic lamina is not distinguishable because the elastic fibers of the intima blend into the heavy elastic layers of the media (Trautmann and Fiebiger 1952). The media is not as dense as in the older animal, with the spaces between the elastic layers filled with metachromatic ground substance. The density of elastic fibers increases through the first year of life, with the ground substance becoming less apparent.

At birth and continuing to about 4 years of age the intima thickens with proliferation of elastic and smooth muscle fibers (Fig. 1.6). There is a thin layer of collagen immediately beneath the endothelium, then the layer of elastic and smooth muscle fibers blending into the media (Krause 1927; Wolkoff 1924). There are fusiform or stellate mesenchymal cells in the intima, which apparently have phagocytic potential. This thickened intima was named the *fasernetzschicht*, or fiber net layer, by Krause (1927).

There is progressive thickening of the walls of the large elastic arteries, certainly ending by 15 years of age. This is partly the result of growth of the vessels and partly that of adjustments to the blood flow (Dahme and Schebitz 1970). The increase of thickness of the wall is particularly obvious in the curving segment of the aorta. The wall can be about 36% thicker in the mature horse as compared to the young animal. The increase in thickness is produced by the proliferation of elastic and interspersed collagen fibers. In older horses there is an increase, as well, in metachromatic ground substance (Krölling and Grau 1960).

At the distal end of the aorta, beginning at about 4–6 years of age, transverse folding of the inner surface of the vessel may appear. This is accompanied by thickening of the wall of the vessel. Histologically, the intima is somewhat thickened. The media remodels with the proliferation of smooth muscle at the expense of the elastic tissue. The latter becomes discontinuous and more and more isolated in islands. At the same time, the elastic tissue of the adventitia devolves to a structureless state [Krause (1933) cited by Dahme and Schebitz (1970)]. The frequency of this aging change was not given. While we have seen this in

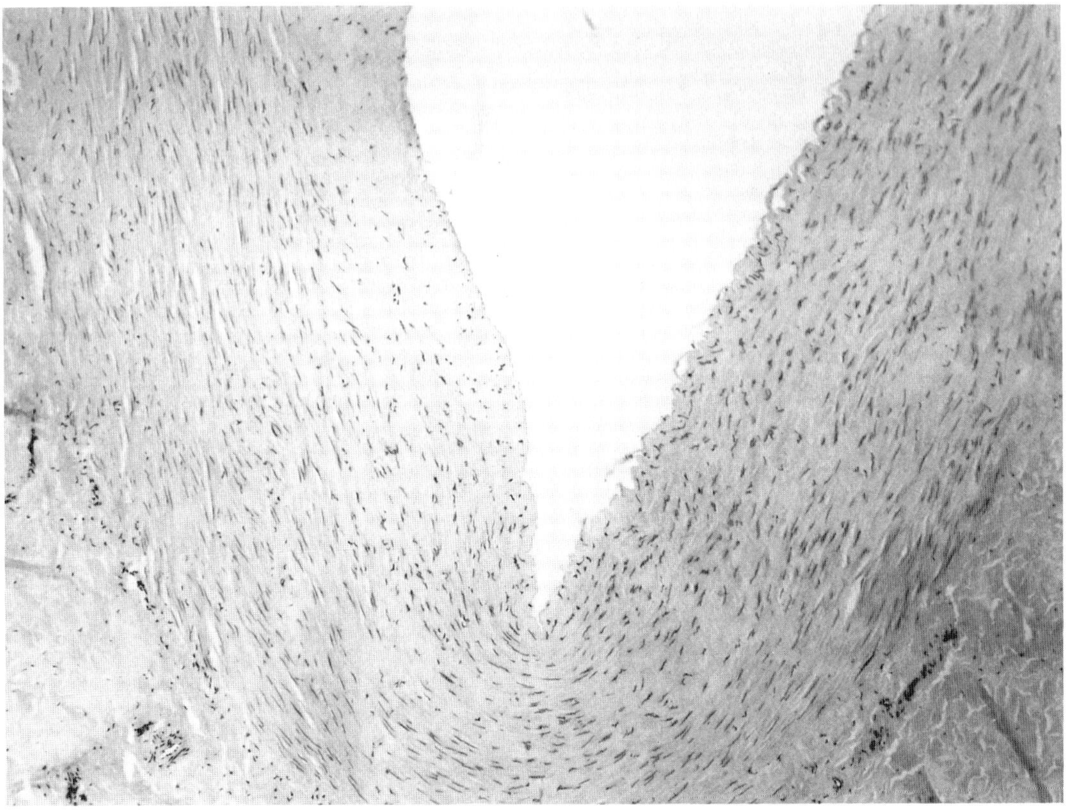

1.6. A plaque of fibroelastosis in a medium-sized artery.

some animals, it is not as striking or common in light horses as in the, presumably, heavy horses examined by Krause.

The status of aging changes in the smaller peripheral arteries is not completely clear. The medium-sized, muscular arteries have a layer of elastic, collagen, and smooth muscle tissue between the endothelium and the internal elastic lamina, a *fasernetz*. This layer is variably thick depending upon the age of the animal and the location of the vessel in the body. It is generally true that this layer becomes thicker with age, but rarely thick enough to compromise the circulation. It is arguable whether this thickening is to be called **endarteritis** (**obliterans**) or if that term should be reserved for truly pathological change, a distinction not easily made. Such thickening related to age occurs in, for example, the celiac artery and its branches as well as in the arteries of the legs. Pathological endarteritis obliterans is not infrequent, being seen in association with a variety of more chronic disease conditions such as abscesses, exuberant granulation tissue, parasitic infestations, and so forth.

The so-called **polster vessels**, arteries or veins (Krölling and Grau 1960), can certainly mimic age-related or pathological thickening of the intima. The thick intima in these vessels is composed of smooth muscle fibers. There has apparently been no systematic study of the occurrence, distribution, or even the existence of such polster vessels in the horse.

Endarteritis

The difficulty of defining pathological endarteritis versus age-related thickening is shown in the work of Köhler (1951) and Bibrack (1963). They found thickening of the intima of the digital arteries, which generally increased in frequency and degree with age (Köhler 1951). Most of their illustrations of intimal thickening and fibrosis are in the range of normal age-related change. Both authors, however, did find marked intimal thickening and, in some cases, thrombotic obliteration of the digital arteries. Bibrack found total obliteration, primarily in the medial digital artery and entirely in cold bloods, in about half of the animals examined. We have not seen this in light horses.

The media of the muscular arteries of the distal parts of the legs are normally thick and prominent, an appearance emphasized by the nearly invariable contracted state of these vessels after death. While we have not seen the extreme obliteration, either by intimal thickening or thrombosis, of the digital arteries reported by Köhler (1951) and Bibrack (1963), we routinely see thickening of the intima of the digital arteries in older horses. As well, elastotic breakup and disappearance of the internal elastic lamina may occur in segments of the digital arteries. The interpretation of lesser degrees of thickening of the intima is difficult. Sections have to be nearly perfectly perpendicular to the intima in order to avoid artifactual appearance of thickening.

In no instance, in our cases or those of Köhler and Bibrack, was there evidence of circulatory disturbance, the collateral circulation being entirely adequate. While those authors suggested causes for the obliterating lesions, the cause(s) was not discovered, and we can offer no useful opinion.

Congenital defects

A basic and seminal reference on cardiac anomalies is Lilleengen (1934).

Cysts

So-called cysts on the atrioventricular valves occur rarely in the horse as compared to other species. Such cysts are entrapped segments of fetal blood vessels that failed to involute properly (Cohrs 1961).

Tricuspid valve atresia

Rooney and Franks (1970) described, among other congenital lesions, two cases of tricuspid valve atresia in 3-month-old foals. Button et al. (1978) described a case in a 10-week-old Arabian crossbred foal, accompanying several other defects. The foal was depressed, in poor body condition with cyanotic mucous membranes. Exercise intolerance, labored breathing, and a grade V/V crescendo/decrescendo murmur were present. Both supravalvular and subvalvular pulmonic stenosis were found at autopsy, together with tricuspid atresia, patent foramen ovale, aplasia/hypoplasia of the coronary circulation, hypoplastic right ventricle, and intraventricular septal defect.

Similar clinical signs and lesions were reported in a 2-day-old Arabian with tricuspid atresia, patent ductus arteriosus, patent foramen ovale, and subaortic interventricular septal defect (Wilson and Haffner 1987).

Incomplete subaortic stenosis

King et al. (1988) described incomplete subaortic stenosis in a mature mixed-breed mare with a history of respiratory distress. There was bilateral hypertrophy of heart at postmortem. A 1.5-cm fibrotic band below a cusp of the valve was not thought to compromise the function of the well-formed aortic valve.

Mitral valve insufficiency

Mitral valve insufficiency following rupture of the chordae tendinae was described in three foals by Reef (1987). Two Thoroughbred foals and 1 Quarter horse foal, 3–8 months of age, had murmurs, jugular pulsation, and other signs of congestive heart failure. In 2 the mitral valve leaflets were thickened, together with jet lesions. One foal had vegetative bacterial endocarditis. Ruptured chordae tendinae were present in all cases. Reef speculated that in 2 of the 3 cases myocardial necrosis played a role in the rupture of the chordae, although no evidence was presented.

Ruptured chordae tendinae were given as the cause of mitral insufficiency in three 4- to 7-year-old horses (Holmes and Miller 1984). There were nodular thickenings of the mitral valve cusps at the points of attachment. In seven other horses with mitral insufficiency, there was minimal fibrosis of the myocardium and a small amount of valvular nodular thickening not associated with rupture of the chordae tendinae or papillary muscle necrosis (Miller and Holmes 1985).

Pulmonary valve stenosis

An uncommon defect is pulmonary valve stenosis. One such case in a 2-day-old Shire foal was reported by Hinchcliff and Adams (1991). There were multiple defects, including pulmonic stenosis and poststenotic dilatation, right heart enlargement, patent ductus arteriosus, and interatrial septal defect.

Ventricular and atrial septal defects

Ventricular and atrial septal defects are more common in horses than congenital valvular defects. Rooney and Franks (1970) considered them among the commonest congenital cardiac defects. They are occasionally found in stillborn foals, but are probably not the cause of death.

Lombard et al. (1983) reviewed the clinical and pathological features of **ventricular septal defects** in six horses 1 day to 2 years old. All had cardiac dysfunction, including murmurs, because of septal defects 1.5–7 cm in diameter. Additional cases of septal defects, alone or in combination with other congenital defects such as pulmonic stenosis, bicuspid pulmonic valve, persistent right aortic arch, tricuspid valve insufficiency, and/or pulmonary atresia, have been reported in a Welsh pony (Critchley 1976), Arabian foals (Vitums and Bayly 1982), a 2-year-old trotter mare (Muylle et al. 1974), and a colt of unspecified breeding (Van Der Linde-Sipman et al. 1979).

Physick-Sheard et al. (1985) reviewed **atrial septal defects** and described a case of persistent ostium primum in a Welsh mountain pony foal. There was cardiac dysfunction, exercise intolerance, grade IV/V pansystolic murmur, cyanotic mucous membranes, and delayed capillary refill. There were multiple cardiac abnormalities, including persistence of the ostium primum, dysplasia of the pulmonic valve, infundibular, subvalvular, and supravalvular pulmonic stenosis, persistent foramen ovale, mitral valve dysplasia, and left ventricular dilatation and hypertrophy. Right to left shunting of blood during life was the obvious cause of clinical signs. The association of atrial septal defects with defective endocardial cushion formation during embryogenesis was discussed, and the authors correlated atrial septal defects with other congenital cardiac anomalies described in the literature.

Hypoplastic left heart syndrome

Hypoplastic left heart syndrome has been reported in two foals (Tadmor et al. 1983; Musselman and LoGuidice 1984). A 2-week-old Arabian crossbred filly had dyspnea and cyanotic mucous membranes. Angiographic studies showed a patent ductus arteriosus. Gross lesions included patent ductus arteriosus and hypertrophy of the left ventricular myocardium, but hypoplasia of the left ventricular chamber and atrial septal defects. The 2-day-old Appaloosa colt of Musselman and LoGuidice was more severely affected with markedly hypoplastic left ventricular myocardium and chamber, hypoplastic aorta, aortic and mitral valve atresia, patent ductus arteriosus, and atrial septal defect.

Tetralogy of Fallot

Much attention has been paid to the tetralogy of Fallot in horses and other domesticated species, attention perhaps excessive for a rare condition. The entity includes pulmonic stenosis, ventricular septal defect, right ventricular hypertrophy, and overriding aorta [Fallot (1888) cited by Prickett et al. (1973)]. Single cases have been reported (Rooney and Franks 1970; Prickett et al. 1973; Borst 1978; Reynolds and Nicholl 1978).

Persistent right aortic arch

Persistent right aortic arch with esophageal stenosis, dilatation, and regurgitation have been described by Bartels and Vaughan (1969) and Petrick et al. (1978). A persistent right aortic arch overrides the bronchus and descends right of midline, with malposition of the aorta relative to the esophagus. The fibrous band formed by the ductus arteriosus, the right aorta, and pulmonary artery forms a vascular ring. This ring causes the clinical symptoms of ineffective swallowing and regurgitation and aspiration of food.

Aplasia of the origin of the left coronary artery

Aplasia of the origin of the left coronary artery (Fig. 1.7) has been seen in several horses (Rooney and Franks 1970). The single right coronary artery provided a branch to the distribution field of the left artery. The lesion did not become apparent until the horses were in training or work, when acute cardiac dilatation, presumably the result of inadequate perfusion, occurred.

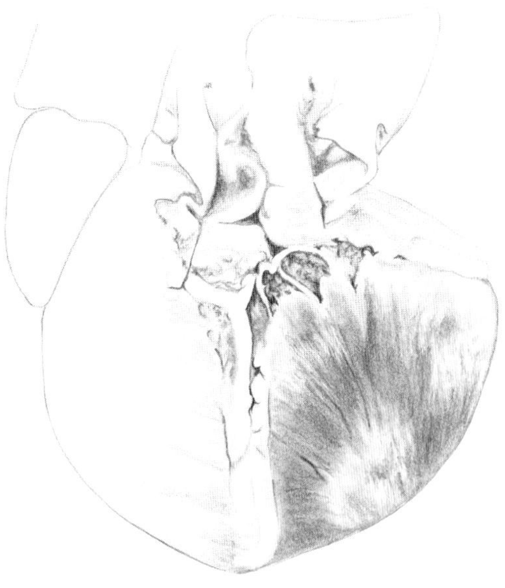

1.7. Aplasia of the origin of the left coronary artery with foci of ischemia in the epicardium.

Medial arterial calcification

Medial arterial calcification is not uncommon in horses. Older animals, especially over 15 years, may show calcification of the media of, particularly, the thoracic portion of the aorta (Krause 1927). This usually appears as scattered, rounded, knotty, or strandlike thickenings, which histologically appear to be calcified elastic fibers. "Mucoid" degeneration, accumulation of metachromatic ground substance, is often said to accompany such changes, but that has not been our experience. Such lakes of metachromatic material do occur with somewhat greater frequency in the elastic arteries of older animals, but there is no clear evidence that this material represents necrosis or relates to dystrophic calcification of the elastic fiber bundles.

Cranley (1983) found discrete plaques of medial calcification about 1 cm distal to the bifurcation in either or both branches of the pulmonary artery in about 9% of a mixed population of 1066 horses. The highest frequency, 27%, was in Thoroughbred horses, reasonably according with our experience.

In light horse foals it is almost routine to find patches of medial calcification in the common carotid artery as it branches into internal and external carotid and occipital arteries. The lesion appears as a corrugated plaque on the intimal surface. While a definitive study has not been done, the lesion apparently disappears with age since it has not been seen in older horses.

Arteriosclerosis/atherosclerosis

Arteriosclerosis/atherosclerosis is essentially unknown in the horse in any site, including coronary and cerebral vessels. Cerebrovascular accidents, "strokes," are invariably incorrect diagnoses. The common lesion of equine vessels is endarteritis (obliterans), primarily as an aging change as discussed earlier.

Widespread, massive calcification of larger blood vessels as well as the endocardium is seen with excessive administration of *vitamin D* and poisoning with *Cestrum diurnum* (Krook et al. 1975).

Aging changes are routine in the ovarian and uterine arteries of mares and are discussed with the ovary and uterus.

Aortic aneurysm

There are two reports of aortic aneurysm in horses (Holmes et al. 1973; Derksen et al. 1981). A 4-year-old hunter gelding with ventral edema and dullness was thought to have profound atrial fibrillation and cardiac failure (Holmes et al. 1973). A dissecting aneurysm of the aorta had ruptured into the left pulmonary artery.

Derksen et al. (1981) found a fusiform dilation of the aortic arch and descending aorta, as well as a bicarotid trunk in a 7-year-old Arabian mare.

Necrosis and rupture of the aorta and pulmonary trunk

Necrosis and rupture of the aorta and pulmonary trunk in four 3-year-old horses (1 stallion and 3 mares; 3 Friesians and 1 Dutch half blood) was reported by Van der Linde-Sipman et al. (1985). All had severe, progressive signs of cardiovascular disease including dyspnea, recumbency, and distress. Two of the horses had well-formed aneurysms between the carotid trunk and the insertion of the ligamentum arteriosum. All four had rupture of the aorta at the level of the ligamentum arteriosum and a transverse rupture of the pulmonary trunk. Microscopic examination showed foci of necrosis, acute inflammation, and fibrovascular proliferation. Lesions were partially calcified in two cases. Hematomas at the sites of rupture of three horses were encapsulated. The investigators commented on the high density of the vasa vasorum at the site of rupture. No cause for the lesions was found although Van der Linde-Sipman et al. acknowledged that the same forces described by Rooney et al. (1967) were probably operative.

Congenital venous aneurysm

A single case of congenital venous aneurysm was reported in a 3-year-old Quarter horse gelding (Hilbert and Rendano 1975). A slowly enlarging mass on the left side of the neck had been present since the horse was a year old.

Varicose veins

Varicose veins in the dorsal wall at the vestibulovaginal junction were the cause of persistent vaginal hemorrhage in four mares and a pony mare (White et al. 1984). The animals were over 8 years of age and multiparous. The cause of the varicosities was not found. We have not seen this.

Cardiovascular disease related to nutrition

Nutritional myopathy caused by deficiency of vitamin E and selenium is recognized in horses and dealt with elsewhere in this book (see Chapter 6, "Locomotor System, General"; Chapter 7, "Fore Leg"; and Chapter 8, "Rear Leg").

Several cases of cardiomyopathy possibly related to dietary deficiencies have been published (Wilson et al. 1976). The cardiac lesions were seen in 3 of 10 foals and horses with suspected nutritional myopathy. Lesions included fragmentation of cardiac muscle fibers and focal myocardial ischemia. The putative nutritional cause was not demonstrated.

Rhythm abnormalities

Atrial fibrillation

Atrial fibrillation is a common disorder of cardiac rhythm, which has been recognized for many years. It is particularly common in horses training for events such as racing and hunting.

Deem and Fregin (1982) reviewed the records of 106 cases of atrial fibrillation. Exercise intolerance was the primary clinical sign in 60% of these cases; dyspnea or epistaxis were present in 25%; and peripheral edema in 12%. Signs of severe cardiac disease, including at least grade III/V murmurs, were found in 12 horses. Contrary to the findings of Else and Holmes (1972d), Deem and Fregin (1982) found no difference between the frequency of atrial fibrillation in horses less than 4 years old and that of those greater than 5 years. In a review of 45 horses with atrial fibrillation, Else and Holmes (1972d) found the highest incidence in horses over 20 years old. Deem and Fregin (personal communication) studied young horses in training while Else and Holmes examined a range of ages.

Both groups agreed that atrial fibrillation was commoner in large horses than in small horses and ponies. Deem and Fregin (1982) found the disease in both Thoroughbreds and Standardbreds, though more often in Standardbreds. Else and Holmes noted that draft horses were far more likely to be affected than horses under 14.2 hands.

Else and Holmes (1972d) found gross atrial lesions in 80% of horses with atrial fibrillation. They described six categories of lesions including patchy or diffuse fibrosis, atrial mural thinning and fibrosis, saccular dilatations known as "ballooning," gross dilatation, and combinations of the above. Microscopic examination showed lymphocytic infiltration and fibrosis with a wide range of severity and distribution. Microscopic examination of the sinoatrial node failed to show any lesions. This differs from Kiryu et al. (1987) who claimed to find fibrosis and inflammation of atrial tissue and the sinoatrial node. Our own observations support those of Else and Holmes. Of the horses with atrial fibrillation studied by Else and Holmes 80% had gross valvular lesions, usually on the left side of the heart.

Deem and Fregin reported autopsy data from 24 horses with atrial fibrillation. They found clinical and gross pathological signs of congestive heart failure in 12, including valvular insufficiency, endocarditis, myocarditis, ventricular septal defects, and pericardial effusion.

The cause(s) of atrial fibrillation has been the subject of intense speculation. It has been shown that atrial fibrillation can occur in the presence of organic cardiac disease, but that such disease is not always present. Else and Holmes (1972) speculated that increased vagal activity predisposed to atrial fibrillation by slowing ventricular contraction, altering the refractory period, and facilitating reentry phenomena. Deem and Fregin (1982) concluded that substantial organic disease was not a factor in most horses since many resume an athletic career following conversion with quinidine sulfate. Reef et al. (1988) reported that horses with organic disease were less likely to convert to normal rhythm with quinidine sulfate. Gelberg et al. (1991) reported pulmonary hypertension (values exceeding 70 mm Hg; normal values less than 26 mm Hg) in four cases of atrial fibrillation in young horses. Lesions in the pulmonary artery ranged from minimal thickening of the tunica media to fibrinoid necrosis. Regional hypoxia associated with the pulmonary hypertension may have rendered the atrial myocardium more reactive.

Paroxysmal atrial fibrillation

A related condition, paroxysmal atrial fibrillation, is rare in horse and humans (Machida et al. 1989). Three of 20 newborn foals had characteristic fibrillation waves on the electrocardiogram shortly after birth. Two of the 3 were weak and ataxic with cyanosis and respiratory distress. Two of the 3 spontaneously converted to normal rhythm within 4 hours of birth, while a third apparently responded to procainamide by converting to normal rhythm.

Idioventricular tachycardia

Miller et al. (1987) recorded a case of idioventricular tachycardia in a 4-year-old Thoroughbred mare. The condition, in which a ventricular pacemaker evolved independently of the normal sinoatrial pacemaker, was detected incidentally. The animal had no clinical signs and raced effectively. Ventricular ectopic beats and partial interference block of normal conduction were noted on electrocardiography. No pathological studies were done.

Sinoatrial block

Sinoatrial block was reported in three 4- to 5-year-old horses by Kiryu et al. (1985). It was characterized by absence of normal P-QRS-T complexes and dropping of complete beats. Two of the 3 horses had retired from racing, and the third from pleasure hacking. All had electrocardiographic evidence of sinoatrial block. In all 3 horses, there was said to be gross focal gray discoloration of the sinoatrial node. Microscopically, lymphangiectasis and myocardial ischemia were found at the sinoatrial node in one heart, and moderate to severe fibrotic lesions were found at the sinoatrial node in the others. Loss of myocardial nerve fibers was shown with histochemical stains. The disturbances in cardiac rhythm were attributed to these myocardial lesions. While facile, these results must be interpreted with care since they have not been corroborated by others despite careful search.

Second-degree atrioventricular block

Smetzer et al. (1969) identified second-degree atrioventricular block in 116 horses in clinics, at an abattoir, and at racetracks. This arrhythmia is characterized electrocardiographically by a normal P-wave not followed by a QRS-T wave. The incidence in horses is 6.4%–15%, depending on the breed (Holmes 1963). Detweiler and Patterson (1972), among others, attributed the condition to increased vagal tone and considered it insignificant. Smetzer et al. reported a higher incidence in Thoroughbreds and Standardbreds than in draft horses. They found arrhythmias and electrocardiographic abnormalities in nearly 25% of Thoroughbred horses. The abnormality was highly labile, sometimes disappearing within 5 minutes of detection in horses at rest. Agreeing with Detweiler and Patterson (1972), Smetzer et al. concluded that second-degree atrioventricular block must be a physiological variant of normal heart rhythm in some horses. In an abattoir study they found no lesions of the sinoatrial node.

Wandering pacemaker

Kiryu et al. (1978) identified five racehorses with wandering pacemaker. This is characterized by shifting of pacemaking activity from the normal sinoatrial node to a focus within the atrium and back. The horses with wandering pacemaker had all competed successfully before being killed for lesions or injuries unrelated to the cardiovascular system. They ranged in age from 3 to 15 years. All had second-degree atrioventricular block. One of the 5 had "discolored" foci in the atrial myocardium and histological lesions of varying severity, including focal atrial fibrosis, edema or fibrosis of atrial arterioles, edema in subendocardial nerve bundles, and lesions in extracardiac vagal and sympathetic nerves. Unfortunately, the authors did not recognize Renaut bodies as normal constituents of horse nerve, misinterpreting them as pathological. Mild degrees of focal fibrosis are not rare in any horse atrium, and edema and fibrosis of arterioles is a problematic description at best.

Multiple atrial dysrhythmias

Gross and histological lesions highly correlated with atrial dysfunction were seen in a 5-year-old Quarter horse with multiple atrial dysrhythmias (Button et al. 1980). Four months after being bitten by a rattlesnake the horse developed severe exercise intolerance and paroxysmal atrial tachycardia, atrial tachycardia with second-degree atrioventricular block, atrial fibrillation, and atrial flutter. Quinidine sulfate and propranolol did not convert the dysrhythmia and seemed to exacerbate it at times. At autopsy, there was myocardial fibrosis and myocytolysis with extensive fibrosis at the sinoatrial node. A mild lymphoplasmacytic epimyocarditis was described. The association of the heart lesions with the rattlesnake bite was discussed, not proved, and problematic.

Toxic cardiovascular disease

Phenylbutazone

Few toxins to which horses are exposed cause cardiovascular disease. Unfortunately, the widely used phenylbutazone may cause vasculopathy at recommended therapeutic doses.

The toxicity of phenylbutazone has been recognized since the drug was introduced. Common undesirable side effects include ulceration of the oral and pharyngeal mucosa and gastrointestinal tract. The drug also causes necrosis of the renal medullary crest and thrombosis of jugular veins. Meschter et al. (1984) studied the lesions in three Thoroughbred geldings given the drug intravenously at 13.63 mg/kg/day for 3 days, 1.5 times the therapeutic dose. One horse received a second regimen 4 days after the first 3-day regimen.

They were killed 4, 7, and 10 days after receiving the phenylbutazone. Ulcers were present in the tongue and gastric fundus and pylorus. There was marked submucosal edema in the duodenum and petechial hemorrhages in the duodenum and jejunum. The renal medullary crest was necrotic in all horses. The jugular veins were thrombosed at the site of injection and along the vessel. Microscopic examination showed endothelial swelling and vascular degeneration in many vessels in several organs and tissues. Sinusoidal endothelial integrity was lost in the liver. Venous hyalinosis and mural degeneration was noted in the renal crest. Vascular damage was seen in segments of the gastrointestinal tract. The pathogenetic mechanism for the observed vascular changes was not defined.

Cantharidin

Panciera (1972) described myocardial failure in horses exposed to toxic amounts of cantharidin in contaminated hay. Severe gastroenteritis, renal failure, and pulmonary edema are seen in horses that consume dried *Epicauta vitatta*, striped blister beetle. Pale, degenerate, or necrotic myocardium is seen in both atria and ventricles. Microscopically, the areas appear ischemic, and there is myonecrosis. See Chapter 14, "Urinary Tract."

Neoplasia

Cardiovascular neoplasms are rare in horses. Jackson (1936) recorded only a single pericardial mesothelioma among 119 equine tumors in the Onderstepoort collection.

Lymphosarcoma

Metastatic lymphosarcoma was described in a 14-year-old Warm blood gelding (Volckart and Loeffler 1978). The animal had second-degree atrioventricular block and supraventricular tachycardia. Gross lesions included nodular lymphosarcoma of the spleen and the myocardium.

Hypercalcemia of malignancy

Complications of lymphosarcoma may also affect the heart and vessels. Two horses with either splenic or mediastinal lymphosarcoma developed hypercalcemia of malignancy with cardiac and aortic mineralization (Mair et al. 1990c). Both horses had cardiac dysfunction. The cause of pathological hypercalcemia in these cases was presumed to be the secretion of calcitonin analogues by neoplastic cells, natural secretion of calcitonin due to malignancy in the kidneys, and renal failure, or a combination of these factors.

Lipoma

Baker and Kreeger (1987) found an infiltrating lipoma of the right ventricular myocardium in a 3-year-old Morgan stallion. There were no signs of cardiac dysfunction. The horse was killed because of an inoperable fracture. There was a spherical 6-cm diameter mass in the right ventricle adjacent to the tricuspid valve and right atrium. Microscopically, it was composed of well-differentiated fat cells arranged in sheets and cords with a connective tissue matrix. Atrophic and degenerating myocytes were present adjacent to the mass.

Lipomas commonly develop from the adipose tissue of the coronary grooves and atria in parallel with the development of lipomas in the mesentery in aging horses. In no case has such a "cardiac" lipoma been the cause of disease.

Mesothelioma

Primary pericardial mesothelioma has been reported only rarely in horses and other domesticated animals (Carnine et al. 1977). Jackson (1936) found one as already noted. Carnine et al. described a pericardial mesothelioma in a 27-year-old Quarter horse with weight loss and a variety of aging lesions. The pericardial sac was distended with approximately 3 liters of serosanguinous fluid. The epicardial surface was studded with small, firm, gray-white nodules, from 1 mm to 5 cm. Similar nodules were found lining the pericardial sac. Microscopically, the tumor was characterized by papillary nodules covered with low cuboidal mesothelial cells. There were no metastases.

Hemangiosarcoma

Birks and Hultgren (1988) reported a primary pericardial hemangiosarcoma in a 22-year-old Clydesdale-Percheron gelding with a history of dyspnea and anorexia. There were 20 liters of serosanguinous fluid in the thoracic cavity. The pericardium was studded with dark red grapelike masses, as were the parietal pleura and left adrenal gland. Histologically the pericardial masses were composed of small, poorly formed vascular channels, typical of hemangiosarcoma. A significant portion of the mass was necrotic.

Cardiovascular diseases with unclassified etiology

Hypertension

There have been few efforts to define or discover hypertension in equids. The virtual absence of arteriosclerotic and atherosclerotic vascular disease and the low incidence of renal disease removes substantial risk factors for hypertension as known in humans. Rugh et al. (1987) and others have reported that horses and ponies with laminitis are hypertensive. In nine chronically hypertensive laminitic ponies, they found left ventricular hypertrophy with increased thickness of the ventricular wall. These reports seem to have led nowhere and have not been confirmed, suggesting, perhaps, technical problems with blood pressure recording rather than hypertension.

Myocardial necrosis

King et al. (1982) described myocardial necrosis in a horse secondary to neural lesions—a condition they called "brain-heart syndrome." Foci of white discoloration of the myocardium were seen in a 2-year-old Quarter horse that had suffered head trauma and died. Microscopic examination of the heart showed foci of myocardial fiber degeneration and mineralization. Two additional cases were found by a retrospective review of pathology records. The significance of these observations remains for future study as the simultaneous occurrence of lesions does not require etiological relationship.

Right atrial ossification

Dystrophic calcification and ossification occur in the right atrium of horses (Stunzi and Teuscher 1970). Cadeac (1897a) cited a number of reports of right atrial ossification, the earliest being by Renault in 1837.

The process appears to begin near one end of the atrium with foci of calcification and bone formation in a heavy, fibrous-tissue stroma. In more advanced cases the entire atrium may be converted to a bony mass covered by epicardium and endocardium. The wall can be 1.5- to 7.5-cm thick with yellowish-white trabeculae of bone on section. Histologically, there may be foci of adipose tissue and islands of cartilage in addition to fibrous tissue and bone.

This lesion is usually seen in older horses, but cases have been reported in a 5-year-old pony and two 5-year-old horses. The incidence is not known. Cohrs and Streich collected 42 cases and added five of their own in 1943. We have seen only three cases in about 15,000 postmortem examinations, primarily of light horses, and it may be that the lesion is commoner in heavy horses.

There are two main etiological theories. Cohrs and Streich believe the lesion is part of an allergic reaction associated with tuberculosis. They believed that more than half of the cases in the literature were probably tuberculosis. They found tuberculous lung lesions in all five of their cases. In the atrium they saw hyaline swelling of the mesenchymal tissues, nonspecific granuloma formation, and endarteritis obliterans. They considered this to be an allergic process with metaplastic bone formation. The lesions, as described, are hardly specific enough to suggest an allergic process.

The second theory is that of Farrelly who felt the lesion was caused by emboli from *S. vulgaris* thrombi in the aorta in the vicinity of the coronary artery orifices. He discussed the role of the arterial

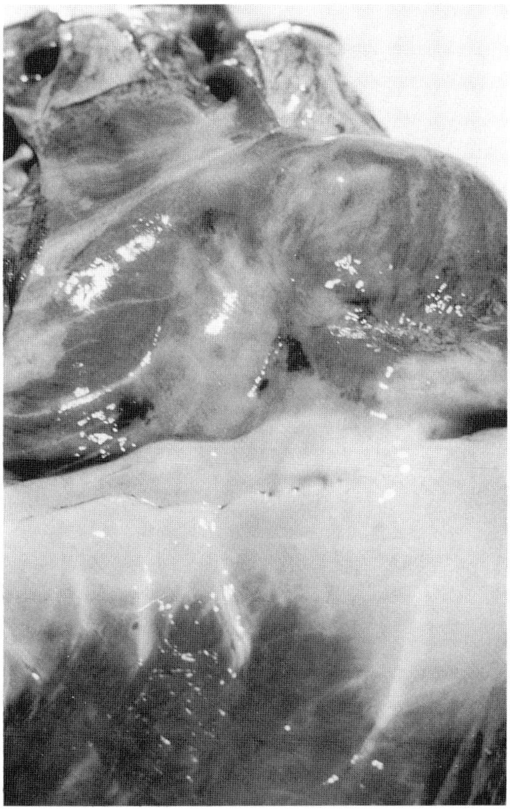

1.8. A focus of infarction and hemorrhage on the right atrium.

pattern of the right atrium in the localization of the lesions (Farrelly 1954).

Two of our cases were fully developed atrial ossification without active lesions. One case, obviously early in development, was an area of pale infarction surrounded by an hemorrhagic border near one end of the atrium. Histologically, there was degeneration of muscle fibers in the infarcted area, with an hemorrhagic, mononuclear cell border, and striking fibrinoid necrosis of muscular arteries. There was no evidence of tuberculosis or of strongyle lesions in the aorta. The cause, then, was not determined (Fig. 1.8).

We think the pathogenesis of these lesions is more reasonably explained by Farrelly's hypothesis. The rarity of these cases correlates well with the rarity of *S. vulgaris* infestations of sufficient severity to involve the proximal aorta. Our case may well have been caused by aberrant larva(e) not seen in the sections.

CHAPTER 2

Respiratory System

Although recognized for thousands of years, equine respiratory disease presents unresolved enigmas. We believe, echoing Cadeac (1897a) and Cohrs (1941c), that there is still confusion in diagnosing and understanding the pathogenesis of many respiratory conditions.

The discussion has been separated into diseases primarily affecting the upper respiratory tract (nares, sinuses, oropharynx, guttural pouches, epiglottis and glottis, and hyoid apparatus) and those of the lower respiratory tract (trachea, bronchial tree, lungs, pleura). Some diseases, of course, affect both portions.

Incidence and epidemiology

Postmortem observations

In a comprehensive review of the incidence of respiratory disease in Hannover, Wirth (1985) found that 13% of all autopsies had respiratory lesions. Her data came from over 3000 cases of various ages and breeds examined between 1933 and 1983. That high percentage is, no doubt, because of the inclusion of herpesvirus (EHV)-1 in foals and the inclusion of strangles.

Incidence of clinical respiratory disease

The incidence of clinical respiratory disease is certainly higher since most horses do not succumb to the usual respiratory pathogens. Several surveys of clinical and subclinical disease have been reported.

Sherman et al. (1977) studied the incidence of viral and bacterial disease in Standardbred racehorses in Ontario for a period of 3 years. Serious outbreaks of upper respiratory disease, sufficient to disrupt racing, occurred once or twice yearly. Serum, bacterial, and viral culture samples were collected from normal and sick horses. The common pathogens from 372 nasal swab cultures were *Staphylococcus aureus* (13.4%) and *Streptococcus zooepidemicus* (11.3%). *Pasteurella multocida* was isolated twice and *Actinobacillus equuli* three times. A number of environmental contaminants, including *Bacillus*, *Neisseria*, *Corynebacterium*, and *Streptomyces* sp. were also isolated. Separate bacterial cultures were collected from each nostril of 152 horses, and the bacterial flora differed between nostrils in over 20% of the horses.

Between 1973 and 1975, 533 viral swabs were obtained. Herpesvirus (EHV)-1 was isolated 10 times (1.8%) and herpesvirus (EHV)-2 72 times (13.5%). Sherman et al. (1977) found that herpesvirus (EHV)-1 samples were frequently obtained from animals with clinical respiratory illness, while herpesvirus (EHV)-2 isolations were from both normal and sick horses. Sherman et al. believed that herpesvirus (EHV)-2 probably was an insignificant pathogen. Equine influenza virus-1 (A equi 1) was isolated 7 times from 182 samples in this 3-year period; equine influenza virus-2 (A equi 2) only once.

Serological conversion, at least a fourfold change in titer, for a number of viruses was assessed. Of the healthy horses, 25% had been exposed to influenza-2. Rates of seroconversion for equine influenza viruses 1 and 2 and herpesvirus (EHV)-1 were found in over 30% of sick animals during epizootics between 1973 and 1975.

A serological study of the incidence of viral infection in racing Thoroughbreds and Standardbreds was done in western Canada (Fretz et al. 1979). Only horses with overt respiratory disease were examined. Peak incidence was at the beginning of the racing season in May and in the autumn. More than 60% of 85 horses with respiratory disease had an initial titer, indicating previous exposure to either influenza-1 or to herpesvirus (EHV)-1. Of the sick horses, 11% had increased titers to equine influenza virus, and 9% developed a convalescent titer to herpesvirus (EHV)-1. As expected, nonvaccinated animals were sicker than vaccinated.

Association of disease with oral pathogens

An association between oral pathogens and those found in lower respiratory infections was suggested by Bailey and Love (1991). They cultured bacteria from the pharyngeal tonsillar surface of 12 normal horses at autopsy. Bacterial cultures were obtained from 14 horses with clinical infection of the lower respiratory tract. Multiple isolates of numerous bacterial species were obtained from both sites, suggesting that some pathogens in lower respiratory infections could have come from the oropharynx. The bacteria included *Eubacterium fossor*, *Peptostreptococcus anaerobius*, black-pigmented *Bacteroides* sp., several species of *Bacillus*, *Fusobacterium* spp., and *Streptococcus equi* subsp. *zooepidemicus*.

Risk factors

Risk factors for the development of equine infectious respiratory diseases have been intensively studied. A brief review of the epidemiology of equine respiratory disease was done by Reif in 1979. Of first importance is an infectious agent in a facilitating environment with susceptible individuals. Infected animals spread infection by aerosol and direct contact. The dynamics of deposition and mechanical clearance of inhaled pathogens was reviewed by Clarke (1987a).

Host immunity

Host immunity is an important determinant of infection. The mature and functional humoral and cellular immune system protects the horse from infectious agents. Foals ingesting adequate amounts of immunoglobulins in colostrum are protected. Secretory immunoglobulin A on mucosal surfaces, especially in the upper respiratory tract, is a major factor in the local response and resistance to infection (Wilkie 1982). It is known that horses have a complex localized immunity in the respiratory system comprising mucosal lymphoid tissue, mucosal immunoglobulin-secreting cells, fixed macrophages, secretory immunoglobulin A, transient immunocytes including macrophages, lymphocytes, and neutrophils, and the mucus barrier itself (Clarke 1987a). Several investigators have shown that there is poor correlation between systemic and local immunity for some important equine pathogens (Galan and Timoney 1985a; Timoney and Eggers 1985). Other factors important in respiratory tract immunity include mucociliary transport of particulate matter from the airways, lysosomal enzymes against Gram-positive bacteria, inhibition of bacterial iron metabolism by lactoferrins in secretions, interferon production and secretion, and complement-associated opsonization and phagocytosis of microbes (Green et al. 1977). Adequate cell-mediated immunity may be particularly important in determining resistance to intracellular pathogens (Wilkie 1982).

Dysfunction of the immune system, failure of passive transfer, the relatively short-lived immunoglobulin A response, and poor secretory immunoglobulin response increase the susceptibility to respiratory pathogens. Adenoviral pneumonia is common in Arabian foals with combined immunodeficiency (see Chapter 18, "Hemolymphatic System"). Foals with failure of passive antibody transfer are at significant risk for pneumonia, gastroenteritis, and neonatal septicemia. We have reported an immunodeficient horse with malignant lymphoma that developed pneumonia (Furr et al. 1992). Another horse with myeloblastic proliferative disease suffered immunosuppression and had pulmonary and systemic aspergillosis (Buechner-Maxwell et al. 1994). Clearly, loss of immune competence significantly increases the risk of respiratory infection. Clarke (1987a) has emphasized that current vaccines and vaccination procedures may not adequately protect against respiratory pathogens, creating a state of "artificial" antigen-specific immunodeficiency. Jakob (1981) noted that viral infection of macrophages impairs function and may impair overall immunity as infected macrophages are destroyed by sensitized lymphoid effector cells. This may be one factor in the development of secondary bacterial respiratory infections.

Age

Reif (1979) cited age as an important risk factor in respiratory diseases. Colostral immunoglobulin transfer has been mentioned. Older animals have usually been exposed to potential pathogens and have immunity based on anamnestic response (except for secretory immunoglobulin A with a notably poor response). The immune response probably declines with age in the horse as in other species, but no specific data has been found.

Intercurrent disease

Intercurrent systemic or respiratory disease may predispose to additional disease. Chronic bronchitis, for example, may delay the clearance of pathogens, allowing multiplication and complicating disease (Allen and Bryans 1986; Clarke 1987a).

Characteristics of infectious agents

Inherent characteristics of infectious agents help to determine their pathogenicity. For example, **antigenic drift** in influenza mxyoviruses occurs readily, so that host immunity and anamnestic response to one viral strain may not be protective for a newly mutated strain. Survival of bacteria and viruses in the environment facilitates their spread. *Rhodococcus equi* prospers in manure-contaminated soil and is a constant environmental contaminant (Barton and Embury 1987). Streptococci are normal inhabitants of the equine oropharynx and readily survive on fomites in the environment. The size of infectious particles are important in determining depth of penetration into the respiratory tract. Smaller particles, lodging deep in the respiratory tract, are better able to establish infection (Clarke 1987a).

Environmental factors

Environmental factors, including season, temperature, humidity and ventilation, and the presence of air pollutants all can have an effect on infectious respiratory diseases. The relationship of ventilation and environment to equine respiratory disease was discussed by Sainsbury (1981) and Clarke (1987a). Sainsbury believed that the incidence of respiratory disease was increasing and that one important factor was large numbers of horses in buildings with less than optimum climatic control. While this may be true, the crowding together of horses for military and other purposes, no matter the housing or lack thereof, has always been a major factor in the epidemiology of respiratory disease. Sainsbury listed acceptable environmental variables for horses:

Ambient temperature	0°–30° C
Relative humidity	30%–70%
Air movement	0.15–0.5 m/sec
Ventilation	0.2–2 m^3/h/kg body weight
Outlet vent area	0.1 m^2/horse
Inlet vent area	0.3 m^2/horse

Sainsbury pointed out that high relative humidity and low temperatures facilitate the survival of respiratory pathogens. Without adequate environmental control, particularly in urban areas, there is increased risk of respiratory damage by high levels of respiratory irritants, such as noxious gases, dust, allergens, molds, and pollens.

Crowding animals for transport is a significant means of spread of respiratory pathogens. Bailey and Love (1991) reported that 64% of horses developing lower respiratory tract infections had been transported shortly before illness appeared.

Upper respiratory system

Nares, nasal cavity, and nasopharynx

Paralysis of the nasal diverticulum

Foerner (1967) described four cases of inspiratory and expiratory false nostril noises in American Saddlebred horses, offspring of a single stallion. There was no pathological description. Surgical obliteration of the opening into the nasal diverticulum eliminated the noises. Cadiot in *Bayer-Fröhner* (1910) mentioned a case seen by Goubeaux in 1848. Mammoli (1960) described a case, but the reference was not found.

The function of the nasal diverticulum in Equidae has, apparently, not been addressed. During inspiration, the entrance to the diverticulum is closed by the action of the *m. lateralis nasi* as it draws the lateral wall of the vestibule of the nasal cavity outward in order to open the vestibule. With relaxation of that muscle, the entrance of the diverticulum opens passively (Colin 1886/1888; Sisson and Grossman 1953). Some fossil horses, *Hypohippus, Archaeohippus*, and *Pliohippus*, have bony fossae as evidence that the nasal diverticulum extended almost to the rostral border of the orbit (Simpson 1951). Apparently, two fossae can be differentiated for paleontological purposes, a dorsal preorbital and a malar fossa (MacFadden 1992). While these fossae suggest that the diverticulum could be an evolutionary remnant, its function, then or now, remains enigmatic. A role in sound production may be possible.

Atheroma of the nasal diverticulum

This is a cystic mass with a firm, elastic capsule and cheesy, caseous content, which develops in the connective tissue of the nasal diverticulum. It usually bulges laterally rather than into the diverticulum and may reach hen egg size. The histological picture is said to be that of cystic sebaceous glandular tissue (Wintzer 1986), but no secure pathological studies have been found.

Nasal amyloidosis

Nasal amyloidosis is peculiar to the horse and uncommon. The nasal vestibule and rostral parts of the nasal septum and turbinates have amyloid deposits in diffuse or nodular form, often reaching considerable size. Ulceration is uncommon. On section the glassy, waxy appearance of amyloid is characteristic. It is deposited around blood vessels, the basement membrane of glands, and within the connective tissue. There may be modest chronic inflammatory cell reaction. This is not part of generalized amyloidosis, and the cause is uninvestigated and unknown (Cohrs 1961; Shaw et al. 1987).

Rhinosporidiosis

This is endemic in India and occurs sporadically in horses, cattle, and humans in South Africa, South America, and the southern United States (Ainsworth and Austwick 1959; Smith and Frankson 1961; Myers et al. 1964). It has not, apparently, been seen in Europe. Masses in the nares are unilateral, polypoid, or sessile. Histologically, sporangia, up to 300 microns, are embedded in a delicate fibrous tissue stroma with macrophages and lymphocytes. Neutrophils and eosinophils may be present in variable numbers. The organism has not been cultured, transmission studies have been negative, and the epidemiology and pathogenesis are unknown (Ainsworth and Austwick 1959).

Mucoid degeneration of the nasal conchae

This was described in 1892 by Sand and exhaustively reviewed in 1962 by Espersen cited by Rubarth and Krook (1968). The latter have demonstrated quite satisfactorily that this is the osteitis fibrosa of nutritional secondary hyperparathyroidism.

Rhinitis

Inflammation of the nasal and turbinate mucosa is virtually unknown as an independent entity. Influenza infection produces histological lesions of erosion and ulceration in the mucosa of the nasal septum and turbinates, but gross lesions are not seen. No pathological studies have been reported with rhinitis virus infections. Catarrhal, purulent rhinitis has been reported with the early stages of strangles infection (Cohrs 1961). Usually, there is only reddening of the mucosa with purulent exudate, but small abscesses or more extensive phlegmonous thickening may be found.

Strangles

This common, highly infectious disease of the horse has been known since antiquity, certainly to the Greeks (Cadeac 1899b). Viborg apparently was the first to transmit the disease by inoculation in 1802 [Viborg (1802) cited by Cadeac (1899b)]. Solleysel (1711) described the clinical disease and may have recognized transmissibility. The name, *Streptococcus equi*, was given to the organism by Schutz in 1888. Strangles is primarily a disease of the young animal, though it is seen at all ages, depending upon exposure experience and immune status. Viborg reported that of 100 cases, 70 occurred before 5 years of age, 20 between 5 and 12 years, and 10 after 12 years.

Experimental infection was, at one time, erratic and difficult. It was eventually shown that *S. equi* cultures in the growth phase were primary pathogens without any helper viruses or other agents being required (Bryans et al. 1964).

Immunity after infection may be incomplete and recurrent infection is not uncommon. There may be several years between significant attacks, however (Cadeac 1899).

As indicated above, the organism enters the nasal passages and causes inflammation, erosions, and small abscesses of the upper respiratory mucosa with early metastasis to the regional lymph nodes. Abscesses develop in the lymph nodes, eventually breaking and draining to the exterior. It appears that treatment with antibiotics before the abscesses break, before sufficient exposure to the immune system, leads to inadequate immune response. As well "bastard strangles," involvement of tissues and organs other than the nasopharyngeal mucosa and regional lymph nodes, may be more common in animals treated with antibiotics before the immune reaction develops. Purpura hemorrhagica is a recognized sequelae of strangles infection and improper use of strangles vaccines.

Herpesvirus (EHV)-1

Catarrhal rhinitis and pharyngitis occur with experimental, intranasal exposure to herpesvirus (EHV)-1. There are hyperemia, edema, and petechiae in the nasopharyngeal mucosa with mucopurulent exudate. The characteristic intranuclear inclusion bodies have not been seen other than in the fetus. The regional lymph nodes may be enlarged and edematous (Gylstorff 1971).

Grass bloom

An outbreak of acute nasal catarrh was reported in horses when grass was in bloom [Walther cited by Hutyra and Marek (1926)]. We have seen no other reports.

Rhinitis bullosa

An epizootic vesicular disease was described by Schnuerer and others (Hutyra and Marek 1926) among army horses in Europe during and after the First World War. There were multiple hemorrhagic foci in the nasal septum and turbinate mucosa. These became gray-red or gray-white, vesiculated, and ruptured to form erosions and small ulcerations. The ulcerations could coalesce to form large, ragged, and deeply eroded areas, on occasion even perforating the nasal septum. Usually, there were no other signs and recovery occurred in 6–8 weeks. The cause was not determined, and the disease is apparently no longer seen in Europe (Wintzer 1986).

Progressive ethmoidal hematoma

This was described by Cook and Littlewort (1974). Cook had seen a suspected case in 1968, and Amman and Fackelman (1971) mention probable cases. There are reports in the older literature (Cadeac 1896) of vascular tumors in the nasal cavity, which were probably this condition.

The lesion is usually encountered in young, working-age horses, but has been seen in older animals. There is difficult breathing and/or nasal exudate. Few postmortem cases have been reported, most reports being of biopsies. Platt (1974) examined material from 10 cases, one of which was the entire head. In the latter, angiomatous lesions were seen in the nasal mucosa and paranasal sinuses, suggesting that the hematoma developed from these preexisting angiomatous lesions. The histological picture was that of the not uncommon angiomatosis in the skin and other sites.

In one postmortem case, we found changes identical to those described by Platt (Fig. 2.1). It is reasonable to propose that so-called ethmoid hematoma is, in fact, a congenital tumor/malformation, **angiomatosis**, of blood vessels in the upper respiratory tract. Indeed, this angiomatosis seems peculiar to the horse, affecting skin, intermuscular connective tissue, and meninges, as well as the upper respiratory mucosa.

Parasites

Linguatula taenioides occur as accidental parasites in the nasal cavity (Cadeac 1896). *Haemopsis sanguisuga*, a leech, was said to be widespread in Europe and particularly in North Africa during the summer months. The parasite is firmly fixed to the mucosa and causes hemorrhages. It can invade any mucous membrane: mouth, nasal cavity, conjunctiva, anus, and/or vulva. We know of no reports in North America.

Sinuses

As already noted by Colin (1888), air leaves the frontal and maxillary sinuses during inspiration and reenters slowly during expiration.

Sinusitis

Considered at length in clinical texts, acute or chronic sinusitis is uncommon at postmortem. The majority of cases are of the maxillary sinuses as a result of infection of the maxillary cheek teeth. It is almost invariably a mucopurulent inflammation with erosion of mucosa and destruction of bone—osteomyelitis—in advanced, chronic cases.

The frontal and sphenopalatine sinuses are rarely sites of infection, and then, by extension from the maxillary sinus or as the result of an external wound in the case of the frontal sinus.

Neoplasia

Benign and malignant tumors of the upper respiratory system are uncommon. Runnells and Benbrook (1941b) examined 156 soft tissue neoplasms of which about 70 arose from the head and nasal passages. These cases were collected in a clinic over a period of 20 years, a very low incidence. Madewell et al. (1976) estimated 15 nasal and 11 sinus tumors per 100,000 patient-years. Comparable estimates for dogs were 65 and 16, respectively.

Squamous cell carcinomas may affect the rostral portion of the nasal passages while adenocarcinoma characteristically arises from the ethmoid mucosa (Fig. 2.2). Squamous cell carcinomas may arise in any of the paranasal sinuses. Benign or malignant soft tissue tumors are usually of fibrous tissue origin, though the varied histological picture of neoplastic growth, invasion, and repair may lead

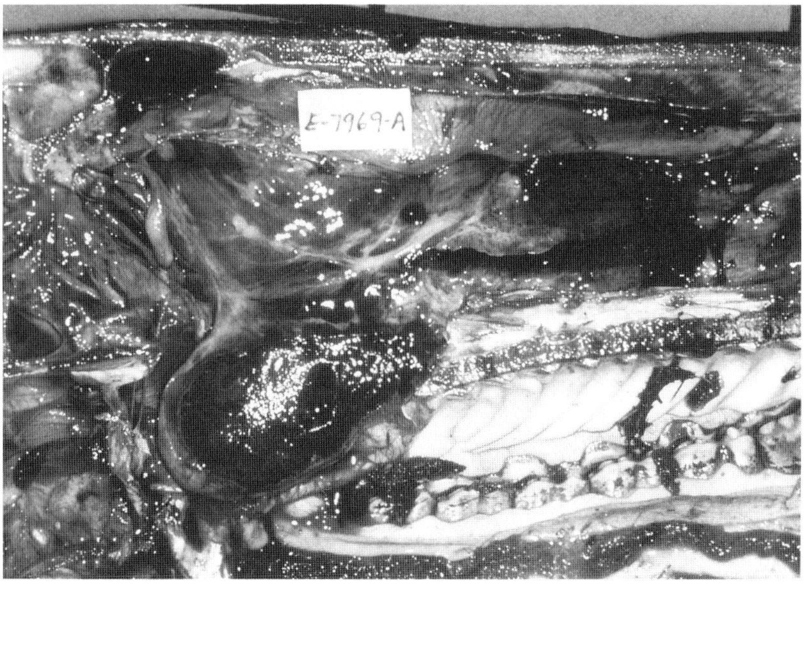

2.1. Angiomatosis of the ethmoid is a congenital anomaly or vascular malformation commonly known as "ethmoidal hematoma."

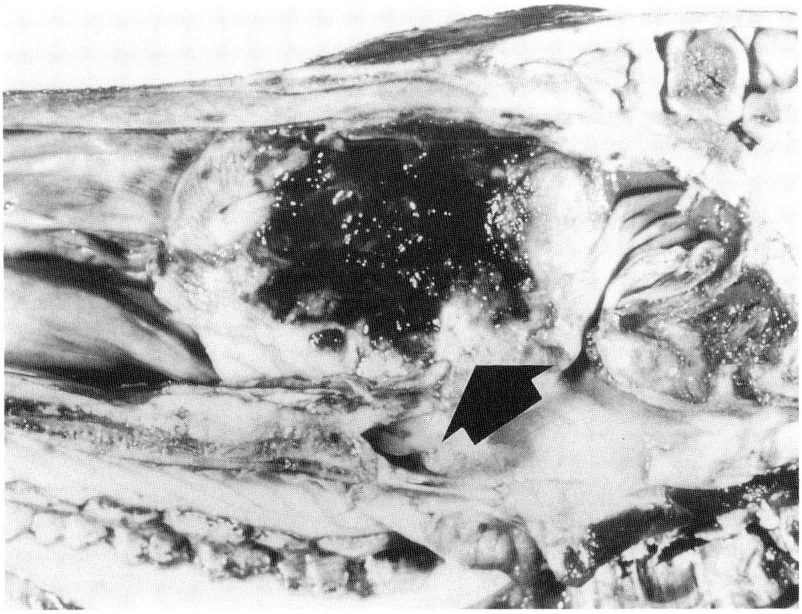

2.2. Squamous cell carcinoma of the nasal passage (*arrow*) must be differentiated from ethmoidal adenocarcinoma.

to a variety of diagnoses (Runnells and Benbrook 1941b; Cohrs 1961).

Carcinomas are more often found in older animals while fibromas/sarcomas may be found at any age; over half of the Runnells and Benbrook cases of sarcoma occurred between 1 and 4 years of age.

The endemic, malignant adenocarcinomas of the ethmoid reported in cattle and horses in Sweden remain an enigma.

Pharynx

There are more clinical entities, real or proposed, of the pharyngeal area than pathological entities to match. Clinical interest is focused in the area because of respiratory noises and inadequate performance putatively associated with inadequate respiration. Several causes of respiratory noise have already been mentioned. It is of interest that such abnormal noises were recorded in Ugaritic hippiatric texts in the 14th to 12th centuries BCE (Cohen and Sivan 1983).

The endoscopist attempts to interpret normal and abnormal function in a system significantly modified by the act of endoscopy. The pathologist attempts to interpret static morphology in terms of necessarily uncertain functional interpretations. Difficulties and differences of interpretation surely follow.

Pharyngitis

Acute and chronic pharyngitis are commonly diagnosed clinically and virtually never seen pathologically. A transient, mild hyperemia and petechiation of the pharyngeal mucosa, **catarrhal pharyngitis**, occurs during the early stages of strangles infection and experimental infection with herpesvirus (EHV)-1.

Purulent exudate may be found lightly adherent to or lying on the mucosal surface in animals with guttural pouch empyema and mucopurulent bronchitis. Histological examination confirms that the mucosa itself is not inflamed.

A trivial, localized inflammation and abscessation may occur in and around tonsillar crypts containing embedded foreign, usually plant, material. Cadeac (1896) described **tonsillar calculi** peculiar to old donkeys. The tonsillar crypts were dilated and contained variable-sized black or gray calculi surrounded by brownish, semiliquid material. Histologically, the lamellated calculus had formed around a fragment of plant material. This is seen in older horses as well, but less often, apparently, than in old donkeys.

Chronic pharyngitis is also called pharyngeal lymphoid hyperplasia or lymphoid follicular pharyngitis. The tonsillar lymphoid tissue of the horse is described in anatomical/histological texts (Zietzschmann et al. 1943; Sisson and Grossman 1953; Krölling and Grau 1960). The diagnosis of chronic pharyngitis in young, working horses has become a veritable icon in the clinical literature (Raker 1976; Robertson 1990). There is no morphological basis for the diagnosis. The lymphoid tissue of the young horse is variably prominent here, as elsewhere in the body, becoming less prominent with age; subjective comparisons among young horses or among populations of young and old horses cannot be made. Attempts to associate pharyngeal lymphoid hyperplasia with infection by herpesvirus (EHV)-2 have been made, but are doubtful.

Biopsies were made of pharyngeal mucosa of a number of horses with a diagnosis of chronic pharyngitis. There were no lesions; indeed, it was not possible, histologically, to separate suspected cases from random controls. Even cases with purulent exudate on the surface had no histological changes. An occasional horse comes to postmortem, for other reasons, with a diagnosis of chronic pharyngitis. Pharyngitis is not found but, rather, a mucopurulent bronchiolitis. This was suggested, as well, by Cadore (1987).

Inflammation of the bronchiolar system is almost always associated with coughing–for example, influenza–while pharyngitis is not. Indeed, suppression of the cough reflex is characteristic of pharyngitis.

Cadeac (1908) described epizootics of pharyngitis. The clinical description, as well as the pathology, are quite different from that considered above. The clinical signs included fever, refusal to eat, difficult swallowing, tenderness on palpation, and extended head. The pharynx was covered by a thick layer of yellowish or greenish mucus containing purulent material, flecks of blood, food material, and large numbers of bacteria. The mucosa was thickened, edematous, and hyperemic with multiple ulcerations. The lymphoid nodules were enlarged, particularly on the base and sides of the tongue. The condition was contagious with recovery in 10 to 12 days. We have seen no example, but this is a clear-cut example of true pharyngitis.

Dorsal displacement of the soft palate

A bewildering variety of soft palate defects has been postulated for wind problems in horses. As well, paralysis of the pharyngeal muscles and collapse of the wall of the pharynx have been proposed. Many of these putative entities have not been confirmed pathologically.

Dorsal displacement, or misplacement, of the soft palate relative to an hypoplastic epiglottis is a reasonable cause of impeded airflow. Whether, as clinical opinion suggests, there are other, morphological, causes for misplacement of the soft palate is problematic. Blythe et al. (1983) examined samples of palatal tissue from horses diagnosed as dorsal palatal displacement as well as normal controls. While they concluded that muscle damage was present, no judgment was made as to the primary or secondary nature of the damage. Indeed, the damage itself is questionable and may not be beyond normal variation. Our own, limited, studies of biopsy material and a few postmortem cases with a clinical diagnosis of palatal displacement have shown no significant changes.

Many of the muscles causing movement of the soft palate and pharyngeal area can be examined on the split head after removal of the pharyngeal mucosa: *mm. palatinus, levator veli palatini, tensor veli palatini*, and pharyngeal muscles (Fig. 2.3). It is apparent from examination of fresh specimens, while the muscle is still responsive to mechanical stimulation, that elevation of the soft palate must be affected by cooperative action of several muscles. The levator alone lifts the middle third of the soft palate, not the caudal third and free border. The tensor seems to tighten only the rostral third. The palatinus does not respond to mechanical stimulation while the pharyngeal muscles, in addition to their other actions, help tense the soft palate. These observations suggest that the levator elevates the entire soft palate when the latter is stiffened by the action of the other muscles (Zietzschmann et al. 1943).

A number of factors can cause functional obstruction of the air flow through the nasopharynx (Raker 1976). It is by no means evident that an elevated position of the soft palate in the standing horse establishes a diagnosis of obstruction of air flow in the moving horse. Even finding such displacement while the horse is moving, for example, on a treadmill, does not establish unequivocally that such displacement is *a* or *the* cause for airway problems while the horse is working in a usual manner. The animal may swallow ("gulp") simply because of the presence of the endoscope, the examiner, and the unusual situation. The term "swallowing hard" when frightened or as a reflex response to a foreign object in the nasal cavity or pharynx is relevant.

Rostral displacement of the arcus palatopharyngicus

This was described by Cook (1974). Deegan and Klein (1987) reviewed six cases in the literature and added four of their own. It has been seen in Thoroughbreds, Haflingers, Hannoverians, and Holsteiners. The condition was sometimes apparent at birth (4 of 10) with inspiratory noise, coughing, and difficult swallowing. Two postmortem cases had malformed thyroid cartilages with bilateral aplasia of the cricopharyngeal muscles. The thyroid cartilages were smaller than normal and misaligned. The rostral displacement of the arcus palatopharyngicus,

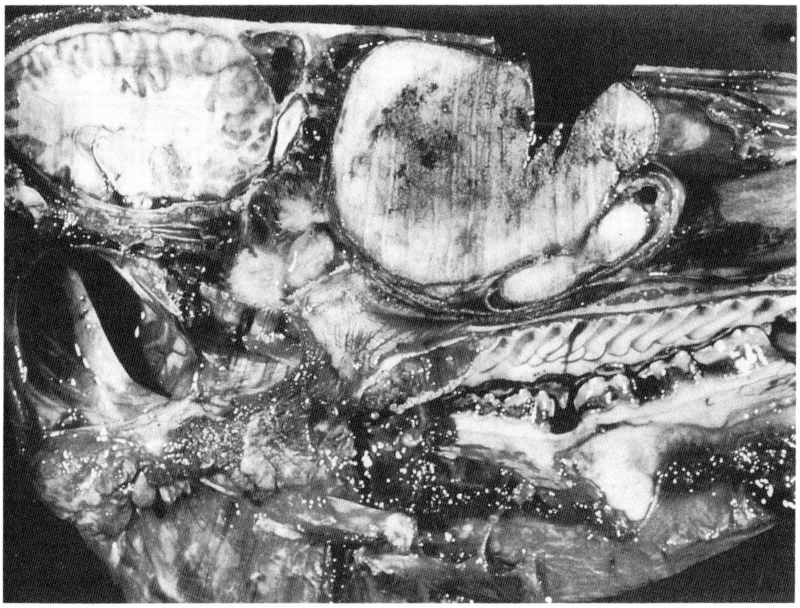

2.3. Muscles controlling the movement of the soft palate and the pharynx can most easily be examined by splitting the skull.

then, appears to be secondary to congenital and/or genetic defects of the laryngeal cartilages.

Malignant lymphoma of the pharynx

Adams et al. (1988a) found three cases of malignant lymphoma with ulcerative pharyngitis in horses 5–15 years old. In all cases, the presumptive diagnosis was pharyngitis and abscessation.

Larynx

Variably extensive calcification and/or ossification of the cartilages of the larynx occurs with age.

Subepiglottic cysts

These congenital cysts, single or multiple and derived from the thyroglossal duct, are almost invariably located just ventral to the epiglottis [Cadiot in *Bayer-Fröhner* (1910); Uberreiter (1937, 1968); Schäper (1939); and Gylstorff (1971)]. They vary from pea to hen egg size with a sticky, mucoid content. The cyst is lined by a simple, cuboidal epithelium with areas of columnar or squamous character. The larger cysts may interfere with normal positioning of the caudal border of the soft palate ventral to the epiglottis and, so, cause noise during inspiration and expiration. These cysts were seen at least as early as 1892 by an unidentified German author (Am Vet Rev 1892/93), and by Degive (1881) and Lesbre (1886) cited by Cadeac (1896). Cadeac published two clear engravings of such cysts.

Raker (1976) mentions cysts in the dorsal wall of the pharynx. There are no other reports, and we have seen no example. They may be bronchiogenic cysts of the same origin as the so-called ear fistula or dentigerous cyst.

Hypoplasia of the epiglottis

This was described by Wilmes and Schneider (1933) and Görnemann (1939) as a cause of expiratory noise during exercise. It has been rediscovered since (Boles et al. 1978). The epiglottis is smaller than normal, without a distinct pointed apex and ends in the upper border of the *plicae aryepiglotticae*. The latter appear to be hyperplastic in some cases. The hypoplasia varies from near normal to very small.

Epiglottic entrapment is cited as a self-standing lesion apart from hypoplasia of the epiglottis. The evidence, however, is that entrapment is always associated with hypoplasia(Fig. 2.4). The epiglottis can be measured on clinical radiographs (Fjeldborg 1987).

The cause of the expiratory noise seems to be incomplete sealing of the oropharynx by soft palate positioning ventral to the epiglottis. During expiration, specifically, the air flow could cause fluttering of the free border of the soft palate as air flowed into the oropharynx and the nasopharynx. Lesser

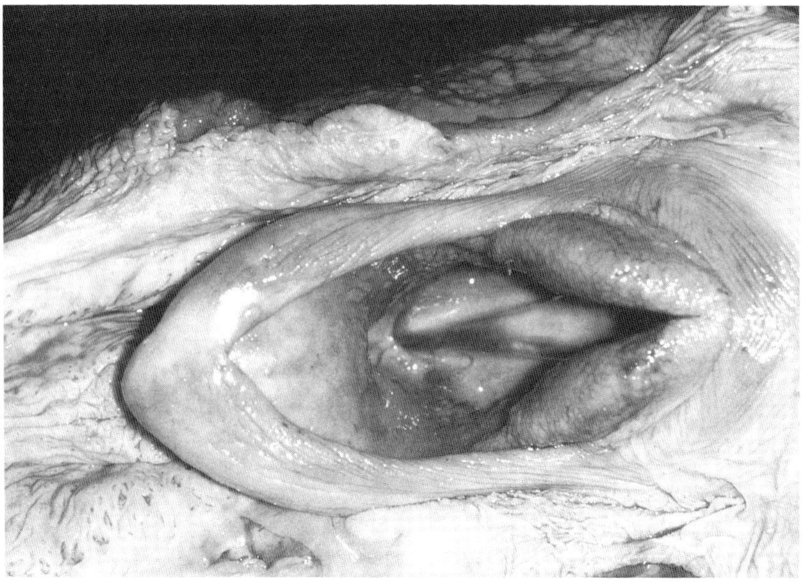

2.4. Entrapment of the epiglottis is usually associated with epiglottic hypoplasia.

degrees of epiglottic hypoplasia might be the basic lesion in so-called dorsal displacement of the soft palate.

A single case of congenital **fusion of the ventral parts of the vocal folds** (web defect) has been reported (Lees et al. 1987). The entire larynx was hypoplastic, including the epiglottis.

Arytenopathy

Indurating ulceration of the dorsomedial aspect of the arytenoid cartilage was briefly described by Joest (1923) (Hutyra and Marek 1926). A case was described by Eeckhout (1905/1906). Dieckerhoff (1890) called the condition **chondritis arytaenoidea chronica** and found no discussion of pathogenesis in the literature. It has been discussed in more recent clinical literature (Haynes et al. 1980; Raker 1976; Robertson 1991). Most cases are seen in young Thoroughbred and Standardbred racehorses (Tulleners et al. 1988). Since these animals are more often examined for upper respiratory problems, the frequency may be deceptive. The descriptions in the older literature were of draft animals.

The pathogenesis and, indeed, the pathology of this condition are unclear, thus the use of the term *arytenopathy*. Reports indicate that an ulcerative chronic inflammatory process is present in young horses and "chondroma" in older horses (Raker 1976). The inflammatory process is said to consist of fibrous tissue, lymphoid, and mononuclear cells with neutrophils in the presence of ulceration. While the cartilage is clearly involved in the inflammatory process in some cases, there is confusion in the literature about the type of cartilage present and its significance. Most of the arytenoid is hyaline cartilage with the corniculate process and vocal process being elastic cartilage. Since the lesion occurs in or at the hyaline/elastic junction, interpretation of changes must take normal cartilage structure into account (Haynes et al. 1980). Elastic cartilage can resemble chondroma on casual examination.

In a few biopsies we have seen chronic inflammation with eosinophils, mononuclear cells, fibrosis, and granulomas with necrotic, eosinophilic centers surrounded by foreign body giant cells. The lesion is reminiscent of equine nodular collagenolytic granuloma (Stannard 1976; Yager and Scott 1985), as well as lesions occasioned by migrating helminth larvae. In other cases chronic inflammation, characterized by lymphoid cells, plasma cells, and macrophages with only scattered eosinophils, was present.

In our specimens, where epithelium was present, there were localized changes of the stratified squamous epithelium. These varied from acanthosis to marked thickening with hyperkeratosis, and/or focal areas of atypia in the stratum spinosum, all associated with chronic inflammatory cell infiltration and/or fibrosis of the underlying connective tissue. The material is insufficient to define the disease process, but there is a suggestion of **leukoplakia**. Such lesions in humans may be precursors of carcinoma in situ and carcinoma and, in one or two cases, we have seen lesions very like carcinoma in situ. Although frank cases of squamous cell carcinoma are uncommon, they have been reported arising in this area of the mucosa of the arytenoid (Wilmes 1938). Montané and Morot (1892) reported a case of squamous cell carcinoma arising from the mucosa of the cricoid cartilage.

McClure et al. (1988) found a significant association between equine lymphocyte antigen A 9 and arytenopathy, although the number of animals was small.

Laryngeal hemiplegia is discussed with peripheral nerves (see Chapter 16, "Nervous System").

Guttural pouch

The guttural pouches are outpouchings of the eustachian tube characteristic of the Perissodactyla. The eustachian tube, as such, was described by Aristotle around 350 BCE (Peck 1979). The pouches are said to be a necessary adjunct to the pharyngeal apparatus of Equidae, allowing normal swallowing to occur (Skoda 1911). Other theories as to the function of the guttural pouches have been proposed, but that of Skoda best fits the available facts (Richter 1923; Gratzl 1934a; Zietzschmann et al. 1943). Skoda based his theory on dissection and direct observation of the pouches in the live horse. Incidentally, Cadeac (1896) credits Lafosse (1790) with an instrument to examine the guttural pouches through the eustachian tube. Heffron et al. (1979a) have reinvestigated pharyngeal function without improving upon Skoda's description. It is generally accepted that air both enters and leaves the guttural pouch during expiration.

The eustachian tubes are formed in the first month of fetal life, and the first outpouching of the guttural pouch is apparent in the third month. During the last third of fetal life, the guttural pouch achieves the proportionate development of the adult (Zietschmann and Krölling 1955).

The pharynx of the Perissodactyla differs from that of other animals. The rostral third of the dorsal wall is directly applied to the skull. The remainder of the dorsal wall and the lateral walls are enveloped by the guttural pouches (Dyce et al. 1987). In the horse, during swallowing, there is considerable movement of the caudal pharyngeal wall rostrally, this movement permitted by the flexible attachment of the pharyngeal wall to the guttural pouches. Skoda argued that this movement is necessitated by the long, narrow pharynx, so that a bolus of food can pass from mouth through oropharynx to esophagus without entering the larynx. Abnormal swallowing can occur with tympany, empyema, or inflammatory disease of the guttural pouches (Gratzl 1934a).

While speculative, it can be suggested that the long, narrow pharynx and the long, narrow, but deep, head developed as the short teeth of the early browsing equids evolved to the long grazing teeth of later equids and Equus.

Empyema of the guttural pouch

Accumulation of purulent material in the guttural pouch usually accompanies strangles infection. While the pharyngeal mucosa and regional lymph nodes are most often affected, infection of the guttural pouch does occur either as primary infection of the mucosa or by extension from abscessed lymph nodes. The thick purulent material cannot readily escape from the pouch and undergoes gradual inspissation, forming multiple balls of caseous purulent material (Fig. 2.5). It is

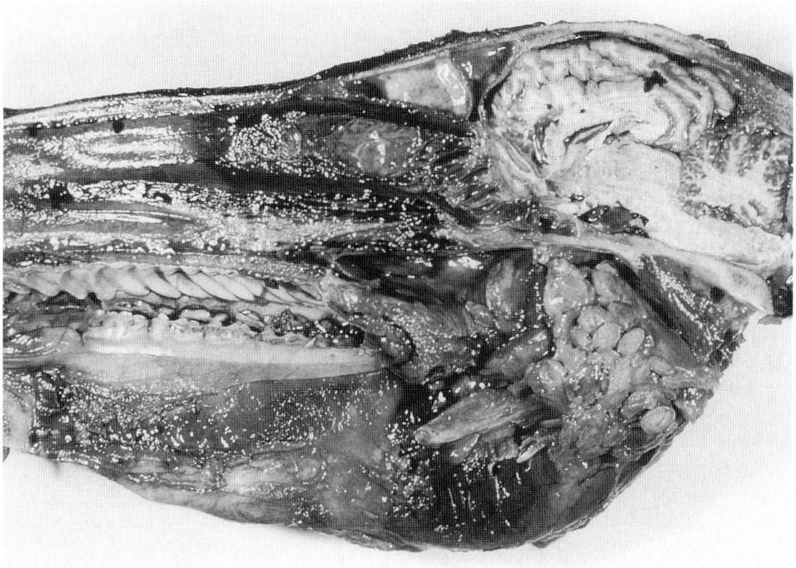

2.5. Inspissated debris in the guttural pouch may form balls of caseous material known as "luftsackstein."

remarkable that an animal may have one guttural pouch full of such caseopurulent material with few, if any, clinical signs, though nasal discharge when the head is lowered and dysphagia are seen. If both pouches are affected, there may be sufficient interference with air flow to cause asphyxia.

Lesser degrees of empyema may be seen in one or both guttural pouches with secondary bacterial infections of the upper respiratory passages. *Streptococcus zooepidemicus* is the common agent. The purulent exudate induced by this organism is characteristically gray and watery and, so, able to clear the pouch more readily than the thick exudate characteristic of *S. equi*.

Mycosis of the guttural pouch

Mycotic infection of the dorsal wall of the guttural pouch was reported in the modern era by Cook et al. (1968). It was recorded prior to that time [Andersson cited by Cohrs (1961); Ridge (1891); Ries (1903); Rivolta (1873) cited by Ries; Hutyra and Marek (1920, 1926); and Bassi cited by Cadeac (1896)]. In Ries's case *Asperillus* sp. was isolated, and the glossopharyngeal and vagus nerves were affected. Mycosis of the guttural pouch is more often seen in young animals in training or work but can occur in horses of any age, including, uncommonly, weanling foals.

The gross lesion is a tough, yellowish, necrotic plaque surrounded by a variably wide hyperemic border situated in the mucosa of the dorsal wall of the guttural pouch medial to the great cornu of the hyoid bone (Fig. 2.6). It is almost always unilateral. Histologically, there is massive infection with hyphal fungi, usually *Aspergillus* sp., with neutrophilic, mononuclear inflammatory reaction. The internal carotid artery, glossopharyngeal, and vagus nerves lie immediately above the lesion. Clinical signs are caused by invasion and destruction of one or more of these structures by the fungi. The wall of the internal carotid artery is invaded by the fungal hyphae, with massive hemorrhages into the guttural pouch. Less commonly, dysphagia is seen because of damage to the nerves. Hemorrhage into the guttural pouch may not be suspected until the animal lowers its head when blood escapes in large quantities, sometimes enough to cause hemorrhagic shock and death.

Aspergillus spp. are ubiquitous in the equine environment and can be cultured from the nasal passages of normal animals. It appears, then, that the pathogenesis is to be sought in damage to the dorsal wall of the guttural pouch by, for example, viruses, which allow secondary fungal invasion. The site of the lesion is a primary impingement point for a stream of air entering the pouch. Plaques of mucosal thickening, squamous metaplasia, may be found here, further suggesting a high rate of exposure to airborne foreign materials.

Tympany of the guttural pouch

Persistent accumulation of air in the guttural pouch is congenital or acquired and uncommon. The acquired case may accompany empyema, inflammation of the mucosa obstructing the pharyngeal orifice and/or the eustachian tube.

The congenital form is more common, though still infrequent. It is usually not recognized in the newborn, appearing before 1 year of age. McCue et al. (1989) reviewed 15 cases in one clinic over 9 years. There was no apparent breed predisposition, but 11 of the cases were fillies, this sex predisposi-

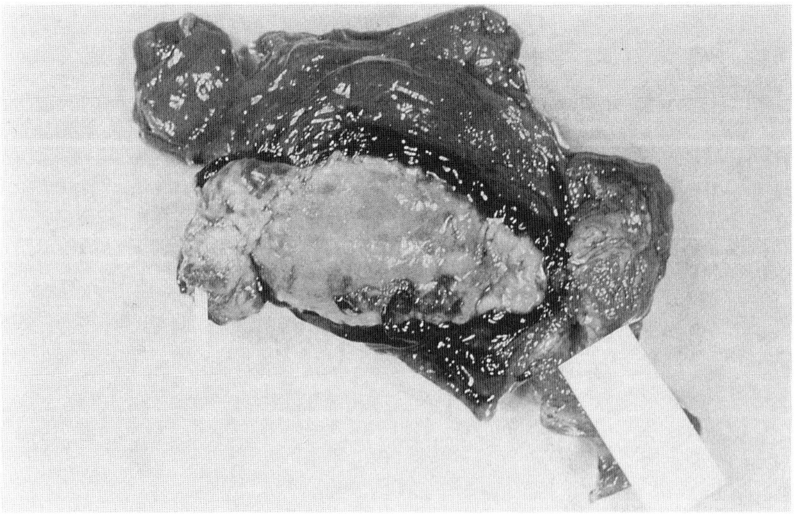

2.6. Guttural pouch mycosis is usually seen grossly as a tough, yellow plaque near the hyoid bone.

tion having been noted by others. Their cases were diagnosed between 1 and 20 months of age.

Gratzl (1934a) mentioned a case of chronic tympany [Conreur cited by Möller (1908)] in which the eustachian tube was fused, not opening into the guttural pouch. The tympany was not corrected by opening the pouch through Viborg's triangle but was corrected when the eustachian tube was split open.

Günther, cited by Zietzschmann et al. (1943), observed that the *m. levator veli palatini* not only raises the soft palate during swallowing but also closes the eustachian tube, preventing accumulation of air in the guttural pouch. The pharyngeal orifice opens during swallowing, but the eustachian tube is closed to the guttural pouch. During swallowing, then, the system operates as it does in animals without a guttural pouch. Results of dissections of fresh specimens agree with Günther's observation. It appears, also, that the *m. tensor veli palatini* contributes to closing the opening of the eustachian tube into the guttural pouch. Gerlach (1894) cited by Cadeac (1896) believed muscle paralysis allowed closure of the opening of the eustachian tube into the guttural pouch, so that air could not escape from the pouch. It is possible for the pharyngeal orifice to be normal while abnormal closure of the eustachian tube would trap air in the guttural pouch. Detailed examination of these muscles and their nerves (glossopharyngeal, vagus, and trigeminal) (Zietzschmann et al. 1943) might be profitable, as well as in putative cases of soft palate dysfunction.

Fracture of the stylohyoid

Healed fractures of the dorsal end of the stylohyoid bone close to the union with the petrous temporal bone are occasionally encountered radiographically and at postmortem (Cook 1970). The petrous temporal bone may be fractured, as well, or involved in the callus of the stylohyoid. While neurological signs may appear (Geiser et al. 1988), the fractures are usually incidental findings. The pathogenesis has not been studied in detail, but sudden ventroflexion of the head on the neck with a sideways, lateral, component (for unilateral fracture) would be required. This movement would be caused by forceful jerking on the reins and is, also, typical of cribbing. Two of Geiser's 3 cases were cribbers.

Lower respiratory system

Diagnosing pulmonary disease

Functional measurements

There have been numerous studies on the physiology of the equine respiratory system. Willoughby and McDonell (1979) reviewed pulmonary function testing and tabulated numerous measurements of function in normal and diseased horses.

Functional residual capacity in normal horses is approximately 45% of total lung capacity (Leith 1976). This decreases in disease with changes in lung elasticity and recoil. With a helium dilution method, 3.99 L/100 kg body weight were found in 8 normal, sedated ponies, and 3.56 liters/100 kg body weight in normal, sedated, larger horses (Willoughby and McDonell 1979). In a horse with chronic pulmonary disease, 10.4 L/100 kg body weight was found (Leith and Gillespie 1971). The functional residual capacity of a horse with an intrathoracic neoplasm was reduced to 3.41 liters/100 kg body weight. While such measurements indicate pulmonary disease, they are difficult to obtain without sophisticated equipment and experience.

Ventilation and pulmonary perfusion can be measured by means of nitrogen washout curves. The principle is that nitrogen is washed out of alveoli more slowly with airway disease (Willoughby and McDonell 1979). Normal horses have end-tidal expired nitrogen concentrations of approximately 2%, while horses with severe, chronic pulmonary disease have 4%–6%.

Analysis of blood gases is useful for detecting pulmonary dysfunction. Measurements in 37 normal horses gave normal pH of 7.38, PaO_2 mm Hg of 83.6, and $PaCO_2$ mm Hg of 42.2. Comparable values in 20 horses with chronic pulmonary disease were pH 7.37, PaO_2 mm Hg 63.3, and $PaCO_2$ mm Hg 47.0.

Rossdale (1979) reviewed neonatal respiratory function and the normal development of the respiratory system during gestation. Most foals have a fully developed system by 300 days of gestation, including adequate surfactant to facilitate lung expansion. Gillespie (1975) measured arterial pH and blood gases in neonatal foals. Seven had mean fetal umbilical artery pH of 7.35, PaO_2 mm Hg of 33.4, and $PaCO_2$ mm Hg of 46.2 before birth. Measurements during birth were pH 7.17, PaO_2 mm Hg 22.6, and $PaCO_2$ mm Hg 72.8. With postpartum breathing, values approached normal physiological levels. The pH in the umbilical artery of seven foals immediately after delivery during spontaneous respiration was 7.26, the PaO_2 mm Hg was 35.4, and the $PaCO_2$ mm Hg was 69.1. Values for normal respiratory function in foals were compiled by Rossdale (1979).

Cytology

Transtracheal aspirates, bronchopulmonary lavage specimens, and mucous secretions are used in the diagnosis of respiratory disease. A number of studies have correlated antemortem cytology with postmortem histological findings. Winder et al. (1989) studied the composition of respiratory mucous secretions in 109 normal and diseased horses. They obtained respiratory secretions from 33 horses prior to slaughter and from an additional 76 immediately after slaughter and compared cytology with histology. Horses with histological evidence of severe chronic small airway disease had copious amounts of mucus, presumably because of goblet cell hyperplasia. There was no significant difference in the amount of mucus in horses with minimal or moderate bronchiolitis as compared to 14 normal horses. The secretions from all normal horses contained exfoliated ciliated epithelium.

Macrophages in secretions showed that specimens were obtained from the lower respiratory tract where such cells predominate. Hemosiderin-laden macrophages were found in horses with pulmonary hemorrhage, and large numbers of macrophages were seen in the respiratory secretions of horses with interstitial pneumonia. There were large numbers of neutrophils in the secretions of moderate and severe chronic bronchiolitis, and significantly increased numbers of lymphocytes in the secretions of horses with severe chronic disease.

Infestation with *Dictyocaulus arnfeldi* caused an increase of eosinophils. Winder et al. (1989) concluded that the type and extent of lung histopathology could not be determined by examination of a single lower respiratory secretion specimen.

Mair et al. (1987a) analyzed lavages from different levels of the respiratory tract in 42 horses and ponies of various ages and breeds. None had overt respiratory disease. Mair et al. found progressive increases in total cell counts in the deeper parts of the lungs. They also found a preponderance of squamous cells in nasal secretions and a larger proportion of inflammatory cells deep in the tract. Horses with chronic pulmonary disease had increased numbers of macrophages in tracheal aspirates (Mair 1987).

The quantity and type of various prostanoid inflammatory mediators secreted by alveolar macrophages and blood monocytes was studied by Watson et al. (1990). These prostanoids play a significant role in a variety of pulmonary and systemic diseases. They compared concentrations of PGE_2, PGF, thromboxane B_2, and 6-keto-PGF_{1a} secreted by cells from 3 normal horses and 3 with chronic pulmonary disease. They also assayed these mediators in bronchoalveolar lavage fluid. The concentration of PGE_2 was increased in bronchoalveolar lavage fluid from all 3 horses with chronic pulmonary disease, and 1 of these horses also had detectable levels of PGF. Baseline prostanoid production in cultured cells was no different in normal horses and those with chronic pulmonary disease.

Diagnostic radiography and ultrasonography

Imaging techniques have become important in diagnosing respiratory tract disease with the development of more powerful machines. Reef et al. (1991) compared sonograms and radiographs of 54 horses with lower respiratory tract disease. They found ultrasonography to be more useful than standard radiography in detecting small amounts of pleural effusions and areas of consolidation. Ultrasonography also allowed better definition of the location of such lesions and the type of fluid present. Adhesions, pleural thickening, and compression atelectasis could be seen with ultrasonography but not clearly with radiography. However, ultrasonography was only useful when lesions were near the body wall. Standard radiographic techniques were superior for localizing and analyzing lesions deep in the thorax.

Viral diseases

The most important viral infections of the equine respiratory tract are influenza, herpesvirus (EHV)-1, adenovirus, rhinovirus, and reovirus. Subclinical infection with viruses has been suspected in poor athletic performance, but there is no evidence (Mumford and Rossdale 1980).

Influenza

This is an acute viral respiratory disease common in young, unvaccinated horses. Immunity of vaccination or prior disease may be only partially protective, and immunity to one virus may not prevent infection by others. Crowding, transportation, and close contact are the usual risk factors. Epizootics occur whenever horses are transported to shows, training, racing, and breeding facilities, and sales (Coggins 1979; Burrows et al. 1982; Powell 1991).

Although the first major epizootics of equine

influenza occurred in Europe in 1956 (A-equi-1), and in the United States in 1963-65 (A-equi-2), there is evidence that A-equi-1 virus was present earlier than 1952 (Goto et al. 1975).

The **infectious bronchitis** described by Waldemann and Schurmann, cited by Cohrs (1941c), was probably influenza as were the several conditions known as: Hoppegärtner cough, grippe, morbus maculosus, bronchite infectieuse ou epizootique, and probably A-equi-1 influenza. Cohrs (1941) said that Waldemann et al. were the first to show that a virus was the cause of epizootic coughing in horses. They transmitted the disease by intranasal instillation to horses, dogs, and cattle but were unsuccessful with rabbits and ferrets. The incubation period was 4–12 days. Hupbauer and Lugomer (1938) isolated a virus, presumably A-equi-1, from an outbreak of epizootic bronchitis in foals. Schurmann (1933) cited by Cohrs (1941c) described the gross and microscopic lesions of infectious bronchitis. He considered it to be a lung disease—bronchitis/bronchiolitis with focal pneumonia. He found lesions in the dorsal part of the diaphragmatic lobe while others found them more often in the apical lobes. Schurmann described the histological lesion as marked infiltration of eosinophils in the subpleural space and around blood vessels and airways. The histological description of infectious bronchitis by Schurmann is remarkably similar to the pneumonia of more recent investigators (Dixon et al. 1992).

Beveridge (1977) cited by Alexander (1982) described the occurrence of human and equine influenza during 12 pandemics in the 18th and 19th centuries. Tumova (1980) reported antibodies to A-equi-2 in human sera from the human influenza pandemic of 1889–1990. Recent major epizootics have occurred in England in 1979, South Africa in 1986, and Western Europe in 1989 (Burrows et al. 1982; Powell 1991). Powell (1991) commented that clinical infection with A-equi-1 is now uncommon and that most cases of influenza are caused by A-equi-2 in the United States.

Classic equine influenza is caused by two type A, single-stranded RNA-containing viruses, designated A-equi-1/Prague/1956 (H7N7) and A-equi-2/Miami/1963 (H3N8). Several substrains of A-equi-2 are recognized: England 79, Fontainebleu 79, and Kentucky 81. The viral genome is transcribed to a complementary messenger RNA through the action of a virally derived reverse transcriptase (Alexander 1982).

The virus is cosmopolitan; only horses in Australia and New Zealand have not been exposed (Alexander 1982). The two viruses are antigenically dissimilar, and infection or vaccination with one does not confer immunity to the other. Like other influenza viruses, they are notorious for antigenic drift (minor variations in antigenicity) and antigen shift (major antigenic variations) because of rearrangement of RNA subunits and surface glycoprotein hemagglutinin and neuraminidase moieties (Coggins 1979). The envelope of the viruses contains lipid, making them susceptible to detergents and disinfectants.

A third equine influenza virus, A/Equine/Jilin/1/89 (H3N8), caused a serious epizootic among horses and mules in Northeastern China in 1989 (Webster and Yuanji 1991). The epizootic was characterized by morbidity over 80% and mortality of 20%–35%. The major causes of death were enteritis and pneumonia. Studies showed the virus had been derived from the avian gene pool, without gene reassortment. There is precedent for this type of viral derivation in the swine influenza epidemic of 1890 and the Spanish influenza pandemic of 1918, both presumably caused by avian-derived influenza viruses.

Experimental infection of horses with human influenza viruses, A2/Hong Kong/1/68 and B/Mass/3/66, showed that these viruses may propagate to a limited extent, for a few days, in nasal epithelium. There was no clinical disease (Kasel et al. 1968; Blaskovic et al. 1969a,b).

The pathogenesis of infection with classic strains of equine influenza virus has been characterized by Coggins (1979). Infection of upper and lower respiratory epithelium follows inhalation of the virus. Viral replication occurs for 48–72 hours in the epithelium, causing acute inflammation, necrosis, and focal desquamation of epithelial cells. Secondary infection of eroded mucosa with bacteria is common. Virus can be detected in nasal swabs in the first days after infection. There is little evidence of viremia. In experimental studies of A-equi-1, Blaskovic et al. (1966) recovered virus from bronchial and cervical lymph nodes and lung up to 7 days after intranasal inoculation.

Local immunity, particularly the secretion of immunoglobulin A, is a key factor in resistance to infection (Coggins 1979). Circulating immunoglobulins are released into the inflamed and eroded mucosa and neutralize virus, aiding recovery.

Influenza is characterized by high morbidity and low mortality. Virtually all susceptible horses develop the disease. Clinical disease is less severe or inapparent in vaccinated and recovered horses. Both viruses can cause disease at the same time, and horses recovering from infection with one virus may become infected with the other. A characteristic hacking and nonproductive cough is frequently present during infection with the A-2 virus. Likewise, there can be fever (104°–106°F) and watery nasal discharge. In the peripheral blood, anemia, lymphopenia, and monocytosis have been noted.

There are few gross lesions. Blaskovic et al.

(1966) described nasal mucosal hyperemia, and Powell (1991) commented that there is increased mucus in bronchi.

Microscopic lesions are confined to the respiratory mucosa, particularly the upper respiratory tract. There is multifocal hydropic swelling, necrosis, and sloughing of epithelium with eventual microscopic erosions, particularly evident on the nasal septum. Inflammatory cell infiltration is light unless secondary bacterial infection occurs. While most adult horses recover without complication, young foals can develop acute, severe bronchitis and bronchiolitis with fibrinous pneumonia. This can be lethal or become so with secondary infection by, especially, *Streptococcus zooepidemicus*. Some horses develop focal interstitial myocarditis or interstitial pneumonia following infection, more commonly in young and old animals.

Brüssler krankheit (Brussels disease) is an infectious bronchopneumonia described in the European literature, which is probably bacterial complication of influenza infection. Cohrs (1941c) describes it as a severe, generalized bronchopneumonia following influenza in which bacterial infection (mixed bacterial flora, primarily streptococci) causes a necrotizing, hemorrhagic pneumonia. It is now uncommon, probably because of antibiotics and vaccines.

Herpesvirus infection

Infection of the upper and lower respiratory tract with herpesvirus (EHV)-1 can cause acute viral rhinopneumonitis. Since the 1930s the disease has been recognized as a cause of abortion in mares. The identification of herpes abortion and respiratory disease did not come until the 1950s when the distinction was made between influenza and herpes infections (Allen and Bryans 1986). The neuropathology of equine herpesvirus (EHV)-1 infection is discussed with diseases of the nervous system (see Chapter 16, "Nervous System"). Infection of pregnant mares with herpesvirus (EHV)-1 causes abortion (Doll and Bryans 1963; Coggins 1979; Allen and Bryans 1986) and is discussed with diseases of the female reproductive system (see Chapter 11, "Female Reproductive System").

The equine herpes viruses are ubiquitous, cosmopolitan, DNA-containing viruses (Matumoto 1965). Respiratory disease and viral abortion have been reported on every continent. The viruses have been isolated from domesticated and feral equids and ruminants (onagers, zebras, and deer) (Powell 1991).

The outer envelope of the virus contains lipid, making it susceptible to lipolytic detergents and disinfectants. In culture, the virus has a characteristic cytopathic effect, forming acidophilic intranuclear inclusions from crystalline viral arrays (Coggins 1979). Some strains of herpesvirus (EHV)-2 produce syncytial cells by fusion. There is convincing evidence that different viral subtypes are more likely to induce either abortion or neuropathy or respiratory disease (Coggins 1979; Allen and Bryans 1986). Most abortions are caused by herpesvirus (EHV)-1 subtype-1, while herpesvirus (EHV)-1 subtype-2 is usually isolated in respiratory infections (Allen and Bryans 1986). These viral subtypes have markedly different DNA fingerprints, sharing only 20% of base pairs as sequence homology (Allen and Bryans 1986). Antibodies to the subtypes do not cross-react completely. The subtypes also differ in their cellular tropisms and ability to penetrate epithelium and enter the circulation. Allen and Bryans found a high degree of genetic variability of subtype-2 isolates not seen in subtype-1 isolates. Indeed, nearly 90% of subtype-1 isolates are a variant identified as *P* (prototype) while the remaining 10% are a variant termed *B* (Powell 1991). Several investigators have proposed renaming the subtypes: herpesvirus (EHV)-1 subtype-1 would retain the designation of equine herpesvirus (EHV)-1 and subtype-2 would be renamed equine herpesvirus (EHV)-4 (Allen and Bryans 1986; Powell 1991). This has not been officially accepted.

Infection is acquired by inhalation with viral replication in the nasal and oropharyngeal mucosae (Allen and Bryans 1986). Neutrophils and macrophages transport the virus to other tissues from the upper respiratory and tonsillar epithelium. Viremia is rarely detected, although Allen and Bryans (1986) stated that subtype-1 was endotheliotrophic and could be present in leukocytes in the circulation. Virus can be recovered in the nasal and oropharyngeal cavities for at least 10 days following infection and has been isolated from leukocytes for 21 days.

As with influenza, herpes causes epizootics and foci of infection when susceptible horses congregate. Hofer (1973) found infection in 79% of Swiss Army remount horses within the first 3 months of contact with a mixed horse population. Infection and clinical signs are more common in the autumn when large numbers of susceptible weanlings are brought together. Doll and Bryans (1963) found that 85% of foals were infected within 8 months of weaning. Young horses under duress are more likely to display clinical signs. Mares coming into contact with infected weanlings may become infected and abort (Bryans and Prickett 1972).

There have been numerous attempts to define a carrier state with equivocal results. Coggins (1979) has suggested a subclinical carrier state in adults. Burrows and Goodridge (1984) found that weaning, castration, and illness appeared to reactivate latent infection in an isolated group of Welsh mountain ponies.

There have been no convincing demonstrations of the activation of latent viruses by administration of corticosteroids (Allen and Bryans 1986; Powell 1991). Immunity following respiratory infection is short-lived (3–5 months); immunity following abortion is only slightly longer. The role of viral antigenic drift and short-lived immunity was briefly discussed by Allen and Bryans (1986).

Clinical signs include pyrexia and serous nasal discharge. Coughing is rare unlike with influenza infection. Fever may last 4–5 days with transient leukopenia and decreased packed cell volume. Weanlings and yearlings typically develop clinical signs of tracheobronchitis; younger foals may develop bronchopneumonia (Prickett 1969; Powell 1991). Secondary infection with such pathogens as *Streptococcus zooepidemicus* can cause purulent tonsillitis and abscessation of the retropharyngeal lymph nodes as well as pneumonia.

Gross lesions include hyperemia of the upper respiratory tract mucous membranes, edema of tonsillar, pharyngeal, and mandibular lymph nodes, and interstitial pneumonitis (Coggins 1979). The interstitial pneumonitis is questionable, the virus seeming to prefer the upper respiratory tract in postnatal animals. The lesions in the aborted fetus are described with the female reproductive system (see Chapter 11, "Female Reproductive System").

Blakeslee et al. (1975) reported that herpesvirus (EHV)-2 could cause respiratory disease since two foals developed chronic pharyngitis some weeks after experimental infection. This is unconvincing and unconfirmed. Antibodies to herpesvirus (EHV)-2 are commonly found in both healthy and diseased horses (Bryans 1968; McGuire et al. 1974a). The role, if any, of this virus in respiratory disease has yet to be established.

Adenovirus

McChesney et al. (1970) showed the pathogenicity of this common virus in suckling Arabian foals. Adenovirus can be isolated from healthy foals and adult horses and is commonly found in the epithelium of the nasal and oropharyngeal mucosae (Powell 1991). It is a DNA virus that, like other adenoviruses, is resistant to inactivation with organic solvents, has a characteristic cytopathic effect on epithelial cells in culture, and resists low pH and temperature (Moorthy and Spradbrow 1978). These characteristics ensure survival of the virus in the environment for prolonged periods of time.

Immunodeficient foals infected with the virus develop a variety of lesions in the respiratory tract, kidneys, conjunctiva, digestive tract, and central nervous system. The foals, whether Arabian foals with severe, combined immunodeficiency or debilitated non-Arabian foals, have nasal discharge, dyspnea, conjunctivitis, fever, diarrhea, and interstitial proliferative pneumonia (Powell 1991). McChesney et al. (1970) described oral ulcers, depletion of lymphoid tissues, discoloration of the cranioventral portions of the lungs, and gritty white foci in the livers, pancreas, and kidneys of a number of infected foals. Microscopically, foci of necrosis and reactive hyperplasia were found in ductular epithelium of the salivary glands and mucosal epithelium of the upper and lower respiratory tract. Characteristic basophilic intranuclear inclusion bodies develop but are not always easily seen.

Equine rhinovirus

Three types of rhinovirus have been isolated from horses, with or without clinical disease. They all belong to the Picornavirus family of viruses with RNA as nuclear material. Equine rhinoviruses grow well in rabbit kidney tissue culture and have a cytopathic effect. They are nonenveloped viruses and moderately hardy in the environment (Powell 1991). Serological investigations show they are widespread. Powell et al. (1974) found serological evidence of exposure in 50%–90% of horses tested at various times and locations in Britain. There is evidence that the virus may localize in the kidneys and be shed in urine.

The importance of rhinoviruses as pathogens has been debated. Coggins (1979) and Powell (1991) consider them of minor import, at least in North American horses. Hofer et al. (1972) reported rhinovirus pharyngitis in remount horses in Switzerland. With clinical, serological, and virological techniques, they found horses with pharyngitis, fever, and rising titers to rhinovirus-1. Epidemiological study showed that young horses seroconverted within 2 months of contact with older horses and that not all developed clinical signs.

Little is known of the gross or microscopic pathology of rhinovirus infection. In a number of reports, it has not been possible to separate putative rhinovirus lesions from those caused by other pathogens such as influenza virus.

Pharyngitis as a lesion of rhinovirus infection is subject to the reservations discussed in the section on pharyngitis.

Equine reovirus infection

Infection of horses and other equids with reoviruses can produce respiratory disease. One such virus, the *orbivirus* causing African horse sickness, causes profound clinical signs with significant mortality. Others, known as equine reoviruses-1, 2, and 3, produce only minor respiratory disease.

African horse sickness is an acute viral disease largely confined to Africa. It is one of the most serious infectious diseases of horses with high mortality during epizootics (Powell 1991). Recent outbreaks in Mediterranean Europe, the Middle East, and the Indian subcontinent have resulted in the death of thousands of horses.

There are nine subtypes of the arthropod-borne, double-stranded RNA reovirus that cause African horse sickness (Powell 1991). Viral types 1–8 are endemic in sub-Saharan Africa where the primary vector, a biting midge, is present. Type 9 has caused epizootics in the Middle East (1959–1961) and in North Africa and Spain (1966–1967). There was an epidemic of type-4 African horse sickness in Spain in 1987. The virus is tolerant of environmental temperature but inactivated in media below pH 6.0 (Lubroth 1987). The virus can also be transmitted by other hematophagous insects like mosquitoes, *Aedes*, *Culex*, and *Anopheles* sp. and by brown dog ticks, *Rhipicephalus sanguineous*.

There is a high rate of exposure in Africa. Bourdin (1978) found that 53% of nonvaccinated horses in sub-Saharan Senegal had complement-fixing antibodies to type-9 virus. Sixty percent of zebra (3/5) and 75% of elephants (>113/150) from endemic areas possessed significant levels of complement-fixing antibodies (Erasmus et al. 1978). Experimental infection of zebra, *Equus burchelli*, showed they are resistant with only mild clinical signs (Erasmus et al. 1978). In zebras, the virus can persist in tissues for over 40 days despite neutralizing antibodies in the serum. The role of the elephant as a reservoir for the virus is unclear. It is likely that centuries of contact between the virus, the biting midge vector, *Culicoides imicola*, and wild equids has produced some selective resistance to the debilitating effects of the virus. The importation of zebras into Spain in 1987 caused an epizootic in which 162 horses, mules, and donkeys died (Lubroth 1987). Antibodies have been found in camels, cattle, dogs, sheep, and goats in Egypt (Awad et al. 1981), but the virus has only been isolated from camels, horses, and dogs (Salama et al. 1984).

There are three clinical forms: pulmonary, cardiac, and systemic. Horses with the pulmonic form have respiratory distress, hyperthermia, and coughing. Most succumb within 3–4 days with pulmonary edema (Lubroth 1987). In the less peracute, cardiac form, edema develops in the intermuscular fascia. Lubarth (1987) and Powell (1991) reported that edema of the supraorbital fossa is characteristic, but not always present. Hydrothorax and hydropericardium occur in the cardiac form of the disease. Petechial hemorrhages and cyanosis of the oral mucous membranes have been seen. In mixed forms of the disease, cardiac, pulmonary, intestinal, and systemic signs can be seen.

Gross lesions can be subtle. There are pockets of yellow, gelatinous edema in the muscles and fascial planes, somewhat more common in the intermandibular space, frontal area of the neck, jugular furrow, and intercostal musculature (Lubroth 1987). Other lesions include ascites, hydrothorax, hydropericardium, hemorrhagic gastritis, congestion of lymph nodes, liver, kidneys, and spleen, pulmonary edema, and occasional myocardial discoloration.

The pathogenicity of other reoviruses is debatable. Thein and Mayr (1974) found antibodies to reovirus types 1, 2, and 3 in 23%, 7%, and 50%, respectively, of 600+ serum samples from Northern European horses with respiratory disease. A few horses had ocular and nasal discharges and coughing. A reovirus type 1 was isolated from a horse that was killed and autopsied. This animal had bronchitis, bronchiolitis, and peribronchitis; it also had secondary bacterial infection with *Micrococcus albus* (Thein and Hartl 1976).

Bacterial diseases

Streptococcal infections

Four species of streptococci cause infection of the lower respiratory tract in horses—*Streptococcus zooepidemicus*, *S. equi*, *S. suis*, and *S.* (*Diplococcus*) *pneumoniae*. The most common pathogen is *S. zooepidemicus* (currently termed *S. equi* subspecies *zooepidemicus*), an opportunistic pathogen causing pneumonia following equine influenza or herpesvirus (EHV)-1 infections (McGee 1969b; Moore and Bryans 1969b; Flores et al. 1984).

S. zooepidemicus was isolated from 56.1% of samples of lung tissue from 40 adult horses, 37 foals less than 1 year old, and five aborted fetuses (Naglic et al. 1982). Other bacteria isolated included *E. coli* (17.1%), hemolytic and nonhemolytic streptococci (17.0%), *Staphylococcus aureus* (9.7%), and *S. equisimilis* (4.9%). Twelve samples (14.6%) were negative. *Streptococcus zooepidemicus* was the only isolate in 26 of 82 samples. The histological lesions were acute, purulent, necrotizing pneumonia with vasculitis, secondary thrombosis, and scattered foci of pulmonary infarction.

In a study of 121 foals, 1–3 months, the most common cause of death was infection with *E. coli* (68/121 foals) (Van der Molen 1979). Many of these foals had lung lesions, as well as systemic signs of septicemia. Ten percent of foals had *Klebsiella pneumoniae* pneumonia, and another 10% had *S. zooepidemicus* or *Corynebacterium equi* pneumonia. Van der Molen noted that older foals were more likely to harbor *S. zooepidemicus*. In our experience *E. coli* is an uncommon pathogen of foals, but not infrequently isolated as a contaminant.

Kanemaru et al. (1985) examined pulmonary lesions in 63 foals. Pneumonia was present in 35 of 63, hemorrhage in 29 of 63, and abscesses in 18 of 63. Twenty-three foals were hypogammaglobulinemic and 21 of these had pulmonary lesions. *Rhodococcus equi*, *E. coli*, *S. zooepidemicus*, and *Actinobacillus equuli* were isolated.

The pathogenesis of *S. zooepidemicus* infection has been examined (Bryans 1972b). The organism colonizes the nasopharynx and adjacent lymph nodes after damage by viral infection. Proliferation in lymph nodes causes the formation of small abscesses, which may be confused with those of *S. equi*. In some cases, a mixed infection with both bacteria can occur (Ford and Lokai 1980). Infection may spread to other nodes and to the lungs, causing bacterial pneumonia and/or pleuritis.

S. equi frequently colonizes the upper portion of the respiratory tract, causing strangles, but infection of the lower tract is uncommon. Sweeney et al. (1987) studied the complications of *S. equi* infection in 235 Standardbred horses at a breeding establishment. Seventy-four horses developed *S. equi* infections in a 9-month period; 15 had complicated infections; and 5 died with pneumonia or pleuritis and pneumonia. In 35 horses with complications secondary to *S. equi* infection Ford and Lokai (1980) recorded 22 deaths (62%) from bacterial pneumonia.

Streptococcus pneumoniae is an important cause of pneumonia, meningitis, and septicemia in humans (Lockley and Wise 1984). The organism has meticulous growth requirements in culture, including an atmosphere enriched with carbon dioxide and medium enriched with purines and pyrimidines (Burrell et al. 1986). Neufeld and Schnitzer (1928) cited by Burrell et al. (1986) said it was pathogenic for horses. Pure cultures of *S. pneumoniae* type 3, and mixed cultures of *S. pneumoniae* type 3 and *S. zooepidemicus* were isolated from nasopharyngeal swabs of healthy horses and those with clinical signs of respiratory disease (Burrell et al. 1986). A higher percentage of horses with clinical respiratory disease had positive cultures. None of the cases were serious, and no horses died. The organism was repeatedly isolated from the nasopharynx of five horses, suggesting that they were carriers. The role of this streptococcus in equine respiratory disease requires study.

S. suis has been isolated from horses and a zebra with polyarthritis, guttural pouch infection, osteomyelitis, pneumonia, and pleuritis (Devriese and Haesebrouck 1992). *S. suis* was isolated from a 10-day-old foal with severe purulent pneumonia and pleuritis. Further studies on this organism are needed.

Rhodococcus equi infection

Rhodococcus (*Corynebacterium*) *equi* infection causes pulmonary abscesses and pneumonia in 2- to 4-month-old foals (Prescott 1987). Two other members of this bacterial family, *Corynebacterium pseudotuberculosis* and *C. pyogenes*, are also equine pathogens, but to a lesser extent than *R. equi*. There are over 100 isolate groups of *R. equi*, filling a variety of ecological niches (Sippel et al. 1968; Barton and Embury 1987). The *Corynebacterium* and *Mycobacterium* genera are closely related members of the family *Mycobacteriaceae* and show similar tropisms and growth characteristics in the lung. In tissue and culture, they are Gram-positive, nonmotile, nonsporulating rods with a tendency to form filamentous aggregates (Sippel et al. 1968). The ability to survive and multiply within macrophages may help the bacterium elude immunological surveillance (Hilledge 1986; Yager 1987). The role of such virulence factors as capsular polysaccharides, cord factor, and phospholipases in some pathogenic strains is under study (Yager 1987; Prescott 1991; Barton 1992).

R. equi is commonly found in the manured soil of premises with infected foals (Barton 1992). It has repeatedly been isolated from the vagina of mares and gut contents of diseased and healthy horses (Smith and Robinson 1981) and in the gut contents of a variety of domesticated and wild herbivores (Prescott 1991). Prescott et al. (1984) found a direct correlation between soil contamination and the time that horses had been on the farms. The bacterium is resistant to inactivation by normal environmental temperatures and may persist on some farms. Typical lung abscesses caused by the infection were seen in an immunocompromised man who came in contact with contaminated dust on one farm (Golub et al. 1967). At least 20 cases have since been reported in immunodeficient humans (Prescott 1991).

The infection is worldwide. The mortality rate in foals, the specific risk group, may approach 80% (Bain 1966; Rooney 1966; Ellisalde et al. 1980). Infection is by inhalation and ingestion (Smith and Robinson 1981; Martens et al. 1982). The disease has been induced by exposure of foals to nebulized aerosols and by intrabronchial and intragastric instillation (Martens et al. 1982; Johnson et al. 1983; Barton and Embury 1987). Earlier speculations of perinatal transmission from infected mares or transmission by nematodes are unproven (Bain 1963). Dewes (1989) reported an association between rhodococcus pneumonia and infection with

Strongyloides westeri in New Zealand. Predisposition to *R. equi* infections after viral pneumonitis or *Streptococcus equi* infections is debatable (Sippel et al. 1968). Barton and Embury (1987) reported a higher incidence in Thoroughbred foals.

Clinical signs include increased respiratory rate, harsh lung sounds, dyspnea, fever, cough, diarrhea, and nasal discharge (Smith and Robinson 1981; Barton and Embury 1987). Signs may develop within 3 weeks of exposure, often when maternal colostral antibodies are declining (Barton and Embury 1987). There are four basic clinical forms. In the peracute form the animal dies virtually without warning. In the second, more prolonged form, the foal is ill for weeks or months. In the third, the chronically affected foal dies suddenly with disseminated pneumonia. The fourth form, which may or may not accompany the respiratory disease, has persistent diarrhea because of lesions of the large intestine. Culture of tracheal aspirates can be diagnostic (Hilledge 1986). Cultural characteristics were reviewed by Prescott (1991). Barton and Embury (1987) believed that elevations in serum ceruloplasmin oxidase activity and copper concentrations had diagnostic value.

In peracute disease the lungs are diffusely consolidated with miliary microabscessation. With more slowly developing disease there are frank abscesses ranging from 1 cm to greater than 6 cm. Some animals, sick for some time, suddenly die. The gross abscesses are accompanied by peracute, miliary dissemination. In all forms the bronchial and mediastinal lymph nodes have similar lesions.

Lesions may also be present in stomach, intestine, kidneys, liver, and lymph nodes, but involvement of the mucosa and lymph nodes of the large intestine is commonest. In experimental cases the bacterium has been recovered from the trachea, lungs, mediastinal lymph nodes, caecal contents, and liver (Martens et al. 1982). Johnson et al. (1983) found pyogranulomatous colitis and anterior hypopyon following intrabronchial instillation of *C. equi*. Hypopyon is uncommon but does occur in natural cases.

Microscopically, the peracute, disseminated disease is characterized by diffuse inflammatory cell infiltration of alveoli and distal airways with striking accumulations of basophilic bacteria in the cytoplasm of macrophages. The prolonged disease has pyogranulomatous bronchopneumonia (Martens et al. 1982; Johnson et al. 1983). There is marked intraalveolar macrophage infiltration. Central areas of necrotic debris are surrounded by a mixed population of inflammatory cells, including macrophages, giant cells, plasma cells, lymphocytes, and neutrophils. Macrophages usually have large numbers of intracellular organisms. The amount of necrotic tissue in the lesions suggests either bacterial toxin and/or release of lysosomal enzymes and free radicals from degenerating inflammatory cells (Sippel et al. 1968; Johnson et al. 1983).

Hyperplasia of the bronchial and mediastinal lymph nodes with aggregations of bacteria-laden macrophages occurs in both naturally occurring and experimental disease (Martens et al. 1982; Johnson et al. 1983).

Tuberculosis

Tuberculosis is, according to the literature and our experience, rare in horses. Innes (1949) cited European authors giving incidence figures from 0.05% to 0.22%. No incidence data has been found for North America.

The portal of entry is almost entirely the gastrointestinal tract, more often the cecum or colon than the small intestine (Godglück 1967). While there may be ulceration of the mucosa at the site of invasion (Godglück; Cohrs 1961), often the colic or mesenteric lymph nodes are involved without gross lesions of the mucosa.

Dissemination of the organism to the spleen, lungs, liver, and serosal surfaces may occur and miliary lesions may predominate in these tissues. In the lung large masses may be present with or without miliary nodules, and the regional lymph nodes are often affected.

In all sites the nodules are gray-white, firm with only rare caseation or calcification. The initial impression might be that of sarcoma. Histologically, there is a cell-rich granulation tissue with epithelioid cells, giant cells, lymphocytic elements, and young fibrous tissue. Tubercle formation is usually not clear-cut, but, rather, there are foci of epithelioid and Langhans giant cells admixed in a diffuse granulation tissue. Mycobacteria may be seen in considerable numbers in some cases and not in others.

Cohrs and Streich (1943) thought that ossification of the right atrium was causally related to tuberculosis. This is discussed with the cardiovascular system (see Chapter 1, "Cardiovascular System").

According to Godglück (1967), the lesions of *M. avium* are the same as those of the human and bovine types. There is an early report of the avian organism causing a Johne's-like disease (M'Fadyean 1918). The large intestine had lesions essentially identical, grossly and histologically, to Johne's disease. There were lesions in the lymph nodes and lungs as well. The organism was readily demonstrated on smears and in sections. There are other reports of generalized or intestinal avian tuberculosis (Mair et al. 1986; Beurgelt et al. 1988; Leslie and Davies 1958; Baker 1973; Merritt et al. 1975;

Anzai et al. 1989; Cline et al. 1991).

Pulmonary osteoarthropathy has been reported with tuberculosis in the horse (Lienaux 1909).

Glanders

This is an ancient disease of the horse, occasionally other animals and human, which, fortunately, is rare in the modern era. Apsyrtos (334–332 BCE) cited by Sarton (1927) gave a clear description of the disease in horses as did Aristotle (330 BCE) cited by Darmstaedter et al. (1908). Transmission from horse to horse was recognized by Labessie de Solleysel in 1711 and from horse to human by Schilling (1821) cited by Darmstaedter et al. (1908).

Cases are still seen in Southeast Asia. The following discussion is based on the older, specifically German, literature. Glanders, an infectious granulomatous disease, is caused by the bacterium *Malleomyces mallei*. The pathogenesis has been the subject of dispute. According to Pallaske (1960) and Cohrs (1961) the evidence is that the source is primarily contaminated foodstuffs and water, with the nasopharyngeal mucosa the portal of entry. Aerosol droplet infection is possible, but probably rare.

The organisms, having gained entry through the nasopharyngeal mucosa, spread to other organs and tissues by lymphatic and vascular routes. The retropharyngeal lymph nodes are regularly affected. It is not known if lesions are produced during the initial invasion of the nasopharyngeal mucosa, but lesions are sometimes found there whether primary or metastatic. The characteristic lesions of the nasal mucosa, lungs, skin, and a variety of other organs are all considered metastatic.

The disease is chronic though Jubb and Kennedy (1985b) indicate that it may be more acute in the donkey.

Gross lesions in whatever site are characteristically nodular with dull yellow, caseopurulent centers. In the nasal mucosa and skin these nodules ulcerate and heal with scarring. In the nasal mucosa the scars are typically stellate. The progressive nature of the disease is indicated by the admixture of small isolated nodules, purulent foci, ulceration, and scarring in the same areas.

In the lung, regularly involved, there may be miliary nodules, which can coalesce, forming large masses involving whole lobules or even lobes. Chronic indurating pneumonia may develop with or without caseopurulent nodules in a sarcoma-like mass of fibrous tissue.

Histologically, the newly formed nodule is a central mass of necrotic debris surrounded by an hyperemic border. In the lung there is a mantle of fibrin around the necrotic center. With progression the necrotic core enlarges and is surrounded by epithelioid cells intermixed with giant cells and an outer mantle of lymphocytic cells.

Lesions with a large necrotic core relative to the thickness of the mononuclear layer have been called exudative, while the inverse has been called productive. With progression fibrous tissue forms around the nodules and may, eventually, fill and completely obliterate the lesion.

The necrotic core was considered quite specific for this infection, though not pathognomonic. Histologically, it consisted of masses of basophilic-staining karyorrhectic nuclei derived from existing tissue cells and neutrophil leukocytes. Particularly notable is the ingestion of karyorrhectic debris by giant cells (Cohrs 1961).

Glanders nodules in the lung are to be differentiated from helminth (ascarid larval) granulomas. In the latter, eosinophils are often present and calcification is a prominent feature. Before calcification, the necrotic centers of parasitic granulomas consist of masses of necrotic eosinophils, which present as an eosinophilic smudge with a fine stippling of hematoxylinophilic, karyorrhectic debris.

Other bacterial and protozoal pathogens

Two cases of pneumonia caused by *Bordetella bronchiseptica* were reported in foals (Koehne et al. 1981). One died with fulminating pneumonia. Gross lesions included pulmonary consolidation and discoloration. There was suppurative bronchopneumonia with aggregation of bacteria, mucus, and cell debris in bronchi and bronchioles. Alveoli were infiltrated with mixed inflammatory cells, and there was focal necrosis and fibrosis. Saxegaard et al. (1971) reported similar findings in a foal.

Saxegaard and Svenkerud (1974) described mixed bacterial pneumonia in a 4-day-old foal. Severe dyspnea and septicemia were seen shortly before death. Grossly, the lungs were mottled dark red and the cut surfaces were dry. There was prominent fibrinous pneumonia with foci of miliary necrosis and neutrophil infiltration. Culture yielded *Actinobacillus equuli*, *Streptococcus zooepidemicus*, and *Pasteurella haemolytica*. Since *A. equuli* was also isolated from the spleen and liver, it was probably the primary pathogen.

Bacterial septicemia and pneumonia in two young Thoroughbred racehorses was associated with isolation of numerous **anaerobic pathogens** (Carlson and O'Brien 1990). *Streptococcus zooepidemicus*, *Fusobacterium necrophorum*, *Bacteroides uniformis*, *Bacteroides mucacae*, *Corynebacterium* sp., *Peptostreptococcus anaerobius*, *B. fragilis* and a species of *Penicillium* were isolated either from tracheal washes or blood. There was radiographic evidence of severe pneumonia in both animals. One horse recovered after antibiotic therapy; the other died. At autopsy, there were several firm, fibrotic masses in one lung lobe, which contained inspissated pus. One mass had eroded the wall of a bronchus and was the source of hemorrhage seen clinically. Severe, fibrosing interstitial pneumonia was diagnosed microscopically. The number of isolates is confusing and anaerobe infection is certainly not usually characterized by fibrosing interstitial pneumonia.

Aerobic and anaerobic cultures of tracheobronchial and pleural fluid aspirates were done on 46 horses with a diagnosis of pleuropneumonia and on 327 horses with pneumonia or pleuropneumonia (Sweeney et al. 1985; Sweeney et al. 1991). (The term *pleuropneumonia* has been used for another, specific, disease of the horse and the terminology we prefer here would be *pleuritis and pneumonia*.)

Anaerobic bacteria were isolated from the 46 horses, most often *Bacteroides* and *Clostridium*. Over 65% of these horses died (Sweeney et al. 1985).

In the larger study of 327 horses, 20% were killed and 5% died. Aerobic pathogens were isolated from 221 of 302 survivors. The isolates included β-hemolytic streptococci, *Pasteurella* sp., *E. coli*, *Enterobacter* sp., and *Klebsiella pneumoniae*. Eighty-one horses had anaerobic bacteria, including *Bacteroides* sp., *Clostridium* sp., and *Peptostreptococcus* sp. The role of the anaerobes is unclear, particularly since well-known aerobic pathogens were also present. Secondary infection or contamination is, at least, to be considered.

In a serological study of *Legionella pneumophila*, the organism of **Legionnaire's disease**, Collins et al. (1982) found 31.4% of 636 horses to have antibodies. Four horses and four ponies, experimentally exposed, developed antibodies (Cho et al. 1983). No clinical signs were seen. Minimal gross and histological lesions were seen in lungs, including focal bronchiolitis and proliferation of alveolar lining cells. The minimal lesions did not resemble the severe fibrosing pneumonia characteristic of Legionnaire's disease in the human and may have been incidental findings.

Mycoplasms have repeatedly been isolated from the respiratory tract of healthy horses and those with acute respiratory disease (Poland 1978). Allam and Lemcke (1975) isolated seven species including *Acholeplasma laidlawii*, *A. oculi*, *A. equifoetale*, *Mycoplasma pulmonis*, *M. felis*, *M. equirhinis*, and an unnamed species. The rate of isolation was approximately 8%. In other studies, isolation rates of 66% from nasopharyngeal swabs were reported (Poland and Lemcke 1978). Only *M. pulmonis* and the unnamed species (N3/N11) were found exclusively in horses with acute respiratory disease: nasopharyngitis and catarrhal pneumonia. Antal et al. (1988, 1989b) isolated mycoplasms from 93.3% of foals with acute respiratory disease, but also isolated *Streptococcus equi* (*equisimilis*) from 62% of these 30 cases. A high percentage of healthy mares carried mycoplasms in the nasopharynx, milk, amniotic fluid, uterus, and vagina (Antal et al. 1989a). Ogilvie et al. (1983) isolated *M. felis* from the pleural fluid of a 7-year-old Thoroughbred suffering from pleuritis. They induced pleuritis in a pony by infusion of a culture of *M. felis* into the thoracic cavity. Since they also isolated *S. zooepidemicus* from the pony, the pathogenicity of the mycoplasma is questionable.

The data of these several investigators do not provide a convincing case for the importance, if any, of mycoplasma in equine respiratory disease.

Two **rickettsialike organisms**, NSDH 91 and NSDH 100, were isolated from the acutely inflamed lungs of two horses in Australia (Moorthy and Spradbrow 1985). Antigenicity and cultural characteristics resembled *Coxiella burnetti*. A role for these organisms in equine respiratory disease is moot.

Pneumocystis carinii was isolated from the lungs of two foals with acute pneumonia (Shively et al. 1974). Both had prolonged respiratory disease and therapy with antibiotics and immunosuppressive drugs. Bacterial pathogens (*Bordetella* sp. and *Rhodococcus equi*) were also isolated. Both cases had necrosis of the respiratory epithelium and growth of organisms in alveolar macrophages. *P. carinii* was considered to be the primary cause of death in one foal, *R. equi* in the other. *P. carinii* is a secondary invader in immunocompromised individuals such as foals with chronic disease of any type.

Fungal diseases

Fungal diseases of the lower respiratory tract are uncommon (Blue et al. 1987; Slocombe and Slauson 1988). Joest (1920) recorded cases of pulmonary mycosis with formation of granulomatous nodules.

Slocombe and Slauson (1988) found 19 cases of invasive **pulmonary aspergillosis** among 7020 case records. Fourteen of the 19 had severe respiratory signs 11 days after start of treatment for salmonellosis diarrhea. Two other horses had malignancies, and two had been treated intensively with immunosuppressive drugs. Eighteen of the 19 horses had foci of hemorrhagic and necrotizing alveolitis with *Aspergillus* sp. fungal hyphae and neutrophil infiltration. Pulmonary aspergillosis associated with leukemia or myeloproliferative disease has been seen by us and others (Blue et al. 1987; Buechner-Maxwell et al. 1994).

Pulmonary histoplasmosis is rare. Marx et al. (1972) observed that disease is rare although exposure is common. Seventy-three percent of healthy horses skin tested with histoplasmin had antibodies. A similar incidence has been found in central Kentucky, again, in the absence of any clinical disease other than an occasional abortion.

Pulmonary histoplasmosis was found in a 2-year-old Trakehner filly with respiratory distress (Cornick 1990). Needle biopsies of the lung and liver revealed chronic cholangiohepatitis and mycotic pneumonia. *Histoplasma capsulatum* was found in pulmonary macrophages and antibodies were present in the blood. Aggressive therapy arrested the disease. Cornick found only 7 cases of systemic histoplasmosis reported in horses; of these, 5 were in animals 2 years old or less. Not all of these cases involved the respiratory tract. Fawi (1971) isolated *Histoplasma farciminosum* from the lungs of two 6-year-old stallions bred in Sudan. Irregular gray-white nodules, 0.5–20 cm, studded the lungs. The histological diagnosis was severe, diffuse granulomatous pneumonia. Fawi hypothesized that the dusty and windy conditions in the Sudan favored inhalation of the common soil saprophyte.

Cryptococcus neoformans is a ubiquitous soil saprophyte like *Histoplasma* and *Aspergillus*. It has an affinity for the central nervous system and the nasopharynx and can cause severe pneumonia. One horse with **cryptococcal pneumonia** developed purulent pleural effusion (Hilbert et al. 1980). At autopsy the lungs were yellow and consolidated. Histological examination showed severe parenchymal destruction, fibrosis, foamy macrophage infiltration, and bronchial and peribronchiolar inflammation. Severe, diffuse interstitial pneumonia was seen in a 1-month-old Arabian horse foal (Ryan and Wyand 1980). There was granulomatous lymphadenitis, but the foal was not considered immunodeficient. In a subsequent pregnancy the mare aborted at 8 months with mycotic placentitis and cryptoccal pneumonia in the fetus.

Pulmonary nocardiosis was found in a 15-month-old Quarter horse colt that had bilateral purulent nasal discharge and weakness (Deem and Harrington 1980). At autopsy, there was an accumulation of dark-red, viscous fluid containing fibrin flakes in the thoracic cavity. There were firm adhesions among the pericardium, visceral pleura, and thoracic wall. The lungs were mottled and discolored and the bronchial lymph nodes enlarged. There were multiple abscesses in the pulmonary parenchyma. Histological examination showed diffuse seropurulent inflammation, abscessation, and vascular thrombosis. The pleura was thickened and inflamed. *Nocardia brasiliensis* was isolated from the lungs.

Although primarily a pathogen of the skin and lymphoid tissue, *Pythium* sp. (*Hyphomyces destruens*), can cause **pulmonary phycomycosis**, as in a 3-year-old Quarter horse mare (Goad 1984). The pleural cavity contained 10–15 L of clear fluid. Fibrin tags were adherent to the parietal and visceral pleural surfaces. Raised nodules, 1–20 cm, studded the pulmonary parenchyma. They had a thick fibrous capsule and contained thick, opaque yellow fluid and sequestered concretions. Typical hyphae of *Pythium* sp. and masses of mixed inflammatory cells were present in the necrotic pulmonary parenchyma. The source of infection was believed to be a wound on the rear leg.

Parasitic diseases

Lungworm

The only notable lung parasite in equids is *Dictyocaulus arnfeldi*. This nematode infests the lungs of donkeys, mules, tapirs, and horses throughout the world (Campbell et al. 1971; Round 1976; MacKay and Urquhart 1979; George et al. 1981; Clayton and Duncan 1981; Lyons et al. 1985). It is especially common in the donkey, which is considered the natural host. A survey of 333 donkeys in 12 studs in Britain found 243 with patent infections while routine fecal analysis gave an infection rate of 26%–46% (Round 1976). Eleven percent of Thoroughbred horses submitted for autopsy in Kentucky in 1 year were infected (Lyons et al. 1985). The horses ranged in age from 1 to 32 years old and were without clinical disease.

Infectious larvae develop from ova on pasture within 3–10 days and can remain viable for as long as 42 days in shaded conditions (Round 1976). Once ingested, larvae pass from the gastrointestinal tract to the lungs by way of the mesenteric lymph nodes and thoracic duct (Wetzel and Enigk 1938). The prepatent period is approximately 39 days, but retardation of development at intermediate larval stages may delay patency. Lyons et al. (1985) found that horses are likely to have prepatent infections, and may not shed ova in feces. Infected horses and donkeys can stay infected for years. Experimental infection indicates that younger animals are more susceptible, especially young foals (Clayton and Duncan 1981). However, Koulikov (1935) and Borovkova (1948) cited by Round (1976), found infections in Russian horses 10–20 years old. Lyons et al. (1985) found infections in 10% of Kentucky Thoroughbred horses 21–25 years old. Infection of horses does not require contact with donkeys, as sometimes proposed, although heavy infections in horses are almost always associated with donkey exposure. Some degree of resistance to reinfection is seen in adult donkeys cleared with antihelminthics (Round 1976).

Observations of natural and experimental lungworm infection show that it is a mild disease in most equids (Soulsby 1965; Round 1976). Donkeys often have large numbers of lungworms without clinical signs. In a few severe cases there may be coughing, increased respiratory rates, and harsh lung sounds (MacKay and Urquhart 1979; George et al. 1981). Increased circulating eosinophils have been seen 3–7 weeks after experimental infection of horses (Round 1976). A review of a number of studies from the early 1900s to the mid-1970s indicated that lungworm infection did not produce serious pulmonary disease (Round 1976). When severe disease was seen, it was in association with epizootics of equine influenza. Cases of generalized unthriftiness or chronic bronchitis were associated with lungworm infection (Campbell et al. 1971; MacKay and Urquhart 1979; George et al. 1981; Lyons et al. 1985).

Parascaris equorum

This small intestinal nematode has a larval stage that migrates through the liver and lung. Soulsby (1965) notes that foals may suffer when heavily infested with the parasite but primarily from the effects of the adults in the gastrointestinal tract. Nicholls et al. (1978) infected pony foals with *P. equorum* infective larvae with transient coughing and nasal discharge 10–14 days after infection. Subpleural edema and hemorrhage were seen in foals killed 11–14 days after infection. Eosinophilic alveolitis, perivasculitis, bronchiolitis, and bronchitis were present microscopically within 11 days as larvae arrived in the lungs. The intense eosinophilia may have been caused by the release of eosinophilic chemotactic factor of anaphylaxis (ECF-A) from mast cell granules. By 23 days postinfection, the infiltrating cells were predominantly lymphocytes and macrophages. Subpleural lymphocytic nodules were present between 23 and 116 days postinfection. Foci of pneumonia in the cranial lung lobes were seen in 6 of 8 experimental foals.

Habronemiasis

Pulmonary abscesses, catarrhal bronchopneumonia, and debilitation were found in a 50-day-old Thoroughbred colt (Bain et al. 1969). Multiple abscesses in the lung, lymph nodes, and gastrointestinal tract were colonized with *Rhodococcus equi*. Larvae of *Habronema* were also found in the lung abscesses. This appears to be the only such case reported.

Ox warble

Infrequently, one finds a striking subpleural hemorrhagic tract. Careful search may uncover an ox warble larva, *Hypoderma bovis*, at the end of the tract; often it is gone. This is commoner in England than in North America. As in cattle the warbles eventually break through the skin on the dorsal midline.

Chronic bronchitis/bronchiolitis

One of the commonest pulmonary diseases of horses is chronic bronchiolitis with or without bronchitis. The disease has been known since antiquity when Aristotle in 333 BCE described the condition [Smith (1919) cited by McPherson and Thomson (1983)]. Hering (1844) cited by Gerber (1989) realized an association between the disease and hay feeding. Cadeac (1897a) published a detailed description of the lesions and clinical signs. He commented on the high frequency of the disease in 4- to 6-year-old horses, and noted that one might see firm white nodules in the lungs. Axe (1906) cited by McPherson and Thomson (1983) associated the disease with certain breeds, advancing age, and contact with damaged fodder. Ackermann (1939) studied 17 cases and believed that heavy work horses were more likely to be affected than racehorses. He attributed this to housing the former in poor conditions and the need to work in foul weather.

It is a disease of synonyms: chronic obstructive pulmonary disease (COPD), chronic small airway disease, chronic bronchitis, chronic alveolar emphysema, chronic pulmonary disease, hypersensitivity pneumopathy, pulmonary emphysema, and broken wind, heaves. We strongly favor the term **chronic bronchitis/bronchiolitis** since that term characterizes the lesions.

Gerber (1973) observed that chronic pulmonary conditions were the most common cause of premature loss in the Swiss horse population. Winder and von Fellenberg (1987) found chronic bronchiolitis to be infrequent in Australia where horses are usually outdoors and more frequent in Europe and the northern United States where horses spend more time stabled.

The clinical signs vary markedly according to the severity of disease. Many horses have a chronic cough and decreased ability to work for weeks or months. Dyspnea and/or forced expiratory effort are seen. Littlejohn and Bowles (1980) listed coughing, rales, nasal discharge, expiratory anal pumping, and forced abdominal expiratory effort as common signs of chronic bronchiolitis in 20 horses. There is no single clinical sign diagnostic of chronic bronchitis/bronchiolitis. Indeed, eosinophilic pneumonitis, bronchopneumonia, chemical airway irritation, parasitic pneumonia, and inhalant allergies may all present with similar signs. Dead space ventilation, regions of high ventilation/perfusion, increased pulmonary artery pressure and pulmonary vascular resistance have been observed (Littlejohn 1980, 1982; Nyman et al. 1991). Alterations in heart rate because of hypoxia are not commonly observed (Littlejohn 1980).

Diagnostic testing is usually inconclusive. Some advocate complete blood counts, serum chemistry analysis, and thoracic radiography (Gerber 1973), while others do not (McPherson and Thomson 1983; Beech 1991). McPherson and Thomson (1983) recommended intradermal skin testing for *Micropolyspora faeni* and *Aspergillus fumigatus*. Halliwell et al. (1979) found such testing unreliable. Schatzmann and Gerber (1972) found many normal horses, without signs of respiratory disease, that reacted to skin testing with mold extracts. Winder et al. (1990) saw an increase in soluble fibrinogen derivatives in the respiratory secretions of 35 of 80 horses. However, the degree of overlap among horses with chronic bronchiolitis and either normal horses or those with other pulmonary diseases was too large for this test to be useful. Mair (1987) found differences in the cytology of tracheal aspirates between horses with chronic bronchitis/bronchiolitis and normal horses, but conceded that similar cellular alterations were also present in bronchopneumonia and interstitial pneumonia. A high percentage of viable neutrophils in the secretions was thought to be a good indicator of chronic bronchiolitis.

The incidence of chronic bronchiolitis in three populations of Swiss horses was studied with a variety of techniques including forced expiration/auscultation, laryngoscopy/tracheoscopy, examination of respiratory secretions, arterial blood gas analysis, history, and physical examination (Bracher et al. 1991). Subclinical, mild or moderately severe chronic bronchiolitis was diagnosed in 73 of 97 horses (81.2%) (group A horses) presented for diseases other than respiratory disease at the Veterinary Institute in Zurich. In a group of 93 healthy Swiss Army horses (group B horses) 58 of 93 (62.3%) had subclinical to moderate chronic bronchiolitis. A third group (group C), those presented to the Veterinary Institute for respiratory problems, had an incidence of chronic bronchiolitis of 100% (113 horses). The incidence of moderately severe chronic bronchiolitis was 10.3%, 20.4%, and 46.9%, respectively, for groups A, B, and C. Severe chronic bronchiolitis was only found in group C horses with an incidence of 13.3%.

Pharyngeal lymphoid hyperplasia was found in 70%–75% of horses examined but did not relate to disease. Indeed, as discussed with pharyngitis, this is not hyperplasia to start with and, so, is not pathological.

Winder and von Fellenberg (1987) studied chronic bronchitis/bronchiolitis histologically in 115 adult horses killed during a 1-year period at Zurich. Of the 115 adult horses, 51.3% were killed for lameness, 17.4% for colic, 9.6% for chronic respiratory disease, 13.9% for a variety of other medical conditions, and 7.8% for unknown reasons. Chronic bronchitis/bronchiolitis was diagnosed histologically in 37.4%. Other pulmonary diseases included interstitial pneumonia (15.6%), eosinophilic pulmonary infiltration (13.9%), pulmonary hemorrhage (3.5%), and bronchopneumonia (2.6%). The average age of 31 horses without pulmonary lesions was 9.5 years and of horses with chronic bronchitis/bronchiolitis was 13.2 years.

McPherson et al. (1978) diagnosed chronic bronchitis/bronchiolitis in 38% of horses presented for respiratory problems and/or chronic coughing in Glasgow. The cases were classified according to partial pressure of arterial oxygen (PaO_2) and maximum intrathoracic pressure changes. They found the incidence of chronic bronchitis/bronchiolitis was highest in ponies, lowest in Thoroughbreds. The disease was seen from 2–15 years of age with the prevalence increasing with age in both horses and ponies. Of 18 horses 11 years or older, 13 had chronic bronchiolitis. Show jumpers and hacks were more likely to be affected than racehorses. McPherson et al. found no correlation of disease with sex, body weight, or season. Many of the animals were housed in inadequately ventilated facilities and/or had contact with moldy hay and straw.

While the risk factors and etiology of this condition have been studied extensively, the pathogenesis is still poorly understood. The frequency increases with age (McPherson et al. 1979). The disease is more prevalent in show jumpers, hacks, and ponies, and decidedly more common in stabled than in pastured animals.

Several lines of evidence suggest that bronchitis/bronchiolitis has an allergic component. First, environmental factors such as poor stable ventilation and exposure to mold in hay and straw have been repeatedly associated with the disease (McPherson et al. 1979). Second, inhalation testing with presumptive allergens such as moldy hay can provoke episodic coughing and dyspnea in horses with chronic bronchiolitis (Gerber 1973). Third, corticosteroids can ameliorate symptoms (Gerber 1973). Fourth, some studies of dermal hypersensitivity have shown an increased 4-hour reaction to a known hay contaminant, *Micropolyspora faeni*.

Reaction to other allergens has, however, been equivocal (Halliwell et al. 1979). Fifth, Derksen et al. (1987) showed pulmonary inflammation and ventilation dysfunction in sensitized ponies following exposure to *M. faeni* antigens, as well as in ponies with chronic bronchitis/bronchiolitis. Finally, Icelandic ponies with haysickness ("heysyki") have high levels of serum precipitins against thermophilic actinomycetes (Asmundsson et al. 1983).

Gerber (1989) proposed a genetic link for chronic bronchiolitis, and Marti et al. (1991) studied 90 German Warm bloods and 42 Lipizzaner horses to establish this link. Their preliminary work in several studs indicated a higher incidence of chronic bronchitis/bronchiolitis in the offspring of affected horses than nonaffected horses. There is apparently no link to the equine major histocompatibility complex (Marti et al. 1991).

While it appears likely that exposure to allergens may trigger a hypersensitivity response, the roles of previous viral or bacterial infections, inhaled irritants, altered pulmonary functional dynamics, defective mucociliary function, the actions of a plethora of inflammatory mediators and inhibitors, and so forth, are complex and the interrelationships poorly understood. A number of investigators have tried to link endogenous and exogenous proteases and protease inhibitor deficiencies to the pathogenesis of chronic bronchitis/bronchiolitis (Matthews 1979; Thomson et al. 1983; Grünig et al. 1986; von Fellenberg 1987), but the results suggest a minor, if any, role.

Gross lesions are variable and related to the severity of clinical disease. McPherson and Thomson (1983) noted that the lungs may fill the chest, fail to collapse, have rib impressions, and appear overinflated and pale pink (Fig. 2.7). Winder and von Fellenberg (1987) attributed the coloration and overinflation to alveolar emphysema caused by bronchiolar plugging with mucus.

Nicholls (1978), cited by McPherson and Thomson (1983), described the histopathology of chronic bronchitis/bronchiolitis in 25 horses. The principal lesion was chronic bronchiolitis with bronchiolar epithelial hyperplasia, goblet cell metaplasia, peribronchiolar lymphoid cell infiltration, and mucus and purulent debris in the bronchiolar lumen (Figs. 2.8–2.10). She believed emphysema was infrequent. She found all of the bronchioles 2 mm or less similarly affected. Interstitial eosinophils were increased in 50% of the cases.

Schoon and Deegen (1983) described the histology of chronic bronchitis/bronchiolitis in 14

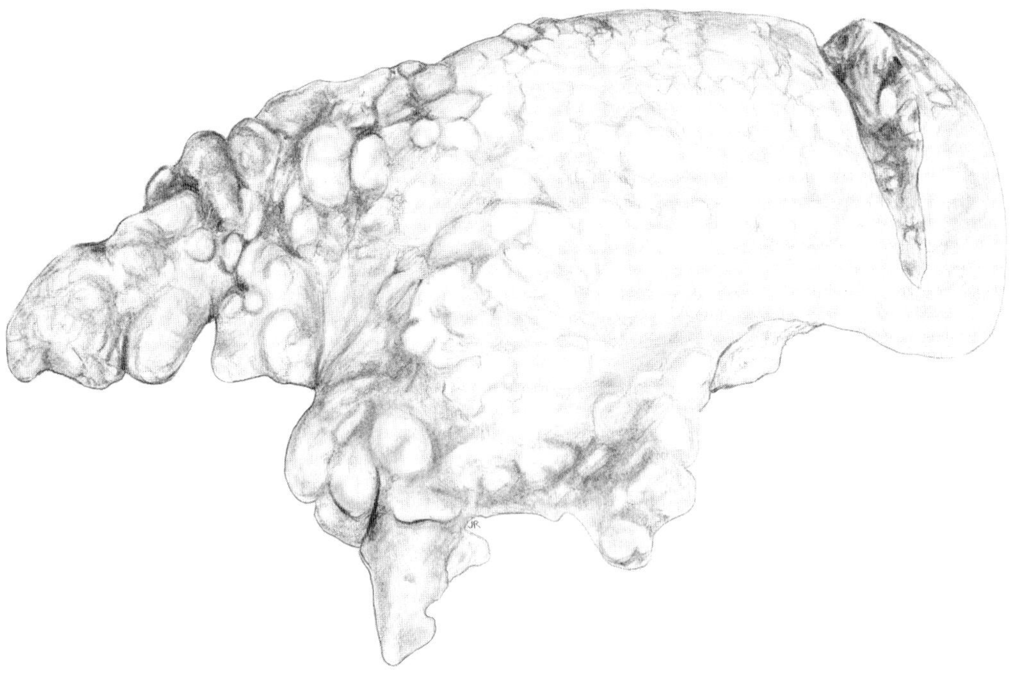

2.7. A portion of the lung from a horse with chronic bronchiolitis. There are extensive areas of atelectasis and pulmonary fibrosis; raised areas are foci of air entrapment.

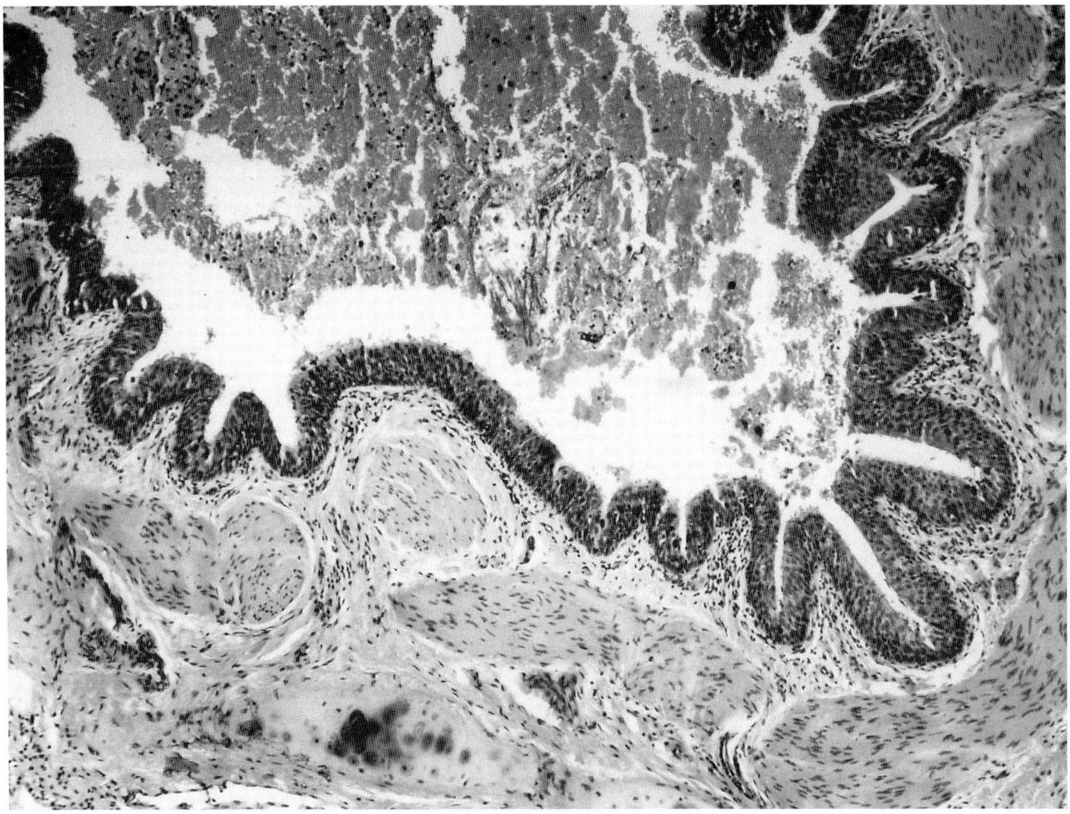

2.8. A bronchiole filled with mucus and cellular debris.

clinically affected horses. Primary lesions included mucus accumulation in bronchioles and bronchi, epithelial cell hyperplasia and metaplasia, goblet cell hyperplasia, epithelial cell desquamation, inflammatory cell infiltration, and hypertrophy of bronchiolar/bronchial musculature. In some cases they also saw peribronchiolar and peribronchial fibrosis and alveolar emphysema. The spectrum of lesions seen in this disease was the result of necrotizing/exudative and proliferative/reparative processes occurring simultaneously.

Winder and von Fellenberg (1987) systematically studied standardized regions of the airways and lungs of 115 slaughtered horses. They described bronchiolar and goblet cell hyperplasia, perivascular and peribronchiolar lymphocytic aggregates, and mucus plugging of bronchioles. Their lesions were more focal and tended to be more prevalent and severe in the caudal half of the lung. Minimal smooth muscle hypertrophy near bronchioles was seen in minimally affected animals. In severely affected animals, lesions were more diffuse, and there was perivascular and peribronchiolar fibrosis, alveolar epithelial hyperplasia, and thickening of alveolar septa with fibrous connective tissue and mononuclear cells. They did not comment on eosinophils. Dilated alveoli, indicative of emphysema, were not seen.

Gerber (1973) commented on the high incidence of bullous emphysema in 21 horses while Nicholls (1978) considered this infrequent. In our experience the frequency of alveolar emphysema is directly correlated with the severity and extent of bronchiolar lesions.

Lungs from 23 horses with chronic bronchitis/bronchiolitis were examined for free and intracellular immunoglobulin using an immunoperoxidase method (Winder and von Fellenberg 1988). The number of cells containing immunoglobulin A and immunoglobulin G increased with increasing severity of disease. Horses with severe chronic bronchiolitis had free immunoglobulin G in the pulmonary interstitium and alveoli. Free immunoglobulin A and immunoglobulin G were found in areas of epithelial cell hyperplasia and metaplasia. Mair et al. (1988) found evidence of increased immunoglobulin A in fluid secretions from horses with chronic bronchitis/bronchiolitis. The role of

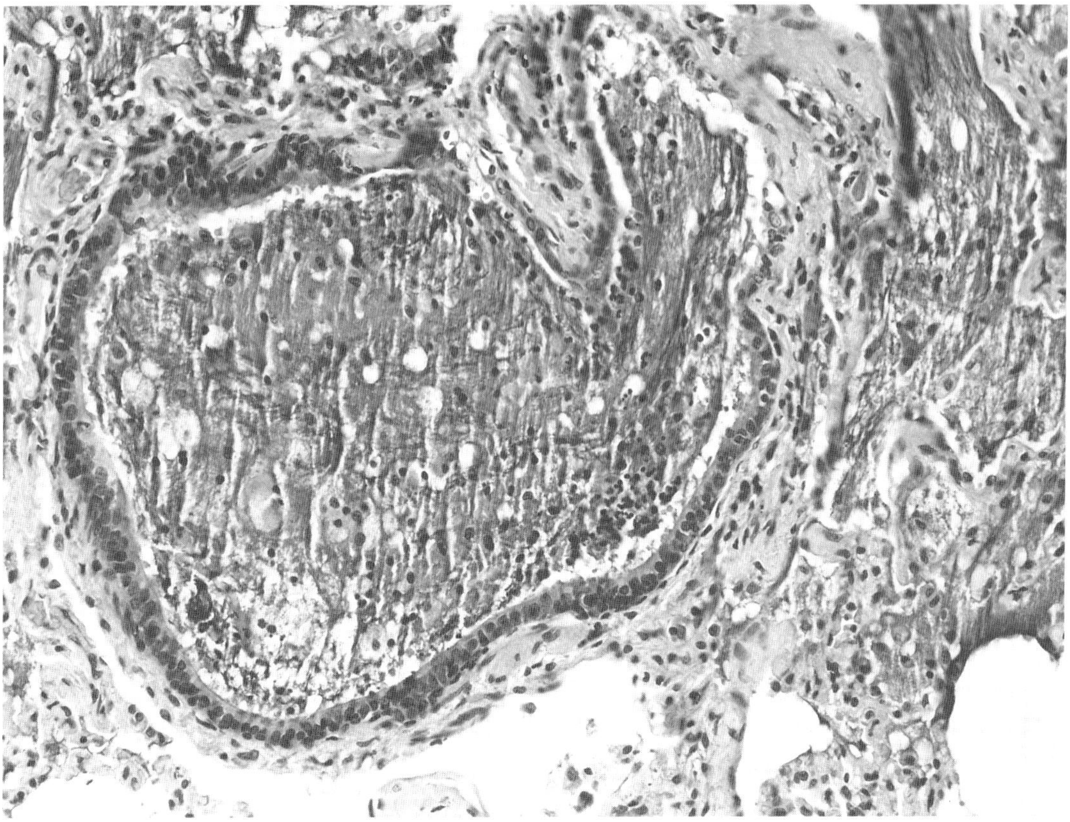

2.9. A dilated bronchiole filled with mucus and cell debris; there is also mucus filling in the adjacent alveoli.

local immunity in the pathogenesis of chronic bronchiolitis is thus suggested but not fully established.

The ultrastructure of the lesions was studied by Kaup et al. (1990a,b). Of 28 horses, 13 had moderate to severe lesions in major airways. These included focal loss of ciliated epithelium, hyperplasia and dedifferentiation of the respiratory epithelium, mast cell aggregations, and the presence of intracytoplasmic crystalloid bodies in interstitial and smooth muscle cells. Significant lesions in bronchiolar and alveolar epithelium included degeneration and dedifferentiation of ciliated and nonciliated bronchiolar epithelium, degranulation of Clara cells, goblet cell metaplasia, and lamellar inclusions in the cytoplasm of epithelial cells. The sloughing of necrotic cells and incorporation of cell debris in luminal mucus was also shown. Such inclusions were also present in alveolar cells together with alveolar fibrosis and cellular necrosis. An increase in the number of Kohn's pores was regarded as an indication of emphysema and loss of alveolar compliance caused by fibrosis.

Alveolar and interstitial pneumonia

Twenty-six cases of an unusual pneumonia, characterized by necrosis of alveolar cells and septal walls, reactive pneumocyte hyperplasia, occasional hyalin membrane formation, and interstitial inflammation have been reported (Ubertini and King 1971; Turk et al. 1981; Buergelt et al. 1986; Winder et al. 1988; Dixon et al. 1992). The animals ranged from 3 days to 15 years old. The clinical signs included acute onset of dyspnea persisting for days or weeks and refractory to therapy. The search for infectious agents, pneumotoxins, dietary intoxicants such as pirella or Crofton weed, or other factors has been unproductive.

Ubertini and King (1971) saw atypical interstitial pneumonia in a 6-week-old Appaloosa foal. At postmortem the lungs were heavy, enlarged, discolored red and gray, and firm. Microscopic features included diffuse congestion, edema, and minimal mixed inflammatory cell infiltration of the interstitium, alveolar septal hyalin membrane formation,

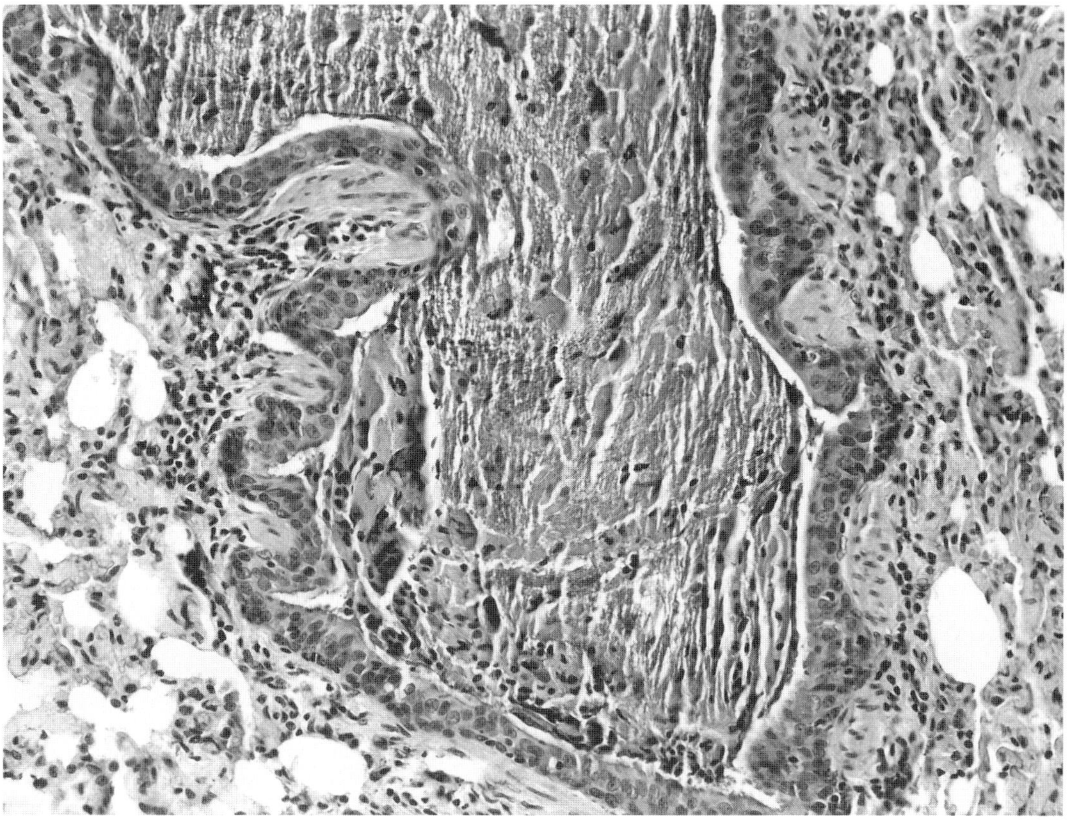

2.10. Squamous metaplasia of the lining of a bronchiole in a horse with chronic bronchiolitis.

and pneumocyte hyperplasia. Multinucleated giant cells were seen in the alveoli. We have seen similar lesions in foals with equine influenza.

Similar lesions were described by Turk et al. (1981) in a 3-year-old Appaloosa mare. The lesions included interstitial and alveolar mixed inflammatory cell infiltration, fibrosis, and pneumocyte hyperplasia. Bronchioles and bronchi were unaffected, save for distortion occasioned by the alveolar and interstitial changes.

Buergelt et al. (1986) found alveolar and interstitial pneumonia in 20 horses in Florida, 14 of which were 6 months old or less. There were Thoroughbreds, Quarter horses, and Arabian horses; 12 colts and geldings; and 8 fillies and mares. Acute, subacute, and chronic cases were seen. No infectious agents were found, and there was no history of recent infectious disease. *Pneumocystis carinii* was identified in lung sections of one horse, and one had an increased titer to equine influenza virus.

Grossly, the lungs were firm, focally discolored, and did not collapse. In acute cases of 3–5 days' duration there was alveolar septal coagulation necrosis and inflammation, exudation of fibrin and other proteins, hemorrhage, and edema. There were fibrin thrombi in some interstitial capillaries in some animals.

In subacute cases (>5 days), hyalin membranes were present on the alveolar septa. Some alveoli were filled with neutrophils, macrophages, and multinucleate giant cells. Pneumocyte hyperplasia produced a glandular, adenomatous appearance.

Chronic cases of 1 or more weeks had adenomatous hyperplasia of alveoli, fibroplasia, and infiltration of the interstitium with a mixed population of inflammatory cells. Some alveoli were filled with cellular debris. Buergelt et al. found bronchiolitis in some of the chronic cases.

Winder and colleagues (1988) described similar cases in a 7-year-old Irish warm blood and a 15-year-old Polish Warm blood. The histological diagnosis in one was granulomatous bronchointerstitial pneumonia; in the other, chronic bronchiolitis and subacute interstitial pneumonia with scarring. The authors believed that a hypersensitivity reaction was responsible for these lesions since there was free immunoglobulin in secretions and infiltrating, immunoglobulin-producing cells in the interstitium.

A Thoroughbred-Arabian with severe, acute eosinophilic interstitial pneumonia was reported by Dixon et al. (1992). It had severe dyspnea, cyanosis, and tachypnea. Bronchoalveolar lavage fluid contained large numbers of eosinophils and mast cells. The pneumonia resolved within 7 days with no residual deficits with corticosteroid therapy.

Pleuritis and pleuropneumonia

Contagious pleuropneumonia

This was a highly infectious scourge of horses until it was eradicated in North America and apparently disappeared spontaneously in Europe. It was a consolidating, multifocal pneumonia. The lungs were dark red-brown and edematous with mucoid exudate in the bronchi and bronchiolitis, progressing to fibrinous and necrotizing pneumonia. The etiological agent(s) or factors were not discovered before the disease disappeared (Cohrs 1961).

Pleuritis

Pleuritis, as a self-standing entity was described by Hutyra and Marek (1920). Recently there has been a rebirth of interest in diseases of the pleura. Byars and Becht (1991) favor the use of the term *pleuropneumonia* for inflammatory lesions of the pleura and adjacent lung parenchyma. They consider that the majority of lesions in the pleura result from direct extension from disease in the lung, save for penetrating chest wounds. While that is true, the lesion in the lung is often focal and small; the term *pleuritis* is useful when qualified and is retained here.

The pleura is a bilayer membrane covering the lungs, visceral pleura, and thoracic cavity, parietal pleura. In horses, the pleura is incomplete at the caudal mediastinum. One layer is composed of squamous epithelium; the other is richly invested with blood and lymphatic vessels (Smith 1979). The pleural fluid is a plasma filtrate. When the pleura is inflamed, the quantity and quality of pleural fluid changes. Smith (1979) notes, for example, that inflammation of the pleura causes increased pleural capillary permeability and an increase in protein-rich fluid, protein greater than 3 g/dL. There is also an increase in the number of cells in the fluid.

Causes of pleuritis and pleural effusion include abscesses, pneumonia, and intrathoracic neoplasms (Raphel and Beech 1982). We have seen a branch of multiflora rose in a bronchus as a penetrating foreign body; other foreign bodies may also cause pleuritis. Raphel and Beech (1992) found that 90 of 122 horses with pleural effusion had either pneumonia or a lung abscess. Of these 90 horses, 51 (57%) died or were killed. No differences were seen in pleural fluid white blood cell count, plasma, or pleural fluid protein, or pleural fluid fibrinogen concentration between survivors and nonsurvivors. At postmortem 33 of the 51 horses had lung abscesses, primarily of the right apical lung lobe. Similar findings were reported by Mair and Lane (1989).

The typical case of pleuritis is a young horse in training or racing/showing that develops an acute, upper respiratory disease with fever and serous nasal discharge. Secondary bacterial infection may follow if the animal is put back to work when the initial, viral episode appears to be over (no discharge, temperature normal, eating normally). Often, after the initial viral infection, the horse is sent home to recuperate. During the trip, or soon thereafter, severe signs appear: fever, inappetence, and signs of pleuritis. One striking clinical sign of pleuritis and pleural effusion is refusal or reluctance to go down a ramp head first, perhaps because of a sense of suffocation as pleural fluid runs forward in the chest. Transportation of horses is a significant risk factor for pleuritis. Seltzer cited by Byars and Becht (1991) recorded transportation in 39.2% of 153 horses that developed pleuritis.

Pleuritis begins on one side, usually the right but may quickly involve both pleural cavities. The prognosis is improved if therapy is begun before bilateral involvement.

At postmortem there is massive fibrinopurulent pleuritis, the severity being related to the duration of the disease. The nidus of infection is usually a focal abscess in the accessory lobe of the right lung, less often in the right apical lobe, contrary to the findings of Raphel and Beech (1982). The abscess is not often discrete, but, rather, a poorly demarcated area of congestion and consolidation with one or more small purulent areas with thin, watery, gray pus. This type of pus is characteristic of *Streptococcus zooepidemicus*, which is the commonest agent. The nidus may be difficult to identify in a given case because of the severe pleuritis.

There are cases of acute pleuritis with massive intrathoracic hemorrhage. The animal is in severe distress and usually dies within hours of onset. At postmortem there is massive bleeding into the lung and pleural cavity.

Culture and histopathological examination often revealed a peracute necrotizing bacterial pneumonia with early inflammatory reaction and large numbers of *S. zooepidemicus*.

The findings are similar to those in horses that die suddenly during a workout or race with massive hemorrhage into the lungs with or without breakout into the pleural cavity. Some of these sudden deaths are simply massive bleeders, while others have the evidence of a peracute necrotizing streptococcal pneumonia, even without a history of upper respiratory disease.

Horses become reinfected with herpesvirus (EHV)-1 and probably have at least minimal lesions of the upper respiratory tract, which could serve as portal of entry for bacterial infection. Clinical signs of such reinfection are few and usually unrecognized.

Smith (1977) studied the pleural effusions of 37 horses, 15 acute and 22 chronic. Diseases associated with pleural effusion included lymphosarcoma (4/37 cases), equine infectious anemia (1/37), pneumonia and abscesses (13/37), intrathoracic sepsis (2/37), pulmonary granulomas (2/37), trauma (1/37), and primary pleuritis (14/37). Seven of the 15 acute cases died or were killed; 24 of 37 cases died or were killed. No age, breed, or sex predilection was found. Acute signs included respiratory distress, colicky pain, fever, and anorexia. The commonest signs of chronic disease were weight loss and anemia. Culture of lung tissue yielded bacteria in 11 of 16 horses studied. Analysis of the effusion itself generally showed markedly increased cellularity and high protein content. The analysis of bronchoalveolar lavage fluid was not diagnostic and the value of such procedures is equivocal (Rossier et al. 1991).

Primary pleuritis, mentioned above, probably does not exist in horses. We have never seen a case at postmortem without either an obvious cause such as a foreign body or large abscess or subtle, difficult to find, abscessation in the accessory lobe. Careful dissection of the lungs, with particular attention to the often overlooked accessory lobe, will dispel "primary pleuritis" as an entity.

Traumatic and mechanical disorders

Tracheal malformation and collapse

Deformation of the trachea, causing respiratory distress and coughing in aged horses, was described by Imlin (1836) cited by Cadeac (1897). Cadeac commented that this may have been the result of tearing of the ligament interannulaire and separation of the mucosa. Gylstorff (1971) described tracheal malformations causing dyspnea. The usual malformation resembles the scabbard of a sword because of flattening of the tracheal rings. The dorsal and ventral walls of the trachea may be virtually parallel. The cause may be stretching of the dorsal smooth muscle as the result of paralysis, overstretching of the elastic tissue of the dorsal trachea, or age-related atrophy of smooth muscle. While a congenital etiology has been suggested for some cases, this is unproven, and we have not seen this in young animals.

Exercise-induced pulmonary hemorrhage

This awkward, pretentious, term refers to the condition of racing horses usually known as **bleeder**. It is common in flat racing Thoroughbred horses and Quarter horses and seen, as well, in Standardbred racing horses and horses that race over jumps. Typically, the horse completes the course, coughs, and bleeds from one or both nostrils.

Bleeding in racing horses has been known since the middle of the 16th century [Markham cited by Robertson (1910)], and was described by Solleysel in 1711. A dominant, sex-limited inheritance was suggested by Robertson (1910), with most cases in horses and geldings. Hillidge and Whitlock (1986) found a higher incidence in geldings than in intact male or female racing Quarter horses. Some studies in Thoroughbreds suggest a male preponderance while others do not (Pascoe et al. 1981; Sweeney et al. 1990). Robertson's opinion was based on bleeding from the nostril while the other reports are based on endoscopic findings, suggesting that bleeding, if not more frequent in males, is more severe, but that was not the experience of Hillidge and Whitlock.

It is accepted that the vast majority of such animals are bleeding in the lung, specifically the dorsocaudal portion of the diaphragmatic lobe. Fiberoptic endoscope examination has shown that more horses bleed into the lung than show bleeding from the nostrils.

The lesion in the dorsocaudal diaphragmatic lobe is a plaque or focal area of marked greenish-brown discoloration laced, in longer-standing cases, with whitish-gray bands of fibrous tissue (Fig. 2.11). Histologically, the discoloration is that of large numbers of hemosiderin-containing macrophages while the fibrous tissue is primarily localized around distorted blood vessels undergoing elastotic degeneration and fibrosis (Rooney 1970). O'Callaghan (1988), as part of an extensive study, showed that longer-standing lesions are neovascularized by the bronchial arterial system. Cases seen at postmortem are recurrent, the animals having bled a number of times. It is, indeed, unlikely if not impossible to recognize a first time "bleeder lesion" at postmortem as will be apparent in the discussion of agonal hemorrhages, below.

The pathogenesis of this lesion remains in dispute in a voluminous, largely clinical, literature. The first question to be addressed is the consistent localization of the lesion in the dorsocaudal part of the diaphragmatic lobe. Observations of lungs of

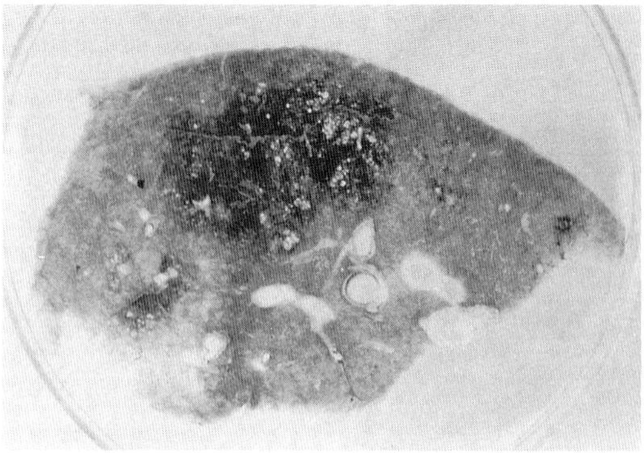

2.11. Section of lung showing bleeding into the pulmonary parenchyma, which is characteristic of exercise-induced hemorrhage.

horses killed for reasons other than pulmonary disease routinely have bleeding in this portion of the diaphragmatic lobe. If the animal dies with virtually no agonal period, there is an increased amount of blood in this area with hemorrhages only seen microscopically. The larger vessels appear normal, and the hemorrhage presumably comes from capillaries. There may be virtually no blood in the bronchi grossly, small amounts being seen in the bronchioles microscopically. With a more prolonged agonal period, there will be gross hemorrhage and streams of blood, admixed with mucus, in the bronchi. These streams of blood extend a variable distance, being found as far cranially as the cervical portion of the trachea. It appears that ciliary transport can move blood from the focus in the diaphragmatic lobe to this point of the trachea in no more than 5–10 minutes after the killing agent has been introduced. That is, blood can be found in the trachea opened within 5–10 minutes after the heart has stopped. With even longer agonal periods, the congestion and hemorrhage involve larger areas of lung, spreading out from the dorsocaudal area.

This is, of course, agonal hemorrhage as a result of asphyxiation. The reason for the more severe asphyxial effect in this portion of the lung is not definitely known. Amis et al. (1984) showed that there is less perfusion and ventilation of the dorsal part of the lung than of the middle and ventral portions. Even though the ratio of ventilation to perfusion is constant throughout the lung, this suggests that the dorsal part of the lung is predisposed to asphyxial damage.

In any event, it is apparent that the dorsocaudal part of the diaphragmatic lobe is the *locus minoris resistentia* for asphyxial hemorrhages in the lung of the horse. Based on this observation, it is reasonable to propose that asphyxiation, of whatever cause, is the final common factor in the pathogenesis of exercise-induced pulmonary hemorrhage (Rooney 1970). While focal chronic inflammatory lesions have been suggested as causes, no convincing pathological evidence has been presented. Indeed, the dorsal portions of the lungs are, in general, less often affected by such lesions than the more cranial and ventral portions, as in all quadrupeds.

Asphyxiation, in racing horses, can have many causes. The unpublished work of Sparks (1968) clearly showed that many horses hold their breath for 30 seconds or more when racing, particularly when leaving the starting gait. One thinks of exhausted (jumping races, specifically) and unfit animals with inadequate, uncoordinated breathing, Standardbred horses with the head and neck held in unnaturally flexed positions, atrial fibrillation, partial or complete laryngeal hemiplegia, pharyngeal lesions, and so forth.

Breathing is coordinated with gait: one respiratory cycle for each stride, 1:1 at the canter and gallop. At the nonracing trot or pace the horse can select a different pattern: 1:2, 1:3, or 2:3 (Bramble and Carrier 1983; Clayton 1991). At the racing trot and pace it appears that the cycle is usually 1:1 or 1:2. With fatigue this regular cycling may be disturbed and cause inadequate pulmonary ventilation. Movement of the abdominal viscera, flexion of the back, and force exerted by the fore legs on the thorax have been suggested as drivers of breathing movement (Bramble and Carrier 1983). Alexander (1989) discounted at least the visceral piston. It seems unnecessary to require more than work done by the usual respiratory muscles, the timing being set by a central nervous system controller.

More generally, horses evolved to travel long distances at moderate velocities, using maximum bursts of speed to outdistance predators. Racing requires such bursts to be carried for longer distances than evolution has provided, with asphyxial bleeding the result. It is of interest that exertional bleeding is said to occur in human athletes, specifically sprint swimmers who may hold their breath for 100 meters.

Pneumothorax

Pneumothorax is rare in the horse and almost always the result of devastating penetrating wounds inflicted by posts, fence rails, and such. Bullet wounds usually seal over rapidly before significant pneumothorax can develop. Pneumothorax must be detected before the pleural cavity is opened; the diaphragm is loose. Careful search usually shows that the diaphragm was nicked or a zealous assistant has stabbed between the ribs or into the thoracic inlet.

July blower

This is an acute dyspnea seen in some foals kept up in boxes during bad, wet weather. It disappears when the foals are turned out, and no pathology has been reported. We have heard of the condition only in Newmarket, England.

Toxic respiratory disease

Ingestion of purple mint, *Pirella frutescens*, caused pulmonary edema in a horse (Lindley 1978). Wilson et al. (1977) and Boyd (1980) indicated that the pulmonary toxicity of this herb followed the metabolism of 3-substituted furans by pulmonary mixed-function oxidases, yielding the proximate toxicant **pirella ketone**. Animals lacking sufficient enzyme systems to detoxify this material develop pulmonary edema and restriction of pulmonary function. Breeze et al. (1984) exposed three adult ponies to synthetic pirella ketone (18 mg/kg in dimethyl sulfoxide). Pulmonary function measurements over 12 days (6 baseline days, 6 days after treatment) had increased respiratory rates, increased peak inspiratory and expiratory flow rates, increased minute volume, and decreased tidal volume. The animals were killed 6 days after exposure. The lungs were congested and edematous. Histological lesions included fluid in the alveoli, hyalin membrane formation, pneumocyte hyperplasia, and hyperplasia of bronchiolar epithelium without airway occlusion.

Silicate pneumoconiosis and pulmonary fibrosis were reported in nine horses in California (Schwartz et al. 1981). Multiple granulomas composed of foamy macrophages, lymphocytes, and plasma cells were distributed throughout the interstitium. The degree of pulmonary fibrosis varied among the cases. Refractile particles were found with foamy macrophages in granulomas. Similar lesions were seen in the bronchial lymph nodes and liver. X-ray diffraction analysis showed the particles contained silicates. Silicates are common in the dry soils of the Monterey peninsula, and the condition appears to only have been reported there.

Dyspnea, cyanosis, and respiratory distress and/or failure were reported in 14 horses accidentally dosed with **flowers of sulphur** (Corke 1981). Two horses died within 48 hours. The lungs had cranioventral consolidation and moderate emphysema. Yellow-tinged froth was present in the trachea and bronchi. There was no microscopic examination.

The oral or intravenous administration of **3-methylindole** causes severe necrotizing bronchiolitis (Derksen et al. 1982; Breeze et al. 1984). Natural exposure to the material is a likely cause of bovine pulmonary disease, but this has not been shown in horses. Indeed, it is unlikely that there is sufficient natural exposure to the material to cause respiratory damage.

Experimental exposure of equids to 3-methylindole has been used to produce chronic bronchiolitis. The lesions are generally limited to respiratory bronchioles where Clara cells show dilation of smooth endoplasmic reticulum within 2 hours of exposure. The cells may become necrotic and slough within 12–24 hours (Breeze et al. 1984). Repopulation of denuded bronchioles occurs within 3 days. Hyperplasia of poorly differentiated cells overlying areas of fibroplasia and lymphocytic infiltration is seen. Within 6 days, bronchioles may be partially or completely occluded, and there is some degree of recanalization in the following days to weeks after experimental exposure. Foci of emphysema were seen in some experimental ponies.

Neoplasms of the lower respiratory tract

Lung tumors are rare in equids. In a survey of 119 primary neoplasms in horses, donkeys and mules, no primary lung tumors were found (Jackson 1936). Monlux (1952, 1953) identified 33 pulmonary neoplasms, including 12 adenocarcinomas and 7 carcinomas. The mean age was 16 years, and tumors were more common in the right lung, especially the diaphragmatic lobe. Sundberg et al. (1987) found no lung tumors among 637 autopsies and 635 biopsies.

Bronchoalveolar adenocarcinoma

Bronchoalveolar adenocarcinoma was found in a 12-year-old Hannoverian stallion in South Africa (Van Rensberg et al. 1989). There was a 4-month history of depression, anorexia, and chronic nonproductive cough. Discrete, 1-10 cm, firm, yellow-white neoplastic nodules were found in the lungs. The bronchial and alveolar architecture was reasonably maintained while cuboidal, ciliated or nonciliated neoplastic cells lined respiratory structures. Myelinoid bodies gave some of these cells a vacuolated appearance.

Cystic mucinous adenocarcinoma

Cystic mucinous adenocarcinoma with multiple metastases and acute bronchopneumonia were found in a 14-year-old Arabian gelding (Schultze et al. 1988). There was a 3-month history of coughing and fore leg lameness. Copious mucopurulent material was present in the trachea and nasal passages, and multiple interstitial masses were seen on radiographs. There were approximately 200 of these masses in the lungs. Histologically there were glandular and ductular formations and eosinophilic mucus. Anaplastic glandular epithelium and goblet cells were present, together with mucous lakes. Metastasis to mediastinal lymph nodes, pleura, diaphragm, and axilla had occurred.

Anaplastic bronchogenic carcinoma

An anaplastic bronchogenic carcinoma was reported by Schultz et al. (1988) in a 21-year-old Appaloosa mare with a 4-week history of pyrexia and weight loss. A partially encapsulated, 8-cm diameter mass was found at the tracheal bifurcation. It comprised several smaller white nodules on the cut surface. Smaller nodules of similar appearance studded the pleural surface. Sheets of poorly differentiated cuboidal cells were present in a matrix of connective tissue and necrotic debris.

Bronchial myxoma

Bronchial myxoma was found in a 25-year-old Arabian mare with intermittent coughing for 2 years prior to presentation (Murphy et al. 1978). A mass bridged the left cranial and caudal lobar bronchi. It was yellow, slimy, and soft and composed of sheets of stellate cells and collagenous fibers in a mass of eosinophilic mucus.

Granular cell myoblastoma

Misdorp and Nauta-Van Gelder (1968) reported four cases of granular cell myoblastoma in a population of 40,000 horses. All four cases were in aged animals, and there was characteristic association of the neoplasm with bronchi. Most masses ranged from a few cm to over 20 cm and were yellow-white. Microscopically, there were closely packed ovoid to polyhedral cells with abundant PAS-positive granules in the cytoplasm. We have seen several of these tumors, in one instance with pulmonary osteoarthropathy.

Several metastatic tumors causing pleural effusion have been reported, including malignant mammary adenocarcinoma (Foreman et al. 1990), ovarian adenocarcinoma (Morris et al. 1985), and malignant hepatoblastoma (Prater et al. 1989). Both metastatic and primary neoplasia of the lung is uncommon in Equids.

CHAPTER 3

Gastrointestinal Tract and Adnexa

- Nutritional enteritis
- Isolated *S. vulgaris* infarction
- Muscular hypertrophy of the ileum
- Impaction of the ileum
- Hemamelasma ilei
- Lymphosarcoma
- Granulomatous enteritis
- Avian tuberculosis
- Eosinophilic gastroenteritis
- Mycobacterium paratuberculosis
- Volvulus, strangulation, and incarceration

Cecum
- Teniae and haustra
- Impaction
- Intussusception
- Rupture

Colon
- Ascending colon
- Descending colon
- Enterolithiasis
- Foreign body obstruction
- Acute/chronic diarrhea
- Equine ehrlichial colitis
- Mucinous enteropathy
- Acorn poisoning

Rectum and anus
- Oxyurosis
- Rupture of the rectum

Neoplasia

Liver
- Aging changes
- Small white nodules
- Infiltrations and degenerations
- Amyloidosis
- Vacuolar and/or fatty change
- Iron fumarate necrosis
- Tyzzer's disease
- Theiler's disease
- Alsike clover poisoning
- Pyrrolizidine alkaloid poisoning
- Purulent cholangiohepatitis
- Vascular cirrhosis
- Fasciola hepatica
- Dicrocoelium dendriticum
- Echinococcus granulosus
- Cholelithiasis
- Neoplasia

Pancreas
- Acute interstitial pancreatitis
- Chronic interstitial pancreatitis
- Carcinoma

Mouth

Vesicular stomatitis

This viral disease is limited to the Western Hemisphere, being enzootic in certain areas of North, Central, and South America. Cattle, pigs, and humans are susceptible as well as equids.

After a 5–8 day incubation there is moderate fever, slow eating, and depression. Reddening of the oral mucosa is followed by formation of nodules inside the lips, alongside the tongue, cheeks, and, occasionally, the coronary band. Clear, watery vesicles develop from the nodules. These form erosions or ulcerations after becoming pustules. The vesicles may contain up to 10 mL of proteinaceous, straw-colored fluid. After rupture, deep, slowly healing mucosal erosions remain. In experimental cases lesions are most extensive on the tongue, suggesting differing cutaneous responses to the virus (Olitsky et al. 1926). The pustules appear 3–6 days after first signs of disease. After a further 4–6 days the pustules rupture and heal. Recovery requires 10 days to 4 weeks (Hutyra and Marek 1920; Blood and Henderson 1963).

The nasal mucosa, tear ducts, and conjunctiva may be involved. Often characteristic vesicles do not appear, the lesions simply drying up to form small necrotic ulcers. In the human, mucosal lesions do not occur, the disease having the clinical characteristics of influenza.

Lesions of the feet have been seen in experimental animals (Cotton 1927). In several horses, vesicles formed on the bulbs of the heels and ruptured, causing lameness. One horse developed extensive lesions of the coronary band and heels and lost the sole. Cotton found an unusual amount of straw-colored fluid in the sheaths of the superficial and deep flexor tendons at postmortem. This was probably secondary to lameness and lack of movement.

Contagious pustular stomatitis

An epizootic vesiculopustular stomatitis of young horses was described in the European literature of the 1800s (Friedberger and Fröhner 1895; Hutyra and Marek 1922). Investigators believed it could be distinguished from horse pox, glanders, and so forth. It was said to be transmissible to horse, cow, human, sheep, pig, and chicken, in that order. The disease in humans was vesicular/pustular, unlike the influenzalike disease of vesicular stomatitis. This was most certainly horse pox (Gillespie and Timoney 1981). (See the next section.)

Horse pox

Horse pox, caused by the cowpox virus, was seen as **grease**, greasy heels, as well as a disease of the oral mucosa and skin: **contagious pustular stomatitis and dermatitis**. The disease has only been seen in Europe and is uncommon (Blood and Henderson 1963). Grease, dermatitis of the plantar surface of the pastern, seen primarily in the rear legs, has other causes, as well (see Chapter 15, "Integument").

In earlier times horses were infected by handlers who had cowpox or had been vaccinated with cowpox virus. Other sources of contagion were horses, cows, or housing in cow stalls. The disease can be limited to the pastern or mouth or spread to the nose and over the surface of the body (Cadeac 1899a–c; DeJong 1917; Hutyra and Marek 1920).

The usual course is 10–14 days but may last up to 3–4 weeks. Pustules appear 3–6 days after onset of first signs of pain and reddish flecks in the oral mucosa. The first lesion is a reddish focus, followed by papule and vesicle formation. The latter may have a depressed, dimpled center. The vesicle is quickly converted to a pustule, which ruptures with scabbing. A scar may remain. The cells of the stratum spinosum undergo vacuolar degeneration as acute inflammation begins in the dermis. Fluid accumulates in the epidermis, forming the vesicle. With infiltration of neutrophil leukocytes into the dermis and epidermis, the vesicle changes to a pustule. After rupture of the pustule, healing is by epithelization. Scar tissue follows severe lesions (Cohrs 1961).

Catarrhal stomatitis

The usual catarrhal stomatitis in the horse is, at first, characterized by dryness and warmth of the mucosa without the significant hyperemia usually seen in other species (Cadeac 1908). There may be slight turgidity as the result of inflammatory infiltration of the submucosal tissues. Diffuse redness and petechiation appears in more severe cases. A gummy layer of grayish-white desquamated epithelium impregnated with mucus accumulates on the top and sides of the tongue. This is stained by food materials and has a disagreeable, putrefying odor. The dryness is soon replaced by an abundant secretion of clear, viscous, normally alkaline saliva as healing progresses.

Agents causing catarrhal stomatitis include white chickweed, mustard, sandwort (*Arenaria serpyllifolia*), and any plant containing parasympathomimetic substances (Cadeac 1908). Various chemical agents, such as carbon disulfide, turpentine, and other horrors of an earlier time, caused variably severe catarrhal stomatitis.

Stachybotryotoxicosis

This has only been reported in Eastern Europe and the Ukraine. The fungus, *Stachybotrys alternans*, grows on straw or hay, producing a toxin in 2–3 weeks, about the time spore formation begins. Signs appear in horses in 1–4 days, with edematous swelling of the lips and inflammation and necrosis of the buccal, gingival, and lingual mucosae. With continued feeding there is leucopenia and thrombocytopenia, followed by a sudden rise in temperature and death (Ainsworth and Austwick 1959; Cohrs 1961; Zakrzewski 1970).

Slobbers

Slobbers is characterized by profuse salivation, the initial stages of catarrhal inflammation not being observed. It is seen in horses grazing pasture with large amounts of white clover (*Trifolium* spp.). It may also be seen with large amounts of red clover. Hay from these clovers does not appear to cause the condition. Since the low-growing white clover appears earlier in the spring than most grasses, epizootics may be seen in horses at that time. The toxic agent is **slaframine**, an alkaloid produced by the fungus, *Rhizoctonia leguminicola*, which infects the clover causing black spot disease (Hagler and Behlow 1981). No pathological studies have been reported, but presumably there is catarrhal stomatitis.

The condition has long been known (Hutyra and Marek 1920, 1926). Cadeac (1908) described a vesicular or exanthematous form associated with exposure to hybrid trefoils. Dadd (1854):

> Slavering horses are frequently met with in farming districts, where clover is used as an article of fodder. There seems to be some peculiar property about the flowers of clover which renders them a source of great irritation to the mucous surfaces and salivary apparatus of the horse.

Insect vesicular exanthema

A vesicular disease of the lips, nose, and adjacent mucosae was described by Cadeac (1905). The lips, nose, and sometimes the skin around the eyes were initially swollen, hot, and painful. In 2 to 3 days these areas vesiculated and sloughed large areas of necrotic skin. Depigmented skin remained after healing.

This was associated with contaminated bedding and believed to be caused by vesicants produced by an insect (*Blaps mortissaga*) and/or caterpillars (*Bombyx* or *Cnethocampa processionnea*). Bassi and Venuta cited by Cadeac (1905) observed the relationship of insects and caterpillars with the condition and reproduced the disease by rubbing the noses of three horses and a donkey with living, but not with dead, *Blaps*. Apparently the caterpillars have cuticular glands that secrete highly concentrated formic acid. *Blaps* secrete an irritant liquid from anal glands (Cadeac 1908). *Blaps mortissaga* cannot be certainly translated to modern terminology, but, apparently, is a member of the *Scarabaeidae* (Cadeac 1908). It may be noted that Zuill mistranslated the cause of this condition as *nettles* rather than caterpillars and beetles (Friedberger and Fröhner 1895).

Teeth

Incidence figures are not available, but comparison of the older and more recent literature suggests fewer dental lesions in the modern light horse population than in the older, predominantly heavy horse population. Ostertag in *Bayer-Fröhner* (1899) found the following for 28,605 horses examined in Berlin, 1892–1896:

Alveolar periostitis (gingivitis)	614
Caries (any opening of pulp cavity)	31
Fracture, incisors	19
Scissor mouth	89
Stepform mouth	178
Waveform mouth	56
Fistula, tooth	81
Split, fractured, tooth	26
Sharp enamel points	726
	1820

The major sources for this section are Cohrs (1961) and Becker (1970). Baker's (1979) thesis on equine teeth was not available for examination.

The aging of horses by their teeth was well known to Xenophon in 370 BCE (Hooper 1936). The evolution of the teeth is of singular importance in the study of equine evolution (MacFadden 1992). The transition from browsing to grazing entailed a transition from low-crowned to high-crowned, hypsodont, teeth of greater height. The greater length of the teeth and the addition of cementum were adaptations to the greater frictional wear of siliceous herbage (Janis 1976; MacFadden 1992). This transition apparently occurred during the Miocene, some 20 million years ago (MacFadden 1992).

Delayed eruption

Premolars

Between 2 and 4 years, there may be **pressure atrophy of the basal ends of permanent teeth P2 and P3 of the maxilla** and, particularly, **P3 of the mandible**. This is suspected because of difficult chewing and painful swelling of the mandible, and is readily confirmed radiographically (Fig. 3.1).

The pressure atrophy may cause fistulation, but, more often, there is marked periosteal new bone formation, which obviates fistulation. The new bone is remodeled once eruption of the tooth occurs.

There are two basic causes (Becker 1970), the obvious one being retention of the deciduous tooth. Less apparent is discrepancy in the growth rates of the tooth and the adjacent bone; that is, the permanent tooth is growing more rapidly than the surrounding bone. Becker considers this a disease of domestication. One can find painful areas over these teeth in animals 1 1/2 to 3 years of age without retention of the deciduous teeth; radio-

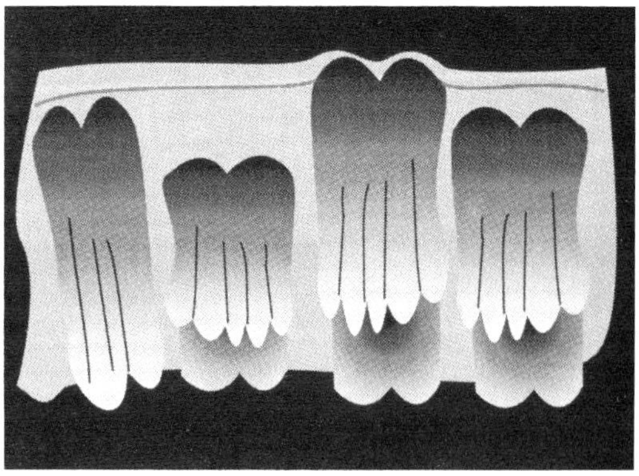

3.1. Schematic drawing of retained permanent 3rd mandibular premolar.

graphs show decreased compact bone at the base of the permanent teeth.

Molars

The larger, longer P2 of the upper jaw results in each pair of teeth contacting its opposite number in the mandible by 3/4 and the next tooth caudally by 1/4.

An important cause of exsuperantia dentium (see below) is improperly timed eruption of the first molars (M1) of the upper and lower jaws. Normally, the first molars erupt at about 9 months. Not infrequently, maxillary M1 erupts at that time, while mandibular M1 erupts some months later. Maxillary M1, then, can overgrow as much as 12 mm or more before the mandibular molar erupts.

Incisors

Becker indicates that eruption of the incisor teeth may be delayed as much as 6 months beyond average in slowly maturing breeds. In the modern Thoroughbred horse delays of eruption of the incisors are not uncommon and can be at least as long as 2–3 years. The situation in other modern breeds is not known. While such delays in eruption of the incisors confuse the determination of age, they cause no pathological changes.

Sharp enamel points

These occur on the outer, buccal, edges of the maxillary cheek teeth and the inner, lingual, edges of the mandibular cheek teeth. Becker (1970) found well over 90% of 32,000 military horses with sharp enamel points.

Leue (1937, 1941), with a clever molograph [Fig. 90 of Becker (1970)], quantitated the excursions of the mandible of horses eating grass, hay, and bran. The excursions were greatest with grass and least with bran. Grass is cut off by the incisors and pushed as small bundles between the cheek teeth by the tongue. Since these bundles tend to cohere, the lower jaw moves fully to one side, so that the buccal edges of the upper and lower teeth are in line and wear uniformly across the masticating surfaces. With concentrates and chopped food materials, no bundles are formed, and the horse must clamp the upper and lower teeth together to hold the food and prevent it falling into the cheeks. Thus, there is less excursion of the lower jaw, and the buccal edges of the upper and the lingual edges of the lower teeth are not properly worn. Chewing is discussed further below.

Wild horses and domestic horses allowed to feed naturally have fewer and less marked sharp enamel points than domesticated horses. Bruner (1941) found no abnormal wearing or enamel points in fossil horse teeth.

Exsuperantia dentium

This is misfitting of the upper and lower cheek teeth. It may take the form of an overgrown maxillary M1 relative to mandibular M1, as described. Congenital excess or absence of teeth may cause misfit, as can brachgnathia and prognathia. Loss of a tooth by fracture or infection entails lack of wear and overgrowth of the matching tooth of the other jaw. Wave and step form are two specific varieties of misfit.

Becker (1970) found 18.8% misfitting teeth in 30,000 cavalry horses. While the cause is apparent in some cases, it often is not, as in the wave and step form. A bow form is occasionally seen with the convexity of one or the other row of cheek teeth matching the concavity of the other row without misfit.

Scissor mouth is a severe misfit with the maxillary rows much wider than the mandibular, allowing overgrowth and abnormal wearing of the teeth. The maxillary cheek teeth normally are about 30% farther apart than the mandibular. Becker found scissor mouth in 0.9% of the 30,000 cavalry horses.

Polyodontie

More teeth than normal are found in 0.5%–4% of horses. These are retained deciduous teeth or true extra teeth such as a fourth incisor or a fourth molar. The practical concern is the role of such teeth in exsuperantia dentium.

Oligodontie

Too few teeth may be congenital failure or acquired loss and is seen in about 1% of horses. Retention or failure of eruption of one or both canine teeth is common in horses. Becker (1970) reported that 25%–30% of mares had canine teeth, but only 2%–3% had all four canines; 99% of stallions had all four canine teeth.

Anomalies of size, shape, and position

A variety of anomalies of size and shape have been reported, as well as improper position of specific teeth. Anomalies may appear alone or with other anomalies, such as polyodontie. The practical importance relates to exsuperantia dentium.

Diastema

The cheek teeth are normally in contact with each other at the masticatory margins. If space(s) is present, either congenital or acquired, it is known as diastema. Food material packed into these spaces is a common cause of gingivitis and inflammatory periodontal disease (Little 1913). Packing of food materials may also be seen as a cause of gingivitis in older horses as the necks of the teeth are exposed and spaces occur between teeth at the gingival margins.

Structural anomalies of the tooth

Hypoplasia, invaginated enamel, maxillary M1

Enamel folds or invaginations surround the *infundibula* of both the maxillary and mandibular cheek teeth. Since senile wearing of the masticatory surfaces begins in the rostral infundibula before the caudal, it is apparent that the rostral enamel folds do not extend as deeply into the tooth as the caudal enamel folds. With normal abrasion, the enamel folds are gradually worn down, so that the dentine comes into wear, and **senile excavation** of the masticatory surface occurs.

With **hypoplasia of the enamel folds** of maxillary M1, the folds are even less deeply invaginated into the body of the tooth than normal. Thus, the complete wearing away of the rostral infundibulum of maxillary M1 begins much earlier than with normal senile wear. The excavation of the dentine begins earlier than normal as **presenile excavation**. In earlier stages the excavation of the dentine is clearly transverse, buccal/lingual, in keeping with the normal motion of the teeth.

Hypoplasia of the enamel folds does not become apparent until sufficient presenile excavation has occurred, usually, according to Becker (1970), in horses over 10 years of age. Senile excavation is not seen until about 18 years of age. If the presenile excavation progresses rapidly, dentine being worn away faster than secondary dentine can form, the pulp cavity may be opened and become infected (see below). Rupprecht (1936), cited by Becker, reported a 10% frequency of hypoplasia of the enamel folds. Cohrs (1961) reported 23%.

Hypoplasia, cementum, infundibulum-maxillary molars

This is a partial, punctate, or, more commonly, complete absence of the cement filling the infundibula of the cheek teeth (Fig. 3.2). It is most frequent in M1, least frequent in M3, and may be seen in any cheek tooth. Buhler (1936) cited by Cohrs found this in 75% of horses. Becker (1970) found only 0.4% among 30,000 horses. Baker (1974) indicated that 43% of horses were affected. Buhler found this more often in the rostral infundibulum, while Becker did not note such a predisposition. It is possible that Buhler did not adequately differentiate hypoplasia of invaginated enamel from cement hypoplasia. In our experience with light horses both infundibula of M1 are most frequently affected, and the incidence would be somewhat less than 50%. Becker's data was based on clinical examination, which could account for his low incidence. Both enamel fold and cement hypoplasia apparently affect horses of all breeds.

Baker (1974) examined the development of the maxillary teeth in fetuses and foals and confirmed

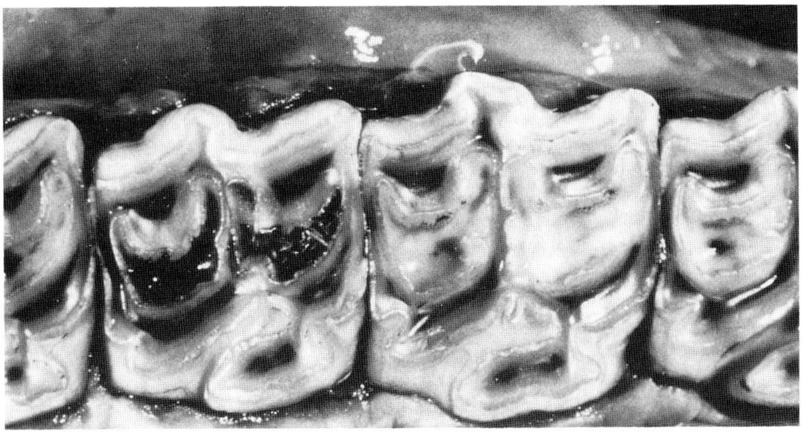

3.2. Cement hypoplasia of the 4th upper cheek tooth. Food material is impacted.

the findings of Joest, cited by Baker. Cementogenesis begins near the occlusal surface as a collar of cement tissue that closes off the infundibulum, extending toward the root of the tooth. This process is incomplete at birth in 43% of cases, which allows food materials to pack the infundibulum, leading to infection as discussed below. Baker indicated that some teeth, which appeared normal on the occlusal surface, had focal necrosis in the deeper part of the infundibulum. In this case bacteria and food materials apparently enter the infundibulum before the cement collar at the occlusal surface closes after eruption of the tooth.

Hypoplasia of the cementum is apparent earlier than hypoplasia of the enamel invagination since manifestation of the latter depends upon wearing of the tooth. With the absence of cement, the infundibulum is open and may be packed with food material. In advanced cases bacterial action in this material opens the infundibulum into the pulp cavity with pulpitis and death of the tooth. The tooth may, then, fracture into several pieces, allowing overgrowth of the opposing mandibular tooth.

It is apparent that differentiation of these two hypoplasias of the masticatory surface can be difficult. In general, with enamel fold hypoplasia, the wearing of the dentine is oriented transversely and food material is not packed into the excavation. In the case of cement hypoplasis the defect is more rounded or oval and often packed with food material. As well, cement hypoplasia may be apparent in younger animals before significant wearing has occurred.

A reason for the high frequency of cement hypoplasia and its specific localization to the first maxillary molar has not been given. There is paleontological evidence that early equids were browsers with no cement on their teeth. As later horses changed from browsing to grazing, the teeth underwent significant changes, including the addition of cement [Matthew and Chubb (no date given); and Simpson (1951)]. Cement hypoplasia, and enamel fold hypoplasia as well, may be atavistic, genetic, or epigenetic, the information for shorter, less folded teeth without cement being retained from ancient times to be expressed, still, in the modern horse. Cement hypoplasia and enamel fold hypoplasia may, then, be genetic diseases of horses per se, not unlike angiomatosis, odontomas, epiglottic cysts, and perhaps other conditions peculiar to equids but not to specific breeds or types.

Porodontie

This is defined as spontaneous opening of the pulp canal of the mandibular molar teeth following failure of secondary dentine formation. Cohrs (1961) apparently used this term both in the specific sense given here, as well as more generally to indicate opening into the pulp cavity of whatever cause, such as cement hypoplasia of the infundibulum. This is only seen in horses, among domestic animals.

Becker reported a 3% frequency among 30,000 cavalry horses. It is failure of formation of secondary dentine said to be caused by pulp "insufficiency" and, more specifically, by inflammation of the pulp. As the tooth wears, secondary dentine must be formed in phase with the wearing. If dentine formation lags as a result of inflammation of the pulp, the pulp cavity will be opened by the wearing. Pulpitis may be the result of the not uncommon gingivitis and periodontal infection and inflammation associated with diastema.

The predisposition of the mandibular teeth to porodontie probably correlates with the common occurrence of periodontal disease in the lower jaw. This, in turn, is a gravity effect, with food materials accumulating here rather than in the upper jaw.

Structural anomalies of enamel

Focal hypoplasia occurs as small pits in the wall of any tooth and may be single or multiple, often in rows or with a honeycomb appearance. The lesions are smooth, white, gray, or brownish.

Structural anomalies of dentine

These minute defects of the dentine cannot be appreciated from the surface. They are said to be congenital or acquired (Becker 1970).

No structural anomalies of the cement have been reported in the horse. **Cement hyperplasia** is common on the body and root of the teeth as a senile change and is, also, seen with chronic periodontal disease.

Caries

Caries has been defined as a localized, usually chronic, noninflammatory destruction of the hard tissues of the teeth. Almost any necrotizing or destructive process involving enamel, dentine, or cementum has been given this name. Becker reported 1% among 30,000 horses. Since, in the horse at least, such destructive processes are almost always associated with predisposing factors that allow the accumulation of food materials, it may be best to refer to those factors with an appended description of necrosis of the specific hard tissue(s) and to avoid the term, caries, altogether.

Tartar/calculus

Becker cites Beier (1915) that 83% of horses have a gray-white, brittle tartar accumulation on the teeth, which is readily removed. It is of no pathological significance. We have not seen it.

Gingivitis, periodontitis, and pulpitis

Baker rediscovered periodontal disease as the commonest dental disease of horses in the 1970s as Ostertag had found in 1899. The frequency increased from 14% in horses 0–3 years old to 60% in horses over 15 years. The initial lesion is gingivitis, usually on the buccal aspect. A triangular pocket is formed by an erosive, necrotizing process. Food materials accumulate in the eroded areas. The lesion becomes progressively larger and invades the deeper-lying periodontal tissues. Inflammation and necrosis may cause the death of the tooth, apical abscessation, pulpitis, and periodontitis. Cement hyperplasia occurs in chronic cases together with localized osteomyelitis. The formation of the pocket is, at least in part, a function of the age-related exposure of the narrow roots of the teeth.

Odontoma

These teratoid malformations of the tooth primordia have not been systematically studied in the horse. Becker (1970), apparently relying on the medical literature, considered them as **simple odontoma**, with several subclasses, and **odontoma multidentiferum proliferans**. The former arises from a single improperly developing tooth, is well differentiated, most common in horses, and does not grow after the birth of the animal. We have not seen this in light horses.

The proliferating, multiple tooth odontoma is most common in 1- to 3-year-old horses and cattle. The mass may be recognized at birth, arising from either the maxillary or mandibular arcades. This, the commonest form in our experience, is characterized by a multicystic or polycystic structure. It has a marked tendency to recur even after apparently complete removal. The mass does not metastasize, but is locally aggressive and continues to grow after birth to considerable, disabling size (Williams 1891/92). It has also been called *odontogenic cyst.*

Other tumors of this area are rare. Benign osteoma may be encountered, even in foals, and is to be differentiated from odontoma.

Choke and teeth

Improper eruption of the permanent teeth, for example, delayed eruption of the premolars, may cause pain when chewing and swallowing of incompletely masticated food and, so, choke. Improper eruption can cause ulceration of the buccal, more often lingual, gingiva with or without infestation by *Gasterophilus* larvae. Periodontal necrosis and ulceration can cause pain and improper mastication in older horses, with choke as a result (see "Esophagus," in this chapter).

Colic and teeth

A relationship between gastrointestinal disorders and disorders of teeth has often been suggested. Leue (1941) used the molograph of Leue (1937) to investigate the chewing pattern of 30 horses with various forms of intestinal obstruction compared to horses with colic caused by ingestion of sand. Anomalies or lesions of the teeth were found in all but one case of obstruction but in no horses with sand colic. While these results may seem too good, the molograph in some form seems a useful tool in assessing chewing function in cases of relapsing and/or recurrent colic.

Fluorosis

Shupe and Olson (1971) described fluorosis in the horse, an animal more resistant to the deleterious effects of fluoride than cattle or sheep. Lesions occur in developing teeth, metacarpal and metatarsal bones, phalanges (particularly at tendoligamentous insertions), mandible, nasal and maxillary bones, and ribs. Dental fluorosis occurs during the period of tooth development, while the bony changes can apparently occur at any time.

The severity of the fluorotic lesions indicates the level of fluoride ingestion during the formation of enamel and dentine. Affected teeth erupt with characteristic lesions such as mottling, staining, hypoplasia, hypocalcification, and excessive rate of wear. Shupe and Olson provided a classification of these dental changes.

Excessive and uneven rate of wear of the fluorotic premolar and molar teeth can cause damage sufficient to lead to infection of the pulp of the tooth and the surrounding bone. Cohrs (1961) indicated that for fluorosis, in general, the skeletal changes are dependent upon the age of the animal and the dose of fluorine. Young animal and high dose cause a ricketslike picture with widening of epiphyseal cartilages and poor mineralization (Jubb and Kennedy 1985). Moderate doses in older animals cause a loss of bone substance, osteomalacia, while lower doses in older animals cause a hyperostotic form of osteomalacia. Obel (1969) describes the latter as a resorption and disappearance of the original compacta of the bone with marked periosteal new bone formation. The latter form appears to be that seen by Shupe and Olsen (1971) and may be the characteristic form in the horse.

Arthrosis of the temporomandibular joint

The temporomandibular joint is unique in that both hyaline articular surfaces are convex, articulating with the concavities of the well-developed fibrocartilaginous articular disk. Such an arrangement provides for a variety of movements in several planes in a joint not subjected to heavy external loading.

Acute and chronic arthritis and arthrosis of the temporomandibular joint have been described (Cadeac 1909; Silbersiepe et al. 1986; Wintzer 1986). Blasse (1909) gave an incidence of 0.05% for all forms of temporomandibular joint damage in the population, while Bartke (1900) reported about 0.1% in military horses. Acute arthrosis was said to be caused by trauma with painful swelling. Acute arthritis was a purulent inflammation, occasionally with fistulation. The articular cartilages were eroded and ulcerated. Cadeac (1909) suggested strangles as one causative agent.

Chronic arthrosis was said to be caused by overuse, that is, trigeminal paralysis of the opposite side, bad teeth causing chewing on one side, and abnormally hard feeds. There is low-grade pain, bony enlargement, and localized muscle atrophy. There is erosion and ulceration of the articular cartilages with perforation of the meniscus and periarticular osteophyte formation (Cadeac 1909). Cohrs (1969) cites Samodjelkin (1920) that ossification of the articular disk (meniscus) of the joint was found in 25% of otherwise normal joints.

Salivary glands

Some features of normal salivary gland function are considered below. The normal radiographic and gross anatomy of the nasolacrimal duct have been described by Latimer et al. (1985), among others.

Calculi

This is the commonest lesion of the salivary glands and is rare at best. It may have been more frequent in earlier times in draft horses. The condition was known in antiquity [Vegetius cited by Leclainche (1936)]. We have seen no example in light horses at postmortem.

The calculus usually forms in the parotid duct near the opening of the duct into the mouth (Cohrs 1961). Calculi weigh between 200 and 600 g though larger have been seen. There is about 10% organic material, 80%–90% calcium carbonate, and about 3% calcium phosphate with small amounts of magnesium, sodium, and potassium (Fröhner 1905; Zakrzewski 1970).

Food may be found in the center of the calculus, and it is presumed that such foreign material is the nidus for calculus formation. Blockage of the duct leads to dilatation and eventual atrophy of the parotid salivary gland, fistula, and/or secondary infection. Cadeac (1896), however, pointed out that calcium carbonate is not a normal component of saliva and believed that it was produced as a result of bacterial fermentation. The role of the foreign body, then, was to transport bacteria into the duct where, producing calcium carbonate, a calculus could form. He further noted that ligation of the duct did not cause calculi to form, supporting his contention that blockage per se was not sufficient to cause calculus formation.

Rarely, there may be atresia of the parotid duct with cystic malformation of the parotid gland [Dietz and Dorn (1957) cited by Zakrzewski]. Pharyngeal pouch cysts occur in the parotid but are rare. Cadeac (1896) mentions calculi in the mandibular and sublingual salivary gland ducts of horses, but they are very rare.

Parotitis

The parotid salivary gland is only rarely involved in strangles or inflamed following trauma. An **epidemic parotitis**, affecting horses as well as other species, has been described (Zakrzewski 1970). The parotid was enlarged with inflammatory edema. The glandular epithelium and ductular epithelium were said to be degenerate. Recovery occurred spontaneously. Berge (1928) and Cohrs (1961) mention this condition and its clinical similarity to mumps in the human. We have seen no cases.

Ranula

These are rare retention cysts arising from blockage of the ducts of the mandibular or sublingual salivary glands on either side of and beneath the tongue. They are oval or sausage shaped, lined by columnar epithelium, and contain mucoid, odorless, yellow-gray or brownish, clear or cloudy fluid (Cadeac 1896; Cohrs 1961; Zakrzewski 1970). The word is from the Latin: *little frog.*

Acute or chronic inflammation of the duct of the mandibular salivary gland in the presence of foreign bodies was described by Cadeac (1896, 1908). The duct was painful, thickened, edematous, and exuded purulent material. This occurred most often, if not entirely, following amputation of the mucosal flaps covering the opening of the ducts into the buccal cavity, due to the mistaken idea that these flaps were abnormal. Such amputation was described and recommended by, for example, de Gray (1639), the supposed condition being known as **barbes** (barbs). Foreign material entered the ducts once the protective flaps had been removed.

Lampas was considered an inflammation of the first bars of the mucosa of the hard palate, just caudal to the upper incisor teeth (Albert the Great 1987). The condition did not and does not exist.

Neoplasia

Tumors, either primary or secondary, are rare. We have seen no case. It is common, as part of the melanosis of older gray horses, to find **melanosis** of both **parotid lymph nodes** (Leblanc et al. 1902). One case of malignant transformation with direct invasion into the cranial cavity was seen in an Arabian.

Gastrointestinal tract

Normal features

We give considerable space to the physical aspects of food intake and processing, insofar as known. While the biochemistry of digestion is obviously important, the physical aspects of digestion are of equal if not greater moment in the pathogenesis of colic in the horse.

Food materials are thoroughly masticated by the side-to-side grinding mechanism of the premolars and molars, the process of mastication shifting from side to side. Leue (1937) studied this mechanism in detail and showed that mastication was most thorough with grass, somewhat less so with hay, and least with materials such as bran and oats.

Leue divided chewing into phases, appearing on his molograph as an elliptical figure (Fig. 3.3). In the first phase, AB, the mouth opens with the mandible moving as far caudally as possible, in order to open the space between the grinding teeth-premolars and molars-as much as possible. The second phase, BC, is cutting and crushing. The mandible swings sideways and upward, so that the grinding teeth on one side cut and crush the raw food or bolus. In the third phase, CD, the grinding teeth close on the food material. It is a quick, powerful movement, the mandible moving dorsally and rostrally. This continues into the fourth phase, DA, with the mandibular grinders sliding inward, axially, on the maxillary grinders. This phase ends with the cut, mashed, and ground food material being propelled into the pharynx by the tongue in preparation for the next mouthful bitten off by the incisors.

Colin (1886/1888) observed that, while masticating on one side, the parotid on that side secreted about 2–4 times as much as the opposite gland. When mastication shifted to the opposite side, the parotid on that side secreted more actively. The mandibular and sublingual salivary gland secretion was not affected by the side of mastication.

Masticated food is mixed with saliva to form a cohesive mash. Meyer et al. (1985) showed that the amount of saliva produced is a function of the duration of feed intake, which in turn is a function of the coarseness of the feed materials. Tree leaves, grass, hay, and a mixed pelleted feed were compared as to duration of intake in minutes per 100 g of dry matter. The time of intake for leaves was about twice that for grass, that for grass twice that for hay, and that for hay twice that for pellets.

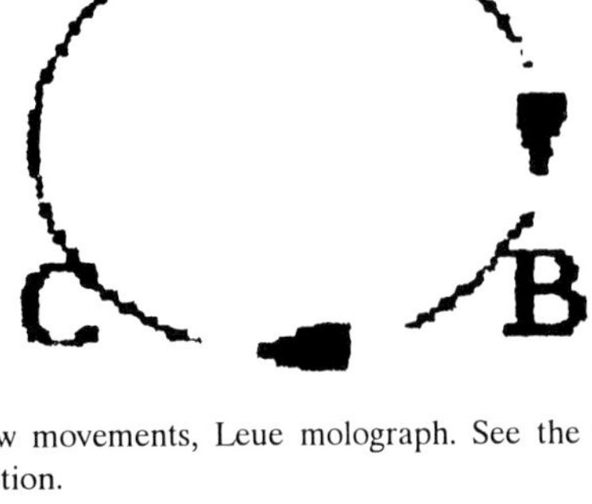

3.3. Jaw movements, Leue molograph. See the text for description.

The amount of saliva produced is a function of the nature of the food materials. The amount produced per 100 g of dry matter was greatest for leaves followed, in order, by hay, grass, and pellets. Saliva production per minute was greatest for pellets followed, in order, by hay, grass, and leaves. The dry matter content of the swallowed boluses of feed, then, varied with the saliva production. The pellets were least moist, while grass, hay, and leaf boluses were nearly the same and about 3 times as moist as the pellet boluses.

Scheunert and Illing (1906) found that, with esophageal fistulas, corn (maize) or oats induced about 2 times their weight in saliva, hay and chopped straw about 2.5 times, and hay alone about 5 times, while fresh grass only induced about 2/3 of its weight of saliva. Smith (1917) noted also that the amount of secretion depended upon the character of the food. Only half of the daily mean secretion occurs with green feeds and only one-third if roots (for example, turnips) are fed. Hay absorbs 4 times its weight of saliva, oats a little more than their own weight, and green feed half its weight (Colin 1886/1888; Smith 1917).

Colin observed that a horse would eat 2.5 kg of hay in about an hour, producing up to 200 boluses and 10 kg of saliva. The same quantity of oats resulted in 40–90 boluses and about 5 kg of saliva. He also studied the digestibility of hay and oats before and after chopping or crushing and found no differences. The importance of saliva is indicated by the following values for "digestive fluids" for a 400-kg horse eating 10 kg of hay per 24 hours, Colin:

saliva	42 kg
gastric juice	5
bile	5
pancreatic juice	5
intestinal juice	10

Dukes (1942) quoted Russian work with a fistulated horse that the empty stomach produced 10–30 L of juice per 24 hours.

Meyer et al. (1985) measured the particle size distribution after chewing and found that chewing grass, hay, and leaves separated the material into large particles (>1.5 mm) and small particles (<0.1 mm and including soluble material). The pelleted feed boluses had a more uniform distribution of particle sizes.

The alkaline food boluses are deposited in layers in the stomach in the order in which they enter. This was described by Ellenberger and his school in the 1800s (Colin 1886/1888; Ellenberger and Scheunert 1910; Sisson 1914; Smith 1917). The layers may appear incomplete to the eye as they undulate through three dimensions. Layering is not apparent in foals before they begin to eat solid food and is, of course, not apparent in the fasting animal. If more food is ingested than the stomach can hold, the pyloric sphincter opens and the ingesta in the pylorus is expressed into the duodenum, providing space for the incoming food materials (Colin 1886/1888; Scheunert and Trautmann 1976). If a horse is excited or worked, the pylorus will close, and emptying of the stomach delayed.

The layers move, as such, through the stomach to the pylorus and into the duodenum (Colin 1886/1888; Scheunert and Trautmann 1976). Peristaltic waves move the ingesta toward the duodenum, but are not vigorous until the pyloric portion of the stomach. Thus, the integrity of the layers of ingesta is maintained without mixing. Casual observation would suggest that ingesta passing along the lesser curvature would exit sooner than ingesta farther away from the lesser curvature. It may be suggested that, in fact, the lesser curvature acts, nearly, as a fixed point or center of rotation with the layer of ingesta rotating around that point. Thus, normally, each layer would reach the pylorus in approximately the same time, since the angular velocity is the same, but the linear velocity at the greater curvature is greater than at the lesser curvature. Colin's observations are not entirely consistent with that hypothesis, but his animals were fasted for 24 hours before feeding a succession of different feeds.

A reason for maintaining the integrity of the successive layers of ingesta has not been explicitly addressed. It appears to subserve specific digestive activity in each feed layer. The layers in the esophageal portion of the stomach are alkaline and undergo carbohydrate digestion by salivary enzymes and enzymes brought in with the feed. Bacterial digestion occurs in the esophageal portion of the stomach as well, breaking down carbohydrate and protein to lower fatty acids, gas, amino acids, and lower breakdown products of amino acids. As the layer of feed moves toward the margo plicatus, hydrochloric acid gradually saturates the mass, changing the pH to neutral, then, acid. With the addition of pepsin, proteolytic digestion begins. There is, apparently, little or no digestion of fat in the horse's stomach. If the duodenum is empty and alkaline, the pyloric sphincter opens. If full and/or acidic, the sphincter is closed. (See "Stomach: Pathogenesis of ulceration," in this chapter.)

There appears to be little information on the motor activity and digestive processes of the young foal, specifically during the transition from a largely milk to natural roughage diet. Alexander and Benzie (1951) showed that gastric emptying time was prolonged in the suckling foal as compared to the emptying time after weaning.

Most, but not all, ingested water bypasses the layered ingesta, moving along the lesser curvature to the duodenum and appearing in the cecum within 15 to 20 minutes. The bypass may be implemented by a functional esophageal groove formed by the muscle bordering the lesser curvature (Krölling and Grau 1960) (see below). Gastrointestinal transit time for fresh grass is about 9–12 hours, while dry roughage may take 3–5 days (Hutyra and Marek 1920).

Colin (1886/1888), in a series of experiments, clearly showed that there is little absorption from the stomach, at least of strychnine and potassium ferrocyanate. He believed, and in vitro studies seemed to confirm, that the mucous blanket prevented absorption in the fundus and the stratified squamous epithelium prevented absorption in the esophageal portion of the stomach. Since it is known that various physiologically active substances can be absorbed through stratified squamous epithelium and, possibly, through mucus, further study would be useful.

The small intestine is often empty. Hay and grass may be present as more or less defined boluses scattered along the length of the intestine. In a fasted animal permitted to graze just before death, grass can be scattered through the small intestine with less obvious bolus organization. Grain, bran, and similar materials are generally scattered through the intestine without bolus formation. Pellets are usually solubilized in the stomach and appear in the small intestine as bran or mash.

This suggests (Rooney 1970) that small intestinal motility may be different for roughage and grain/bran type ingesta; that is, bolus/large particle versus nonbolus/small particle. Roughage appears to move rapidly through the small intestine to the cecum as variably coherent boluses in as little as 30 minutes. Readily soluble nutrients are removed and cellulose is quickly moved to its site of digestion. Bran and grain, on the other hand, are not formed into boluses and move more slowly, allowing for digestion of soluble sugars, proteins, and fats by the enzymes of the pancreas and intestine. Cannon (1911) commented, after Cohnheim: "The greater length of the small intestine in herbivorous animals compared with carnivorous . . . is possibly associated with the greater rapidity of movement of plant food and the necessity of digesting out the valuable contents from cellulose surroundings."

These observations are compatible with experimental observations that the amount of fiber is a critical factor in determining how much soluble carbohydrate is removed during passage through the small intestine (Argenzio et al. 1974; Argenzio 1975). The larger the amount of soluble carbohydrate, grain, as opposed to roughage, the more such carbohydrate will reach the cecum and colon. The digestive enzymes produced by the pancreas and small intestine are destroyed when the ingesta enters the cecum.

Cannon (1911) showed that carbohydrate, fat, and protein had different resident, or passage, times in the stomach of cats. While not directly applicable, this is consistent with the concept of differential movement of food materials in the gastrointestinal tract.

The water balances of the large intestine are of critical importance in the horse. The large intestine alone must reabsorb a volume of water approximately equal to the total extracellular fluid volume during a 24-hour period (Argenzio 1975).

At postmortem the water content is greatest in the cecum and ventral colon, decreasing steadily through the dorsal colon to the anus, in a nearly uniform gradient. This is certainly the case with animals at pasture. Animals on dry forage are similar, although the cecal content may be somewhat drier than that of the ventral colon. In animals fed considerable amounts of concentrates such as grain and pellets, the **water gradient** is present, but the ingesta overall is drier. These observations agree with those of Meyer (1990).

Disorders of the large intestine, such as exhaustion shock, salmonellosis, infarction, and torsion, are, in part, characterized by loss of the water gradient, the content of the large intestine being fluid from end to end. As well the gradient is lost with diarrhea of whatever origin, large intestine or otherwise, whether septicemia, proximal enteritis, ascarid infestation, or so forth.

It has been said that all diarrhea of horses originates in the large intestine. While that may be overstated, it is true that all diarrheas are associated with the loss of the water gradient of the large intestine. The proximate cause of diarrhea may be derangement of the water balance mechanism of the large intestine even though the initiating lesion is distant from the large intestine. Barker and van Dreumel (1985) provide a lucid discussion of the pathogenesis of diarrhea.

If the postmortem is done immediately after death of the animal for reasons unrelated to the gastrointestinal tract, little or no free **gas** will be found. Within a matter of minutes gaseous distension of the large intestine is apparent. While it is customary to consider this as postmortem gas formation, the early onset in the large intestine suggests that it is the normal gas formation that was going on during life. The gas accumulates because of failure of the absorptive and dissipative mechanisms (Dyce et al. 1976). This initial gaseous distension is quickly overwhelmed by true postmortem gas formation involving the small intestine, stomach, and descending colon, in addition to the large colon and cecum. Although subjective, the normal gas does have a grassy odor, less objectionable than the putrefied, sewer smell of postmortem gas.

The composition of intestinal gas [Cadeac (1896) after Pinner] was carbides of hydrogen, 49 parts per 100; nitrogen, 42 parts per 100; and carbonic acid, 8 parts per 100. Small quantities of hydrogen and hydrogen sulfate, hydrogen phosphate, and methane were also present. Ammonia and volatile fatty acids were also present in the large intestine. Phillis (1976) indicated that colonic gases, in general, comprised 40% carbon dioxide, 50% nitrogen, and 10% methane, hydrogen, and hydrogen sulfate. The odor of postmortem gas is, in part at least, that of hydrogen sulfite.

It is apparent that there is a balance of ingesta, water, and gas in the lumen of the gut controlled by the absorptive and secretive mechanisms of the gut wall. In the normal horse, on grass pasture, the cecum and ascending colon have a gradient of ingesta/water with little or no dead space. That is, the lumens of the cecum and ascending colon are adjusted to the amount of ingesta. Although less obvious with the descending colon, the same is generally true, with the lumen very small in the absence of ingesta.

The **abdominal cavity** includes all structures within the visceral peritoneum: liver, spleen, gastrointestinal tract, and pancreas. The kidneys and adrenals are retroperitoneal. The **peritoneal cavity** is the potential space between the visceral and parietal peritoneum, the opposing surfaces separated by the serous fluid secreted by the peritoneum (Sisson and Grossman 1953). The peritoneal space is, however, dynamic, and a consideration of those dynamics may be of assistance in understanding certain gastrointestinal disorders.

For a short time after death, before the accumulation of natural and postmortem gases within the gastrointestinal tract, air rushes into the peritoneal cavity when the cavity is opened; that is, the pressure within the peritoneal cavity is below ambient. This may be explained by the diaphragm bulging forward into the thoracic cavity, the flanks sagging laterally, and the viscera settling on the dorsal wall. During life, contraction of the diaphragm lowers the pressure within the pleural cavity and increases the pressure within the peritoneal cavity. No measurements are available, but the pressure within the peritoneal cavity may reach ambient during inspiration. As the diaphragm relaxes during expiration, raising intrapleural pressure, the intraperitoneal pressure tends to decrease below ambient. Since there should be equilibrium of pressure between the gastrointestinal lumens and the peritoneal cavity, these pressure changes occur in the former as well.

The changes in intraperitoneal pressure may be unique to equids. While no data is available, it may be suggested that the pressure changes are a function of the very large thoracic cavity of horses as compared to other species. It would, obviously, be of interest if the tapir and rhinocerus, two other members of the Perissodactyla, have such pressure variations. Movement of the abdominal viscera, a visceral piston, has been suggested as an aid to respiration and a reason for one-to-one entrainment of stride and respiratory frequency at the gallop. Alexander's (1989) analysis, however, was not consistent with such a mechanism.

Normally, the fluctuations of intraperitoneal pressure do not imply the appearance of dead, actual, space in the peritoneal cavity. In the starved animal, the amount of ingesta decreases, and the animal becomes "tucked up." The abdominal cavity decreases in volume, so that the peritoneal space remains constant and potential only. In the fattening animal, the reverse, of course, occurs. The desirability of preventing dead space is that dead space would permit excessive movement of one part of the gastrointestinal tract relative to another. That is, a portion of gut could occupy a position it would not normally occupy.

There are several states in which dead space can occur. The first is atrophy of the right lobes of the liver, which is often associated with torsion of the ascending colon or incarceration through the epiploic foramen. The second is loss of tone of the abdominal muscles, so that the muscles cannot adjust the size of the abdominal cavity in response to changes of "fill." Such loss of tone may be associated with age or with prolonged periods of obesity and/or overfilling of, specifically, the cecum and ascending colon. A third, and special case of the second, is the postpartum broodmare. Immediately after foaling, dead space may appear as the uterus is involuting. In the multiparous older mare loss of tone of abdominal muscles certainly occurs. Torsion of the ascending colon is commoner in broodmares and in the postpartum period (see "Ascending Colon: Torsion," in this chapter).

A fourth predisposing factor we take as genetic, that is, tall, large, Warm bloods such as Trakhener and Westphalian, which apparently suffer from displacement of the ascending colon into the nephrosplenic space more commonly than smaller breeds. In such predisposed animals even marginally inadequate abdominal muscle tone could allow dead space. If this scenario is combined with the tendency in the modern era to use concentrates, pellets, and so forth, at the expense of roughage, there is less gut fill and further predisposition to dead space.

The importance of roughage during the evolution of the horse has been pointed out by Janis (1976). The horse is basically a fiber-eating animal, adapted to coarse stemmy grasses such as timothy, rather than to leafier feeds such as alfalfa. It is undoubtedly no accident, as discussed later, that torsion of the entire ventral colon has increased markedly in the modern era of pellets, alfalfa hay, and improved pastures. An association of various forms of colic with lucerne (alfalfa) is often encountered in the older European literature. It may well be that the undoubted nutritional value of alfalfa is counterbalanced, in the horse, by inappropriate physical character.

A possible and partial scenario for the high frequency of gut malpositions in the horse may be outlined. If segmental ileus occurs, whatever the cause as discussed with the specific entities, gas accumulates in the affected segment. As the gas accumulates, the pressure within the segment increases and the segment expands. Since the peritoneal cavity is a closed system, the expansion can only proceed so far before pressure within the peritoneal cavity increases to balance that within the segment and no further expansion occurs. In the horse, the pressure within the peritoneal cavity decreases during expiration, so that the segment can expand during expiration. This is a nonequilibrium situation developing as a result of the intraperitoneal pressure changes.

Nickel et al. (1960) give the following lengths (in meters) for the gastrointestinal tract. Colin (1886/1888) reported comparable values.

overall	25–39
small intestine	19–30
duodenum	1–1.5
jejunum	17–28
ileum	0.7–0.8
large intestine	6–9
cecum	0.8–1.3
ascending colon	3–4
descending colon	2.5–4

There are values for the capacity of the different parts of the tract, but these are highly variable and offer no assistance in pathological evaluation. Cecal capacity, for example, is reported to vary from 16 to 68 L. Colin reported the following average values (in liters), presumably for larger horses:

stomach	17.96
small intestine	63.82
cecum	33.54
large colon	81.25
descending colon	14.77

Gastrointestinal motility

The animal dying a natural death rarely, if ever, has gastrointestinal movement. The following observations were made shortly after killing. Alexander (1952a), Argenzio et al. (1974), and Sellers et al. (1984) have done in vivo studies of gastrointestinal motility. It is unfortunate that such studies as are available on motility, digestion, water balance, and so on, have been done in animals fed under domesticated husbandry conditions, rather than under more natural grazing, free range conditions. However difficult to carry out or evaluate, the horse's gastrointestinal tract evolved under the latter conditions, and this is the normal baseline required for understanding the gastrointestinal diseases of domestication (Janis 1976; Clarke et al. 1990).

The *stomach* does not move, and movement cannot be elicited by mechanical stimulation (Smith 1917) in the absence of the external nerve supply, specifically the vagus. The *small intestine* is always moving and may continue to do so for about 30 minutes. The jejunum is somewhat more active than either duodenum or ileum. Segmenting and pendular movements are readily seen, and short peristaltic rushes may occur. Colin (1886/1888) reported that antiperistalsis was common and normal in the small intestine of the horse. We have seen this only as pendular movements. Mechanical stimulation induces movement. The *large intestine* is usually moving or can be induced to do so by pinching either the wall or the vessels. The reaction to the former is immediate, while the reaction to the latter may be delayed some seconds (Colin). The cecum, ventral, and dorsal colon make segmenting movements, which propagate for a short distance. The motility of the cecum and colon usually disappears 15 minutes or so before that of the small intestine.

The descending colon does not move, and mechanical stimulation is rarely effective. Colin said, and we concur, that cold air increases the frequency and amplitude of the intestinal movements.

Gastrointestinal motility is a function of (a) intrinsic myenteric rhythm—the interaction of myenteric and submucosal plexuses and smooth muscle, and (b) extrinsic autonomic nerves. Given that the extrinsic autonomic control would be immediately disrupted after death, it is apparent that the motility of the stomach and descending colon are strongly dependent upon extrinsic control. This is shown, as well, by vagal transection, which causes atony of the stomach (Colin 1886/1888; Phillis 1976). In the human and some animals it has been shown (Wingate 1992) that the intrinsic plexuses and smooth muscle of the entire intestinal tract operate virtually as an independent entity, without necessary external autonomic neural action. This is evidently not true for the stomach and descending colon of the horse.

The cecum and ascending colon are less dependent and the small intestine least dependent upon extrinsic autonomic control. Since long peristaltic rushes are not seen in the small intestine after death, however, it is probable that extrinsic control is necessary for coordination of such movements. The long-distance propagation of the segmenting movements of the cecum and ascending colon, as well, appear dependent upon extrinsic coordination.

The motility of the rectum is externally controlled by a defecation center in the medulla (Phillis 1976). Loss of extrinsic neural control, for example, neuritis of the cauda equina, causes paralysis of the rectum. The reason for significant extrinsic control of the descending colon proximal to the rectum is unclear. Indeed, a reason for the considerable length of the descending colon is not clear. Water reabsorption is the usual function ascribed. Argenzio's data for ponies, however, shows that about 90% of the water entering the cecum and ascending colon from the ileum and by transmural flux is reabsorbed before reaching the descending colon. This leaves only a small quantity of water to be reabsorbed by a descending colon that is as long as the ascending colon. Alexander's (1950) study indicated that a barium meal remained longer in the right dorsal and descending colon than in any other portion of the gastrointestinal tract. The question remains open.

Obstipation

Obstipation of the intestinal tract often occurs at the anatomical narrowings of the gut lumen. That these areas are, indeed, related to slowing of movement of ingesta has been summarized by Argenzio (1975) from marker studies. Normal retention of ingesta appeared to be controlled by barriers at the pylorus, the ileocecal junction, the cecocolic junction, the pelvic flexure, and the transverse colon. The fact that impactions and obstipations occur at these junctions, however, should not be attributed to anatomical narrowing, but to improper function of those junctions, whatever the specific cause(s) in a given case.

Rigor

All motility is lost as the intestinal tract goes into **rigor**. Rigor is quite obvious in the small intestine, considerably less so in the large. It disappears rapidly, the intestinal wall becoming flabby. Color changes are largely a function of the status of the circulatory system. The circulatory system is failing during the agonal period, and blood is shunted about passively by active and passive movement of the intestinal tract.

Rigor squeezes blood passively into the mucosal folds and tips of the villi. As rigor wanes, dependent loops of small intestine, in particular, will fill with fluid and mucus as hemolyzing blood is diffusing out of the autolyzing vessels. Hyperemia, diffuse reddening, may be distinguished as (a) true inflammatory, present before the agonal period, (b) agonal, developing during and as a result of events in the agonal period, or (c) postmortem, as a result of autolysis.

Inflammatory hyperemia

Inflammatory hyperemia, whether of serosal or mucosal surface, is in the form of multiple, fine petechiae. **Agonal hyperemia** is a diffuse, bright red coloration as the result of pooling of blood in paralyzed small vessels. Discrete petechiae are not apparent. **Postmortem hyperemia** is characterized by distinct aborization of blood vessels with diffuse, dirty-reddish staining of the immediately adjacent tissues. Beyond postmortem hyperemia, autolytic changes become pronounced and the term *hyperemia* is no longer appropriate. Obviously all of these changes can be present at the same time and interpretation may be difficult.

Blood vessels, lymphoid tissue

Asteroid bodies

The intramural arterial vessels of the intestinal tract, as well as other sites, often have a unique histological appearance. Small, basophilic masses are present in the intima of small submucosal muscular arteries with or without thickening of the intima. These were clearly described by Bollinger (1869). They stain positively for calcium/phosphates and are known as **asteroid bodies** (Fig. 3.4). They are not seen in the fetus or very young foal. The evidence suggests that they are dystrophic calcified foci as a result of the migration of *S. vulgaris* (Bollinger). Aberrant migrations may account for the presence of these asteroid bodies in such locations as the middle cerebral artery, lung, kidney, and other sites. (See Chapter 1, "Cardiovascular System.")

Media of submucosal arteries

The media of many submucosal arteries has a lacy, open-work, even vacuolated appearance (Fig. 3.5). There is no stainable lipid, glycogen, or metachromatic material in the spaces. It is certain that this is normal for small muscular arteries of horses. The appearance is reminiscent of the spaces in the media of the arteries in the amnion and allantochorion, except that the spaces in those vessels are filled with metachromatic, basophilic

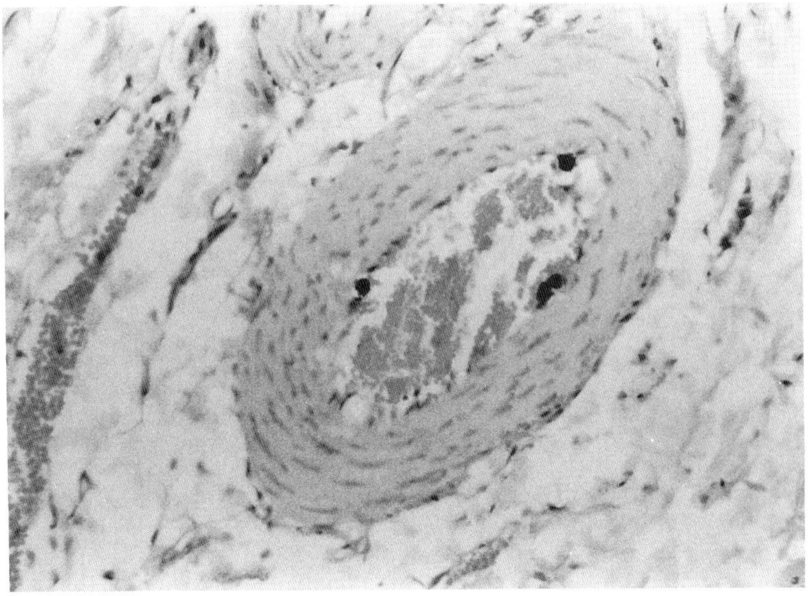

3.4. Middle power, H & E of asteroid concretions in the intima of an intestinal submucosal artery.

material. It is seen most frequently, or obviously, in the gut, but may be encountered in any small artery anywhere in the body, an exception being the muscular arteries in the distal parts of the legs. These latter vessels have a strongly developed, thicker media than average for vessels of similar luminal size in other parts of the body, and "vacuolation" is uncommon.

Macrophages

Macrophages containing necrotic debris and/or hemosiderin are often present in the subepithelial lamina propria at the tips of villi of the small intestine and between the openings of the colonic glands (Barker and van Dreumel 1985). Macrophages phagocytize normally senescent epithelial and, perhaps other, cells in this area. This process of normal removal of senescent cells occurs in most tissues, being particularly obvious in the equine intestine and in the germinal centers of the spleen and lymph nodes. It has been given the name **apoptosis** (Kerr et al. 1987). The variable but always small amounts of hemosiderin are normal. Iron beyond requirement is stored in the mucosal epithelial cells and lost from the body when these cells die and are shed.

Wundernetz (rete arteriosum)

Dobberstein and Hartmann (1932) studied the *wundernetz* (rete arteriosum) described by Franck (1883). This is a network of anastomosing branches of the dorsal and ventral colic and medial and lateral cecal arteries surrounding the corresponding veins. It is well illustrated in Cohrs (1961) and easily demonstrated in the postmortem room. The network is more marked for the colic than the cecal arteries and becomes denser approaching the pelvic flexure. Dobberstein and Hartmann (1932) also pointed out the numerous anastomotic vessels between the dorsal and ventral colic arteries through the mesocolon. They emphasized the protective effect of this richly anastomotic cecocolic circulation in light of the high frequency of verminous arteritis and low frequency of verminous infarction.

While the *wundernetz* could have evolved in the face of the threat of *Strongylus vulgaris*, it probably evolved to serve a physiological function. That is, the higher pressure arterial system forms a network around the veins, serving as an auxiliary, peristaltic-type pump, assisting venous return to the portal vein. That is compatible with the lesser anastomotic network around the shorter cecal veins, and the increased density of the *wundernetz* around the distal segments of the very long colic veins. Snyder et al. (1989a,b) and Dart et al. (1991a,b) have redescribed the *wundernetz* for the ascending colon and cecum, and have added information on the microcirculation.

Lymphoid nodules, usually solitary, are found throughout the gastrointestinal tract both in the lamina propria and the submucosa. In the young animal they are usually not apparent grossly in the stomach and small intestine, but are obvious in the cecum and large intestine. After about 1 year of age all lymphoid tissue aggregations are smaller and the nodules are no longer apparent grossly in the large intestine. Peyer's patches are infrequently seen

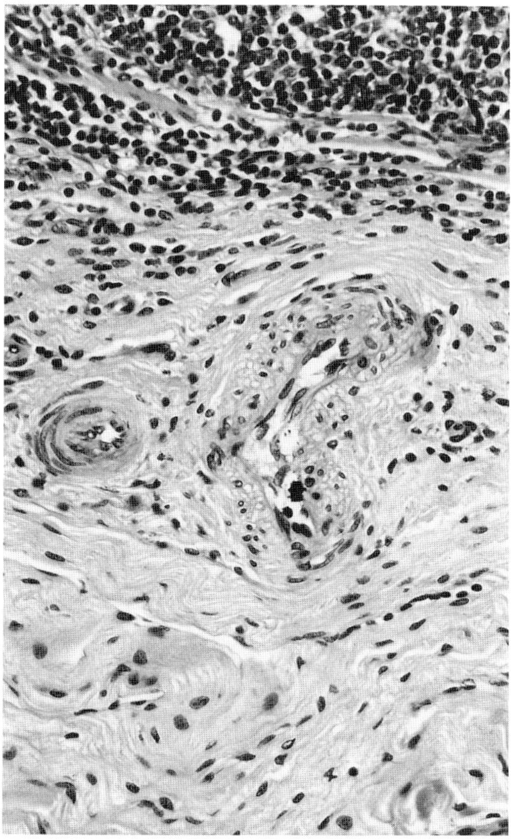

3.5. Middle power, H & E of intestinal submucosal artery with lacy, loculated media.

grossly and histologically and are not as well developed as in other species, being essentially loose aggregations of solitary lymphoid nodules. The apex of the cecum of the young animal, however, does have dense masses of nodules that qualify as Peyer's patches. Intestinal glands within lymphoid nodules in the submucosa, common in cattle and swine, are rarely evident and, then, in the submucosa of the apex of the cecum (Krölling and Grau 1960) (Fig. 3.6). Even here, there are few submucosal glands despite extensive disruption of the muscularis mucosae, and they rarely penetrate as deeply as in, for example, cattle. The lymphoid tissue of the gut first appears in the 4-month fetus (Zietzschmann and Krölling 1955).

Statistics of colic

Most data on the epidemiology of colic in horses—morbidity, mortality, age, and environment—was found in the older literature though there is interest in more recent literature (White et al. 1991). Colic, as a clinical disease at least, was known to Aristotle (Leclainche 1936).

The morbidity for all forms of colic was about 5%–6% of the total population. The mortality rate was about 0.5%. For all cases of colic, the mortality rate was about 10%. Tennant et al. (1972) reported an about 33% mortality rate among 453 cases of colic. Fatal colic was about 35% of all deaths (range, 15%–50%) for different venues: Germany, Berlin, Sweden, Denmark, and Switzerland (Dobberstein and Dinter 1942; Wirth 1985). Huskamp (1982) reported that, of cases for which surgery was completed, 87.7% survived, a mortality of 12%. An owner survey in North America, Morris Animal Foundation (1991), showed 28 deaths from colic among 1102 horses, about 2.5%, while fatal colics represented about 36% of all deaths. Estimations of colic morbidity, in one part of North America, suggested frequencies between 0.19 and 0.39 cases per horse-year (Uhlinger 1991a). European data indicate that in the early 1900s about 50% of all clinic cases were colic. In Prussian military horses colic was 11% of all illness. The difference was

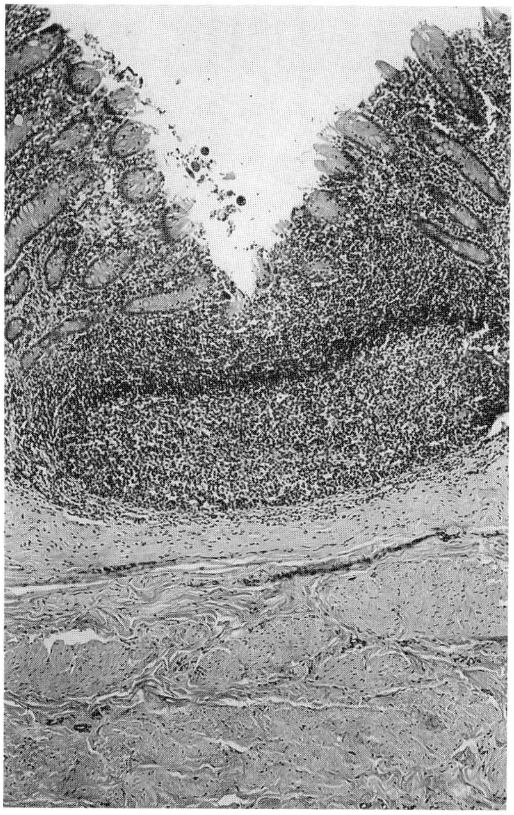

3.6. Lower power of apex of cecum with Peyer's patch (accumulation of lymphoid tissue).

attributed to better care, better reporting, and inclusion of all cases of illness in the data for military horses, as opposed to civilian horses for which many illnesses would not be recorded. The data is in overall agreement with earlier statistics of Friedberger and Fröhner (1895). It is apparent that the morbidity and mortality rates for colic have changed little over the years.

Gutmann in *Bayer-Fröhner* (1899) reported on volvulus of the small intestine and torsion of the cecum and colon. In the Prussian army, 1890–1894, there were 2168 cases of colic, with about 43% being gut displacements. In the veterinary clinic at München, 1876–1894, there were 361 colics, of which 56.2% were gut displacements. The data for the army, München (Munich), and the Vienna pathology department, 1850–88, are summarized in Table 3-1.

Dobberstein and Dinter (1942) examined the monthly frequency of different fatal colics in Berlin. While there were some differences among the different forms, overall the highest frequencies were in the summer months—June, July, and August—with a second, considerably smaller, increase during November, December, and January. February, March, April, and May had the lowest overall frequency of fatal colic. Wirth (1985) found a similar incidence. The obvious conclusion is that the highest frequency of fatal colic was in those months when *Strongylus vulgaris* is active, although it is not suggested that verminous infestation is the only cause of fatal colic. Feed and feeding practices as well as verminous activity are to be considered in the pathogenesis of colic. In a given case, for example, thromboembolism of the cecum and colon, verminous lesions may be entirely responsible. In many cases both the type of feed and verminous activity may be involved.

Parasites

Parasites and parasitic disease are discussed here since the large strongyles, in particular, are associated with many forms of gastrointestinal disease.

Large strongyles

The life cycles of *Strongylus spp.* are summarized, together with a discussion of some of the lesions produced by these lethal parasites. The large strongyles are the most important parasites of the horse and *Strongylus vulgaris* is the most important of the group.

The larvae of *S. vulgaris* were apparently recognized in Roman times (Werk 1921), and it would appear that strongyles have been with the horse throughout its evolution. There are four species: *S. vulgaris*, *S. edentatus*, *S. equinus*, and *S. asini*. The last has been reported only in donkeys and wild equids in East Africa and Eastern Europe (Drudge 1985), and little seems to be known of its biology and pathogenicity.

Epizootology

This discussion is largely taken from Drudge (1985). The life cycles of the large and small strongyles are direct, with no intermediate host or vector being required. Sexually mature adults reside in the large intestine; the females lay eggs, which pass into the environment with the feces. The eggs require a period of development before becoming infective larvae, with favorable moisture and temperature conditions of about 1 week. The infective larvae are enclosed in a thin, protective sheath and are actively motile on the herbage. Since they do not feed, their life span is limited to the amount of food material stored in their intestinal cells. During the grazing season the infective larvae may remain viable for several months. In temperate climates the larvae can overwinter.

Younger infective larvae, with abundant stored food material, are more vigorous than older larvae and, so, more infectious. That is, they move up the blades of grass more actively and are thus more likely to be ingested by the grazing animal. In temperate regions the infection rate is greater during the spring and summer months. This variation may not be apparent under tropical and subtropical conditions.

Infection of the grazing animal is by chance

Table 3-1. Number of cases of volvulus of the small intestine and torsion of the cecum and colon

	Colon torsion	Cecum torsion	Descending colon torsion	Small intestine volvulus
Prussian Army	354	34	7	309
München	118	0	3	40
Vienna	433	29	8	490

Source: Gutmann in *Bayer-Fröhner* (1899).

ingestion of larvae migrating randomly on the herbage. Compensating for the low chance of achieving transmission, the average female large strongyle produces about 5000 eggs per day. The small strongyles produce fewer eggs, less than 100 for the smaller species and several hundred for the larger.

Strongyles infect horses of all ages, exposure of foals beginning as soon as they begin to nibble grass. There is no antenatal transmission. Fatal cranial mesenteric parasitic arteritis is seen as early as 21 days after birth.

Time for maturation varies with the species as follows: *S. vulgaris*, 6 1/2 months; *S. equinus*, 9 months; *S. edentatus*, 11 months; and the small strongyles from 5 to 10 weeks, according to species.

Strongylus vulgaris

The behavior of ingested larvae has been described by Enigk (1950). The infective larvae cast off their protective sheaths during the passage through the stomach and small intestine. Exclusive milk feeding appears to inhibit this process, but the precise mechanism of exsheathment and the role of modifying factors is not known.

Third-stage infective larvae penetrate the mucosae of the ileum, cecum, and ventral colon and move into the submucosa. Development to fourth-stage larvae occurs in the submucosa on the 4th to 5th day. The fourth-stage larvae invade arterioles in the submucosa to begin their migration. These arterioles have neither external nor internal elastic laminae.

Fourth-stage larvae migrate in the intima against the blood flow. The endothelium is damaged and fibrin, inflammatory cells, and thrombi mark the pathways of the larvae as thin, meandering threads or tracks in/on the intima. Within 8 days these migrating larvae reach the larger vessels, some as far as the ileocecocolic artery. By 11 days the cranial mesenteric artery and aorta contain larvae. The migration reaches its height about the 19th day and declines thereafter.

There is disagreement as to larval migration *on* or *in* the intima of the arterial vessels. The question is moot and difficult to decide based on spontaneous case material since the intima of the smallest arteries is only composed of endothelium and an internal elastic membrane. The head of a larva destroys the endothelium and is pressed firmly against the intact internal elastic membrane (Enigk 1950). The caudal end of the larva lies on intact endothelium, within the lumen, with a thin, coating layer of fibrin. In larger arterial vessels, the intima is composed of endothelium, a thin layer of subendothelial connective tissue, and the internal elastic lamina. In these vessels the larvae seem to migrate in the subendothelial connective tissue, destroying the endothelium, but not penetrating the elastic lamina. Endothelium quickly regenerates after the passage of the larvae, the characteristic *tracks* comprising fibrin and mononuclear cells covered by regenerated endothelium.

Morgan et al. (1991), however, saw disruption of the internal elastic lamina in 95% of cranial mesenteric arteries and branches, in agreement with Deorani (1966). They believed that physical damage, release of inflammatory mediators, elastases from stimulated macrophages, and hydrodynamic effects were all responsible for the intimal lesions. They classified the verminous arteritis as chronic-active and chronic. *Chronic-active* lesions were characterized by edema, mixed inflammatory cell infiltration with eosinophils and neutrophils predominating, and extensive fibrin deposition. Degenerating larvae in arteries strongly correlated with intensity of eosinophilic infiltration. *Chronic* fibrosing lesions were characterized by intimal fibrosis, smooth muscle and intimal hypertrophy/hyperplasia, and fewer inflammatory cells.

Verminous arteritis

Fourth-stage larvae elicit a fibrinous inflammatory reaction in the cranial mesenteric and ileocecocolic arteries—verminous arteritis (Fig. 3.7). The larvae molt from fourth to fifth stage from the 90th day postinfection onward. It is not clear why the inflammatory reaction in the ileocecocolic and cranial mesenteric arteries is of greater magnitude than in the smaller vessels. There appear to be two possibilities. First, that the molt from the fourth to fifth stage releases products that induce a greater reaction than the physical presence of the larvae alone. Second, it may simply be that there are more fourth- and fifth-stage larvae in a given area of the larger arteries with appropriate inflammatory reaction.

Aref (1984) suggested that larvae sense the curvature of the vessel wall as they migrate and are "reluctant" to make sharp turns. The larvae shuttle up and down in the ileocecocolic and cranial mesenteric arteries, not making the turns into the aorta or the branches of the cranial mesenteric artery. This continuing shuttling, damaging and redamaging the intima, could be a third mechanism for enhancing the inflammatory reaction. With large numbers, however, it is obvious that at least some larvae overcome their reluctance to turn and enter the aorta as discussed below.

The more severe inflammatory reaction can involve all layers of the arterial wall, no longer being limited by the internal elastic membrane, with resulting thickening and/or aneurysmal dilatation of the vessel. It is quite incorrect, however hallowed

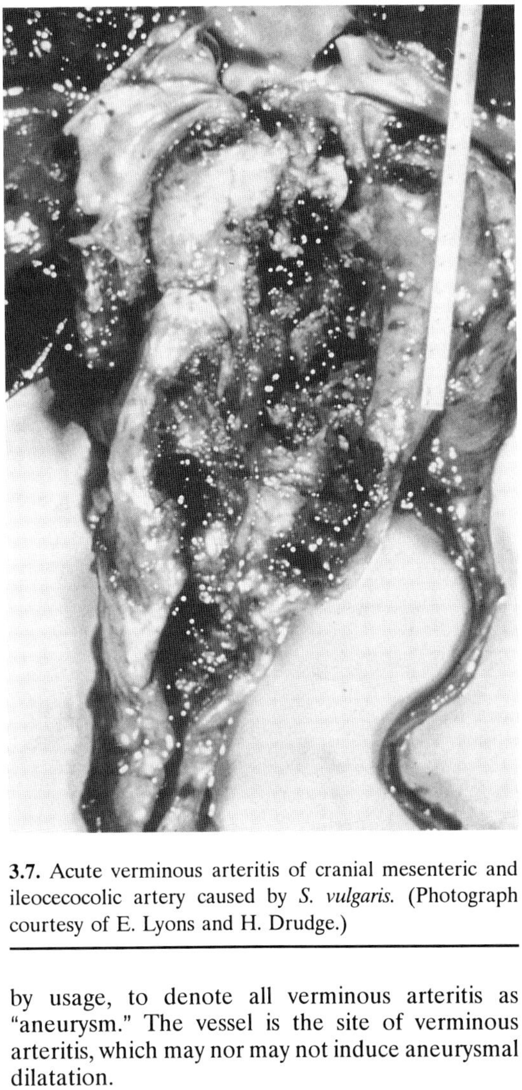

3.7. Acute verminous arteritis of cranial mesenteric and ileocecocolic artery caused by *S. vulgaris*. (Photograph courtesy of E. Lyons and H. Drudge.)

by usage, to denote all verminous arteritis as "aneurysm." The vessel is the site of verminous arteritis, which may nor may not induce aneurysmal dilatation.

The fifth-stage larvae are driven or washed to the wall of the cecum and colon, forming pea-sized nodules in the wall. At varying times the larvae penetrate the mucosa into the lumen and become mature after a prepatent period of 6–6 1/2 months.

Fourth-stage larvae may continue migrating beyond the cranial mesenteric artery, with intimal tracks comprising fibrin and mononuclear cells radiating out from the cranial mesenteric artery into the aorta as far as the coronary arteries, the renal arteries, celiac artery, internal iliacs, and so forth. The conditions for such migration beyond the cranial mesenteric are not known. At least one factor would appear to be numbers and rate of infection. The more larvae present, the greater the probability of migration beyond the cranial mesenteric. The available "housing" in the cranial mesenteric may be full, the larvae overcome their turning reluctance and continue on, looking for a place to undergo the molt to the fifth stage. During such migration, vessels may be temporarily or permanently occluded by thrombi in many parts of the body, particularly the abdominal cavity, leading to fatal and nonfatal colic, infarction of the spleen, and cirrhosis of the liver, as discussed with the several organs. The frequency of thrombosis is about 93% in the cranial mesenteric and ileocecocolic arteries, 5% in the celiac artery, and 2% in the caudal mesenteric and renal arteries [Hutyra and Marek (1926); compatible with our experience prior to the advent of modern anthelmintics].

Hemamelasma ilei

Hemamelasma ilei have been described by Enigk (1951a) as infarction and healing caused by thrombi in the vessels (Fig. 3.8). It is apparent that these blackish areas develop only in the antimesenteric quadrant of the ileum and always involve the serosa, rarely penetrating the outer muscularis. This suggests the alternative hypothesis that fourth-stage larvae invading the mucosa of the antimesenteric quadrant may not find the major vessels coming from the ileocecocolic artery and, so, wander in the serosa of the antimesenteric quadrant until destroyed by host defense mechanisms. Hemamelasma is discussed further with the ileum.

The lesions produced during the course of the migration of *S. vulgaris* are described below.

Infarction of the small intestine

This entity does not appear to have been recognized in the older literature and scarcely noted in more recent times (Rooney 1970; Pauli et al. 1971). A horse may acquire a massive infestation

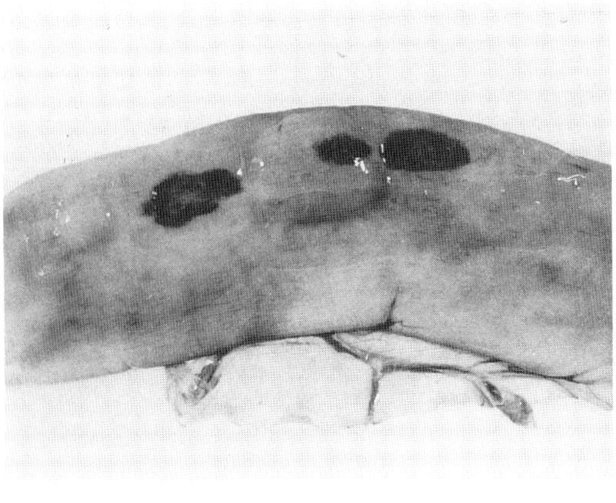

3.8. Hemamelasma ilei: ileum.

of *S. vulgaris* infective larvae experimentally or by grazing heavily infected pasturage. Such massive infestations occur, for example, when animals are grazed in heavily populated areas around show barns, racing stables, and sales arenas. About 10 days after grazing, the animal has signs of severe colic, which is rapidly fatal or surgical.

At surgery or postmortem a variable portion of the mid to distal jejunum and/or ileum is infarcted (Fig. 3.9). The segment is distended with fluid, green or gray-green, and sharply demarcated by hemorrhagic borders from the proximal dilated normal segment and the distal collapsed normal segment. Splash hemorrhages are common in the mesentery of the affected segment. There may be no active verminous damage in the cranial mesenteric artery.

Careful dissection, with low-power magnification, of the jejunal arteries reveals multiple thrombi in which fourth-stage *S. vulgaris* larvae may be found. It appears that if large numbers of larvae are ingested in a short period of time, they invade not only the ileal and cecal mucosae, but more proximal portions of the jejunum. As if in a traffic queue, the larvae at the end of the queue simply do not wait to reach the ileum and cecum, but invade the mucosa where they are at a given time after ingestion. Drudge and Lyons (1986) have produced such jejunal infarctions experimentally in worm-free ponies given between 800 and 9000 infective larvae.

Pauli et al. (1971) discussed infarction of the small intestine, primarily the distal jejunum, caused by *S. vulgaris*. They believed the embolization occurred from proximal—thrombus in the ileocecocolic artery—to distal, in the jejunal arteries, in the same manner as embolization in the cecal and colic arteries. That was not true in our cases.

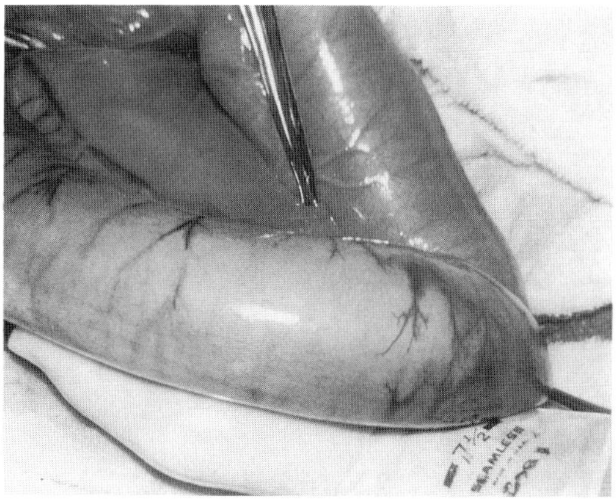

3.9. Infarction of the jejunum. Photo taken during surgery.

Thrombotic disease

This is an uncommon entity (Rooney 1970). The clinical history is of sudden, severe illness with shock. The clinical signs are essentially identical to those of exhaustion shock. At postmortem the cecum and ascending colon are diffusely and uniformly muddy red and filled with liquid, sometimes blood-tinged ingesta. There may be just-perceptible to moderate edema of the mucosa and submucosa. The ileocecocolic artery is tightly and completely plugged with a friable, brownish-yellow mass of fibrin containing numbers of fourth-stage larvae.

The changes in the large intestine are those of the earlier stages of exhaustion shock and torsion of the colon. It appears that the formation of the massive fibrin thrombus—many larvae arriving at the cranial mesenteric artery in a short time—shuts off the blood supply of the cecum and colon as a sudden, single event. Ileus, shock, and death occur before morphological evidence of ischemic necrosis develops.

While the fibrin thrombus is easily found, the changes in the large intestine can be masked or rendered equivocal by postmortem change. The postmortem diagnosis is most confidently made when the examination is done soon after death.

Thromboembolic disease

This is the well-known and described classic form. The older literature (Dobberstein and Dinter 1942; Hutyra and Marek 1920) indicates that about 5% of all colic-related deaths were thromboembolic infarction of the cecum and/or large intestine. White (1987) found 3.5% among 2385 cases of fatal and nonfatal colic. The cecum and ventral colon are most severely affected, but any portion, with the exception of the descending colon, may be involved (Figs. 3.10–3.11). The first part of the descending colon is supplied by the middle colic artery, which arises from the cranial mesenteric proximal to the ileocecocolic artery. The verminous thrombus is usually in the ileocecocolic artery, distal to the origin of the middle colic artery.

There is frank segmental necrosis: green, gray, and white, with clearly demarcated hemorrhagic borders. Multiple emboli are present in the related medial and lateral cecal, dorsal and ventral colic arteries. The parent thrombus in the ileocecocolic artery may be quite small, with evidence of breaking away of the emboli. The thrombi in this artery are either sessile, with less chance of embolization, or pedunculated, teardrop shaped, with greater risk.

Thromboembolic disease of the celiac, caudal mesenteric, and renal arteries, as well as the end of the abdominal aorta, does occur, though much less

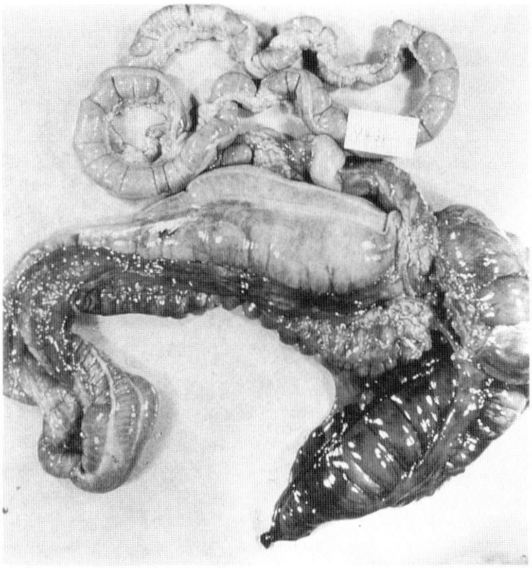

3.10. Infarction of cecum and ventral colon in experimental *S. vulgaris* infestation of a pony.

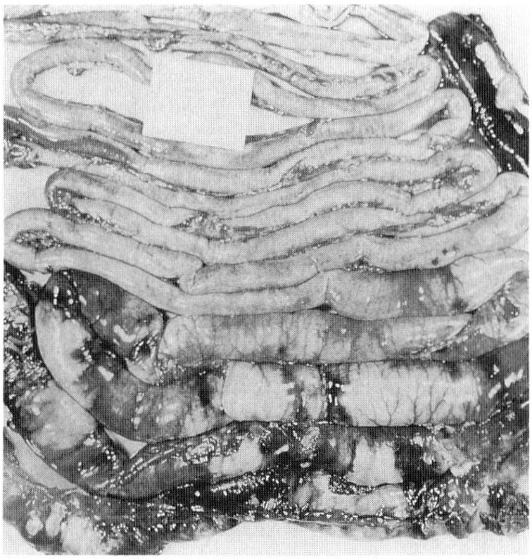

3.11. Infarction of the small intestine. The duodenum and first part of the jejunum (*above*), are normal, while infarction becomes progressively more severe in distal jejunum and ileum.

commonly than in the cranial mesenteric artery. Celiac, renal, and terminal aortic thrombosis is considered later with the respective areas supplied by those arteries. Thrombosis of the caudal mesenteric artery is least common and, of course, causes infarction of the involved portion of the descending colon.

Miscellaneous

The role of *S. vulgaris* and the other large strongyles in causing abscesses, ulcerations, and transient colic is discussed elsewhere in this book. Pathological study (Rooney 1965) and anecdotal epidemiology have shown that the frequency of nonfatal colic, as well as volvulus and the various incarcerations and strangulations, is greatly reduced when stringent deworming programs are in effect. There is little reason to doubt that migration of large strongyle larvae, particularly *S. vulgaris*, causing transient ischemia and ileus, is a major factor in both nonfatal and fatal colic, quite apart from the thrombosis and embolism described above.

Poynter (1960) pointed out the high frequency of fibrin tracks in the intima of the aorta and its several branches as a result of vulgaris larval migrations. It is probable that larvae pursuing these migrations and passing into smaller arteries are the cause of such entities as volvulus, gas colic, and so on. Several examples are shown below with consideration of specific organs.

S. vulgaris "septicemia" of foals

A striking syndrome occurs in foals first exposed to *S. vulgaris* either naturally or experimentally. The animal has clinical signs like, if not identical to, those of acute bacterial septicemia (Enigk 1950; Drudge 1985). At postmortem of both spontaneous cases and experimental, worm-free pony foals, the cellular reaction to migration of larvae through the wall of the intestine and in the cranial mesenteric artery is almost entirely neutrophils. Subsequent larval invasions are met by mononuclear cells, lymphocytes, and eosinophils, characteristic of an immune reaction. The earliest naturally occurring cases of fatal verminous arteritis of the cranial mesenteric artery are in foals 21 days of age. With subsequent exposures similar clinical signs can be observed though eosinophilia in the peripheral blood picture replaces the neutrophilia of first-time exposure.

It is apparent that immune mechanisms are at work in *S. vulgaris* infections. Only limited work has been done with the techniques of modern immunology (Drudge 1986). Most deaths occur in young horses and in horses only sporadically exposed to large numbers of infective larvae. It appears, then, that repeated exposures maintain some degree of resistance to the migrating larvae. The presence of lesions in horses of all ages indicates that age resistance per se is not a large factor.

Strongylus edentatus

Third-stage larvae penetrate the mucosa of, principally, the cecum and ventral colon and travel within 2 days to the liver via the portal circulation (Wetzel and Kersten 1956; McCraw and Slocombe 1974, 1978; Drudge 1985). They migrate through the liver, leaving white foci and whitish, tortuous tracks. In naturally occurring cases the foci and tracks are particularly evident on the parietal surface of the right lobe of the liver, less so on the middle and left lobes, and are uncommon on the visceral surface of any lobe (Fig. 3.12). In experimental cases lesions were found in all lobes, presumably because of the large number of larvae inoculated. These foci and tracks are composed of mononuclear cells and eosinophils, later replaced by fibrous tissue. Characteristically, there is a necrotic core of eosinophils in which larvae or larval remnants may sometimes be found.

The larvae molt to the fourth stage within the liver about 16 weeks after infection. Eventually they leave the liver, primarily via the right hepatorenal ligament, to enter the subperitoneal tissues of the right flank and/or the cecum. In the flank the larvae are readily seen in edematous, blood-tinged pockets of fluid. The larvae induce similar lesions in the submucosa of the cecum before exiting as adults into the cecal lumen. The time from initial infection to appearance of adult worms in the cecal lumen, the prepatent period, is 11 months.

The above description is based on experimental infections and accords with what is seen during routine postmortem examinations. In addition, in the experimental cases, multiple, enlarged hemorrhagic lymph nodes were present on the serosal surfaces of the cecum and ventral colon. The lymph nodes had eosinophilic tracks, large numbers of eosinophils, giant cells, and intact or disintegrating larvae. Similar changes were found in the omentum and, to a lesser extent, in the lungs. The experimental infections were with larger numbers of larvae than encountered in naturally occurring infections. The changes in the lymph nodes, omentum, and lungs are rarely seen in naturally occurring cases. As suggested for similar "overdosing" with *S. vulgaris*, it may simply be that so many larvae are present that the pathways available for migration are jammed, and the surplus larvae migrate randomly until destroyed by host reaction.

In heavier naturally occurring infections, there is considerable involvement of the liver as well as the right flank and, to a lesser extent, the left flank. Plaques of scar tissue long remain in Glisson's capsule of the parietal surface of, particularly, the right lobe of the liver. An occasional case of chronic fibrosing pancreatitis is caused by *S. edentatus* larvae, though most are caused by *S. equinus*.

Larvae remain in the liver for about 9 months and exit via the right hepatorenal ligament to gain the head of the cecum. It is not clear if the larvae normally migrate into the subperitoneal tissue and, then, transperitoneally into the cecum and ventral colon, or if these subperitoneal larvae are lost. It

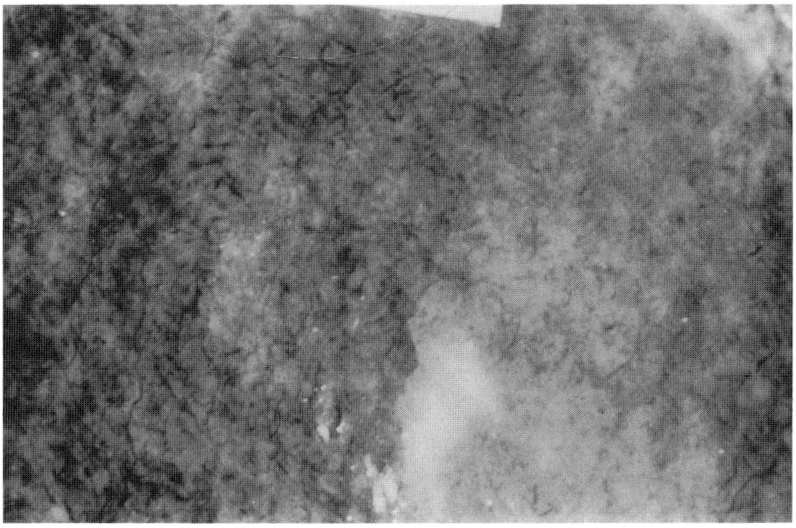

3.12. *S. edentatus.* Massive infiltration of the liver in experimental infection. With survival many of these infiltrations become scars. (Photograph courtesy of E. Lyons and H. Drudge.)

has been suggested that the larvae migrate from the hepatorenal ligament directly to the cecum (McCraw and Slocombe 1974). On the other hand, no evidence of destruction and granulomatous reaction has ever been seen in the lesions of the flank, indicating that it may be part of the normal migratory pathway.

Strongylus equinus

S. equinus is much less common than the other two large strongyles. Infective larvae penetrate the wall of the ileum, cecum, and ventral colon (McCraw and Slocombe 1985). Within 2 weeks postinfection they have molted to the fourth stage within the submucosa, muscularis, and serosa of the gut. Some larvae are present with minimal inflammatory reaction, while necrotic eosinophilic masses distinguish other foci. It is not clear whether the latter are induced by death of larvae or by the sheaths discarded during molting. Grossly, larval activity is indicated by raised hemorrhagic foci or whitish nodules in the serosa of the ileum, cecum, and colon.

Larvae reach the liver via the peritoneal cavity as early as 8 days postinfection. They wander in the liver for as long as 17 weeks. The lesions are identical to those of *S. edentatus*. The pancreas is invaded at least by the 7th week with maximum numbers of larvae recoverable at 17 weeks. The molt to the fifth stage occurs about 15 weeks, with preadults present in the wall of the ventral colon at 30 weeks, and adults in the lumen at 40 weeks. The larvae may wander extensively off course in experimental infections, granulomatous changes being found in the lung, flanks, diaphragm, and omentum. As noted for *S. edentatus* infection, this is not seen in naturally occurring cases and is no doubt a function of the numbers of larvae administered. The pancreatic lesions are discussed with the pancreas.

Small strongyles

These are among the commonest equine parasites and may be present in very large numbers. Some 40 species have been recognized.

The larvae of small strongyles only migrate within the mucosa and submucosa of the cecum and large colon, limiting their potential for producing disease. The larvae may encyst in the superficial parts of the mucosa without tissue reaction, or penetrate deeply into the lamina propria and submucosa, inducing granulomatous nodules. Rupture of these nodules into the lumen causes small ulcerations. One species, *Triodontophorus tenuicollis* (LeRoux 1924; Drudge 1985), accumulates in large numbers [500 worms in one ulcer (LeRoux)] in craterlike ulcerations in the dorsal colon. The parasite appears to cause, rather than just colonize, the ulcer.

Adult small strongyles live in the interface of the ingesta and mucosa, unattached to the mucosa, with only a few species attaching to the mucosa and taking blood.

A definite clinical and pathological syndrome is associated with the small strongyles (Blackwell 1973; Chiejina and Mason 1977; Mirck 1977; Ogbourne 1978; Jasko and Roth 1984; Giles et al. 1985). Larvae ingested in a given year may encyst as inhibited third-stage forms in the mucosa of the cecum and colon. In the late winter and early spring these larvae transform to the fourth stage and migrate *en masse* into the lumen of the cecum and colon. With sufficient numbers a clinical syndrome occurs, characterized by intermittent, persistent diarrhea, anorexia, mild colic, loss of weight, leucocytosis (not eosinophilia), hypoalbuminemia, and low fecal egg counts. At postmortem the walls of the cecum and colon are edematous, as is the mesocolon, and there may be thickening, focal nodular formations, and patchy ulceration of the mucosa. Histologically, there is mononuclear cell and eosinophil infiltration of the mucosa with numerous encysted and free larvae. While the precise cause of the loss of inhibition is not known, it is probable that the adult worms in the lumen are dying off, releasing the larvae for migration and development to the adult stage.

This syndrome has been reported in the United Kingdom, Russia, and the Netherlands, with only one case reported in North America (Jasko and Roth 1984).

Tapeworms

Anoplocephala perfoliata is seen regularly in moderate numbers near the ileocecal orifice in the cecum (Fig. 3.13). Drudge and Lyons (1986) found infestation of 54% of Thoroughbreds at postmortem in Kentucky. In 1920 Hutyra and Marek found tapeworm infestation in 55% of horses autopsied for their study, with 80% of those infestations being *A. perfoliata*. *Anoplocephala magna* is seen infrequently in small numbers in the distal jejunum and ileum. *Paranoplocephala mamillana* is very rare in North America.

Horses with chronic, debilitating disease, particularly older horses, may have heavy infestations, with *A. perfoliata* completely covering the cecal mucosa as well as being found in large numbers in the small intestine. Such debilitated animals may, either simultaneously or separately, have heavy infestations with *Parascaris equuorum*, age-related resistance having been lost. It is doubtful, or at least not established, that the moderate numbers

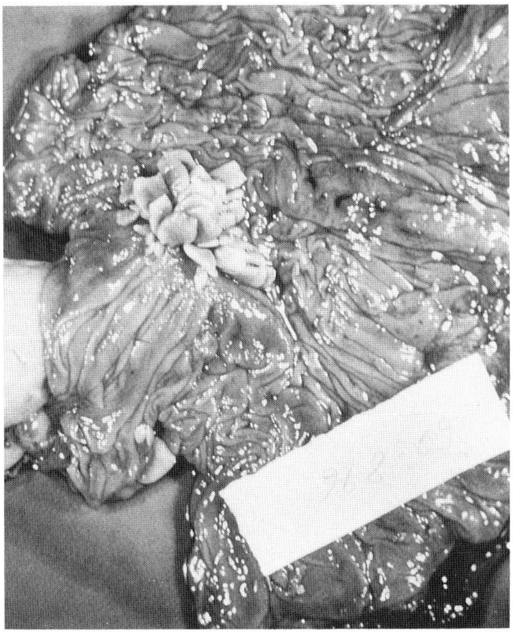

3.13. *Anoplocephala perfoliata* around the ileocecal orifice.

of tapeworms regularly seen in horses have any deleterious effects.

Esophagus

Lesions of the esophagus in light horses are uncommon. Migrating *Hypoderma bovis* larvae cause marked, yellow, gelatinous edema around the esophagus. Massive ulceration of the distal third of the esophagus may be seen with acute gastric dilatation, presumably the result of passive regurgitation of stomach contents. Similar ulceration is seen in chronic or recurring choke.

Obstruction

Deegen et al. (1976) reviewed the literature and reported 98 cases of **choke** over an 8-year period. They found a higher frequency in young horses, up to 5 years of age, and in old horses, over 10 years of age. They believed that abnormalities of dental development were responsible for inadequate chewing of food materials in young animals, while aging changes in the dentition were responsible in the older animals (see "Teeth," earlier in this chapter). *Gasterophilus* can cause significant ulceration of the lingual gingiva of the upper cheek teeth. Several cases of choke have been associated with such, presumably painful, lesions. These problems are compounded by the type of food material, such as dry, finely chopped sugar beets, which would be inadequately chewed and quickly swallowed. Erosion and ulceration of the esophagus as a result of pressure necrosis eventuated, in untreated cases, in stricture of the esophagus.

Fine, often barely perceptible, linear erosions may be present in the esophagal mucosa in cases of undefined **chronic diarrhea**. Histologically, the epithelium shows nonspecific necrosis with a mild infiltration of inflammatory cells in the submucosa and mucosa.

Idiopathic muscular hypertrophy

Muscular hypertrophy of the esophagus has been reported in the horse (Schmidt 1937; Cohrs 1961; Schulte 1970) but is certainly rare. We have seen no cases in light horses. The inner, circular layer of muscle is greatly thickened proximal to the esophageal hiatus, reaching 3 cm or more in contrast to the normal 1 cm. Most of the thoracic portion of the esophagus can be affected. Diverticula are rarely found in association with the thickened esophagus.

The esophageal muscle is skeletal until about the base of the heart where it becomes smooth muscle. From there to the cardia of the stomach it steadily increases in thickness. The wall of the intrathoracic part of the esophagus of the horse is thicker than that of other domestic species. It may be suggested that the thicker wall, and so muscular strength, is an adaptation for propelling boluses through the relatively longer, low-pressure chest cavity and into the higher-pressure stomach lumen. Since hypertrophy of the muscular wall is *prima facie* evidence of increased work, the pathogenesis, in a given case, is to be found when the reason for increased work is found. Improperly masticated feed materials, such as bran, pellets, and chopped roots, are less efficiently propelled from esophagus to stomach (Schmidt 1937).

Peristalsis of the esophagus is controlled via the vagus nerves. If the nerves are cut, the control of the proximal, striated muscle is permanently lost, while the distal, smooth muscle regains intrinsic motility and can generate peristaltic waves in response to distension by food. These observations were made by Cannon (1911) for several species and not, specifically, the horse. In general the posttransection peristaltic waves are less efficient than normal, and food material may remain in the esophagus until there is sufficient accumulation to distend the wall and initiate a peristaltic contraction. The conditions would appear favorable for the development of muscular hypertrophy of the distal part of the esophagus, suggesting examination of the vagus innervation in any case of muscular hypertrophy of the esophagus.

Dilation and diverticula

Dilated segments of esophagus are usually found with chronic choke and the strictures induced by such choke. A congenital case has been described by Rohrbach and Rooney (1980).

False or pulsion **diverticula** have been seen (Cohrs 1961), apparently the result of rupture of, or perhaps congenital defect in, the muscularis of the thoracic portion of the esophagus. They are very rare, and we have seen no case.

Stomach

The normal esophageal mucosa of the stomach is whitish gray and sharply demarcated from the fundus by the margo plicatus. In the foal, before ingestion of solid food, the esophageal mucosa is often partially or completely covered by a tough, brownish-yellow layer, which can be peeled away—the stratum corneum of the stratified squamous epithelium (Fig. 3.14).

The normal fundic mucosa is pinkish gray and slimy, with a finely cobblestoned surface giving way to a smoother and grayer pyloric mucosa. The slimy appearance is caused by a variable, usually considerable, amount of clear, viscid mucus. The mucus becomes progressively cloudier and more viscid with autolytic change, often appearing as a virtual pseudomembrane stained with food pigments.

There are two pyloric sphincters in the horse between which is the **antrum pyloricum**. According to Krölling and Grau (1960), this antrum is probably present because of the absence of the gallbladder. The antrum fills with ingesta when the proximal sphincter is open and the distal sphincter closed, while the antrum empties when the distal sphincter is open and the proximal closed. Thus, only a small portion of the stomach contents enters the duodenum at any given time. This is thought to occur because the bile only flows into the duodenum in a dropwise manner (Krölling and Grau). The antrum pyloricum and the two sphincters are described by Nickel et al. (1960): the proximal sphincter as **musculus sphincter antri pylori** (not noted in *Nomina Anatomica Veterinaria* 1983) and the distal **musculus sphincter pylori**. The two sphincters and the antrum (*Pförtnersac*) are also shown by Zietzschmann et al. (1943). While the function of the antrum and sphincters is speculative, there may be eventual relevance for the pathogene-

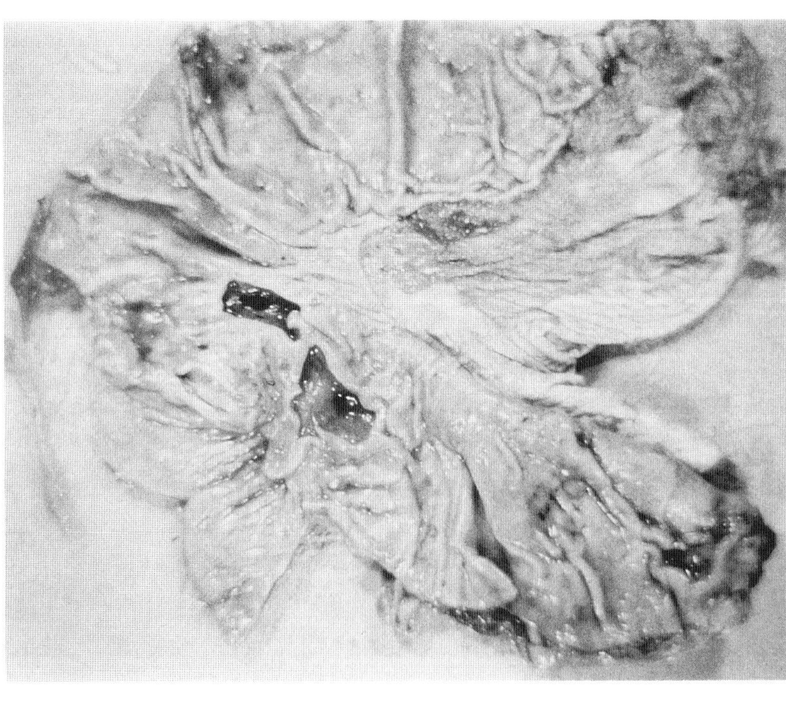

3.14. Stomach of a foal. The normal stratum corneum partially coats the esophageal portion of the stomach. There are several fundic ulcerations, one of which had perforated.

sis of lesions of the stomach and duodenum.

The orientation of the musculature of the cardia of the stomach (Zietzschmann et al. 1943; Nickel et al) led Krölling and Grau to speculate that the muscular branches flanking the lesser curvature of the stomach could form a furrow or channel, functioning as an esophageal groove. Such a functional channel, if it occurs, would help water to bypass the stomach.

There may be variable numbers of fibrous tags and shaggy roughening of the serosal surface of the stomach, as well as other tubular viscera. These increase in frequency and numbers with advancing age. This is superficial fibrous tissue proliferation of the serosa without significant infiltration of inflammatory cells. In younger horses with, for example, chronic gastritis, chronic musculofibrous hyperplasia, or chronic cecal impaction, these tags can be present in considerable numbers and localized to the affected areas. It is probable that inadequate movement, not to say periods of total ileus, is involved in their genesis. The more diffuse distribution in old horses may be a function of general depression of gastrointestinal activity with age. There is no evidence that these tags represent healed peritonitis. Fibrous tags on the parietal surface of the liver can have a different origin (see "Liver," in this chapter).

Gastric ulceration

Erosions and ulcerations, often accompanied by irregular islands of cornification, are common in the esophageal portion of the stomach, particularly adjacent to the margo plicatus at or near the lesser curvature. These ulcerations may be focal, appearing as elevated whitish nodules with ulcerated centers, or may be larger, irregular, or confluent areas of epithelial loss. On average, the numbers and extent of these lesions are marginally less in the winter months, although present in all seasons. Hammond et al. (1986) found such ulcerations in 80% of Thoroughbred horses in racing or training and in 52% of horses out of training for at least a month. The ulcerations were more extensive and severe in the horses in training and racing. In their venue, Hong Kong, *Gasterophilus* spp. are not present.

Gasterophilus intestinalis larvae are certainly the initiating cause of many ulcerative lesions at the margo plicatus, specifically the nodules with ulcerated centers. *Draschia megastoma* routinely involve the fundic mucosa immediately adjacent to the margo plicatus (Fig. 3.15). In foals, sharp foreign material, such as sand, may be a factor (Rooney 1964). In many cases it is not clear why the ulceration is present. Since these lesions occur primarily in the esophageal portion adjacent to the margo plicatus, the area where the transition from alkaline to neutral/acid reaction occurs, the cause may be sought in disturbance of this transitional region by feed and feeding practices. The Hong Kong results imply but do not establish "stress" as a factor, as will be seen.

Histologically, with erosive lesions, there is loss of the outer layers of stratified squamous epithelium with infiltration of the submucosa and epithelium by neutrophils, mononuclear cells, and eosinophils. With ulceration into the submucosa there is amorphous, necrotic debris in the base of the ulcer, with chronic inflammatory cell infiltration and fibrosis. No etiological agent has been seen with special stains. While eosinophils suggest parasitic involvement, eosinophils are not at all uncommon in considerable numbers in virtually any chronic inflammatory process in the horse. Occasionally, one of these ulcers perforates, particularly in foals, causing fatal peritonitis (Rooney 1964).

Erosions and ulcerations of the fundic and pyloric mucosae have been seen in seriously ill foals under prolonged antibiotic and steroid therapy (Rooney) (Fig. 3.14). Perforation of such ulcers is not uncommon. Phenylbutazone has been implicated as a cause of ulceration of the fundic and pyloric mucosa of foals, but does not seem to be as ulcerogenic in older horses. The drug has been implicated as a cause of ulceration of the distal portion of the right dorsal colon in older horses (Simmons et al. 1990). This is of interest in light of

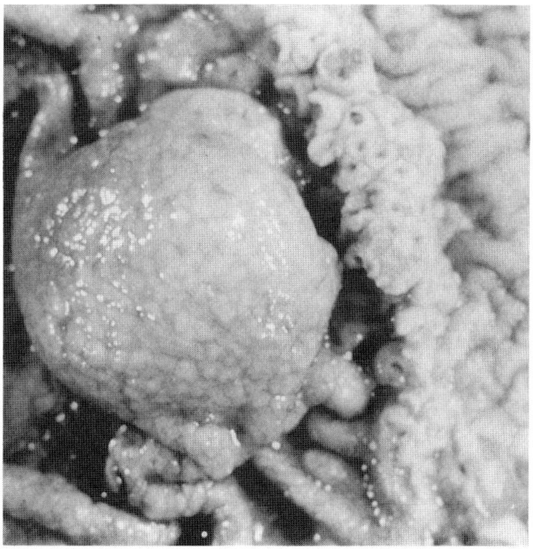

3.15. *Draschia megastoma* nodule adjacent to the margo plicatus. (Photograph courtesy of E. Lyons and H. Drudge.)

the ulceration of the right dorsal colon related to one species of small strongyle, *T. tenuicollis* (LeRoux 1924), as well as the observations of Cadeac (1896), Alexander (1962), and Argenzio (1975) that the concentration of phosphate increases from proximal to distal colon. Alexander also noted that the concentration of potassium increases in the same manner. Lesions in the intestinal tract caused by *Erlichia risticii* are also more frequent in the right dorsal colon.

Gasterophilus nasalis may be found in considerable numbers in the pylorus and first part of the duodenum. They are less common in North America than *G. intestinalis*. While damage is done to the mucosa, this damage does not persist or become confluent as appears to be the case with *G. intestinalis* in the esophageal region. *Gasterophilus hemorrhoidalis* is rarely seen.

Foal ulcer syndrome

A specific ulcerative syndrome of young foals was first seen in the late 1970s in North America (Acland et al. 1983). This is massive ulceration of the esophageal portion of the stomach on the lesser curvature with or without ulceration of the proximal portion of the duodenum. Although the lesions in the stomach appear to be most frequent and severe near the margo plicatus of the lesser curvature, the entire esophageal portion may be involved, with, in some cases, near total loss of the stratified squamous epithelium (Fig. 3.16). Ulceration of the duodenum is less common and may be related to failure of the sphincter actions of the pyloric antrum.

Histological changes are nonspecific. In recent years (1989–1993) the frequency of the condition seems to have decreased. The cause is unknown. As is suggested below, early grain feeding may be a factor. Severe ulceration of the esophageal portion of the stomach, particularly at the lesser curvature, is seen in foals with foreign bodies (for example, plastic trash bags) lodged in the pylorus and duodenum, with consequent delayed emptying of the stomach.

Pathogenesis of ulceration

As indicated above there are two basic types of ulceration of the stomach in horses: the more common ulceration of the esophageal portion at or near the margo plicatus, and the less common ulceration of the fundic and pyloric mucosa. The latter would seem clearly duress-related, whether the duress be disease or such agents as phenylbutazone. The pathogenesis of such ulceration in horses, as in other species, is undefined. Ulceration of the esophageal portion of the stomach does not appear to be duress related and it is suggested below that it is, in fact, related to dietary factors, with the obvious exception of gasterophilus lesions.

As pointed out by Clarke et al. (1990) bolus feeding of horses causes numerous definable and possible physiological changes from normal, normal

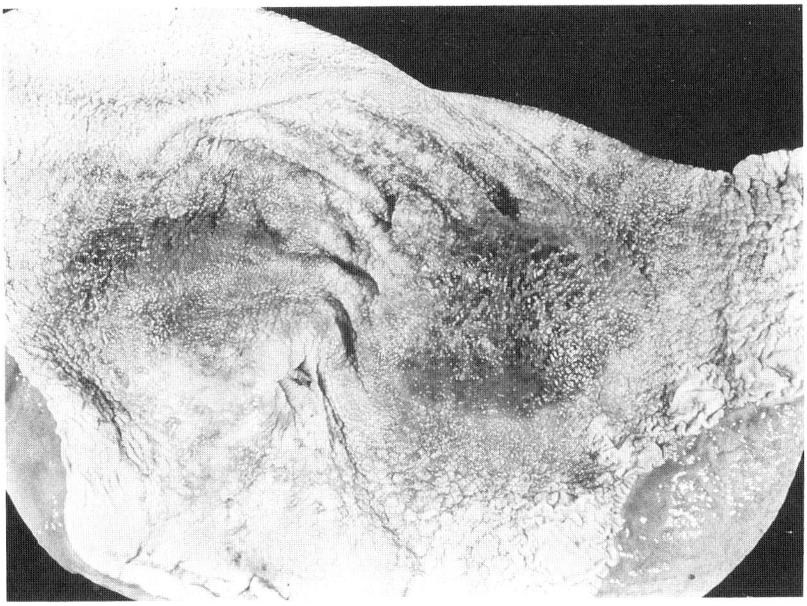

3.16. Massive ulceration of the stomach of a foal. (Photo courtesy of Helen Acland.)

being defined as the horse that eats ad lib throughout a 24-hour period. A major difference between wild horses that eat natural foodstuffs and those fed foodstuff provided by humans is that, apart from bolus feeding, the former subsists almost entirely on roughage, while grain and concentrates are added for the latter. For the adult horse with nonclinical ulceration at or near the margo plicatus, the following scenario is proposed. A meal of grain/concentrate, rich in digestible carbohydrate (starch), is ingested and deposited in a layer in the stomach. Digestion begins with the salivary amylases together with bacterial action, producing short chain fatty acids. As the layer of grain moves toward the margo plicatus, it becomes more acid, the buffering capacity is compromised, and the bacterial population shifts to lactic acid producers instead of short chain fatty acid producers. The increase in acidity is more rapid than normal because starch is rapidly broken down by lactobacilli, and these lactic acid producers proliferate at the expense of the short chain fatty acid producers. As well, the rapid drop in pH is lethal to the latter organisms. Since the layer moves as already described, less linear movement along the lesser curvature than along the greater curvature, the mucosa of the lesser curvature has a longer exposure to the increased acidity. The higher than normal acidity in the region of the margo plicatus, specifically, the lesser curvature, may be the cause of the ulcerations so commonly found in this area. Once the layer of grain has passed distal to the margo plicatus, it is in a normally acid environment, and ulceration is not to be expected. The localized ulcerations caused by *G. intestinalis* could, in addition, serve as a *locus minoris resistentia* for acid action. It has been shown in a number of species (though not specifically for the horse) that the higher the concentration of carbohydrate in the stomach, the slower the emptying time, providing a longer time for the above mechanisms to operate (Usry 1989).

This pathogenesis is essentially that of rumenitis and ulceration in grain-fed cattle. Although epidemiological evidence is not available, it may be suggested that the massive ulceration seen in foals is related to early grain feeding, specifically creep feeding or allowing foals to eat with the mare. The larger, greedier foals should be predisposed, and this does seem to be the case. Both a high percentage of grain in the diet and bolus feeding would appear to be major factors in ulceration of the esophageal portion of the stomach both in adult horses and foals. Some aspects of this pathogenesis have been suggested by Barker and van Dreumel (1985). In the foal the prolonged emptying time of the stomach (Alexander 1950), together with grain supplementation, may be relevant, an observation consistent with the ulceration that occurs when the pylorus is occluded or partially occluded by a foreign body. The Hong Kong experience, already cited, may be explained by the shift from a high grain to predominantly roughage diet when horses were removed from training and racing, rather than to the suggested decrease of "stress."

Gastritis

Gastritis is uncommon but not unknown.

Acute catarrhal gastritis

Acute catarrhal gastritis is characterized by excess mucus and multiple, fine petechiation of the fundic and pyloric mucosae (Fig. 3.17). The only known cause of acute gastritis in the horse is infestation with *Trichostrongylus axei*, most often seen in horses grazing with cattle and sheep

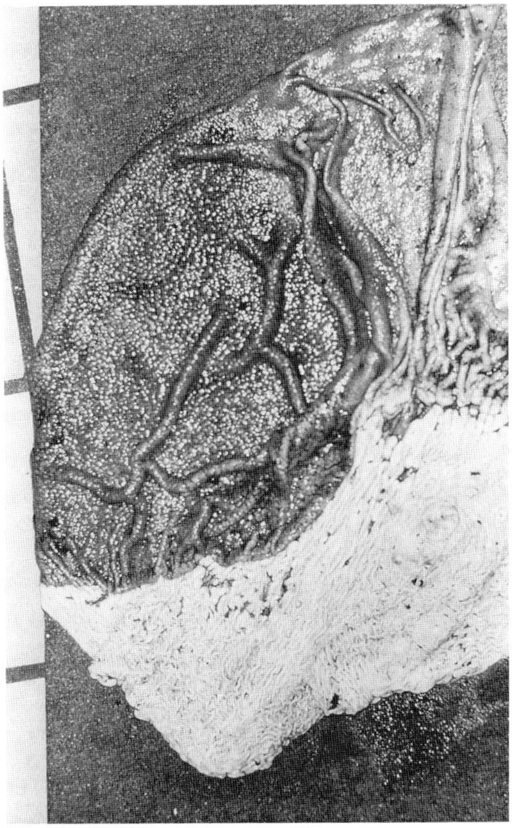

3.17. Acute gastritis involving the portion of the fundus to the right. There are multiple ulcers in the esophageal mucosa adjacent to the margo plicatus. The two conditions have no necessary relationship.

Britton 1939). There may be no specific clinical signs, gastritis being found incidentally at autopsy. *T. axei* may be recovered in the absence of gross evidence of disease. Britton (1939) believed that *T. axei* caused chronic gastritis, but his cases were complicated by infection with *Habronema* spp. Roth and Christensen (1942) also believed that *T. axei* caused chronic gastritis, but they studied mixed infections and gave no evidence to specifically incriminate *T. axei*. Leland et al. (1961) too believed chronic gastritis to be related to *T. axei* infestation, but, again, the presence of habronema was not controlled.

Chronic gastritis

Chronic gastritis is somewhat more common than acute gastritis, particularly in warm climates, such as the southern United States and Mexico, and was reported many years ago by French veterinarians (Hutyra and Marek 1926). It is characterized by patchy reddening and a marked increase in the coarseness of the cobblestone appearance of the fundic mucosa, often progressing to frank nodular formations (Fig. 3.18). Histologically, the lamina propria is heavily infiltrated with mononuclear cells, lymphoid cells, and variable numbers of eosinophils. The submucosa is less involved. The gastric glands undergo metaplasia to largely mucous cells with, occasionally, worms present in the glands. The cause of such chronic gastritis, in our experience, is infestation with *Habronema muscae* and/or *H. majus*. Hodgkins, cited by Hutyra and Marek, was apparently of the same opinion. Britton (1939), Roth and Christensen (1942), and Leland et al. (1961), as noted above, believed that *T. axei* was the cause of chronic gastritis, and this was apparently observed in France as well (Hutyra and Marek). It may be, then, that both parasites are capable of producing chronic gastritis, but that *T. axei* is the principal cause of acute gastritis. Our experience, however, is that trichostrongyles can be absent with chronic gastritis, while habronema are never absent.

Drudge and Lyons (1986) reported an infestation rate in central Kentucky of 38% for *H. muscae* with no *H. majus*. Despite the high rate of infestation chronic gastritis is rare in this area, the infestations being light compared to those found in more southerly areas.

Chronic gastritis can cause nonspecific signs of weight loss, poor haircoat, and general unthriftiness. One case presented as hypocalcemic tetany, temporarily responsive to intravenously administered calcium. It was proposed that the chronic gastritis impaired calcium absorption, with resulting hypocalcemia and tetany.

Single nodules of considerable size with a central, apical hole are found in the fundic mucosa adjacent to the margo plicatus. These are caused by *Draschi megastoma*. The worm burrows into the submucosa and elicits a granulomatous reaction with large numbers of eosinophils. The worm is usually not found, its location marked by a caseous core of degenerate eosinophils. While impressive, these lesions seem to be of no clinical significance.

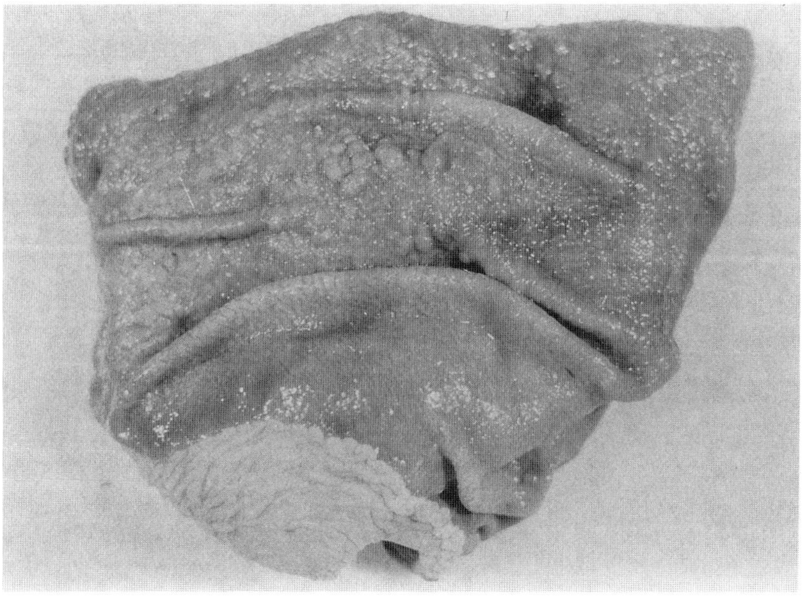

3.18. Chronic gastritis, *Habronema*. Esophageal mucosa and margo plicatus are at bottom. The cardiac and fundic mucosa is normal adjacent to the margo plicatus (though decomposed). The fundic mucosa becomes progressively thicker and more cobblestone toward the pylorus.

Drudge and Lyons (1986) reported an infestation rate of 62% for this parasite in Thoroughbred horses in central Kentucky.

Acute gastric dilatation

This condition, quite unique to equidae because of their inability to vomit, has been long known. The almost invariable outcome is rupture of the stomach and the postmortem diagnosis readily made. Seven to 10% of all cases of colic were acute dilatation. Of note, most cases of acute dilatation occurred in the summer (Hutyra and Marek 1920; Dobberstein and Dinter 1942).

When the abdomen is opened, ingesta is free in the peritoneal cavity, particularly in and around the greater omentum. When free ingesta is encountered, the prosector should examine and note its distribution in the peritoneal cavity. The ingesta is dense at and near the site of rupture, spreading and thinning, fan or flowerlike, through the peritoneal cavity.

This permits initial determination of the rupture site and may suggest modifications in the exenteration in order to display the pathological process most effectively. It may be noted that this is readily done with the postmortem procedure described, considerably less so, if at all, when the animal is on its side.

The site of rupture is almost invariably the greater curvature. The tear is longest in the serosa, somewhat less so in the muscularis, and least in the mucosa, which bulges out through the tear. The mucosal bulging may not be as apparent with advanced autolysis. After the initial failure, the tear may veer off to one side. It is important to distinguish between ruptures as the result of gas pressure and perforations as the result of ulceration, carcinoma, and so forth. In the latter case the lesion is generally discrete and rounded or elliptical.

Acute gastric dilatation causing death before rupture is less frequent, but does occur and presents diagnostic difficulty. Postmortem gaseous distension is routine, and the diagnosis cannot be made on that basis alone. Careful examination of the greater curvature shows slight to moderate tearing of the serosa with petechiae and/or small extravasations of blood. As well, splitting and tearing of the outer layers of the muscularis may be present together with fine, linear hemorrhages (Lindt 1970).

The proximate cause of acute dilatation and rupture is ileus of the stomach. This may be caused by events in the stomach itself or as the result of anatomical or functional ileus of the duodenum.

Overeating fermentable materials is one of the common causes. The animal, usually a young one, gains access to desirable foods and overeats. *S. vulgaris* migrations and thromboses of the left gastric and/or gastroepiploic arteries can be found in some cases where overeating is not implicated. Often, but not invariably, there will be evidence of verminous arteritis in the celiac artery, as would be expected.

Despite the ileus that must, to some extent, accompany acute or chronic gastritis, carcinoma, and severe gastric ulceration of foals, gastric rupture is not seen. Perforation is more probable, at least in the latter two cases. Obstruction of the duodenum, either anatomical or functional, causes acute gastric dilatation. The anatomical strictures are obvious and usually caused by indurated ulcers or abscesses. Functional ileus of the duodenum is problematic. In a few cases, parasitic thromboses have been found in the arteries supplying the duodenum—jejunal, gastroepiploic—with the presumption of anoxic ileus.

Gastric dilatation is a feature of grass sickness and so-called duodenitis/proximal enteritis, in the latter case an example of functional ileus of the duodenum and proximal jejunum.

Neoplasia

Neoplasia of the stomach is uncommon. While lymphosarcoma, leiomyomas, and adenocarcinoma have been seen, most are squamous cell carcinomas arising from the esophageal mucosa (Lindt 1970; Barker and van Dreumel 1985).

Squamous cell carcinoma presents as a cauliflowerlike mass bulging from the esophageal mucosa, usually ulcerated, scirrhous, and well demarcated. The animal may be destroyed before metastasis occurs. Metastasis is by direct implantation on the liver, spleen, diaphragm, and any peritoneal surface. Distant metastasis, to the lung for example, is uncommon. The implantation metastases resemble mesothelioma, not unequivocally reported in horses, as well as the metastases of undifferentiated pancreatic carcinoma. The primary tumor has the usual characteristics of a squamous cell carcinoma. The metastases may be less differentiated.

Small intestine

Only small amounts of ingesta are regularly in the lumen of the small intestine, and are virtually never in the ileum. The mucosa is grayish tan with a considerable quantity of clear, watery mucus in the lumen and adherent to the mucosa. As in the stomach the mucus becomes cloudy and thickened with autolytic change.

Meckel's diverticulum and the mesodiverticular band

Meckel's diverticulum is a remnant of the omphalomesenteric duct, and the mesodiverticular band is a remnant of a vitelline artery (Zietzschmann and Krölling 1955). The former is located about a meter proximal to the ileocecal junction (Fig. 3.19). In the horse it is, if present, usually an about fist-sized spherical pouch on the antimesenteric border of the intestine. The blind end may have a fibrous string attached to the umbilicus and can cause strangulation (Grant and Tennant 1973). Larger diverticula may become impacted with ingesta and perforate (Cadeac 1896; Sprinkle et al. 1984). A mesodiverticular band can persist in the same area and cause strangulation and volvulus (Freeman et al. 1979). Meckel's diverticulum occurs in about 1 of 3000 horses. There is no data on mesodiverticular bands, but they are rare.

Catarrhal enteritis

Catarrhal enteritis is common in foals with bacterial septicemia, whatever the inciting organism.

Enteritis in adult horses is rare with the exception of the so-called **duodenitis/proximal jejunitis syndrome**, which, perhaps, represents about 1% of all clinical cases of colic. It acts clinically as acute ileus and obstruction of the proximal portion of the small intestine. At postmortem the lesion is distension of the duodenum and proximal jejunum with a brownish or brownish-red fluid. The serosal surface has multiple petechiae and ecchymoses (Fig. 3.20). The mucosa is intensely hyperemic with gross erosions rarely apparent. Histologically, there is catarrhal enteritis with necrosis of the epithelium of the villous tips, hyperemia, hemorrhage, and mild edema of the lamina propria. There is a variable infiltration of neutrophil leukocytes. White et al. (1987) reported similar findings in 20 cases.

While duodenitis/proximal jejunitis was not so named in the older literature, it is apparent that enteritis of undetermined origin as a cause of fatal colic has been seen for many years (Cadeac 1896). Dobberstein and Dinter (1942) reported about 0.8% of all fatal colic cases as enteritis of unknown cause, with similar findings in earlier reports. Horses of all ages were affected, but there were more younger horses affected than for colic in general. Johnston and Morris (1987) found more than half of their cases to be less than 10 years old. Dobberstein and Dinter indicated that there were more cases in the hot summer months. Sojka (1991) said that more cases were seen in the southern United States, but gave no details. Johnston and Morris found a higher frequency during the warmer months. As already noted, however, the frequency of all forms of colic is higher during the warm months. The cause is not known.

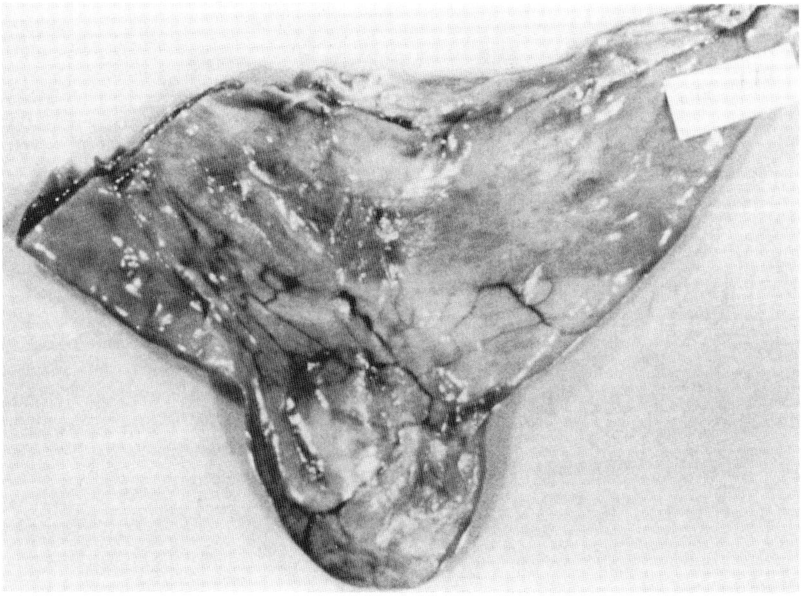

3.19. Meckel's diverticulum, incidental finding.

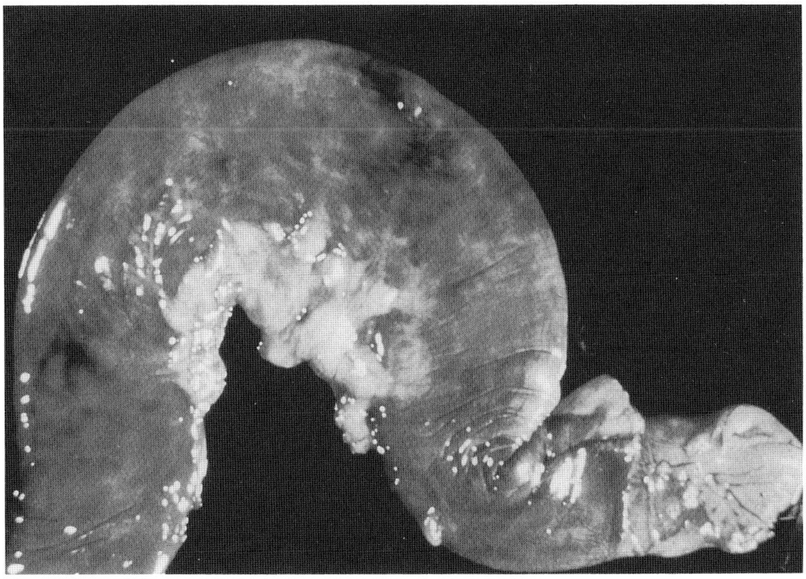

3.20. Distended, discolored proximal jejunum in duodenitis/ proximal jejunitis syndrome.

Ascarids

Ascarids occur in foals and, in sufficient number, can cause marked hyperemia if not enteritis. Perforation does occur, probably as the result of ileus, obstipation, and subsequent necrosis of the intestinal wall. Heavy infestations with ascarids may be found in old and/or debilitated horses, even sufficient to cause death. As with *R. equi* and *A. perfoliata* in older animals, the immune system has been disabled, and infestations and infections characteristic of the immunologically naive reappear.

Strongyloides

It is not unusual to find an incidental, limited, mild to moderate catarrhal enteritis at postmortem of young foals. The duodenum and proximal jejunum have hyperemia, slight mucosal edema, and punctate hemorrhages. This is caused by either *Strongyloides westeri* or the coccidium, *Eimeria leukarti*. In the former case the adult worms are not seen grossly but can be found in sections with their heads buried deeply in the intestinal glands. While there is a vascular reaction—hyperemia, hemorrhage, and edema—inflammatory cells are often no more numerous than usual in the intestine. Light infestations of adult worms are also found histologically in the absence of gross lesions.

S. westeri is transmitted through the mare's milk to the foal. After a period of egg-laying in the foal, immunity develops, ending the infestation by about 6 months of age. Apparently mares harbor somatic stages of the worms in their tissues for years, being the source of infection for foals each year (Drudge and Lyons 1986).

Eimeria

Eimeria leukarti does not cause catarrhal enteritis unless present in large numbers. They are usually found incidentally as large, thick-walled oocysts, without inflammatory reaction, in the subepithelial tissues of the villi. Wetzel (1967) described diarrhea, loss of weight, and occasional deaths caused by this parasite in horses. Enteritis was present and characterized by infiltration of eosinophils, mononuclear cells, and occasional neutrophils. We have not seen a case.

Nutritional enteritis

It has long been recognized that unusual feed materials and sudden changes of feed can be associated with acute, less often chronic, intestinal malfunction. The clinical signs are variable and include depression, hyporexia, and constipation followed by diarrhea, foul-smelling feces, and variably severe signs of colic (Hutyra and Marek 1920, 1926; Wintzer 1986). The feeds implicated are usually high in soluble carbohydrates (as compared to forage and hay), such as beets, turnips, bread, potatoes, large amounts of molasses and/or bran, and beet tops. Spoiled hay and grains as well as rice, wheat, and rye grains have been implicated. Rye, specifically, has been associated with acute laminitis as well as gastroenteric malfunction (Hutyra and Marek).

There may be increased amounts of mucus, hyperemia, and petechiae in the mucosa of the small and large intestine. More often the increase of mucus is equivocal and the hyperemia difficult to consider pathological. The characteristic changes are fetid, watery content of both small and, particularly, large intestine, together with general dehydration. In more protracted cases there will be evidence of inanition: loss of fat, serous atrophy, small liver, and mild, usually microscopic, fatty infiltration of liver, adrenals, and kidneys.

We have little or no experience of this condition at postmortem. There have been suggestions that it is a clostridiosis, but without evidence. Disruption of the normal bacterial flora is probable, however difficult to define. The mortality is low, and the diagnosis based on clinical history, slender postmortem evidence, and absence of specific etiological agents. There are some resemblances to grass sickness.

Isolated S. vulgaris infarction

Three specific entities have been observed in the duodenum, jejunum, and the large intestine, which form a pathological entity or complex.

1. Solitary nodules, often with an apical orifice, may be found bulging into the lumen from the submucosa. They contain caseous or caseopurulent debris expressible through the orifice. Strongyle larvae have not been found in these nodules, but the histology is that of a parasitic granuloma.

2. A discrete, chronic, indurated ulcer anywhere in the duodenum or jejunum, rarely ileum, as well as in any part of the large intestine. The lesions may be found incidentally or be the proximate cause of stricture and colic. They apparently arise from earlier, nonperforating infarctions caused by *S. vulgaris* larvae (Fig. 3.21).

3. A focal infarct of the mucosa (Figs. 3.22–3.24). In the small intestine or descending colon it can cause obstipation. There is a bolus of dry, mucus-coated ingesta, with dilated intestine proximal to and collapsed intestine distal to the site of obstipation. When the viscus is opened and the bolus removed, a nearly rectangular area of intense hyperemia, often with central grayish-white necrosis, is seen in the mucosa of the mesenteric quadrant of the gut. Histologically, this is infarction with thrombotic material in the submucosal arteries and/or small arteries in the immediately adjacent mesentery. As well, there is infiltration of mononuclear cells and, often, eosinophils.

This focal infarction, caused by *S. vulgaris* migration, may be the cause of the first two lesions, as well. The infarction is small, not devitalizing gut in sufficient amounts to be immediately life threatening. It does, however, breach the mucosal defenses, allowing the development of either ulcer or abscess. At the time of infarction with ileus and obstipation in the small intestine or descending colon, a nonfatal colic episode occurs. Fatal colic

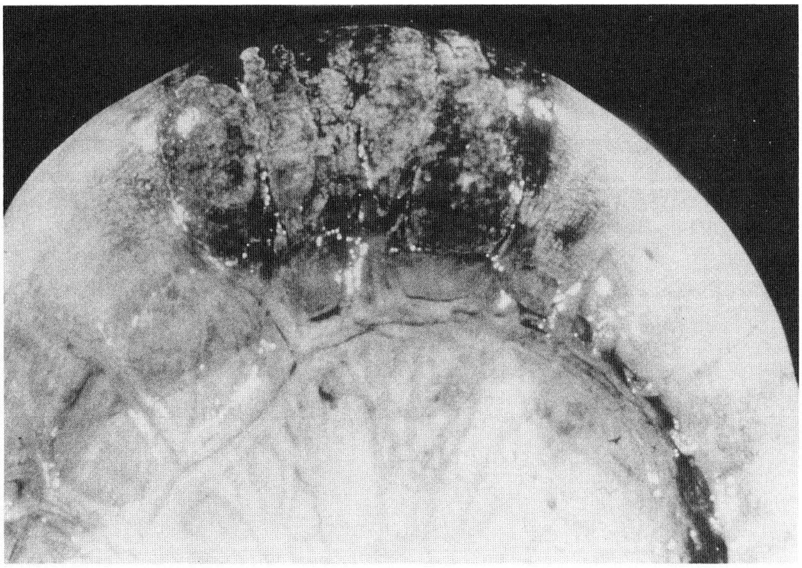

3.21. Focus of intense hyperemia and hemorrhage verging on infarction of the small intestine, *S. vulgaris*.

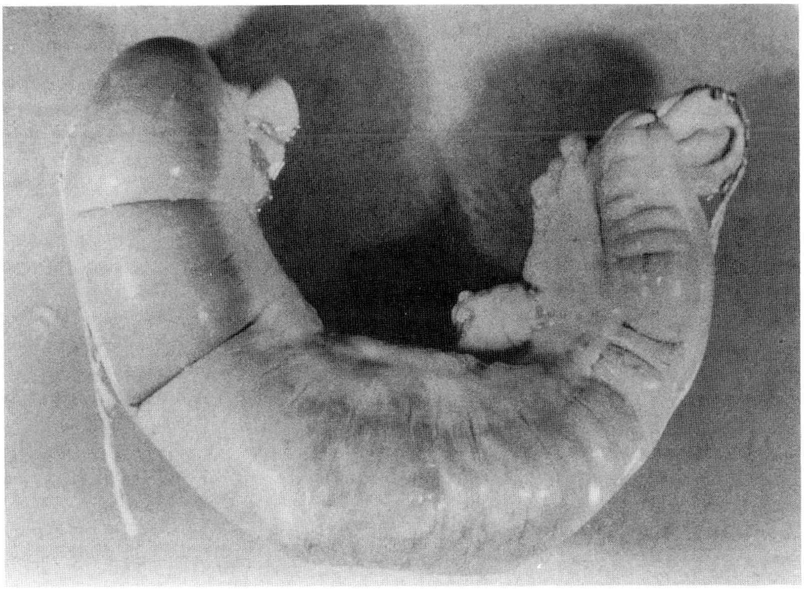

3.22. Impaction of the descending colon.

may occur months later as a result of anatomical or functional stricture caused by the abscess or indurated ulcer.

Muscular hypertrophy of the ileum

The ileum is normally thicker and more hose-like than the jejunum because of the thick circular muscle coat. The lumen is narrow, and the mucosa forms long folds. Schummer (1953) considered the function of the equine ileum. The cecum contains gas, often under considerable pressure during contractions. The heavy muscular wall and mucosal folds of the ileum provide for sealing the usually empty ileum, so that reflux of gas and ingesta from the cecum to the ileum does not occur. As well, the passage of ingesta from ileum to cecum must be against a pressure gradient, so that strong peristaltic activity is required of the ileum. One envisions a

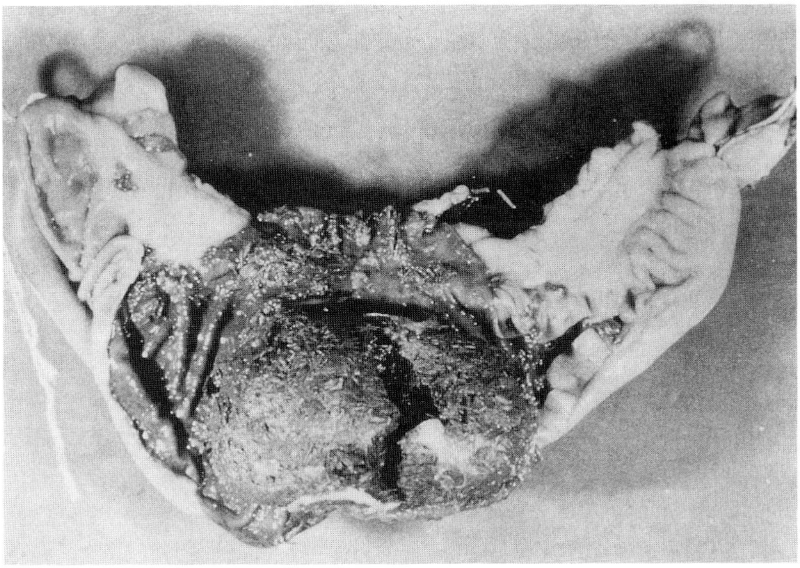

3.23. Figure 3.22 with the colon opened to show the impacted bolus.

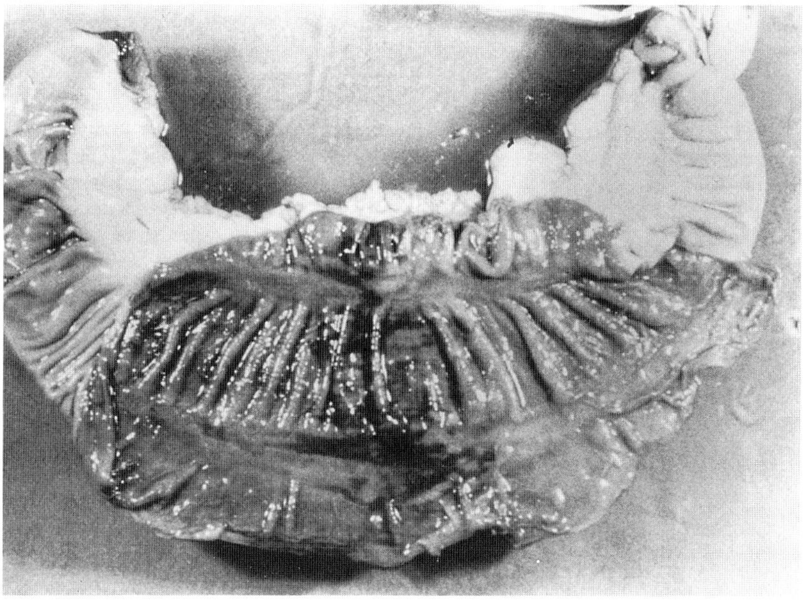

3.24. The bolus removed revealing an elongate focus of hemorrhage with a pale center in the mucosa, infarction, *S. vulgaris.*

peristaltic wave propelling material from the jejunum, through the ileum, and into the cecum, with the ileal lumen closing serially behind the moving mass of ingesta, preventing backflow of cecal ingesta into the ileum. A sphincter in the usual sense, is not present at the ileocecal orifice, the muscular ileum subserving that function.

Idiopathic muscular hypertrophy of the ileum has been reported by Schulte (1950), Cohrs (1961), Godglück (1967), Rooney and Jeffcott (1968), among others. It is uncommon, about 1% of fatal colics (Dobberstein and Dinter 1942; Steenhaut 1988). In a few cases stenosis, just distal to the hypertrophied area, was found as the result of scarring of mucosal lesions. This was attributed to the irritation of short-cut chaff or buckwheat straw (Hutyra and Marek 1926). In most cases no anatomical stenosis was apparent.

Rider (1932) reported muscular hypertrophy, apparently of the entire small intestine, in six ponies used in coal mines. Diverticula, protrusions of mucosa through the muscularis, were found in the mesenteric border. The cause was not determined. Five were Icelandic ponies and one a Shetland. Cohrs (1961) noted that diverticula are frequently found together with muscular hypertrophy of the ileum. Godglück (1967) defined these mucosal herniations through the muscularis as **false diverticula**. He noted that **true diverticula**, all layers of the intestine involved, could occur in horses with intestinal calculi and large quantities of sand in the gastrointestinal tract.

Chaffin et al. (1991) reported 10 cases. There was no apparent breed or sex predisposition, and the animals ranged from 5 to 18 years. Diverticula were present in 5 cases and hemamelasma ilei in 8. In a second report Chaffin et al. (1992) apparently added 1 case: 11 cases, 5 involving ileum only, 2 a segment of jejunum only, 2 jejunum and ileum, and 2 involving the entire small intestine. Diverticula were present in 1 jejunum and all 5 cases of hypertrophy of the ileum. Schulte (1950) reported 2 cases with diverticula, suggesting that damage caused by migration of strongyle larvae could be involved in the pathogenesis. Infestation of the cecum with *Anoplocephala perfoliata* has been suggested as causative, but those infestations are common, while muscular hypertrophy is not.

Impaction of the ileum

Dobberstein and Dinter (1942) found impaction of the ileum in about 11% of fatal colics. Huskamp (1982) had ileal impaction in about 9% of his surgical colics. Steenhaut (1988) encountered 1.3% among 151 surgical cases. Parks et al. (1989) reported 75 cases, but did not give the incidence. They stated that the condition was more common in certain areas such as the southeastern United States, and that Arabians and females were predisposed. Ileal impaction has been rare in our experience with Thoroughbred and Standardbred horses in Kentucky and the eastern United States and always associated with marked hemamelasma ilei.

Dobberstein and Dinter (1942) felt that improper feeds, such as finely chopped straw, could be a factor. They reported that this colic, as others, was more common in horses kept under urban conditions than in country horses. Parks et al. (1989) believed that fine consistency coastal bermuda hay was a factor in their area. Clarke et al. (1990) also suggested a relationship between fine or finely chopped feeds and ileal impaction. Both Dobberstein and Dinter and Parks et al. found that the frequency of ileal impaction increased up to middle age, about 10 years, and decreased thereafter. Dobberstein and Dinter noted that 75% of their cases occurred between May and October, although, again, the frequency of all colics is greater during these months.

In light of Schummer's (1953) description of the function of the ileum and observations of Argenzio (1975) and Alexander (1962), several suggestions can be offered for the pathogenesis of impaction of the ileum, hypertrophy of the ileum, volvulus, strangulation, and intussusception. Ischemia caused either by migrating strongyle larvae and/or by feed materials can be the initiating factor(s).

With ischemia of the ileum causing sudden ileus there can be volvulus, intussusception, or strangulation as a loop of jejunum bursts through the ileal mesentery. If the ischemia develops less rapidly and less completely, there could be inadequate propulsion of ingesta through the ileocecal orifice into the cecum, allowing ingesta to pile up in the ileum. Berry et al. (1986) showed depression of the motility of the ileum with exposure to either live or dead *S. vulgaris* larvae. Alexander (1952b) demonstrated that the ileum is very sensitive to anoxia.

Ischemia may also be involved in the pathogenesis of muscular (work) hypertrophy of the ileum. Chaffin et al. (1991) found hemamelasma ilei in 8 of their 10 cases. A general consideration is that the ileocecal junction is supplied by the ileal artery and nerves and the cecal arteries and nerves and that loss of neurovascular coordination, induced by ischemia or other factors, is the important factor for muscular hypertrophy and, perhaps, ileal impaction as well. (See "Cecal impaction" in this chapter.)

The reports of Dobberstein and Dintner, Parks et al, and Clarke et al. suggest that larval-induced ischemia need not be the only cause of impaction of the ileum, inherently fine food materials, such as bermuda hay or finely chopped roughages, being implicated.

Argenzio (1975) and Alexander (1962) found a marked accumulation of bicarbonate in the ingesta during its passage through the small intestine. The pH increased almost linearly from the stomach to reach values of 7 or more in the ileum (Colin 1886/1888; Smith 1917). The ingesta entering the cecum, then, was alkaline, one might say in preparation for buffering volatile fatty acids produced in the large intestine. Alexander (1962) likened this to the buffering action of saliva in the forestomach of the ruminant. The mechanism for this increase of bicarbonate in the ileum is not known (Argenzio 1975). One can but speculate that improper, too low, pH of the ileal contents could cause depressed motility, neurovascular incoordination, and ileal impaction. Surgeons might be interested to determine the pH in impactions of the ileum, at least, if not in impactions in every case.

As already suggested for colics in general, interaction of feed materials and verminous activity could be involved in any given case. For example, depressed motility of the ileum caused by transient ischemia of *S. vulgaris* larval migrations could allow piling up of fine feed material in the ileum, which could not be properly expelled into the cecum once normal motility returned.

Hemamelasma ilei

The infectious larvae of *S. vulgaris* invade the mucosa and submucosa of the ileum to find their way into the more distal jejunal arteries and the ileal artery as they migrate to the cranial mesenteric artery. It appears that those larvae that enter the vascular system of the mesenteric quadrant of the ileum proceed without impediment toward the cranial mesenteric artery. Those larvae that enter the vascular system of the antimesenteric quadrant, or fail to enter the vessels at all, apparently are delayed and subject to the action of defense mechanisms. The acute reaction to these larvae is marked greenish edema with hemorrhage, primarily in the serosa of the antimesenteric quadrant (Fig. 3.8). With progression the lesion becomes an elevated serosal plaque of greenish-black fibrous tissue, infiltrated with hemosiderophages, mononuclear cells, and eosinophils. Rarely, a portion of larva may be found in the lesion; polarized light can be helpful. This is known as **hemamelasma ilei**. Enigk (1950) offers a different explanation for the pathogenesis of these lesions.

Hemamelasma ilei is invariably found with intussusception of the ileum into the cecum. Several cases of impaction of the ileum were associated with severe hemamelasma ilei. Hemamelasma are also found, on occasion, in the jejunum as well as the ileum. Several foaling mares have died of peritonitis following rupture of the jejunum through such a hemamelasma, a *locus minoris resistentia*.

Lymphosarcoma

Lymphosarcoma of young horses seems to have some preference for the ileum, perhaps because of the normally higher frequency of lymphoid nodules in the ileum. Grossly, the ileum is enlarged and stiff with white masses infiltrating the submucosa and mucosa. Histologically, the lymphosarcoma is composed preponderantly of large, lymphoblastic type cells. Achilles found sarcomas, presumably lymphosarcomas, in the intestine of 0.2% of horses slaughtered in Leipzig (Hutyra and Marek 1926).

Granulomatous enteritis

This condition, largely though not entirely restricted to Standardbred horses, was described by Rooney in 1970. Cimprich (1974) reported 10 cases, 9 in Standardbreds. Lindberg (1984) added additional cases and said that the disease had been known for many years in Scandinavia. Younger animals seem more often affected by this chronic, debilitating disease characterized by intermittent diarrhea and/or colic. At postmortem the small intestine, particularly the ileum, is the site for nodular thickening of the lamina propria, submucosa, and serosa, often with adhesions to intestine or abdominal wall (Fig. 3.25). The lesions are firm, white, and often ulcerate into the ileal lumen. There may be involvement of the large intestine. The regional lymph nodes are enlarged, meaty, and edematous. Histologically, there is chronic, granulomatous enteritis with lymphocytes, mononuclear cells, and occasional eosinophils and multinucleated giant cells (Fig. 3.26). There is widespread villous atrophy. The microscopic changes are more widespread in the intestine than the gross lesions suggest. The regional and other lymph nodes (Lindberg 1984), are the site of lymphoid hyperplasia, as well as focal or diffuse infiltration of mononuclear cells. The cause is not known. (See the next section.)

Avian tuberculosis

Avian tuberculosis has been reported in horses (M'Faydean 1918; Leslie and Davies 1958; Mair et al. 1986; Beurgelt et al. 1988; Cline et al. 1991). The clinical signs and lesions in the intestinal tract are essentially identical to those described for granulomatous enteritis. It is unclear whether granulomatous enteritis and avian tuberculosis are the same disease in horses. Special techniques are necessary for culture, and stainable organisms may be difficult to find in tissue sections in a given case. Avian tuberculin is unreliable.

Eosinophilic gastroenteritis

Pass and Bolton (1982) and Lindberg et al. (1985) have described eosinophilic gastroenteritis, affecting both Thoroughbreds and Standardbreds. Lesions are found anywhere in the gastrointestinal tract, including esophagus, stomach, small and large intestine, as well as pancreas, bile duct, lymph nodes, and skin. Thickened mucosa was infiltrated by mast cells, lymphocytes, plasma cells, macrophages, and eosinophils. There were foci of caseation necrosis with central eosinophilic cores surrounded by eosinophils, giant cells, and other mononuclear cells. This condition may be that described in earlier literature as chronic catarrhal enteritis (Godglück 1967).

The histological lesions are essentially those described for helminth larval migrations in the liver and pancreas, equine nodular collagenolytic granu-

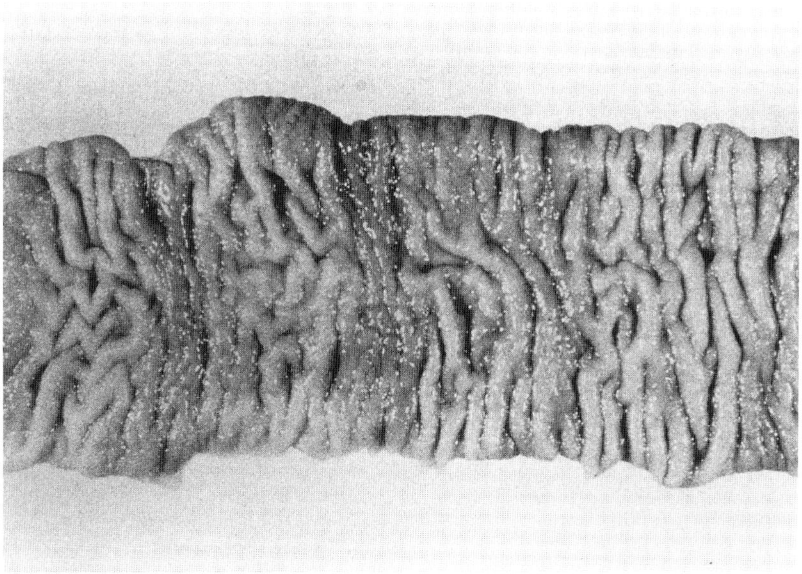

3.25. Marked thickening of the mucosa of the distal jejunum in granulomatous enteritis. A few less-involved patches are present among the thickened folds.

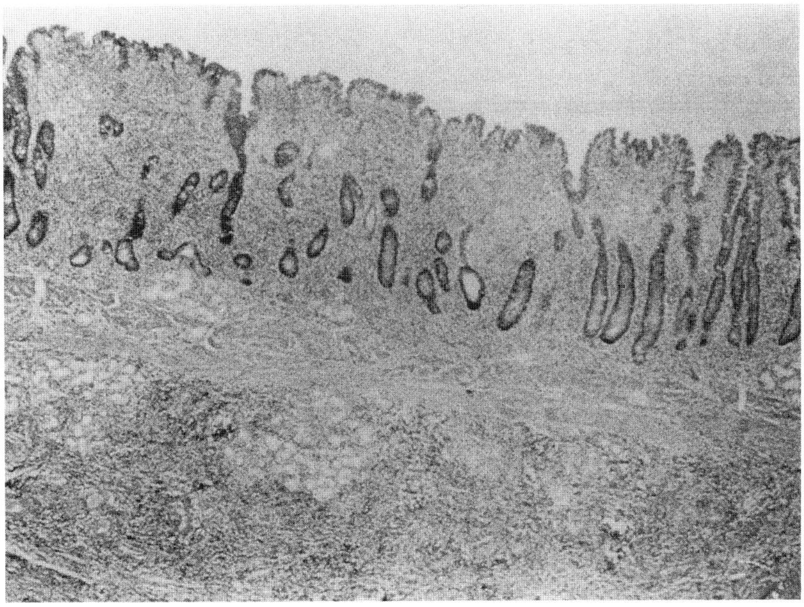

3.26. Low power of Figure 3.25 showing the infiltration of the mucosa with mononuclear inflammatory cells.

loma, some cases of arytenopathy, and the putative myositis related to sarcosporidia. While identity of lesions does not demand identity of etiology, at least a common final pathological pathway involving immune mechanisms seems probable. Sarcosporidia would appear good candidates. Pass and Bolton (1982) made an intensive but negative search for parasites. They injected material into the duodenum and ileum of one horse and produced serosal lesions, but discounted them as nonspecific.

Mycobacterium paratuberculosis

Johne's disease has not been reported as naturally occurring in equids. Eveleth (1943) found a number of horses positive by the johnin skin test, but there were no lesions at postmortem. Larsen et al. (1972) exposed young foals to the organism intravenously, intragastrically, and by contact and produced characteristic gross and microscopic lesions identical to those seen in cattle.

Volvulus, strangulation, and incarceration

These all involve the small intestine, although rare cases of volvulus of the descending colon have been mentioned (Keller and Horney 1985). About 5% of all colic deaths were caused by strangulation and incarceration (Dobberstein and Dinter 1942). Huskamp (1982) found these conditions in about 12%–13% of surgical colics. Volvulus was 6%–7% of all cases of fatal colic (Dobberstein and Dinter), and 5% of all cases of colic undergoing surgery (Huskamp). White (1987) found 4.3% among all cases of fatal and nonfatal colics. Among 98,249 cases of colic in Prussian army horses, 1.7% were volvulus.

As already noted the frequency of virtually all (the exceptions are noted below) of these conditions has declined precipitously with the advent of effective helminth control.

Volvulus

This is twisting of the small intestine around the mesenteric axis. It appears immediately upon opening the abdominal cavity as corkscrew coils of dark red small intestine (Fig. 3.27). The twisting may be in either direction and 180 degrees or more. The distal extent of the twisting has always been the jejunal-ileal junction, in our experience. Dobberstein and Dinter (1942) indicate that the ileum is not so frequently included. The proximal extent is variable, occasionally extending as far as the duodenocolic ligament, that is, the entire jejunum.

Careful examination of blood vessels in many cases has shown consistent evidence of *S. vulgaris* activity, although it may not be possible, in a given case, to point to a specific lesion as directly responsible. Those comments apply as well to strangulation and some cases of incarceration.

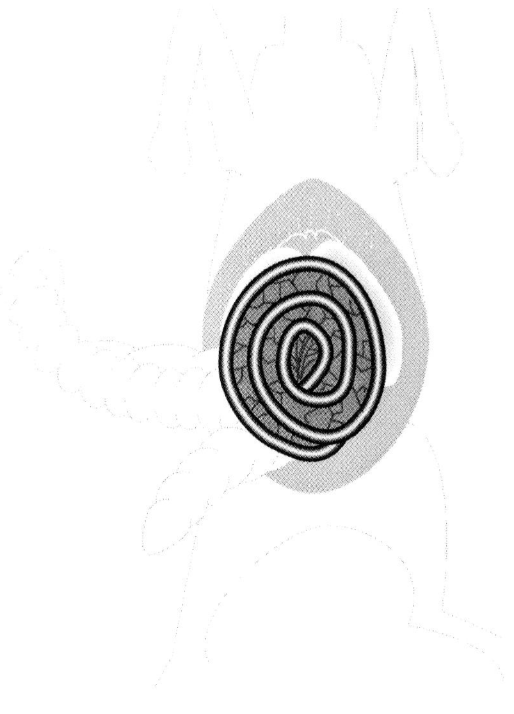

3.27. Schematic of volvulus of the small intestine in situ.

Strangulation

This is a loop of intestine tying a knot upon itself without rupturing the mesentery. This may occur any place in the small intestine, but is most frequent in the distal jejunum and ileum.

Incarceration

This is entrapment of a loop of small intestine through a rent in the mesentery, usually the distal jejunum and ileum. While it appears that tearing of the mesentery and entrapment of gut occur as a single event, in some cases the rent is older with smooth, rounded edges. Such healed rents in the mesentery are found incidentally at postmortem, indicating that they occur without necessarily entrapping gut.

Kopf et al. (1979) suggested that mesenteric rents occur as the result of transient intussusception. This would seem unlikely in view of the rarity of intussusception per se in the adult horse. A more general pathogenesis suggests segmental ileus occasioned by strongyle larval migration, with a peristaltic wave "stumbling over" such a segment and tearing the mesentery.

Special incarcerations

With the possible exceptions of splenorenal incarceration, gastrosplenic incarceration, and incarceration through the lesser omentum, these special incarcerations are not related to *S. vulgaris* migrations.

Epiploic foramen

This is incarceration of a loop of small intestine through the epiploic foramen, primarily in older horses (Fig. 3.28). It is usually but not invariably associated with atrophy of the right lobe of the liver. Such atrophy is accompanied by an increase in size of the foramen, and that is predisposing. The gut usually breaks through the greater omentum into the omental bursa, proceeding through the foramen from medial to lateral. The blackish-red, distended loop of intestine is apparent in the cranial quadrant of the abdomen on the right side immediately upon opening the abdominal cavity. Herniation of the loop of intestine from lateral to medial has also been described (Cohrs 1961; Huskamp 1982), but is much less common. In the 1900s about 0.2% of all colic deaths were epiploic incarcerations (Hutyra and Marek 1920). Huskamp found epiploic incarceration in 8.4% of all cases submitted for surgery, suggesting an older population. Steenhaut (1988) encountered 4.6% among his surgical cases.

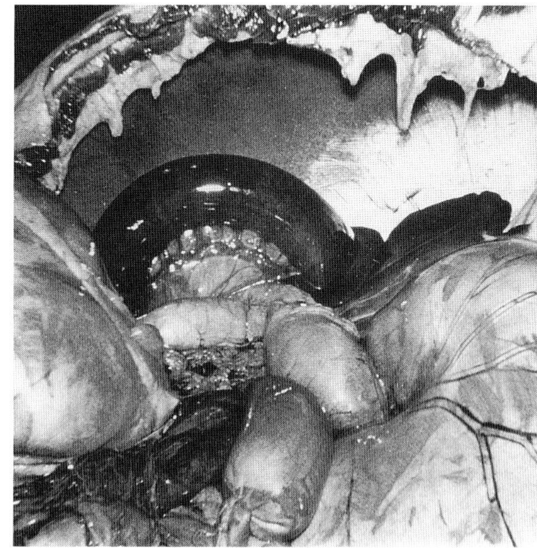

3.28. Incarceration of the jejunum through the epiploic foramen.

Lesser omentum

Incarceration of small intestine through the lesser omentum between the lesser curvature of the stomach and the liver is rare. Incarceration within the omental bursa has been described (Cohrs 1961). We have seen no case.

Gastroplenic ligament

Three cases of incarceration have been seen, one of which was the pelvic flexure of the large intestine and the others, jejunum. Yovich et al. (1985b) reported five cases, noting that the distal jejunum or ileum was incarcerated. It is difficult to understand how the ileum could be involved, given the usual anatomical definition of *ileum*.

Diaphragmatic hernia

These have long been known [Cartwright (1828) cited by Smith (1976)]. They are congenital or acquired. The congenital form is a smooth opening in the left dorsal part of the diaphragm. Acquired, traumatic, ruptures of the diaphragm may affect any portion, particularly the tendinous part of the diaphragm and the musculotendinous junction. Wimberly et al. (1977) reviewed 18 cases. The pathogenesis must be related to excessive abdominal pressure, whether generated by internal or external factors. Of all colic deaths in Prussian military horses, 0.4% were related to diaphragmatic hernias (397 cases in 98,248 fatal colics) in the late 1800s and early 1900s (Hutyra and Marek 1920). Huskamp (1982) had 5 cases among his 785 surgical colic cases (0.6%). Krause (1930/31) reviewed 54 cases, in which 1 congenital case was associated with agenesia of the left kidney. Steenhaut (1988) found about 1% among his surgical cases.

Although it would appear obvious, **postmortem rupture** of the diaphragm is frequently misinterpreted. This rupture occurs in the diaphragm adjacent to the xiphoid cartilage. While the edges are ragged and torn, there is no hemorrhage. Antemortem ruptures in this area have not been seen. There are many case reports of diaphragmatic hernia in the older literature. While some are bona fide acquired or congenital hernias, many, inadequately described, may have been postmortem ruptures.

Scrotal hernias

These occur occasionally in stallions, but appear to be uncommon in light horses.

Umbilical hernia

Congenital umbilical hernias are not uncommon, specifically in Thoroughbred foals. They are treated surgically and do not come to postmortem except as incidental findings (see Chapter 12, "Neonate.")

Herniation through persistent **urachal duct** tissue and the **falciform ligament** have been reported (Cohrs 1961). Herniation may occur through postsurgical adhesions, but it is moot whether these are to be called hernias or incarcerations.

Incarceration by lipomas

Lipomas of the mesentery, and epicardial fatty tissue, occur in older horses and increase in frequency with age. When such fatty masses reach sufficient size, they become pedunculated and undergo ischemic necrosis and calcification. Eventually the long, thin pedicle ties a half-hitch around a loop of jejunum and incarceration occurs (Fig. 3.29). Together with incarceration through the epiploic foramen, it is a common cause of fatal colic in the older horse. These tumors were recognized in horses at least as early as 1829 [Goodwin cited by Smith (1976); Mègnin (1878) cited by Cadeac (1893); and Aulage (1891)].

Splenorenal incarceration

This may be considered either a displacement or an incarceration of gut into the space formed by the left kidney, the splenorenal ligament, the head of the spleen, and the sublumbar tissue. The small intestine, descending colon, or left dorsal and ventral colon may be entrapped (Cohrs 1961). Entrapment of the left dorsal and ventral colon is apparently most common, the displacement occurring either from cranial to caudal or between the left abdominal wall and the spleen (Hutyra and Marek 1920, 1926; Huskamp 1980, 1982). Huskamp found splenorenal incarceration in 9.9% of his surgical colics. Steenhaut (1988) found 4.6%. The condition appears to be commoner in large, 4- to 8-year-old geldings of Warm blood or draft type (Huskamp and Kopf 1980). It is uncommon in other breeds.

The pathogenesis is unclear. Splenic engorgement with blood is usually present, and it is possible that ventral displacement of the spleen provides the pathway for displacement between the spleen and the lateral abdominal wall. It is equally possible, and more probable, that the splenic engorgement occurs after the entrapment. Carlström (1926/27) overfilled the stomach with water in living horses after tying off the duodenum and produced

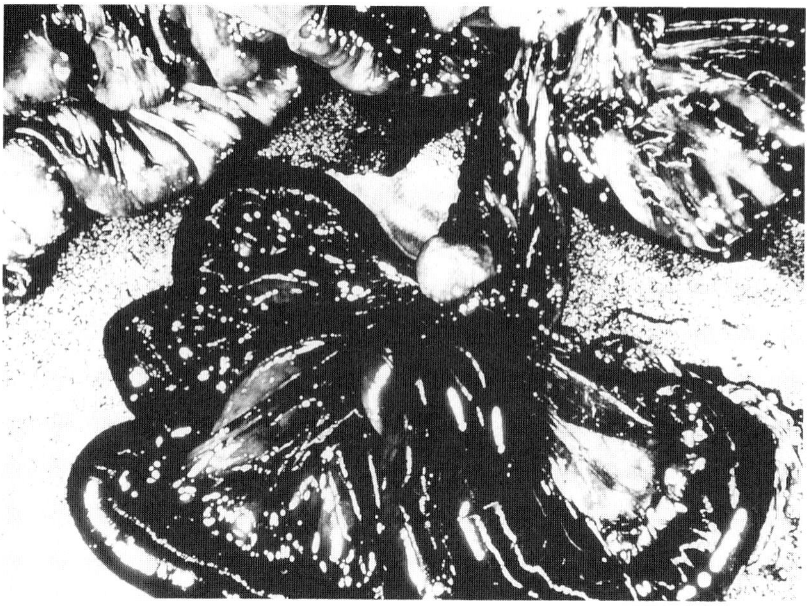

3.29. Lipoma strangulation of the jejunum.

splenorenal incarceration. Ventral displacement of the stomach and spleen probably provided the pathway for displacement. The role of dead space as a predisposing factor for gut displacement has been discussed elsewhere in this chapter (see "Gastrointestinal tract: Normal features," above).

Intussusception

Intussusception of the jejunum is most frequent in suckling foals (Fig. 3.30). Intussusception of the ileum into the cecum can occur at any age but is most frequent in younger horses, about a year of age (Cadeac 1896; Ford et al. 1990). In our experience ileocecal intussusception almost invariably occurs in the presence of marked hemamelasma ilei. Occasionally, there is an intussusception of the descending colon and/or rectum in postparturient mares, with tearing of the mesocolon and significant hemorrhage.

Agonal intussusception of the small intestine is common in young foals and usually differentiable from the antemortem lesion by the absence of significant signs of vascular stasis and inflammation. Intussusception with moderate stasis and petechiation, intermediate in severity between obvious agonal intussusception and obvious severe intussusception, may be the cause of illness and death, that is, shock causing death before marked signs of stasis in the affected intestine. The diagnosis is problematic but may be correct in any given case.

True intussusception occurs at any point in the jejunum and often is multiple. Not infrequently it is double, with the first intussusception providing the segmental ileus for the second, overlapping intussusception. In most cases no precipitating cause is found, though ascarids and/or evidence of *S. vulgaris* migration may be present. One is left to postulate immature neural controlling mechanisms as the important predisposing factor, consistent with

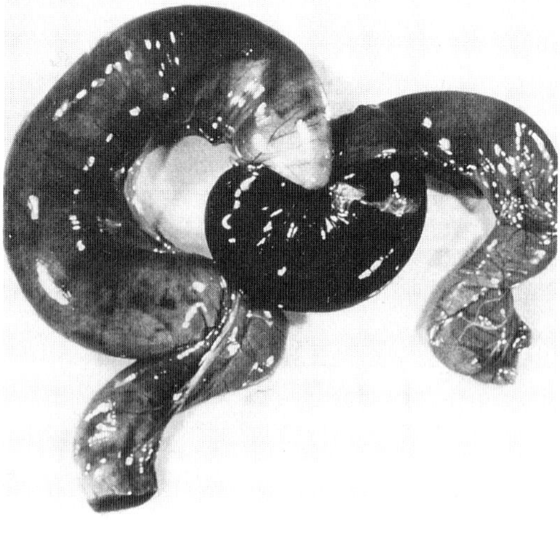

3.30. Intussusception of the jejunum of a foal. In fact, this is a double intussusception, the first forming the area of ileus for the development of the second.

the observation of Laplace (1972) that irregular neuromuscular activity was commoner in the small intestine of younger pigs than older. (See Chapter 12, "Neonate.")

Cecum

Teniae and haustra

The cecum and colon are characterized by concentration of the external layer of the muscularis into bands or **teniae**. These are largely composed of elastic tissue in the cecum and ventral colon, largely muscular in the dorsal colon (Burns 1992), and almost entirely muscular in the descending colon (Sisson and Grossman 1953). The cecum and colon form haustra demarcated on the luminal side by **plicae semilunares ceci (coli)**. If the teniae are removed the haustra disappear (Zietzschmann et al. 1943). This is easily demonstrated by tensing the descending colon and transecting the teniae, particularly the one in the mesenteric border. The haustra provide a greater surface area for a given length of intestine. It appears that the teniae evolved with the development of haustra and, together with the active circular muscle layer, maintain the haustra (Jacobshagen 1937).

The variation in relative amounts of elastic and smooth muscular tissue in the several parts of the cecum and colon has not been helpfully addressed (Burns 1992). The relative increase of muscle vis-a-vis elastic tissue in the dorsal and small colon suggests a need for active adjustment of haustral size, as compared to the passive maintenance of haustral size characteristic of the cecum and ventral colon. A reason for such need is not immediately apparent.

Impaction

There is a considerable European, specifically German, literature (Hallmich 1939) on chronic cecal impaction. The frequency has decreased in the modern era. Dobberstein and Dinter (1942) found 17.6% of all fatal cases of colic between 1922 and 1940 to be chronic cecal impaction. Huskamp, writing in Germany in 1981, recorded only 0.4% among his cases of surgical colic. Steenhaut in 1988 found about 1%. Campbell et al. (1984) reported 21 cases in Florida over a 3-year period, but gave no incidence data. Our autopsy experience with North American light horses from 1960 to 1991 accords with that of Huskamp.

Older horses are more commonly affected than younger. There is an increase in the amount and dryness of the cecal content, together with increased thickness of the circular layer of the muscularis. The submucosa may be fibrotic, and the entire cecum is leathery and stiff. Fibrotic tags on the serosal surface are common. When many cases were seen, over 70% died of peritonitis after rupture of the cecum.

The pathogenesis is unclear (Cohrs 1961). Gratzl (1934a,b) believed that cramping contractions of the musculature between the base and body caused impaction in the base, specifically the cupula, so that the latter folded over on the lesser curvature, impeding the outflow of ingesta from the cecum through the cecocolic orifice into the right ventral colon. He cited an in vitro study of Ellenberger (1917) in which water was run into the cecum through the ileum. The cecum filled with water that did not escape through the cecocolic orifice. The head of the cecum folded over more and more on the lesser curvature as the cecum filled. While this speaks to his hypothesis, it also suggests that muscular activity is necessary for emptying through the cecocolic orifice, and that loss of such activity (see below) is the causative factor in impaction of the cecum and the eventual muscular hypertrophy caused by such impaction.

Dyce et al. (1976) studied the normal transport of ingesta and gas through the base of the cecum and the cecocolic orifice into the right ventral colon. Ross et al. (1986) provided additional observations. Emptying through the cecocolic orifice was accomplished by contraction of muscles of the cecal base, isolating a mass of ingesta in the cupula and raising its floor, so that the cecocolic orifice opened passively. The mass of ingesta followed an essentially sigmoid pathway from the cupula into the right ventral colon. The contraction of the muscles of the base of the cecum raised the floor of the cecum because of the connective tissue attachments of the base to the sublumbar area. These observations essentially confirmed those of Gratzl, but showed that his cramping contractions were, in fact, normal.

Gratzl (1934a,b) reported a marked increase in the number of cases of chronic cecal impaction associated with an economic crisis and widespread use of automotive transportation, conditions leading to poor feeding and care of horses. It might be suggested that heavy food materials accumulating in the cecum and, specifically in the base, would act against the muscular work that raises the floor of the cupula, inhibiting or preventing opening of the cecocolic orifice. "Heavy food materials" is vague. More properly, one could say food materials that are not readily and rapidly broken down to a finer mash within the cecum, remaining in agglomerated, dense masses, not as readily moved by contraction of the cecal muscles.

Some additional light may be thrown on the pathogenesis by consideration of experimental infection of worm-free ponies with *S. edentatus*. Infection with large numbers of larvae induced marked thrombosis and fibrosis of the neurovascular complexes of the medial and lateral cecal vessels. The cecal veins are the route for *S. edentatus* larvae from the cecal mucosa to the liver (McGraw and Slocombe 1974, 1978). Accompanying these lesions was marked musculofibrous hypertrophy/hyperplasia of the cecal wall: fibrosis of the submucosa and increased thickness of the circular muscle layer.

Based on these findings ischemia appears to be at least one cause of chronic cecal impaction, but it cannot be said that massive cecal vascular disease is always or even often the cause. It does seem to be the case that failure of emptying through the cecocolic orifice is the basic pathogenetic mechanism, whether purely mechanical or caused by ischemia.

Ross et al. (1986) suggested that a pacemaker somewhere in the cecum initiated contraction of the body, propelling ingesta into the base and cupula and, hence, through the cecocolic orifice. The lateral cecal artery, with its accompanying nerves, provides a dorsal branch to the base and cupula of the cecum and to the first part of the right ventral colon as well as the ventral branch to the body and apex of the cecum. The pathway for such a putative pacemaker, then, may be sought in the dorsal branch of the lateral cecal artery and nerves, which supply the area concerned with cecocolic emptying. Disruption of the activity coordinated along this pathway may be the pathogenesis for one form of chronic cecal impaction.

An additional factor, quite apart from consistency of ingesta or verminous ischemia, is the microbial digestive processes in the cecum. The cecal and colonic content is normally buffered to near neutral pH. If a large quantity of rapidly fermentable substrate is presented to the cecum, the production of volatile fatty acids and gas would be expected to increase markedly as in the stomach of the horse and in the forestomachs of ruminants. The volatile fatty acids lower the pH. This, together with the greater availability of carbohydrate, would encourage lactic acid production, further depressing the pH. The lower pH, then, could be associated with depression of cecal motility and eventual impaction (Argenzio 1975). This scenario has already been adduced as an explanation for the pathogenesis of gastric ulceration and may well apply here as well, the pH dropping sufficiently to induce partial atony of the cecum but not ulceration. In that regard the stratified squamous epithelium of the stomach is susceptible to pH-related damage, while the epithelium of the fundus and pylorus are normally exposed to lower pH values. Similar resistance may be true for the cecal mucosa even though it is normally not exposed to a low pH.

Intussusception

Intussusception of the cecal apex into the body and intussusception of the cecum partly or wholly into the right ventral colon are rarely seen (Wintzer 1986; Huskamp 1981). We have not seen a case.

Rupture

Rupture of, particularly, the head of the cecum may be seen as the terminal event of chronic cecal impaction. Rare case reports indicate that external trauma of sufficient magnitude can cause rupture of the cecum (Piot-Bey 1912).

Rupture of the cecum occurs in the postparturient mare. The rupture is in the middle third of the medial surface and may be obscured by the cecocolic ligament. The mucosa bulges out through the ruptured muscularis and serosa, characteristic of rupture by increased luminal pressure. While the precise sequence of events is not known, it is apparent that large increases of abdominal pressure during foaling are relevant. Retroflexion of the cecum into the pelvic cavity during foaling could permit pressure sufficient for rupture (Rooney 1970). Such retroflexion of the cecum occurs normally; at least, it is found on occasion at postmortem without pathological change.

Colon

Ascending colon

Congenital Defects

Atresias

Atresia ani and atresia coli are among the commoner congenital defects of horses, though rare even then, with a frequency in the population of about 0.4% (Nappert 1992). No breed predisposition has been reported. Atresia coli usually involves aplasia of the pelvic flexure of the ascending colon. Occasionally, hypoplasia of this area is seen as a segment of narrow, hoselike colon. Some with such hypoplasia had survived for a considerable time with intermittent bouts of obstructive colic. This is to be differentiated from chronic obstruction with musculofibrous hyperplasia.

Hultgren (1982) and Vonderfecht et al. (1983) described a congenital, no doubt genetic, defect of the small intestine and colon in overo foals. These foals have white hair and pink skin, sometimes with pigmented patches. They show colic soon after birth. The ascending and descending colon and rectum lack both myenteric and submucosal ganglia and are narrow, pale, and inactive. Ganglia are also missing in the ileum and at least part of the jejunum, but present elsewhere.

Salmonellosis

Salmonellosis is an enzootic/epizootic disease of young foals. Once introduced to a farm, the organism tends to persist and infect successive crops of foals. Salmonella can also cause serious illness and death in older horses otherwise under duress because of illness, surgical procedures, and so forth (Hansen et al. 1971; Bryans 1972a). It is important as a persistent contaminant of veterinary hospitals and clinics. *Salmonella typhimurium* and *S. enteriditis* are the usual species, though others have been incriminated in individual outbreaks.

Peracute: These occur in the early phases of an outbreak. Death is within hours of onset of clinical signs. The serosa of the large intestine is severely hyperemic with fine, freckling petechiation. The mucosa of the large intestine, particularly cecum and ventral colon, is intensely hyperemic and even hemorrhagic, while ingesta is thin, watery, and yellowish or blood-tinged (see Fig. 3.34). The other organs and tissues show nonspecific signs of septicemia.

Acute: Similar changes with grayish focal necrosis of the solitary lymphoid nodules of the large intestine. These progress to abscessation and ulceration. Mucosal hyperemia and hemorrhage is less diffuse and more localized to the necrotic nodules. Systemic signs of septicemia become less obvious with more prolonged disease.

The histological lesions are as the gross findings in the peracute case. In the acute case severe degenerative, necrotizing changes are seen in the lymphoid nodules with large numbers of neutrophils. A characteristic but inconstant change is thrombosis of submucosal venules and veins. Focal proliferation of reticuloendothelial cells in the liver is not usually found, though Baumann and Gratzl (1931) found such foci in 3 of 6 adult horses dying of salmonellosis.

In protracted cases there may be fatty degeneration of the liver and renal tubules. Multiple foci of myofiber degeneration and necrosis, cloudy swelling, fatty change, and dystrophic calcification may be found in the heart. These appear grossly as white or yellowish flecks and streaks in the myocardium.

Rhodococcus equi infection

This disease is described with the respiratory system (see Chapter 2, "Respiratory System"). While not invariable, involvement of the large intestine in *R. equi* infections is common. Intractable diarrhea is the predominant clinical sign. The organism localizes initially in the solitary lymph nodules of the mucosa and submucosa with focal inflammation and caseopurulent necrosis. The cecocolic lymph nodes are invariably involved with caseopurulent necrotizing inflammation.

Torsion

Torsion of the cecum or descending colon is rare; we have not seen a case.

There are two forms of torsion of the ascending colon: **partial** and **complete**. The first, extensively described in the older literature (Cadeac 1896; Drechsler 1958), is torsion of the left dorsal and ventral colon with the limits at the sternal and diaphragmatic flexures (Fig. 3.31). This was, apparently, the main type of torsion recognized prior to about 1960. The frequency varied, by author, from 0.1% to 7% of all cases of colic (Dobberstein and Dinter 1942). Since 1960 no more than a dozen cases of this type of torsion have been seen in over 10,000 autopsies, primarily light horses. Those dozen cases were all seen before the advent of modern anthelmintics.

Huskamp (1981), in a population of Warm bloods and light horses, found 2.3% partial torsions as compared to 17.2% total ascending colon torsion among 785 cases of surgical colic. Snyder et al. (1989a,b) indicated that 11%–17% of surgical colics involved the entire ascending colon. Of 57 cases of torsion of the colon, 1 involved only the left dorsal and ventral colon. Steenhaut (1988) found partial torsion in 4.5% and complete torsion in 3.3% of his 151 cases in Belgium. White (1987) gave 10.6% of all colics for torsion and displacement of the large colon combined. Reeks (1911) mentioned this type of torsion and did not mention complete torsion.

In our dozen cases, histologically confirmed verminous emboli were in the dorsal and ventral colic arteries at the sternal/diaphragmatic flexures.

In the 1960s an occasional case of torsion of the entire ascending colon was seen at postmortem (less than 1% of the autopsy population) primarily in older horses. In recent literature torsion of the colon is often referred to as volvulus. While not incorrect, we prefer the term, torsion, avoiding confusion with volvulus of the small intestine. At postmortem the ascending colon was distended with

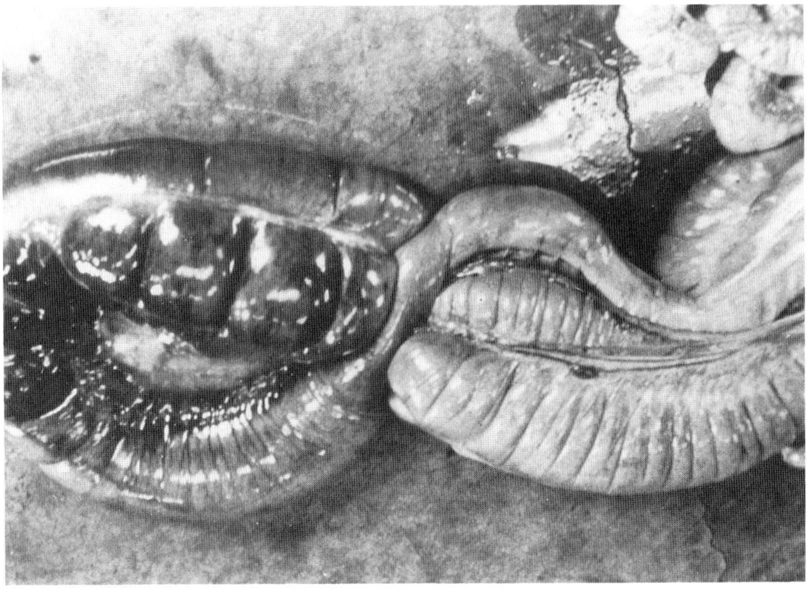

3.31. Torsion of the colon at the sternal-diaphragmatic flexure.

fluid and gas and appeared bluish, cyanotic, on the serosal surface. The limits of the torsion were the origin of the right ventral colon and the right dorsal colon. The mucosa was intensely hyperemic with blood-tinged moderate to severe submucosal edema. The gross and microscopic picture was identical to exhaustion shock with, of course, the absence of torsion in the latter. There was no correlation with verminous arteritis, thrombosis, or embolism. Atrophy of the right lobes of the liver was present in many but not all cases.

Since the 1960s, the frequency of torsion of the entire ascending colon has increased, particularly in broodmares and larger horses (Huskamp 1981). Huskamp reported that in broodmares torsion often coincided with change from winter feeding to early, lush spring pasture. Snyder et al. (1990) reported 42 broodmares (21 postparturient), 8 stallions, and 7 geldings in 57 cases. Seventeen cases occurred in the spring, 24 in summer, 11 in autumn, and 5 in winter. Harrison (1988) had 73 mares among 122 cases; 31 were pregnant or had foaled within 10 days. The status of the other 42 was not given.

The predilection for older broodmares and large horses indicates that sufficient dead space is available for torsion to occur. That is obvious in the broodmare soon after foaling and could occur, somewhat less obviously, in the older mare and horse with the gradual loss of tone of abdominal muscles, age-related atrophy of the right lobes of the liver, and a low-fiber diet. The immediate event would appear to be the presence of considerable quantities of fermentable materials in the ventral colon. The dorsal colon is normally drier than the ventral and with less fermentable content. The production of gas at a greater rate than can be absorbed or moved down the tract would allow the ventral colon to rise on the medial side of the dorsal colon and turn clockwise (rear view) around the dorsal colon. Intermittent grazing, sudden change from hay to lush, fertilized grass pasture, or feeding of fermentable materials—all as opposed to natural free range grazing—would entail greater intake per unit of time and contribute to overproduction of gas. Basically, predisposing is the shifting of the diet from natural, coarse-fiber, stemmy grasses to pellets, alfalfa hay, and the finer flora of so-called improved pastures with the consequent decrease in fiber intake, gut fill. As Janis (1976) has clearly demonstrated, the horse evolved as a coarse-fiber-eating animal, and the basic, predisposing factor for this form of gut malposition is dead space, in part a function of the physical nature of the food materials. The received wisdom of timothy hay may not suit modern nutritional theory, but it certainly suits the evolutionary biology of equids.

Epidemiological studies of broodmares with torsion of the colon in central Kentucky found no relationships with estrogen content of pasturage, a variety of weather factors, type of pasture plants, or grain feeding (Moore et al. 1991; Yenne et al. 1991; Dreesen 1991; Boudinot et al. 1991). These studies did not address the considerations given above.

Another displacement of the ascending colon was described by Reeks (1911). The pelvic flexure was folded upon itself or, less frequently, twisted upon itself. There was significant congestion and hemorrhage. We have seen no example or other reports. Reeks believed this to be distinct from impaction, but impaction would seem the reasonable, if unrecognized cause.

Descending colon

Dart et al. (1991a,b) reviewed 102 cases of abnormalities of the descending colon. Arabian horses, ponies, American Miniature horses and animals over 15 years of age were more commonly affected. Enteroliths were more common between 5 and 10 years and not seen in animals 2 years or less. Impaction and strangulating lipomas were commoner after 15 years. There is further discussion with specific entities, elsewhere in this chapter.

Impactions

Impactions are commonest in the large intestine. As with chronic cecal impaction, the frequency of such impactions seems to have decreased in the modern era. Dobberstein and Dinter (1942) reported about 15% of all cases as impaction of the large intestine, while Huskamp (1981) reported only about 2%, including sand colic. White (1987) reported 7.3% of all fatal and nonfatal colics as impaction of the large colon. Our experience in North America accords with that of Huskamp in Germany.

The pelvic flexure of the ascending colon and, particularly, the right dorsal/transverse colon junction are the common sites of impaction. There are two clinical syndromes. The first is the single or acute/subacute impaction, which resolves with medical and/or surgical treatment and rarely comes to postmortem. The second is the chronic or, more accurately, recurring form, which eventually does come to postmortem because of owner despair or rupture and peritonitis.

At postmortem the site of impaction is defined by the enlarged viscus proximal and collapsed viscus distal to the site of impaction. If rupture has occurred, it is always proximal to the site of impaction. In the acute or subacute case the wall of the colon is of normal thickness. In the recurring case the wall of the colon proximal to the site of impaction is thickened by musculofibrous hypertrophy/hyperplasia for a variable distance. This is a true *work hypertrophy*. It is a characteristic change, recognizable both at surgery and at postmortem. The serosal surface appears whiter than normal and may have fibrous tags. The wall is palpably thickened. In some cases there may be little impacted ingesta present, the musculofibrous hyperplasia having become self-standing. Histologically, the circular muscle layer is thicker than normal. The submucosa and mucosa are often somewhat thinned with fibrosis of the submucosa. The muscularis mucosae are not thickened.

Several factors are to be considered in the pathogenesis of any given case of acute or subacute and recurring impaction of the large intestine. Rarely, a definite stenosis of the gut is found as the cause. In the very young foal this may be an *atresia coli* or *aplasia coli* of the pelvic flexure of the ascending colon. *Hypoplasia coli* of the pelvic flexure has been seen. In one remarkable instance, an 11-year-old mare with such hypoplasia had a history of recurring colic since a foal.

In most cases of impaction the cause is not so apparent. Interesting epidemiological observations have been made by Dobberstein and Dinter (1942) and Dobberstein (1950), incriminating the unnatural feeding of city horses as compared to the more natural feeding of horses in the country (Janis 1976). There seems to be little doubt from this and the observations of many others over many years that feeding controlled by humans is the major factor in impactions of the large intestine.

Pastured horses, however, may develop impactions. Migrating *S. vulgaris* larvae cause transient ischemia with impaction/obstipation as the obvious clinical sign. Usually, cases of impaction of the pelvic flexure and transverse/dorsal colon come to postmortem long after the initiating event, and such signs of larval activity as may be present cannot be certainly established as the cause of ischemia, ileus, or impaction. The case is somewhat stronger at the pelvic flexure where verminous granulomatous masses may be present in the mesocolon, though not always associated with impaction.

The important local sites for ileus are the duodenum, ileum, pelvic flexure, and transverse/dorsal colon. In the duodenum, ileum, and transverse colon, the vascular supply comes from two separate sources. That is, the duodenum receives its arterial supply from the gastroepiploic branch of the celiac artery proximally and the first jejunal branches of the cranial mesenteric artery distally. The ileum receives its supply from the last jejunal artery and the ileal artery, a branch of the ileocecocolic artery. The transverse colon/dorsal colon is supplied proximally by the middle colic branch of the ileocecocolic artery, while the distal supply is from the caudal mesenteric artery. The pelvic flexure is the site of end-to-end anastomosis of the dorsal and ventral colic arteries.

While these anatomical considerations, of themselves, do not explain ileus, one may suggest circulatory events relevant to ischemia and ileus which are flagged by these *vascular borderlands*. An additional consideration for the right dorsal/transverse colon junction are the physiological differences and susceptibility of this area to a specific small strongyle lesion, phenylbutazone, and *E. risticii* infection as already discussed.

Dobberstein and Dinter found 0.7% of all cases of colic to be **impaction of the descending colon**. Other earlier authors found similarly low frequencies. By contrast Tennant et al. (1972), in California, reported a frequency of about 9% among 453 cases, half in Shetland ponies. They, also, found a higher frequency in the winter and early spring, unlike most forms of colic.

Sand impaction

Sand is a clear cause of impaction, primarily in the right dorsal/transverse colon but, occasionally, in other parts of the large intestine. It is seen in areas with sandy soils under such conditions as overstocking, drought, and feeding on the ground.

Enterolithiasis

This condition decreased in Germany as the number of working horses decreased (Keller 1957). It may be true that fewer horses meant fewer cases of enterolithiasis, but horse numbers, in North America at least, are probably as large as ever and, in some areas at least, the frequency of enterolithiasis is not trivial.

The enterolith is almost invariably at the junction of the right dorsal/transverse colon (Cadeac 1896). They are variable in size and characterized by concentric layers on section. It has been suggested that each layer represents a meal. Fürstenberg, cited by Cadeac (1896), recognized an enterolith with 720 layers and, assuming two meals a day, arrived at an enterolith age of 360 days. Cadeac warns, however, that such age determination may not be completely accurate.

A number of etiological factors have been suggested:

1. Horses working for millers and bakers had a high incidence (Keller 1957).
2. The modern, cultivated oat has no hairs on the hull, and these hairs apparently served as a matted nidus for enterolith formation (Cohrs 1961).
3. Most horses today are for pleasure and/or have considerable monetary value unlike the roughly cared for draft horse of earlier times. The idle farm horse often roughed through the winter on very poor quality feed. In the spring and summer, the draft horse often went long periods without water, and marginal or frank dehydration was not uncommon. Such dehydration could, at least in principle, predispose to enterolith formation.

Blue (1979) reported 30 cases of enterolithiasis in California, about 7% of all colics. This may be compared with the frequency in Prussian military horses (1895–1914) of 2.5% of all fatal colics, 0.27% of all colics, and 0.013% of all horses (Keller 1957). In most of Blue's cases the enterolith lodged in the transverse colon. He suggested alfalfa hay as a possible factor, alfalfa hay being common in California and the southwestern part of the United States. Alfalfa hay, however, is commonly used for horses in many other areas.

Lloyd (1987) provided a thorough review of enterolithiasis, specifically in high-risk California. Arabian horses were at greater risk than other breeds and most cases were 9 years of age or older. The enteroliths were always magnesium ammonium phosphate hexahydrate, *struvite*, as Colin had observed in 1859 (Cadeac 1896; Fröhner 1905). Lloyd suggested that a foreign body nidus was required, as noted by earlier authors (Colin 1886/1888; Cadeac). In the case of the millers' horses, bits of the grindstone used for milling were incriminated. The hairs on oat hulls were another nidus.

Hutyra and Marek (1926) and Barker and van Dreumel (1985) suggested that the major source of the magnesium phosphate was grain. Normally, the phosphate in grain is ionized in the stomach and the phosphate absorbed in the small intestine. Nonionized magnesium phosphate, reaching the large intestine, combines with ammonia produced by the bacterial digestion of protein to form magnesium ammonium phosphate. Feeding large amounts of grain may, therefore, be a factor in enterolithiasis. "Large amounts" is relative, of course. If the grain were ingested over a period of time, gastric digestion and ionization of phosphate could proceed apace. Taken as two discrete bolus meals a day, however, an overload of nonionized magnesium phosphate could be delivered to the large intestine.

Hintz and Snyder (1992) indicated that enterolithiasis was more common in California and in the southern United States with Arabians and Morgans at greatest risk. These geographical and breed frequencies are unexplained, but the former may be related to availability of the required nidus and heavy grain feeding. None of the North American studies appear to have included search for the nidus.

Foreign body obstruction

Foreign bodies are infrequent causes of obstruction. Usually the foreign material obstructs the right dorsal colon at the junction with the transverse colon or the transverse colon itself. Baling twine is a common culprit. When recycled automobile tires were used for fencing material, horses developed an appetite for the rubber with obstruction of the right dorsal and/or transverse colon the result.

Acute/chronic diarrhea

This is a poorly defined condition, most often but not exclusively seen in younger horses in training or work. Foals are not affected. Typically, only one animal is affected. There is sudden illness with fever, depression, and mild or severe diarrhea. The animal may die within 48 hours or appear to recover, only to have diarrhea for weeks or months. Some horses have the persistent or chronic diarrhea without an acute history. The feces vary from soft cow manure to watery, from day to day, and are consistently abnormal.

The predominant postmortem finding is watery, fetid ingesta throughout the large intestine with occasional petechiae in the mucosa. The remainder of the intestinal tract is unremarkable, with the exception of fine, linear erosions in the distal third of the esophageal mucosa. There are nonspecific lesions of shock in the acute cases. The histological findings are not remarkable. Bacteriological, virological, and toxicological studies have been negative. Attempts have been made to implicate intestinal protozoa without result.

The acute disease resembles Potomac fever, but laminitis has never been a feature, as it is in Potomac fever, and persistent diarrhea has not been reported with Potomac fever. This condition is seen year-round. The erosive lesions of the large intestine reported in Potomac fever have not been seen, and there is no description, for Potomac fever, of the nearly pathognomonic esophageal erosions. Some cases thought to be this condition in the past, were, no doubt, Potomac fever. There remain, however, cases without explanation.

Equine ehrlichial colitis

Equine ehrlichial colitis, Potomac horse fever, is an acute diarrheal disease. It caused an epizootic in Maryland and Virginia in 1979 (Ziemer et al. 1987) and has occurred for a number of years in the Middle Atlantic States with some cases in New England and the Midwest. It has not been reported outside the United States.

The disease appears in summer and early autumn, suggesting an arthropod vector(s) (Morris et al. 1988). Searches for vectors have been unprofitable. The causative organism, *Ehrlichia risticii*, grows in monocytes but is rarely seen in smears of peripheral blood. It has antigenic identity with *E. sennetsu*, the cause of human rickettsiosis in Southeast Asia (Holland et al. 1985). The organism grows in monocyte culture enclosed in a cytoplasmic vacuole. Cultured organisms have substantial pleomorphism by electron microscopy (Holland et al. 1985).

There are fever, anorexia, depression, laminitis, edema of the legs, and acute, profuse diarrhea. Experimental cases developed fluctuating fever within 3–12 days and diarrhea within 9–15 days. Dutta et al. (1988) reported acute diarrhea in 73% of experimental horses. Transient leucopenia followed by leucocytosis occurs during febrile episodes. Animals with diarrhea may have nonspecific hemoconcentration with elevated packed cell volume and relative increases of plasma proteins. Morris et al. (1988) found altered hemostatic parameters interpreted as evidence of hemostatic activation. The mortality is about 10%–30% (Holland et al. 1985; Dutta et al. 1988).

There are no gross lesions except nonspecific loss of fluid gradient in the large intestine. The microscopic changes have not yet been adequately defined, but the organism apparently prefers the dorsal colon.

Mucinous enteropathy

This uncommon condition, of unknown cause, has been described in horses and other domestic animals in Europe. We have not seen a case, the description being that of Cohrs (1961), also cited by Godglück (1967).

The condition is seen after feeding spoiled or lodged food materials, after "rich" meals, and after chilling. The content of the ileum, cecum, and colon is abundant, watery, foul smelling, thin, yellowish or brown with tenacious masses of mucus, which appear like pieces of skin, tubules, or cylinders 1/2 to 1 m, even up to 8 m, in length. The mucosa is swollen and reddened, often with hemorrhages. While this looks like fibrinous colitis, the masses are almost entirely mucus.

Acorn poisoning

This has been reported in horses less often than in other species (Duncan 1961; Anderson et al. 1983). It usually appears as acute severe gastrointestinal disease following ingestion of oak leaves or acorns. In one case there were increased quantities of pleural and peritoneal fluid and marked edema of the mesentery and the gastrointestinal tract from stomach to rectum. There were hemorrhages and ulceration of the mucosa, becoming progressively more severe in the cecum and colon. The kidneys were pale and swollen and the adrenals hemorrhagic. There was congestion and edema of the lungs.

Histologically, the intestinal lesions were characterized by necrosis and sloughing of epithelium and thrombi in the submucosal vessels. The adrenals had multiple infarcts. The kidneys had segmental nephrosis of the proximal convoluted tubules with cellular and hyaline casts. The renal lesions were less extensive than seen in, for example, cattle with acorn poisoning (Anderson et al. 1983).

The cause is thought to be tannin or its metabolites. Some chronic cases have been seen and mildly affected animals may recover.

Rectum and anus

Oxyurosis

Pinworm infestation of horses is common throughout the world and in horses of all ages. There are two pinworms, *Oxyuris equi* and *Probstmayria vivipara*. The latter, known as the minute pinworm, is the smallest nematode of the gastrointestinal tract and multiplies without leaving the host. It causes no lesions (Wetzel 1967; Drudge and Lyons 1986).

Oxyuris equi third-stage, infective larvae are ingested, pass to the cecum and ventral colon, and may be found for the first 3 to 8 days deep in the mucosal glands. The glands are somewhat enlarged with flattening and necrosis of epithelium, mild hyperemia, and minimal inflammatory cell infiltration. The larvae molt to the fourth stage and fasten to the mucosa in order to feed, exciting, at most, a minimal inflammatory reaction (Wetzel 1967).

Adult, gravid females emerge from the anus after a 4 1/2- to 5-month prepatent period. Rupture of the females releases eggs and gelatinous substances to the perineum, inducing intense pruritis with characteristic tail rubbing and hair loss.

Rupture of the rectum

Tearing or rupture of the rectum occurs during foaling and during manual examination. The tear is invariably in the ventral quadrant and near the pelvic inlet. Tearing during foaling may be direct, as a foot of the foal rips out the dorsal wall of the vagina and vulva and the ventral wall of the rectum and anus. It may also be indirect, the tear occurring only in the ventral wall of the rectum. A possible mechanism is discussed below.

Rupture of the rectum during manual examination is not common. While the pathogenesis may seem straightforward, attempts to tear the rectum in the fresh carcass show that it is not. The arm in the rectum is a necessary but not sufficient cause. No studies have been reported on this phenomenon and the following is hypothetical. As discussed elsewhere in this chapter, rupture of the intestine, particularly the cecum and colon, is usually the result of impaction or obstipation of some duration. The rupture occurs just proximal to the site of obstruction and/or work hypertrophy of the muscle of the gut wall. This suggests an area of ileus with accumulation of large quantities of gas, with eventual rupture in the antimesenteric border. As with rupture of the stomach and the urinary bladder of foals, rupture of the rectum almost invariably begins with tearing of the serosa, followed by the muscularis and mucosa, and this is *prima facie* evidence of excessive pressure within the viscus as the cause of the rupture.

A pathogenesis is suggested for rupture of the rectum during foaling and during rectal examination. The anal sphincter opens, allowing air to be drawn into the rectum (ballooning the rectum), and closes again either on itself or around the examiner's arm. The generally lower than ambient pressure in the peritoneal cavity is predisposing. The rectum now contains a pocket of air. A peristaltic wave passing from the descending colon to the rectum suddenly raises the pressure within this pocket and rupture occurs. As well, peritoneal pressure builds up with contraction of the abdominal muscles (straining), adding to the increase of pressure within the rectal air pocket. The same pathogenesis is proposed for indirect rupture of the rectum during foaling, with the exception that air is entrapped in the rectum as part of the straining of delivery. Preventing complete, sealing closure of the anus around the examiner's arm would appear advisable.

Neoplasia

We have seen few tumors, benign or malignant, in the gastrointestinal tract of light horses. The following is taken largely from the compilation of Dobberstein and Tamaschke (1969).

Benign or malignant tumors of the small intestine and large intestine are rare. Myxomas and myxofibromas have been described in the small intestine, colon, and rectum. Chondromas have been described in the small intestine and cecum. Hemangioma cavernosum has been seen in the mesocolon. Leiomyomas have been found in the small intestine. Polypoid adenomas of the mucosa, apparently mainly in the large intestine, have been seen. We have not seen any of these conditions in over 10,000 postmortem examinations of light horses. Lymphosarcoma is discussed elsewhere (see "Small intestine: Lymphosarcoma" in this chapter).

Adenocarcinomas represent about 4% of all carcinomas of horses. They are said to occur most commonly in the large intestine, only about 20% having been encountered in the small intestine. We have seen only one adenocarcinoma in the small intestine of an aged Standardbred stallion.

Liver

The fetal liver is larger relative to body size than that of foal or horse. It undergoes degenerative changes with placental insufficiency as described with abortion. Extramedullary hematopoietic foci are common, though never numerous to the naked eye. They are small, yellowish-white rectilinear foci. Megakaryocytes are rarely seen.

Within the first few months after birth, fine, fibrous tags often appear on the parietal surface of the liver, particularly on the left lobe but on the middle and right as well, **perihepatitis filamentosa** (Cadeac 1896; Cohrs 1961). Some may be attached to the diaphragm and/or have arisen there. These have been found in apparently early stages of development as thin, fluid-filled outpouchings from the surface of the liver. Histologically, there is fluid accumulation in fine, saclike outpouchings between the peritoneum and Glisson's capsule. A few strands of fibrin may be present. These sacs undergo fibrosis—the grossly apparent fibrous tags. The cause is unknown. There is no evidence of inflammation. They have been called serous cysts, Kelly (1985), but really are not cysts.

These fibrous tags are to be differentiated from more numerous, shaggier tags associated with plaques of fibrosis of Glisson's capsule caused by the migration of *Strongylus edentatus* and *S. equinnus*. These lesions are more common on the parietal surface of the right lobe.

Cohrs (1961) mentioned congenital cysts in the liver of foals; we have seen no case. Van der Luer and Kroneman (1982) reported biliary atresia in a foal. The horse does not have a gall bladder, as already recognized by Apsyrtus 340 BCE cited by Darmstaedter et al. (1908) and by Aristotle 384-322 BCE cited by Leclainche (1936).

Aging changes

Atrophy of the right lobes of the liver is common in older horses, varying from modest reduction to near total absence. The atrophy regularly proceeds from the distal, ventral border proximally. As atrophy proceeds there is compensatory hypertrophy/hyperplasia of, particularly, the left lobe. Histologically, there is simple loss of hepatic parenchyma, with collapse and consolidation of connective tissue before it, too, disappears. During the collapsing phase, the histological picture could be mistaken for cirrhosis. There are dense, amorphous bodies in the liver cords and macrophages, the **apoptotic bodies** described by Kerr (1971) in mild ischemia of the liver.

The cause of the atrophy is not known. Study of the intrahepatic branches of the hepatic artery showed intimal thickening by fibrous tissue with elastotic degeneration of the internal elastic lamina, the usual endarteritic, aging changes in the peripheral vessels of horses. The changes were no more numerous or marked than in normal liver lobes. Blanc (1895) cited by Cadeac (1896) said that the blood in the portal vein follows a nearly linear path into the left and middle lobes, while the portal branches to the right lobe make right angle turns, suggesting to him a predisposing, "less active," flow of blood.

Kitt (1900) suggested the cause to be pressure by the head of the cecum and the large colon. The right lobe of the liver does not reach the ventral body wall, while the left and middle lobes more nearly do so. One may think, then, of tension over the years as a relevant, or even primary, factor, tension being as effective as compression in compromising circulation and causing atrophy.

Hemosiderin in Kupffer cells increases in amount in a nearly linear manner with age after about 10 years (Pallaske 1960). At the same time, the connective tissue in portal spaces increases irregularly and there may be patchy and modest accumulations of lymphoid and/or other mononuclear cells. Often there is an increase of fibrous tissue, often hyalinized, around the central vein (Klaus and Mathias 1958; Cohrs 1961).

These changes are nonspecific, age related, and to be differentiated from present disease. For example, hemosiderin and accumulations of cells in the portal spaces are lesions of equine infectious anemia, and fibrosis of central veins has been described with pyrrolizidine toxicity and incorrectly called venoocclusive disease (Kelley 1985).

Soft, friable, pigmented calculi can be present in variable numbers in the extrahepatic biliary passages. They are of no known significance and often present in old and/or cachectic horses. There are no relevant histological findings. (See "Cholelithiasis," below).

Chiaravalle and Aramburu (1942) studied bile excretion in 10 horses. There was continuous bile flow in the fasting animal, which increased with feeding. The specific gravity was 1.010, and the amount produced varied among animals from 1900 to 5900 mL per 20 hours. Colin (1886/1888) indicated that horses secrete bile continuously, but irregularly, at about 250 mL per hour.

Small white nodules

Small white or gray nodules are often present in the liver parenchyma and, in larger, fibrotic form in the liver capsule. The more characteristic of these lesions, in the earlier stages, are caused by the migration of the larvae of *S. edentatus*, less often, ***S. equinnus***, and, in foals, ***Ascaris equorum***. They are found anywhere in the liver, most numerous in the right lobe with edentatus. They may appear grossly as small white or greenish-brown foci. Histologically, there are tracks of necrotic, homogenous, eosinophilic debris with variable numbers of bordering mononuclear cells and intact eosinophils. As these lesions age, as the larvae move on or die, fibrous tissue replaces the necrotic debris, and a small mass of scar tissue remains, perhaps with a few mononuclear cells. Calcification is uncommon. At this stage, the cause is larval migration by inference.

The characteristic residua of *S. edentatus* migration are plaques of fibrous tissue in Glisson's capsule. They appear to persist for a considerable time after larvae are no longer present, particularly on the parietal surface of the right lobe.

Infiltrations and degenerations

The various infiltrations and degenerations of the liver of other species are found in the horse, as well. Fatty infiltration, however, is uncommon no matter the nutritional or disease status of the animal. Fine droplet fat can be stained in hepatocytes in most horses, but large droplet fatty change/degeneration is nearly restricted to ponies. Normal Shetland ponies have more large droplet stainable fat in hepatocytes than horses. With hyperlipidemia of ponies, the liver is grossly fatty with rounded margins.

Amyloidosis

Amyloidosis of the liver, and other organs, is not uncommon in horses used for antitoxin and antivenom production, but rare otherwise. The pathogenesis involves repeated stimulation of serum amyloid A protein, a segment of which, amyloid AA, when deposited on basement membranes, forms the insoluble, fibrillary, β-pleated amyloid (Maxie 1985).

Arndt (1928) reported amyloidosis of the liver in 2% and 4% of horses slaughtered in Moscow and Kazan, of the former U.S.S.R., respectively. The liver was soft and friable, unlike the usual descriptions of firm, hard consistency. Often hematoma and rupture occurred. No explanation for the high frequency in these areas was found. Most cases have been associated with some type of chronic, debilitating disease process (Cadeac 1896). We have not seen amyloidosis in light horses, other than rare cases of nasal amyloidosis.

Vacuolar and/or fatty change

Centrilobular vacuolar and/or fatty change, progressing to single cell necrosis, is seen in livers of horses with severe anemia and acute anoxemia. The fresh liver has central, ill-defined pale areas. Acute equine infectious anemia, red maple poisoning (Tennant et al. 1981), onion poisoning (Pierce et al. 1972), and postparturient hemorrhage in mares are examples.

Centrilobular vacuolar degeneration has been seen in horses dying during **halothane anesthesia**. This has been reported in untoward deaths of humans with halothane, but the specificity of the lesion in the horse is doubtful and probably related to severe anoxemia (inadequate ventilation).

Iron fumarate necrosis

Massive necrosis of the liver was seen in neonatal foals following ingestion of iron fumarate in a feed supplement (Swerczek and Crowe 1983; Acland et al. 1984). The supplement was given in the first hours after birth with death within 24–48 hours. Mullaney and Brown (1988) studied the disease in experimental ponies. There was periportal or massive necrosis of hepatocytes, cholestasis, proliferation of bile ducts, fibrosis, and inflammatory cell infiltration. The liver was smaller than normal, markedly affected areas being dark red-brown and somewhat elevated. Acland et al. (1984) reported generalized lymphoid necrosis and the presence of Alzheimer type II cells, clumps of enlarged pale nuclei with indistinct or absent cytoplasm, in the cerebral cortex of all their cases.

These *leberglia* were reported, particularly in the cerebral cortex and caudate nucleus, with liver disease, by Dobberstein in 1926. He also found loss of ganglion cells and focal degeneration of white matter. Additional observations were made by Stenius (1941).

While this specific iron fumarate toxicity no longer occurs, it provides a striking example of the rapidity with which liver damage can occur, and an even more striking example of the rapidity of the response of young liver to damage. Marked regeneration of hepatocytes and fibrosis were seen in livers of foals that had ingested the iron only 24 hours previously.

There is some evidence that excessive iron intake in older horses can cause clinically relevant liver damage qualitatively identical to, but quantitatively less severe than, in foals. This is usually iatrogenic, the result of iron overdosing by horse trainers. Additional work in this area is required.

Tyzzer's disease

Tyzzer's disease, caused by *Bacillus piliformis*, is a sporadic, highly fatal disease of foals, at least in North America and Great Britain (Swerczek et al. 1973; Pulley and Shively 1974; Whitwell 1976). The foal, about a month of age, is usually found dead, but clinical signs of depression, fever, and icterus may be seen. The liver is enlarged with multiple areas of dark red and yellow-white necrosis, often with an overall greenish hue (Fig. 3.32). The hepatic lymph nodes are enlarged and edematous. Histologically, there is multifocal coagulation necrosis with remarkably little inflammatory reaction. The filamentous organisms are found intracellularly and extracellularly at the periphery of the necrotic foci. Special staining may be necessary. The organism has not been cultured.

Tyzzer's disease has been reported in many species, particularly rodents. The epizootology in foals is not known but probably related to rodent infestation. Swerczek (1977) said mares become inapparent carriers, shedding the organism in the feces. No data was provided, and the observation has not been confirmed.

Theiler's disease

This was first described by Theiler (1919), who produced it inadvertently in horses with early versions of African horse sickness vaccine. Since that time single cases and virtual outbreaks have been seen in horses injected with materials of horse tissue origin, such as tetanus antitoxin, pregnant mare serum. The morbidity is low but the mortality 100%. The disease is often referred to as **serum hepatitis**, an unhelpful and unetiological avoidance of the innocent eponym.

The clinical course is almost invariably fulminating and violent: liver–brain syndrome. Some animals may be found dead with suspicion of lightning strike. The carcass shows acute toxemia: dark, tarry, nonclotting blood; dull, dark yellowish discoloration of tissues; and an enlarged, engorged spleen. There may be striking contusions and lacerations and even fractures because of the violent clinical course.

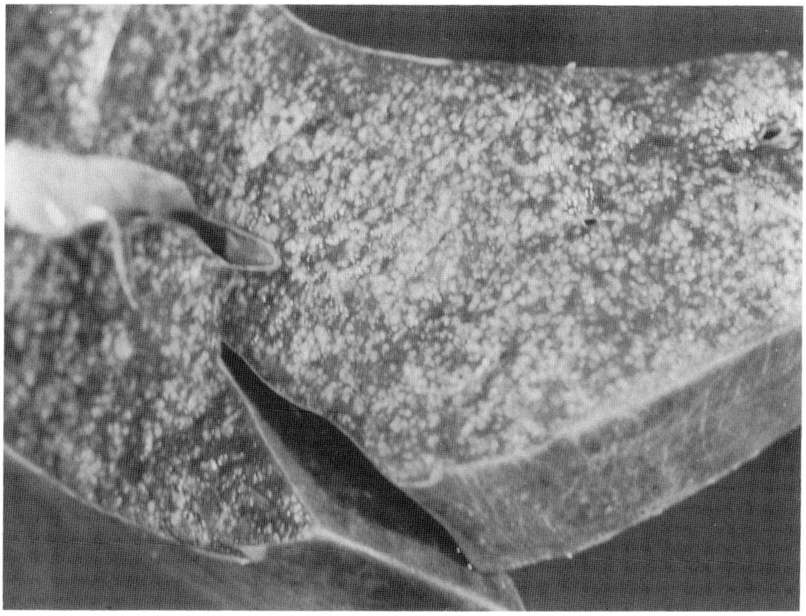

3.32. Tyzzer's disease in a foal.

The liver is enlarged, with the lobules demarcated by a whitish or yellowish color. Ill-defined areas of hemorrhage may be apparent with a distinct greenish cast from massive release of bile pigments. Histologically, there is necrosis of virtually every hepatocyte in all parts of the liver. A few, vaguely normal cells may be present adjacent to the portal spaces. Sinusoidal integrity is destroyed, and blood is admixed with the necrotic hepatocytes (Fig. 3.33).

Alsike clover poisoning

This has been reported infrequently (Schofield 1933; Hjärre and Carlström 1933). We have seen several cases in the Middle Atlantic States. Apparently, the alsike clover, *Trifolium hybridum*, pasture or hay must be ingested over a considerable time. Clinical signs are nonspecific: slowly progressive loss of weight, inappetence, colic, and icterus. Only rarely does the liver–brain syndrome develop in the late stages. The condition has been reproduced experimentally by feeding alsike clover.

The liver is enlarged, pale, and tough in consistency. The cut section has a mottled appearance caused by dense, gray-white bands of fibrous tissue outlining individual liver lobules. The histological picture is biliary cirrhosis. In less severe cases there is striking proliferation of bile ducts with normal epithelium in the portal spaces, with minimal to moderate proliferation of fibrous tissue. In more advanced cases portal spaces are linked by proliferating bile ducts and, particularly, fibrous tissue. The proliferating tissue gradually constricts, but does not invade the lobules.

Pyrrolizidine alkaloid poisoning

The pyrrolizidine alkaloids are the toxic principles of a number of plants, including *Senecio* and *Crotalaria,* as the common causes of liver disease in horses in North America. Liver disease of this type

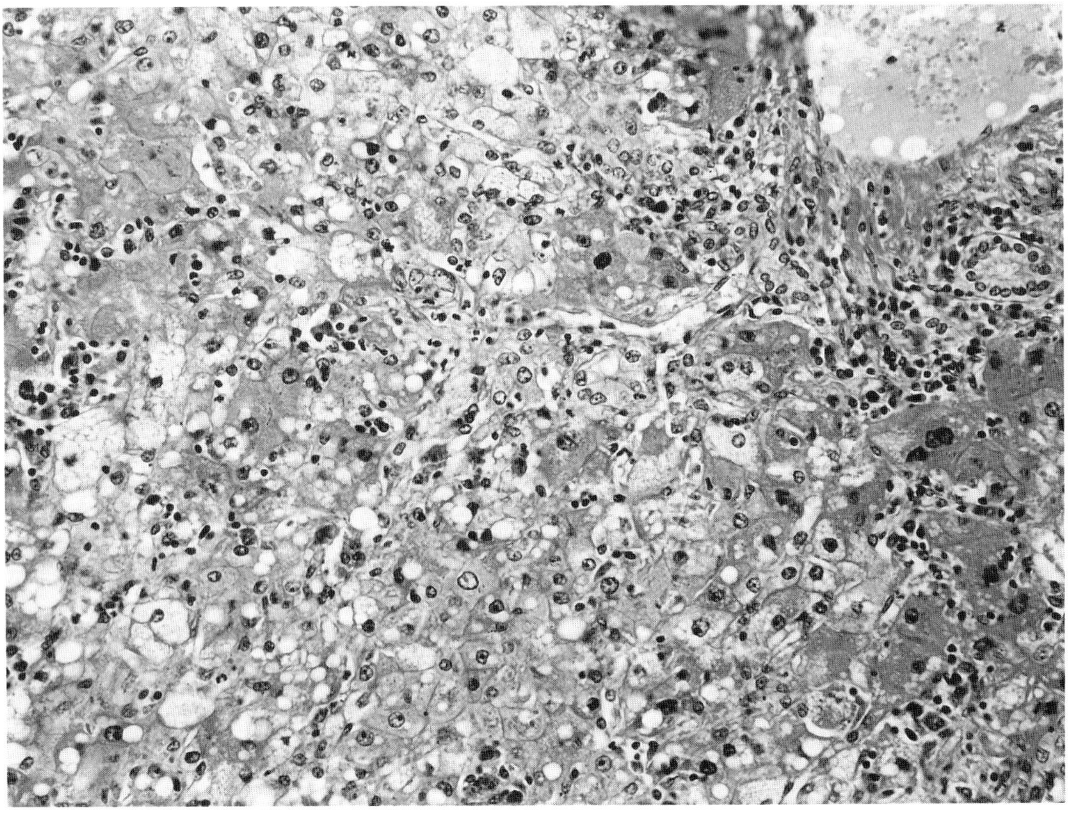

3.33. Middle power, H & E of Theiler's disease of the liver. There are virtually no viable hepatocytes, only shattered remnants adjacent to portal triads.

has been seen all over the world and has a long and venerable history (Jubb and Kennedy 1970).

The plants are generally unpalatable and only eaten if more desirable food stuffs are limited. The clinical signs are those of the **liver–brain syndrome**: mania, incoordination or sleepiness, depression with head pressing, walking in circles, and tenesmus. Death occurs soon after onset of clinical signs. Clinical evidence of disease appears some weeks or even months after the ingestion of the toxic material.

At postmortem the liver lesions are related to the duration of disease and amount of material ingested. With heavy exposure, short duration, the liver may be enlarged with multiple whitish, lobular discoloration. With longer duration the liver is cirrhotic and smaller than normal. The cut surface is laced with fibrous tissue with lobules of lighter than normal color.

Microscopically, there is a variable pattern of centrilobular necrosis, focal areas of striking enlargement of hepatocytes (megalocytosis), and portal fibrosis (Fig. 3.34). The enlarged hepatocyte is many times larger than normal, with pale cytoplasm and nucleus. There is mild or moderate proliferation of bile ducts and infiltration of mononuclear cells in the portal spaces. Fibrosis of the central veins, so-called venoocclusive change, has been reported, but this is a nonspecific aging change. Changes in the brain are of the same type as those described by Acland et al. (1984) in foals with iron fumarate intoxication and in other forms of liver disease described by Dobberstein (1926).

Enzootic liver disease has long been known in many parts of the world under a variety of regional and descriptive names. While it is probable that most of these conditions are caused by pyrrolizidine alkaloid-containing plants, that does not appear to have been established in all instances. Krage (1942), for example, reported acute centrilobular liver necrosis in horses in East Prussia associated with ingestion of a fungus, *Dothidella trifolii*, which causes disease of white, red, and Swedish clovers. Some outbreaks did not appear to have this association, and Krage suggested that other factors might be involved, perhaps pyrrolizidine alkaloids.

Moldy corn poisoning by *Fusarium moniliforme* is primarily a disease of the central nervous system. In some outbreaks, however, toxic hepatic necrosis, not unlike that caused by the pyrrolizidine alkaloids, has been observed. It appears that smaller amounts of the mycotoxin affect the nervous system, while larger amounts affect both the nervous system and the liver.

Purulent cholangiohepatitis

This is uncommon and, in our experience, most often found on histological examination without specific clinical signs of hepatic disease. Many of our cases were encountered in horses dying with exhaustion shock, the hepatic lesion being one of two or more stressing factors.

Usually, there are no gross lesions, but there may be an impression of multifocal, whitish, exag-

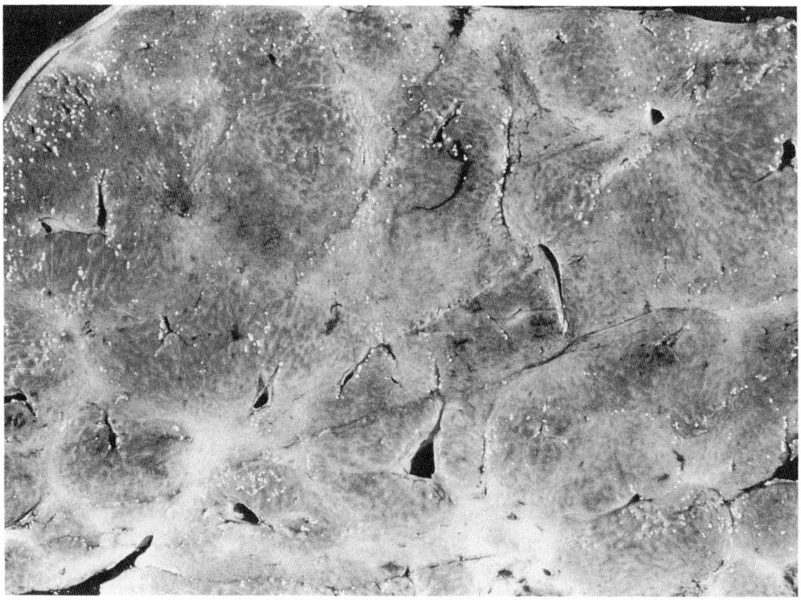

3.34. Cirrhosis of the liver caused by pyrrolizidine alkaloid, *Crotalaria.*

geration of the portal triads. Histologically, the bile ducts in the portal areas are distended, with purulent debris with a light infiltration of mononuclear, rarely neutrophilic, cells in the surrounding tissue. There may be slight fibrosis of the portal triads and variably distributed bile canalicular stasis within the liver lobules. No gross or microscopic lesions have been found in the extrahepatic bile ducts.

Routine culture of the liver is rarely done and has been noncontributory. Special stains have not shown organisms. The cause is unknown. **Chronic active hepatitis**, so-called (White 1991), has lesions similar to, if not identical to, those just described.

Vascular cirrhosis

Although rare, verminous thrombosis of the hepatic branch of the celiac artery does occur and is associated with atrophy and fibrosis of the liver with attendant clinical signs. Rubarth (1967) also described such thrombosis of the hepatic artery.

Fasciola hepatica

The frequency of liver fluke infestation in horses in North America is not known. We have seen no case in over 10,000 postmortem examinations in the eastern half of the United States. Ingested larvae penetrate the wall of the duodenum and migrate transperitoneally to penetrate the liver capsule. The larvae wander in the liver for some time, leaving tracks in their wake like those of *Strongylus edentatus* and *S. equinus*. They eventually enter the bile ducts to become egg-laying adults. The bile ducts are mechanically dilated by the presence of the flukes, with moderate catarrhal inflammation of the mucosa and minimal fibrotic thickening of the wall. There is at least partial obstruction of bile flow, the bile becoming thick and gummy. Occasional larvae do not reach the bile ducts, becoming encysted in whitish foci in the liver parenchyma. The larvae are found in a greasy, brownish mass within a thick fibrous capsule (Cohrs 1961; Wetzel 1967).

The hepatic lymph nodes are enlarged and hyperplastic with dilated sinuses containing enlarged reticuloendothelial cells, eosinophils, and phagocytosed bile pigments.

Dicrocoelium dendriticum

This small fluke lives in the bile and pancreatic ducts of many animals. Cadeac (1896) said it was not uncommon to find it (*Distoma* spp.) in small numbers and without significant lesions in the biliary tract of horses. In the ass, on the other hand, they can be as serious and numerous as in sheep. We have not seen these parasites in horses in North America.

Echinococcus granulosus

Infestation with this larval tapeworm is rare in North America. We have seen only a few cases in horses imported from Ireland and Great Britain. It is not rare in Great Britain; Cranley (1982) reported that 50% of slaughtered horses had echinococcus lesions in the liver. The gross cysts are characteristic, and the lesions are those seen in other species (Cohrs 1961; Wetzel 1967).

Cholelithiasis

Bile pigment agglomerations in the biliary tract are not uncommon, particularly in older horses, and of no pathological significance. True biliary tract calculi, with liver disease and clinical signs, are uncommon (Van der Luer and Kroneman 1982; Traub et al. 1982; Johnston et al. 1989). A number of cases in the older literature are cited by Cadeac (1896) and Rubarth (1967). Averons (1896/97) reported a case with postmortem findings. The clinical course is characterized by intermittent, usually mild, colic, fever, icterus, and elevation of serum γ-glutamyltransferase (Johnson et al). Hepatic encephalopathy is seen in some cases (Traub et al). Clinical disease, usually in older horses, is not to be expected unless the calculi obstruct the common bile duct. In these cases there is low grade, ongoing damage to the hepatic parenchyma with portal fibrosis, proliferation of bile ducts, bile stasis, and variable inflammatory cell infiltration. The liver may be either enlarged or somewhat atrophic with distinct lobular markings.

The cause is not known, but regurgitation of ingesta into the common bile duct has been suggested (Johnson et al. 1989), leaving regurgitation unexplained.

Neoplasia

The older literature is summarized by Cadeac (1896). We have seen no tumors, other than lymphosarcoma, in the liver. **Cavernous hemangioma** has been described, often in association with angiomatosis of the skin (Messow 1952/53).

Adenomas

No adenoma deriving from hepatic cells has been reported. One simple adenoma arising from the biliary tract has been mentioned [Kitt (1923) cited by Dobberstein and Tamaschke (1969)].

Carcinoma

These are rare, with no more than 1.5% of all tumors of horses arising in the liver (Dobberstein and Tamaschke 1969). Only cholangiocell carcinomas have been seen.

Lymposarcoma

Liver involvement occurs with generalized lymphosarcoma.

Pancreas

Pancreatic disease is uncommon in horses. There are three entities: acute and chronic interstitial pancreatitis and pancreatic carcinoma. Calculi have not been seen or reported in the pancreatic ducts. Lesions of the pancreatic islets and insulin-dependent diabetes have not been reported (see Pituitary in Chapter 4, "Endocrine System"). Colin (1886/1888) indicated that pancreatic secretion was continuous, though not uniform, in the horse, amounting to about 250 mL per hour.

Acute interstitial pancreatitis

Acute interstitial pancreatitis is caused by the migration of *Strongylus equinus* or *S. edentatus*. The larvae migrate in the interstitial connective tissue, causing hemorrhage, edema, and reddish discoloration of the parenchyma (Fig. 3.35). Interstitial edema, pooling of blood, and blackish discoloration are routine postmortem changes and not to be mistaken for interstitial pancreatitis. Larvae may be recovered by careful dissection. Histologically, the specific lesion is a core or tract of largely amorphous eosinophilic material with dottings of basophilic debris. Intact eosinophils and mononuclear cells surround these tracts. Rarely, a section of larva may be encountered. Clinical signs have not been seen with acute interstitial pancreatitis, the lesion only encountered incidentally at postmortem.

Chronic interstitial pancreatitis

Chronic interstitial pancreatitis is easily recognized as firm, hard masses of fibrous tissue with few remaining lobules of partially intact pancreatic tissue (Fig. 3.36). Histologically, the cores and tracts described above are laced through a mass of mature and maturing fibrous tissue. There are scattered foci of mononuclear and lymphoid cells.

Clinical signs of progressive weight loss with normal or increased appetite are usual. Sometimes there is focal or multifocal alopecia and, rarely, severe, intractable pruritis [Siedamgrotsky (1878) cited by Cadeac (1896); and Hutyra and Marek (1920, 1926)]. The skin lesions are nonspecific: edema, focal hemorrhages, and infiltration of mononuclear cells around small blood vessels. The cause of the skin lesions is not known, but may be essential fatty acid deficiency. Despite the severity of the lesion, pancreatic islets remain intact, or, at least a sufficient number remain functional, so that diabetes mellitus has not been seen. Diabetes mellitus occurs in horses with adenomas of the intermediate lobe of the pituitary gland in the absence of lesions of the pancreatic islets. (See Chapter 4 "Endocrine System.")

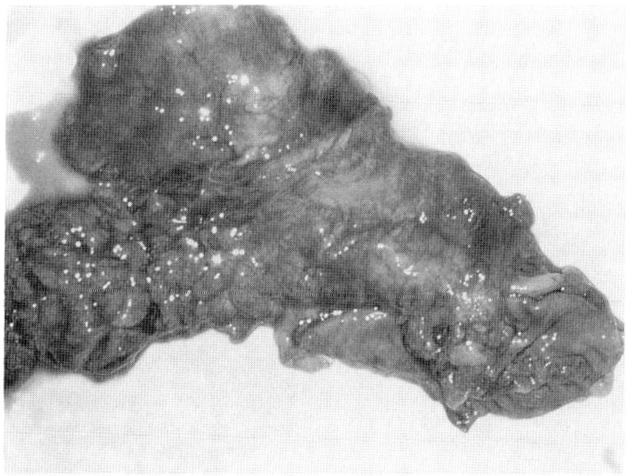

3.35. Acute pancreatitis caused by migration of *S. equinus.*

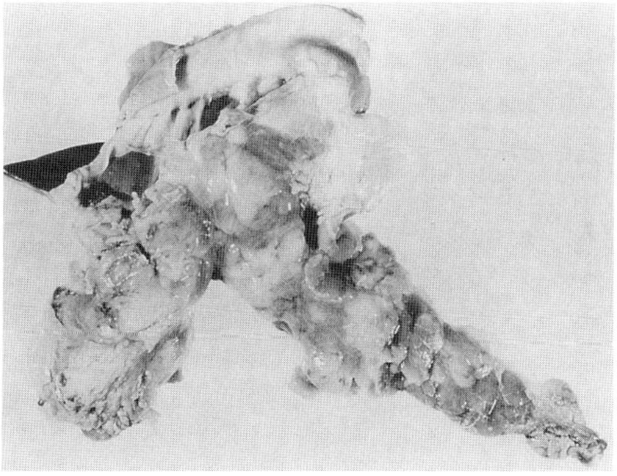

3.36. Chronic pancreatitis, *S. equinus.* Some reasonably normal lobules remain.

Carcinoma

Pancreatic carcinoma is rare and almost entirely in aged horses. In our cases the clinical history was only old age and loss of weight. Within the abdomen, there were numerous firm, white and confluent implantation metastases scattered over the visceral and parietal peritoneum. Careful examination showed the tumors characteristically "flowering" from the area of a no longer identifiable pancreas. Histologically, the tumors comprised anaplastic round cells with rare evidence of tissue organization. The diagnosis is provisional and based on gross findings. Histochemical examination in two cases was not contributory.

The undifferentiated character of pancreatic carcinoma is mirrored, in a sense, by the unusual histological appearance of the normal equine pancreas. While the pancreatic islets are clearly demarcated, the acinar configuration of the exocrine pancreas is far from as clearly defined as in other species, even suggesting neoplasia on casual examination.

Balozet and Chainet (1937) reported an undifferentiated carcinoma in a 15-year-old cryptorchid. Kerr et al. (1982) reported, in a donkey, a case of scirrhous, well-differentiated pancreatic adenocarcinoma that had undergone squamous metaplasia. Church et al. (1987) reported cases in a pony and in a Thoroughbred, both scirrhous adenocarcinomas in younger individuals. They suggested that the tumors had arisen from duct epithelium rather than acinar epithelium. These differentiated tumors are probably of duct origin, while the old horse anaplastic carcinomas arise from acinar epithelium. No cases of benign neoplasia have been seen or reported.

CHAPTER 4

Endocrine System

Thyroid

Clinically important disease of the thyroid gland is uncommon in horses. "Colloid goiter" occurs in fetuses and newborn foals of mares on excessive iodine intake (Baker and Lindsey 1968; Drew et al. 1975). The thyroid glands of these fetuses and foals are markedly enlarged (Fig. 4.1), and colloid poor. The acinar epithelium is flattened, endothelioid, but there are a number of acini or portions of acini that are hypertrophic and/or hyperplastic. The thyroglossal duct is enlarged and polycystic. As discussed by Baker and Lindsey, excess iodine intake by the mare blocks the fetal thyroid gland, inducing epithelial hypertrophy and hyperplasia followed by colloid goiter.

Hypothyroidism

The deficiency of thyroid hormone delays maturation of cartilage to bone (Looser 1929). The foal, characteristically, appears normal at birth, with the exception of thyroid enlargement and a dry, brittle haircoat. At birth the foal escapes the iodine blockade, and the thyroid gland returns to normal appearance, and probably activity, within the first month. The delay of ossification can, however, lead to crushing and collapse, particularly of the small tarsal bones, as weight bearing begins (Rooney 1969). This is discussed with osteochondrosis (see Chapter 7, "Fore Leg").

Hyperthyroidism

Hyperthyroidism has been suggested as a cause of clinical problems, but there is no evidence that this occurs in horses. Schlotthauer (1931) examined the thyroid glands of 100 horses, average age 18 years, and described a variety of changes. No breeds were recorded. There were no sex differences. He found adenomatous lesions in 37 horses, a frequency in this older age group consistent with our experience.

It is moot if the "adenomatous change" is to be considered adenoma or hyperplasia. The lesions are usually pale, whitish or tan foci, which may or may not cause enlargement of the thyroid (Fig. 4.2). Microscopically, these foci consist of masses of thyroid epithelium of normal appearance, poorly demarcated from the surrounding normal thyroid tissue. There may be pressure effect on the surrounding tissue, bespeaking the expansive growth of the focus (Trautmann 1924; Pallaske 1960). An occasional focus has papillary characteristics in some areas. There appears to be no endocrine activity, and no evidence of malignant transformation has been seen. Indeed, carcinoma of the thyroid is extremely rare (Groth 1968).

Dysharmonie

The thyroids of older animals have variably marked pigmentation of the acinar epithelium and

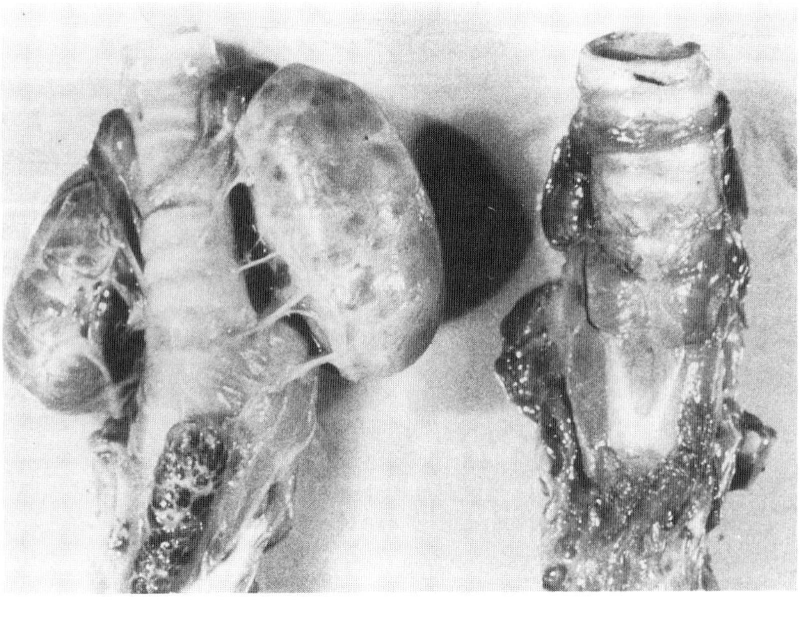

4.1. Colloid, iodine-deficiency type, goiter in an aborted fetus (*left*) compared to age-matched control (*right*).

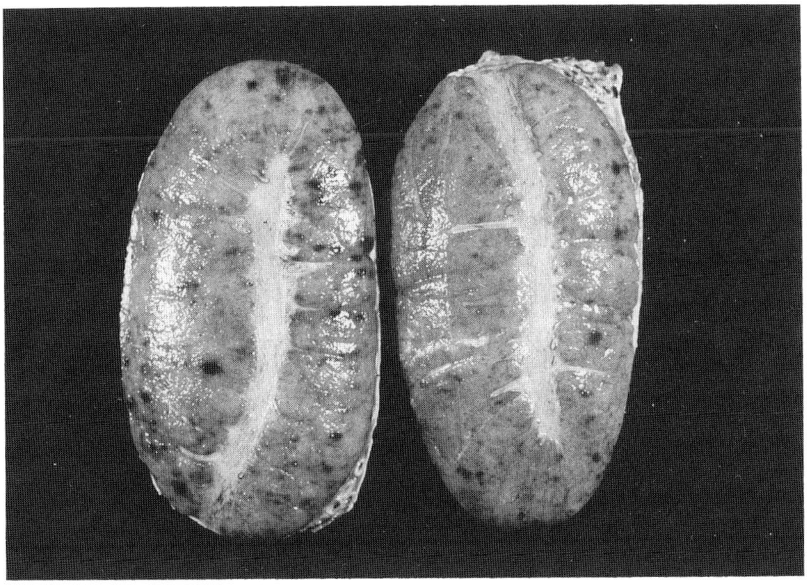

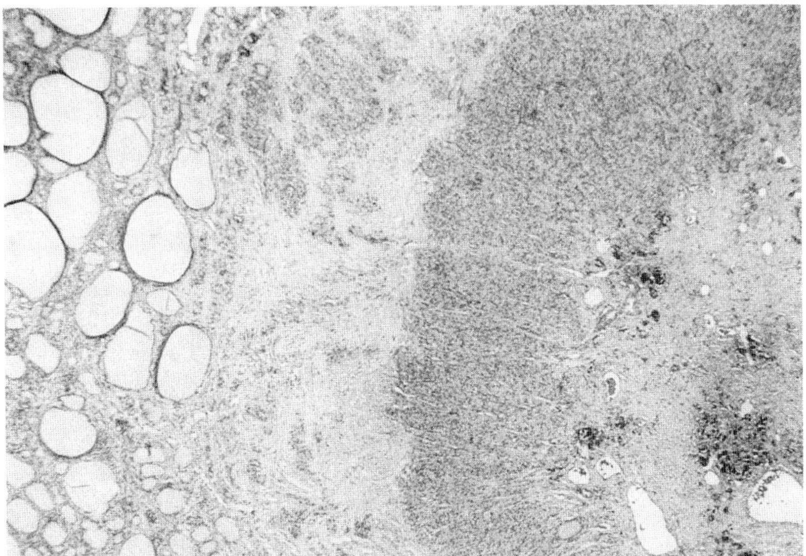

4.2. Adenoma, adenomatous hyperplasia of the thyroid of an old horse.

"dysharmonie"—marked variation in acinar size, as well as variation in height of acinar epithelium from acinus to acinus and within a given acinus. These changes increase, qualitatively and quantitatively, with age. Schlotthauer thought they might have clinical significance, but they are routine findings in the older horse without clinical correlation. Abbott and Prendergast (1934) and Dimock et al. (1944) believed that only somewhat more than half of the thyroids they examined were normal, the others having hyperplastic or colloid goiter. This is certainly incorrect. The colloid content varies considerably from region to region, as does the appearance of the acinar epithelium in the normal equine thyroid, particularly in older animals, as indicated. As with endocrine glands in general, physiological correlations cannot safely be based on morphology alone.

Parathyroids

Parathyroid III is usually about 15 cm from the first rib, near the bifurcation of the carotid artery. Parathyroid IV is usually found on the dorsomedial aspect of the thyroid, embedded in connective tissue about 1 cm from the thyroid, rarely in the thyroid itself. Both glands are about pea size, gray, yellow, or brownish, flattened or pyramidal, sometimes lobated, and firmer than adjacent lymph nodes. The parathyroids are enlarged in nutritional secondary hyperparathyroidism—and easier to find.

The parenchymal cells are generally arranged in perivascular rosettes and are large with rather small, dark nuclei, in contrast to other species (Krölling and Grau 1960). The basic cell is the "chief cell," occurring in either a light or somewhat smaller and darker form. "Oxyphiles" are larger than chief cells.

They have a granular, somewhat eosinophilic cytoplasm and small, sometimes shrunken nuclei. Various transitions between these cell forms may be present. The "water clear cell" is as large or larger than the oxyphile, with no stainable cytoplasm. It appears only with hyperparathyroidism. The other cell forms apparently represent different degrees of functional activity. So-called "syncytial giant cells" may be seen, particularly in older animals. They appear to form by fusion of chief cells and have densely eosinophilic cytoplasm and small dark nuclei (Krölling and Grau; Capen 1985).

Microscopic, colloid-containing cysts are occasionally encountered. While these may arise from displaced thyroid tissue, most may be of branchial pouch origin, partially lined by ciliated epithelium (Krölling and Grau 1960). It is doubtful if true neoplasms have been seen in equine parathyroids. See, also, nutritional hyperparathyroidism (Chapter 6, Locomotor System, General).

Adrenal

Telangiectasia

The adrenal gland rarely has lesions of primary pathological significance. It is important to recognize the variably numerous normal cortical nodules that contribute to the growth and replacement of the cortex (Elias 1948). These have often been misdiagnosed as nodular hyperplasia (Fuchs 1959), an undefined entity in the horse. The outer part of the cortex is called the "zona arcuata" because of the arch arrangement of the cell cords. Yellowish-brown lipofuscin pigmentation is common in the zona reticularis, increasing with age (Fuchs 1959).

Accessory adrenal cortical tissue, small brownish nodules, is occasionally seen in the tunica vaginalis or near the ovary. Accessory adrenals, with both cortical and medullary components, have been reported once (Matthias 1968).

On section the normal adrenal cortex is usually a tan-gray, shading to yellowish. Histologically, there is a moderate amount of stainable lipid in the cortex. The amount of lipid is decreased in acute conditions such as septicemia, toxemia—Selye's alarm reaction—and in animals with long-term, chronic disease—Selye's stage of exhaustion (Fuchs 1959). The amount of lipid appears to increase in conditions intermediate between the two—the stage of resistance of Selye (1950). These distinctions are interesting and definable in the absence of autolysis.

The marked accumulation of fat, characteristic of inanition and metabolic disease in other herbivores, is rarely seen in horses with the exception of obese ponies in which fat accumulates without reference to state of health or disease. With septicemia and toxemia (for example, gastrointestinal malpositions), there is usually marked hyperemia and hemorrhage. Mononuclear cell accumulations may be found in the cortex or medulla, sometimes associated with equine infectious anemia. Neoplasia is rare. Pheochromocytomas do occur in the medulla, but without clinical signs. Small islands of cortical cells are normally present in the medulla (Fuchs 1959). True telangiectasia may occur near the corticomedullary junction in older animals, but is uncommon and the appearance more often artifact in decomposed and/or roughly handled glands.

Folger (1909) reported an astonishing 46 tumors among 300 adrenals examined, 11% in the medulla. He called these "hypernephromas" with the histological structure of the zona arcuata. While most of these were probably the growth nodules described by Elias (1948), several of the drawings were of masses of considerable size, which may have been pheochromocytomas. Certainly, we have seen no such frequency of neoplasia in any part of the equine adrenal.

Autolysis and artifact

It is important to recognize autolytic and artifactual change, by far more common than lesions. The adrenal, particularly some hours after death, is easily damaged by handling. The cortex tears away from the medulla, mimicking cystic change or telangiectasia. Histologically, the cells of the fasciculata shrink and crumple and the pericapillary spaces fill with postmortem fluid, spurious edema, and necrosis. Squeezing artifact, while less common than in the adrenals of small animals, does occur. These are areas of mashed-together cortical cells with apparent nuclear pyknosis, suggesting infarction. While hemorrhagic infarcts may be suspected in some cases of purpura hemorrhagica, postmortem pooling of blood is apt to give the same appearance. Occasionally, there is true septic infarction in septicemias of foals. Although *S. vulgaris* thrombi and emboli occur with some frequency in the renal arteries, they have not been seen in the adrenal arteries or gland.

Platt and Whitwell (1971) found adrenal cortical infarction in pony and donkey foals with steatitis. The cause was fibrinoid necrosis of arterial vessels, a lesion characteristic of vitamin E/selenium deficiency.

Turning-out syndrome

Adrenal insufficiency has been suggested on clinical grounds as a cause of "poor racing performance," as well as the "turning-out syndrome." The latter constitutes loss of condition, nervousness, and intermittent diarrhea in horses turned out to pasture after long periods under human control (racehorses, primarily). There is no morphological or physiological evidence implicating the adrenal cortex as a cause of either poor performance or the turning-out syndrome. Indeed, there have been no reports of pathological findings in horses with either of these syndromes. Postmortems of a number of horses, said to be afflicted with these conditions and dying or destroyed for other reasons, have shown no relevant changes.

Pituitary

The functional cytology of the pars distalis of the pituitary of the horse has apparently not been studied systematically. The cytology, in general, may be found in Krölling and Grau (1960) and Capen (1985).

Hyperplasia/adenoma

The pituitary of the horse is virtually free of lesions, with the exception of hyperplasia/adenoma and cysts of the intermediate lobe (Fig. 4.3). The frequency and size of the hyperplastic/adenomatous changes in the intermediate lobe increases with age (Potel 1968). With encroachment on the caudal lobe of the pituitary and the hypothalamus, diabetes insipidus, diabetes mellitus, and retention of haircoat (improperly: hirsutism) occurs. Most intermediate lobe masses, however, are found incidentally at postmortem. Eosinophilic and basophilic adenomas and craniopharyngioma have been mentioned in the literature (Potel). We have seen a single case of craniopharyngioma. It is doubtful that eosinophilic and basophilic adenomas occur in horses.

Diabetes insipidus can be explained by the encroachment of the enlarged intermediate lobe on the neurohypophysis, either directly or by compromising the neural pathways from the hypothalamus. The pathogenesis of diabetes mellitus associated with intermediate lobe adenoma is unclear (Tasker et al. 1966; Baker and Ritchie 1974). The pancreatic islets are normal. Merritt (1983) suggested that ACTH or growth hormone could be produced in excess and, so, give rise to diabetes mellitus. That seems unlikely since both of those hormones are produced by the uninvolved "pars distalis."

The pathogenesis of retained haircoat, overgrowth of hair, and failure to shed in the spring, is obscure. One can only note that the pituitary and/or hypothalamus are involved in the cyclical shedding and growth of hair.

Kroon and van der Plank (1931) reported proportionate dwarfism in inbred Friesian horses.

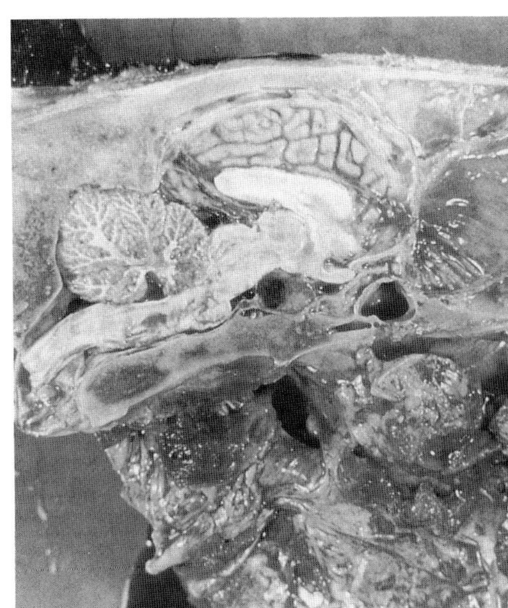

4.3. Adenoma of the intermediate lobe of the pituitary gland in an old mare.

The condition appeared to be a simple recessive character. The pituitary of the one foal examined at postmortem was reported to be atrophic and contain large numbers of acidophilic cells, the opposite, perhaps, of what would be expected.

Hamori (1983) described a lethal chondrodystrophy in ponies associated with particoloring. No anatomical or pathological studies appear to have been reported on these animals. Hamori briefly described a chondrodysplasia in Shetland ponies. The smaller than normal ponies had complete ulnas and fibulas, an atavism. The condition is hereditary and apparently a simple autosomal recessive (Hermans 1970; Wintzer 1986). There are several examples of dwarfism in the fossil record (MacFadden 1992), suggesting that this genetic information is still extant in the pony population, at least.

Pineal

Senile pigmentation, fibrosis, and calcification have been observed in the pineal (Cohrs 1961; Potel 1968). Two pinealomas have been reported, one in a zebra and one in a horse by Potel. We have seen no lesions in light horses. Routine examination may be indicated in mares, in particular, in view of the role of melatonin in reproduction.

CHAPTER 5

Eyes and Ears

Diseases of the eye

General

Soundness examinations

Diseases of the eyes are common in horses as in other species. Affected animals may be reluctant to work or may bump into objects, readily calling attention to visual defects. Some horses with ocular disease shake their heads repeatedly (Lane and Mair 1987). Gelatt (1982) lists blindness, strabismus, corneal opacities, heterochromic irides, equine recurrent uveitis, cataracts, errors in refraction, floaters, and optic neuritis/atrophy as sufficient causes to fail a horse in a soundness examination.

A number of texts deal with comparative and equine ophthalmology, many with color photographs of ocular lesions (Gelatt 1981). A symposium on large animal ophthalmology in 1984 is still current and useful (Moore 1984). Two journal supplements are devoted entirely to equine ocular diseases (Barnett et al. 1983, 1990). There is a comprehensive bibliography, 1819–1989 (Startup and Tatum 1990).

Preparation of specimens

Utmost care is needed in preparing the eye and surrounding tissues for pathological examination. Some diseases, such as glaucoma, are dynamic, and since eyes are rarely removed during the course of the disease for pathological examination, only the burned-out remnants of the disease remain for study.

The eye must be immediately fixed in Bouin's or Zenker's fluid in order to preserve delicate eye tissues. For large horse eyes, the sclera is pierced at the ora serrata with one or two small gauge hypodermic needles to allow fixative to run into the interior of the globe, while it is immersed in fixative. Rough handling will certainly detach the retina from the layer of pigment epithelium at the cell cytoplasm of the inner nuclear layer, making retinal examination difficult and of limited value. Many pathologists lack experience in trimming fixed eyes and may create artifacts sufficient to confuse diagnosis. Care should be taken to examine anatomic relationships during trimming, especially when malpositioning has contributed to disease (lens luxation and glaucoma, for example). The trimming and sectioning of the lens is particularly vexing, and in most cases the lens is not well preserved for examination. *The most rewarding examination of the eye is done in the living horse, before the eye is removed for pathological examination!*

Inflammation and infection

Cornea, conjunctiva, nictatans, and nasolacrimal duct

Keratitis is one of the most common ocular diseases of horses, accounting for 40% of ocular disease according to Rebhun (1979). Trauma is of major importance in many cases of keratitis and keratoconjunctivitis (Kern et al. 1983). The cornea is the most anterior segment of the globe, coming in contact with considerable amounts of debris thrown up as horses are running or working. Horses also damage the face by bumping into objects, particularly within buildings. The face may be injured by blows intended to vent human or horse anger. The cornea may be abraded, lacerated, or punctured with subsequent inflammation.

Tears and defects in nasolacrimal apparatus

Decreased tear production, or alteration of tear composition, may increase the risk of keratitis (Munger 1984). Tears act as lubricant and wash fluid for the cornea and the conjunctiva, entrapping and removing debris, and preventing accumulation of microorganisms. Secretory immunoglobulin A, white cells, and lysozyme in tears are important defenses against microbes (Kern et al. 1983). Inflammation of the lacrimal glands may alter the quantity and composition of tears. In our experience, keratoconjunctivitis sicca ("dry eye") is uncommon in horses.

Defects of the nasolacrimal ducts

Defects of the nasolacrimal ducts may compromise tear delivery and function. Stenosis, atresia, and obliteration of the opening of the nasolacrimal duct cause overflow of tears. The causes of nasolacrimal obstruction include congenital malformations of the duct, foreign bodies lodged in or near the duct, inflammation, or compression by the growth of tumors, such as sarcoids (Fig. 5.1), squamous cell carcinoma, or melanoma. Purulent conjunctivitis may localize in the nasolacrimal sac, causing dacryocystitis and nasolacrimal fistulae (Silbersiepe et al. 1986). Parasitic infections can interfere with tear production and discharge (see below).

Keratoconjunctivitis can be caused by infection with viruses that proliferate in epithelial cells, such as herpesvirus (EHV)-1 (Riis 1981). The incidence is low, however, given the frequency of this virus in the population.

Keratoconjunctivitis was found in 7 Thoroughbred horses; equine herpesvirus (EHV)-2 was isolated from 1 foal (Thein and Bohm 1976). The foal and its mare had elevated antibody titers. Six

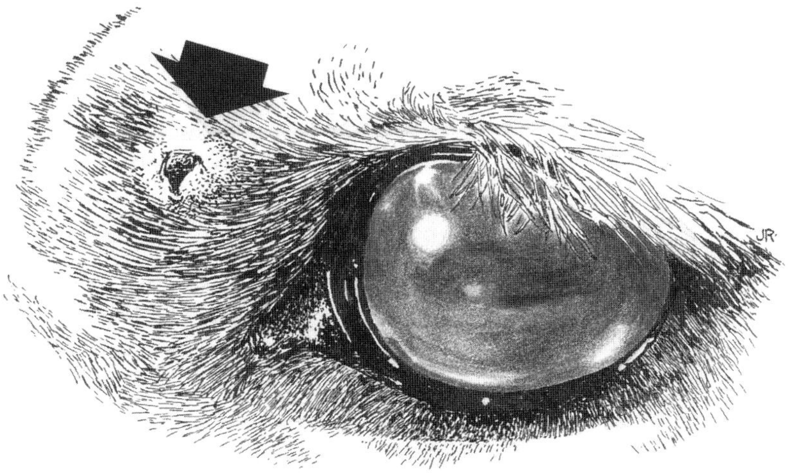

5.1. The growth of a small sarcoid (*arrow*) near the medial canthus of the eye leads to partial obstruction of the nasolacrimal duct and epiphora.

cases of unilateral ulcerative or punctate keratitis, presumed caused by herpes, responded to antiviral medication (idoxuridine), but the virus was not isolated (Matthews and Handscombe 1983c). Miller et al. (1990) isolated herpesvirus (EHV)-2 from the eye of a 5-year-old Thoroughbred with keratitis and corneal edema.

Horses with equine viral arteritis virus often have conjunctival and corneal inflammation (Whitley and Gelatt 1981). Intense hyperemia of the conjunctivae is a clinical hallmark of this disease. Purulent conjunctivitis caused by adenovirus infection of the epithelium has been reported in Arabian foals with combined immunodeficiency (Studdert 1978).

Keratoconjunctivitis or conjunctivitis is not an uncommon complication of such diseases as influenza and strangles. Hughes and Pugh (1970) reported infectious keratoconjunctivitis caused by *Moraxella* sp. (not *bovis*), though this is not a major cause of these conditions in horses.

The normal and pathological flora of the conjunctiva has been intensively studied (Whitley and Moore 1984). Reovirus-3 (Ralph strain) has been isolated from normal foals, but is apparently nonpathogenic since experimental inoculation does not cause ocular disease (Conner et al. 1984). Species of *Corynebacterium*, *Staphylococcus*, *Bacillus*, *Streptomyces*, and 10 other bacteria were isolated from 56% of normal horse eyes (Whitley and Moore 1984). Others found bacteria in up to 97% of normal conjunctivas (Lundvall 1967; Cattabiani et al. 1976; Whitley et al. 1983). *Chlamydia psittaci* was isolated from 5% of the nasal and conjunctival swabs of 300 horses (Mair and Wills 1992). This is obviously a normal inhabitant since there were no signs of respiratory or conjunctival disease. Inoculation of the organism into the conjunctival sacs, nasal cavity, or bronchi of six ponies produced no clinical disease, although the organism was recovered weeks later, and all ponies produced antibodies.

Fungi are also common in the normal flora. Eastwood, cited by Whitley and Moore (1984), found 28 genera and 111 species of fungi in the conjunctival sacs of 216 normal horses. The common species isolated in several studies were *Aspergillus*, *Alternaria*, *Penicillium*, *Fusarium*, and *Absidia* (Lundvall 1967; Eastwood 1969; Riis and Smith 1975). Samuelson et al. (1983) cultured *Aspergillus* from the conjunctival sacs of 95% of 111 horses. Differences in geographic distribution, seasonal occurrence, conditions of husbandry, and methods of isolation and culture influenced the types of bacteria and fungi found.

The flora of diseased eyes, especially those treated with antibiotics and corticosteroids, differed from that of healthy eyes (Moore et al. 1983; Whitley and Moore 1984). Common isolates from horses with ulcerative keratitis and conjunctivitis included species of *Streptococcus* (44% of eyes sampled), *Pseudomonas* (27%), *Enterobacter* (24%), *Staphylococcus* (13%), and *Klebsiella* (11%) (McLaughlin et al. 1983; Whitley and Moore 1984).

Streptococcus viridans was isolated from the corneas of 13.5% of 249 horses with ulcerative keratitis (Higgins et al. 1984; Silva-Curiel et al. 1990). This species of *Streptococcus*, usually considered nonpathogenic, may simply be an opportunistic invader of devitalized corneal tissue. Species of *Pseudomonas* are particularly important since they secrete proteases that severely damage the corneal stroma (Gelatt 1974; Rebhun 1981; Moore et al. 1983).

Severe ulcerative keratitis was caused by mixed bacterial and *Aspergillus* infections, possibly because of the selective effects of antibiotics and corticosteroids on ocular flora, corneal collagen synthesis, and tear production and composition (Moore et al. 1983; Kern et al. 1983). Peiffer (1979) described 6 cases of keratomycosis. *Aspergillus* was isolated from 3, *Fusarium* in 2 and *Cladosporium* in the other case. The clinical course of 11 cases of keratomycosis was described by Beech et al. (1983), and 11 additional cases were described by Joyce (1983).

Grossly, keratitis is highly variable, depending on the inciting cause, duration, segment of the cornea involved, growth of microorganisms, and therapy. With simple keratitis, there may be focal opacification of the cornea at the site of inflammation. Defects in the corneal epithelium predispose the cornea to invasion by opportunistic or pathogenic microorganisms, the inflammatory response being more intense and extensive with diffuse corneal cloudiness. Characteristically, there is congestion of the conjunctiva and, in severe cases, congestion of the sclera. Defects in the surface are shown by staining with fluorescein dye. Ulceration through the layers of the cornea may allow accumulation of debris in the ulcer crater. Infection with herpesvirus causes focal, punctate keratitis (Matthews and Handscombe 1983c). In severe cases, ulceration reaching Descemet's membrane, the pressure of the aqueous in the anterior chamber causes bulging of the membrane with immediate danger of rupture. In chronic keratitis, vascular and fibroblastic elements infiltrate and form easily recognized organized opacities on the corneal surface. In protracted, severe cases of keratomycosis, infection may extend to the anterior uveal tract.

Peripheral corneal ulcers

An unusual variant, peripheral corneal ulcers, was described in five horses (Dice and Cooley 1990). Corneal ulceration occurred at the corneolimbal junction and spread outward and toward the center of the cornea. None of the horses had a history of trauma.

The microscopic appearance is variable, depending principally on the duration of the keratitis and the presence of a pathogen. In simple cases of trauma and viral or bacterial infection, the lesion may be limited to necrosis of the corneal epithelium and infiltration with inflammatory cells. In more complex or serious cases defects may penetrate through the epithelial layer into the corneal stroma. Colonization with bacteria such as *Pseudomonas aeruginosa*, which secrete proteases, may lyse the stroma. Mixtures of debris, necrotic cells, bacteria, and inflammatory cells are seen. Fibroblastic and vascular proliferation occurs in chronic lesions with large, healed defects. Focal corneal abscesses may occur.

Microscopic lesions with keratomycoses include erosion of the corneal epithelium, stromal necrosis and inflammation, abscess formation, and deep penetration and growth of fungi. Anterior uveitis and conjunctival infection and inflammation by extension have been described (Kern et al. 1983). Scar formation is recognized microscopically as zones of fibrosis and neovascularization.

Peripheral corneal ulcers appear somewhat different than other ulcers. Microscopically, they penetrate the cornea from the most superficial layers of the epithelium and stroma to midstroma (Dice and Cooley 1990). Folding and lipping of the epithelial edge of the ulcer was seen in most cases. The ulcer bed may be extensively infiltrated with lymphocytes and plasma cells.

Eosinophilic granulomata

Eosinophilic granulomata of the membrana nictatans have been reported with habronemiasis in the southern United States, although the parasite is rarely found in sections (Joyce et al. 1972). Large lesions may irritate the cornea with predictable corneal edema, inflammation, and scarring.

Uveal tract

The uveal tract is the vascular system of the globe. It comprises the iris, ciliary body, and choroid. There are three important inflammatory diseases: equine recurrent uveitis, lens-induced uveitis, and uveitis associated with onchocerciasis. A unifying scheme for the pathogenesis of uveitis was given by Matthews and Handscombe (1983c). Ocular trauma of sufficient severity may cause uveitis as well as other lesions.

Equine recurrent uveitis

Equine recurrent uveitis is the commonest cause of blindness in horses and the most common inflammatory disease of the eye, after keratitis. The acute lesions include iridocyclitis, chorioretinitis, and optic neuritis. The recurring inflammatory episodes cause progressive disease and irreversible lesions (Cook et al. 1983).

Recurrent uveitis has been known at least since the Greek veterinarian Apsyrtos described it in the fourth century BCE. Synonyms include *periodic ophthalmia*, *recurrent ophthalmitis*, *recurrent iridocyclitis*, and *moon blindness* (Gelatt 1982; Hines 1984; Jubb and Kennedy 1985). These terms refer to the characteristic relapsing nature of the disease, relapses occurring at irregular, or roughly monthly, intervals. Despite intensive studies of pathology and etiology, the disease is still not completely understood.

It has been estimated that equine recurrent uveitis affects up to 10%–12% of the horse population (Cross 1969; Gelatt 1982) but the British Equine Veterinary Association survey of 1965 found it in only 0.09% of the horse and pony population, cited by Matthews and Handscombe (1983c). The disease appears to have relationships with geographical areas, housing, and husbandry, but there has been little or no investigation of these aspects of the epidemiology.

Three clinical forms are recognized: acute, subacute/quiescent and chronic/relapsing. In general, horses suffer an initial acute attack with the iris and choroid infiltrated predominantly by neutrophils. This is followed by a clinically quiescent period during which there is progressive tissue damage and infiltration of lymphocytes and plasma cells. Periodically, there are flare-ups of inflammation, primarily mediated by lymphoid cells. Grossly, there may be corneal edema, conjunctival and sclera congestion, aqueous flare and hypopyon, cataract and synechia formation (Gelatt 1982). Choroiditis and chorioretinitis are common. Protracted or repetitive bouts of inflammation lead to circulatory compromise, atrophy and scarring of the retina and optic nerve, endophthalmitis, and collapse of the globe (phthisis bulbi). Altered lenticular nutrition, lens luxation, and synechia may lead to cataracts and glaucoma (Cook et al. 1983). Collapse or shrinkage of the globe allows accumulation of debris in the socket and secondary inflammation (Gelatt 1982).

Many causes have been proposed. Jones (1942) suggested an hereditary predisposition as well as riboflavin deficiency, neither of which had been substantiated. Heusser et al. (1948) reported an association with infection by *Leptospira*. Other organisms, including *Brucella* sp., *Onchocerca cervicalis*, *Streptococcus* sp., *Toxoplasma gondii*, equine herpesvirus (EHV)-1 and parainfluenza, *Chlamydia psittaci*, mycoplasms, *Strongylus vulgaris*, and some species of fungi, have been suggested. Hypersensitivity reactions to antigens present in infectious organisms or in ocular structures have been proposed (Matthews and Handscombe 1983c). At present immune-mediated processes and infection with *Leptospira pomona* and *Onchocerca cervicalis* appear to be of importance in the pathogenesis of the disease.

There is little doubt that, based on the available evidence, leptospirosis is one, if not the only, cause of uveitis in horses. There have been repeated observations that leptospirosis in humans is a cause of uveitis (Weil 1886; Hines 1984). Gelatt (1982) found that 70%–95% of horses with recurrent uveitis had serum agglutinins to leptospiral antigens, confirming earlier work by Rimpau (1947) and Morter et al. (1969) cited by Hines (1984). Ponies experimentally infected with *Leptospira pomona* developed recurrent uveitis within 12–24 months (Williams et al. 1971). The intravitreal injection of leptospiral antigens elicited strong inflammatory responses, with some evidence of cross reactivity between uveal and leptospiral antigens (Wood and Davis 1950; Williams 1973). Higher levels of leptospiral antibodies are found in the aqueous humor than in sera of affected horses, suggesting local production by sensitized cells (Witmer 1954). The organism has been isolated from the eyes of horses with leptospirosis and bilateral uveitis. Vaccination with leptospiral bacterins apparently reduced the number of new cases of recurrent uveitis on farms with a high incidence (Roberts 1969).

Some data, however, are inconsistent with a simple role for leptospirosis in this disease. For example, many normal horses have antibodies to leptospiral antigens. While some surveys show 30%–50% of horses with serum agglutinins, only about 10% of horses develop recurrent uveitis (Roberts 1969). Few horses experience systemic disease with leptospiral infection, despite the rather high rate of exposure suggested by antibody surveys. Hines (1984) noted that the inflammatory response seen in experimental uveitis differs from that in the naturally occurring disease. In experimental disease, acute inflammatory cells are present. In natural cases, aggregates of lymphoid cells in the ciliary body and iris are considered highly characteristic.

Infection of the eye by *Onchocerca cervicalis* also causes uveitis and has been cited as a cause of recurrent uveitis. **Onchocerciasis** is a significant cause of human ocular disease worldwide (Attenburrow et al. 1983). Fifty to sixty percent of the equine population in some geographical areas have antibodies against this filarid parasite (Lloyd and Soulsby 1978). An incidence of 14%–24% was found in horses at an abattoir in England (Mellor 1973), but Attenburrow et al. (1983) only found 2.3% using skin biopsy isolation techniques.

The clinical, gross, and microscopic features of equine onchocerciasis have been described (Cello 1971; Schmidt et al. 1982; Attenburrow et al. 1983; Munger 1983). The acute inflammatory response includes hyperemia of the anterior segment and conjunctival vasculature, chemosis, and corneal opacification. A wedge-shaped plaque of disorganized, hyperplastic, and inflamed corneal epithelium and stroma, oriented from the limbus to the center of the cornea, is considered the characteristic corneal lesion of the disease (Munger 1983). Conjunctival lymphoid aggregates are common (Cook et al. 1983; Munger 1983). In more severe cases, acute anterior uveitis with aqueous flare has been seen. More advanced and degenerative changes in long-standing cases include cataracts and synechiae, choroidal sclerosis, and retinal depigmentation and detachment (Attenburrow et al. 1983).

Recovery of the filarid from the eyes of horses with recurrent uveitis is not sufficient to establish it as a cause of the disease (Gelatt 1982). Horses with retinopathy and conjunctival depigmentation caused by infection with *O. cervicalis* did not have uveitis (Schmidt et al. 1982). Treatment with diethylcarbamazine citrate kills microfilaria and induces marked ocular inflammatory reaction, including anterior and posterior uveitis (Cello 1971; Schmidt 1982). Attenburrow et al. (1983) noted, however, that horses did not develop ocular inflammation following ivermectin treatment. Munger's (1983) hypothesis that dead microfilaria were a potent antigenic stimulus for recurrent bouts of uveitis is called into question by the latter results.

Various other immune-mediated processes have been proposed as the cause of acute and recurrent uveitis (O'Connor 1981; Hines 1984). The uveal vasculature and the vasculature of the kidney and choroid plexus are similar in structure and function. A high flux of fluids and filtration of plasma occur in all three sites. In the kidney, the structure and function of the filtration apparatus facilitate the deposition of circulating immune complexes—soluble combinations of antigens and antibodies. A similar mechanism has been proposed for the uveal vasculature in recurrent uveitis, but there is a lack of morphological evidence: presence of immune complexes, in situ deposition of antigen, and complement activation.

An immune-mediated pathogenetic mechanism would explain how a variety of organisms like *Leptospira*, *Onchocerca*, or viruses, altered structural proteins, and so on, could incite disease. As in the kidney, immune-mediated inflammation could be a common pathway for damage to uveal structures. This mechanism might also explain the recurrent nature of the disease. The initial inflammatory insult to the uveal tract, or other segments of the eye, could degrade normal structural proteins or induce cross reactivity to antigens in the eye, some of which might normally be sequestered from immunological surveillance. These antigens could induce specific antibodies that would either bind in the eye or circulate to the uveal filtration apparatus. The immune complexes could then stimulate further inflammatory response and antigen production, the cycle recurring until no more eye-derived antigen was available (that is, phthisis bulbi). Efforts to produce recurrent uveitis by induction of sensitization with retinal S-antigen in complete Freund's adjuvant were equivocal in 14 ponies (Hines et al. 1992).

Lens-induced uveitis

Lens-induced uveitis may be a consequence of penetrating ocular trauma or cataract liquefaction. Lens proteins are normally enclosed within the collagenous lens capsule early in fetal life and have only limited contact with immunocytes. The avascularity of some portions of the eye and the blood-aqueous barrier help to maintain a state of "immunologic blindness" to certain ocular antigens (Hines 1984). When the lens capsule is damaged or a mature cataract dissolves, lens proteins enter the aqueous and vitreous humors, inciting an acute inflammatory reaction. Jubb and Kennedy (1985) note that lens proteins are weakly antigenic and stimulate B-cell but not T-cell reaction.

Retina and optic nerve

Rebhun (1983) suggested that the structure of the chorioretinal blood supply predisposes this area to lesions of both the choroid and retina; retinitis alone is rare. Lesions tend to be more common in the nontapetal retina (Rebhun 1983).

Chorioretinitis

Chorioretinitis has been seen with upper respiratory infections, septicemia, and trauma (Rubin and Woodard 1974; Gelatt 1979; Rebhun 1983). Punctate foci of depigmentation and hyperpigmentation in the retina accompany a variety of inflammatory cells (Rebhun 1983). Rebhun (1983) described a distinctive chorioretinitis with a band of depigmentation below the optic disk in the nontapetal retina. Retinal edema, vasculitis, peripapillary inflammation, and optic neuritis have been reported in recurrent uveitis (Rebhun 1983).

Exudative optic neuritis

A primarily exudative optic neuritis causing sudden blindness in German horses was described by Roesti (1941) cited by Rebhun (1983), but has not been reported elsewhere. Bayer (1878), cited by Platt et al. (1983), gave brain disease, hemorrhage, infectious disease, purpura hemorrhagica, poisoning, and diabetes as causes of optic neuritis in horses. Retinal and optic neuropathy have been described in association with toxoplasmosis, Borna disease, and trypanosomiasis (McDonald and Cleary 1970; Rubin 1974; Saunders and Rubin 1975).

Granulomatous optic neuritis

A single case of granulomatous optic neuritis was described in a 10-month-old Australian Thoroughbred (Slatter and Huxtable 1983). A segment of the optic nerve rostral to the optic chiasm was swollen and discolored. Histologically, there was extensive infiltration of lymphocytes, eosinophils, macrophages, plasma cells, and a few giant cells, together with necrosis, hemorrhage, and fibrinoid vascular necrosis. Other lesions included nonsuppurative leptomeningitis and retinal degeneration.

Adnexal inflammatory lesions

Ocular habronemiasis

Ocular habronemiasis has been reported (Glaze 1983; Moore et al. 1983). The migration of larvae in the medial canthus and conjunctiva induces an ulcerative, granulomatous conjunctivitis, and focal dermatitis. The lesion may be filled with mucus, debris, mixed bacterial flora, and inflammatory cells (Moore et al. 1983). Yellow, raised conjunctival plaques and "sulphur granules" are considered characteristic of habronemiasis (Moore et al. 1983). Invasion of the lacrimal duct and periductal tissue has been reported. Rapid progression and seasonal occurrence are helpful in differentiating these lesions from periocular squamous cell carcinomas.

The parasitic filarid, *Thelazia lacrimalis*, may inhabit the tear ducts and cause conjunctivitis and keratitis. According to Lyons et al. (1980a,b), this parasite infests the eyes of 30% of the horses in the United States, only rarely causing clinical disease (Moore et al. 1983). Horses less than 3 years old are more susceptible (Lyons et al. 1980). *Thelazia lacrimalis* can also be found within the eye itself, as well as in the lacrimal gland and ducts, where it causes a chronic inflammatory reaction (Silbersiepe et al. 1986). Conjunctivitis caused by *Thelazia californiensis* has been reported (Grant et al. 1973).

Riis (1981) reported mild blepharitis associated with *Demodex equi* in the margin of the eyelid. Disease caused by this parasite is apparently rare, although infestation is not uncommon.

Congenital and developmental

Ocular dermoids

Ocular dermoids are foci of differentiated skin, usually with hair, on the limbus, sclera and cornea. They are uncommon. An hereditary predisposition has been noted in a few related Quarter horses (Joyce et al. 1990). While small dermoids are usually inconsequential, the impingement of hair on the cornea or conjunctiva can cause irritation and keratoconjunctivitis.

Corneal leukoma

We have seen several cases of corneal leukoma, a variably colored, usually white, rarely dark, accumulation in the cornea. Although it may be a residuum of inflammation, trauma, or corneal ulceration, it can also be a congenital anomaly. The lesion could be confused with the corneal changes in recurrent uveitis.

Corneal band opacities

Corneal bands or sickle-shaped opacities, are about 1–1.5 mm in width, double-contoured, and usually located on the inner surface of the cornea adjacent to sharply circumscribed thinnings of Descemet's membrane. Inflammatory cells are rarely present. Band opacities are not uncommon and may be either congenital or the result of inflammation (Walde 1983a). Sickle-shaped opacities occur on the lateral or medial border of the cornea in more or less marked form in almost all horses, and are of little functional consequence.

Congenital iris hypoplasia

Joyce et al. (1990) reported congenital iris hypoplasia in related Quarter horses with ocular dermoids and cataracts. Erikkson (1955) reported hypoplasia of the iris in Belgian horses: a stallion and 65 progeny. The pupil was dilated, rounded, and unresponsive to light. The animals were photophobic (Joyce et al. 1990; Ueda 1990). The edge of the lens can be visualized in such animals, which is not possible in normal horses. Histologically there is a substantial reduction in size and differentiation of the iris (Joyce et al. 1990).

Cysts of the iris

Cysts of the iris occur on either the front or back surface of the iris, more often on the back. There was an incidence of 4.4% in Thoroughbred horses in one study [Szutter cited by Silbersiepe et al. (1986)]. Ciliary body cysts, 1–10 mm in size, have been reported in ponies (Dziezyc et al. 1990). Iridial cysts may be either uveal or stromal and are generally spherical, with a variable amount of pigmentation (Matthews and Platt 1990). Stromal cysts are more common in heterochromic irides.

Granula iridica

Granula iridica, or hyperplasia of corpora nigra, is not uncommon in the horse (Mathews and Platt 1990). If large enough they may interfere with vision, though that is uncommon. They are not preneoplastic.

Cataracts

Cataracts are unilateral or bilateral areas of opacification in the lens. In horses, as other species, both congenital and acquired forms are found. Leclainche (1936) says that cataracts were seen in horses and successfully operated upon in antiquity—BCE.

Congenital cataracts are not uncommon, usually as suture line cataracts on the anterior or posterior cortex (Walde 1983b). The causes are largely unknown. Whitley et al. (1983) stated that persistence of embryonic vasculature, parturient trauma, prenatal foal and maternal nutrition, infectious agents, and heritable factors had been proposed but not established. Malformation of the iris and congenital cataracts are heritable as an autosomal dominant trait in some families of Belgian and Thoroughbred horses (Ericksson 1955; Slatter 1981). Three of 82 Thoroughbred foals, 1-30 days, had posterior polar cataracts with prominent Y-sutures in one study (Koch et al. 1978). Beech et al. (1984a) described congenital nuclear cataracts in 11 of 16 related Morgan horses and 3 unrelated Morgan horses. The mode of inheritance was not determined. Histological examination of lenses from affected animals has rarely been done. Cataracts, ocular dermoids, and iris hypoplasia were reported as an autosomal dominant in a group of Quarter horses (Joyce et al. 1990).

Cataracts may be acquired in several ways. Traumatic damage to the lens covering and recurrent uveitis are common causes (Whitley et al. 1991; Dziezyc et al. 1991). Any disease process that alters lenticular nutrition will predispose the lens to cataract formation, and, so, cataracts may occur with glaucoma or panophthalmitis. Irradiation, altered nutrition, and toxins are thought to be factors, although none of these has been proven. Ocular neoplasms together with cataracts have been reported (Davidson et al. 1991).

Senile lenticular sclerosis, common in older dogs, is uncommon in horses, according to Severin (1974), but is known in horses 20–45 years old (Silbersiepe et al. 1986). A lenticular degeneration known commonly as "**Berlin rings**" is a not uncommon form of sclerosis of the lens (Silbersiepe et al. 1986) and may cause visual impairment.

Grossly, cataractous lenses are focally and irregularly discolored, with irregular mottling and zones of opacity. Focal opacity may be at the edge of the lens, equatorial cataract, or in the center, nuclear cataract. Distortion of lens size and shape may result in displacement of the lens from the zonular fibers. Progressive degeneration of the lens, specifically liquefaction of the lens substance, is important in determining the extent of lens deformation and luxation. Lenses that lose connection with suspensory fibers can move away from the vitreopatellar fossa, occlude the pupil, and cause glaucoma. Liquefaction and rupture of the lens releases lens proteins into the aqueous and vitreous, inducing uveitis.

Microscopic lesions are variable. Gelatt (1982) states that equatorial vacuole formation is an early lesion of cataract formation. Disruption of the lens capsule, degeneration of lens cells, and liquefaction of lens substance are seen in good histological sections. Inflammatory cells may be present in lens-induced uveitis.

There are a number of reports of removal of cataracts (Whitley et al. 1991; Dziezyc et al. 1991). Sequelae or complications of such surgery include acute and chronic keratopathies, adherent synechia, uveitis, endophthalmitis, and phthisis bulbi (Whitley et al. 1991). Corneal edema and infection have also been reported.

Persistent pupillary membranes

Persistent pupillary membranes are remnants of embryonic vasculature. In 144 foals persistent free-floating tags were found in one or both eyes of 47 foals (Latimer et al. 1983). When not free-floating, these membranes may attach to the cornea or lens with focal opacification.

Microphthalmia

Microphthalmia, or reduced size of the globe, is not common. One case was reported in a survey of 82 foals, 1–30 days (Koch et al. 1978). It may only be appreciated by measurement of the cornea (Latimer et al. 1983). Normal corneal size in 144 foals, 5 days to 20 weeks old, was 26.1 mm in the horizontal plane and 19.8 mm in the vertical plane (Latimer et al. 1983). A case of bilateral microphthalmia in a 1-week-old Thoroughbred filly was reported (Dziezyc et al. 1983). The eyes were covered with pigmented, nonkeratinized squamous epithelium, had remnant lenses, retinal dysplasia, and optic nerve atrophy. Similar lesions were reported in two Quarter horse foals (Mosier et al. 1983). More cases of microphthalmia occur than the literature indicates, but the frequency is not known. Infectious agents may induce this congenital defect in humans and other species, but none has been identified as a cause of microphthalmia in horses.

Colobomas

Colobomas are congenital defects in which a portion of the normal eye is missing because of failure during the closure of the embryonic fissure during embryogenesis [Willcock (1985) cited by Jubb and Kennedy (1985)]. The failure of orderly fusion of the fissure results in loss of continuity in the neurosensory membrane, pigment epithelium, and optic nerve. Defects occur in any segment of the eye, but are commonest in the retina, iris, and optic nerve. Colobomas are frequently seen in a constellation of ocular defects, which may include excavation of the optic disc, detached retina, and retinal dysplasia or atrophy. Irregular pigmentation of the tapetum has been reported. Colobomas are rare in horses, but not uncommon, according to Matthews and Handscombe (1983a); no data is given for either viewpoint. Cause or causes are not known.

Traumatic and mechanical

Traumatic lesions are very common and adequately dealt with in clinical and surgical texts.

Glaucoma

Glaucoma, a dynamic disease characterized by increased intraocular pressure, is uncommon in horses. This may be a function of the anatomy of the iridiocorneal angle. There is a well-developed capillary cleft, supported by a strong pectinate ligament and associated vascular channels with little likelihood of collapse (De Geest et al. 1990). Smith et al. (1988) reported normal intraocular pressure (23.5 mm Hg) and normal aqueous humor flow (0.88 μL/min/mm Hg) in ponies. These normal pressures and flows are significantly higher than in humans or dogs.

There are many causes of glaucoma in horses and other mammals, including congenital malformations of the iridiocorneal (drainage) angle or lens, inflammatory diseases altering the production and drainage of aqueous humor, cataracts causing movement of the lens and occlusion of aqueous humor drainage, neoplasms, and ocular trauma. Clinical distinctions are made between primary and secondary forms of the disease. Primary glaucoma is increased production of aqueous humor or decreased drainage without other disease. This has not been reported in horses. Secondary forms accompany ocular disease or trauma (Gelatt 1982; De Geest et al. 1990). Davidson et al. (1991) described secondary glaucoma in a horse with uveal melanoma, cataract, and keratitis. Glaucoma is rarely seen in equine recurrent uveitis; indeed, in recurrent uveitis there is gradual loss of globe shape because of decreased intraocular pressure and lenticular and vitreal degeneration (Miller and Whitley 1987).

Astigmatism

Astigmatism is said to occur in horses. According to Gotz cited in Silbersiepe et al. (1986), 30% of horses were found to have pathological astigmatism. In 80% the condition was bilateral, in 20% unilateral, and the author considered the defect to be relatively severe in two-thirds of horses with the defect. About half of the horses were *myopic* and were the more so, the more severe the astigmatism. Trevoert cited in Silbersiepe et al. (1986) found myopia and astigmatism to be interrelated, occurring mostly in Cold bloods in Belgium. Hamori (1983) reported this in Hungary as well. We have not yet found the clinical and examination details of these observations.

Entropion/ectropion

Defects in the anatomy of the eyelids can lead to entropion (infolding of the lid) or ectropion (outfolding of the lid). Trauma to the eyelid with eventual formation of scar tissue or neuromuscular damage can lead to these lesions. Some cases are congenital and seen with some frequency, not reported, in Thoroughbred and Standardbred foals. In one survey of 144 Thoroughbred, Standardbred, and Saddlebred foals, 5 days to 20 weeks old, only one foal had entropion (Latimer et al. 1983), but in our experience this frequency is too low. With entropion vibrissae may contact and abrade the cornea, causing superficial keratitis. The pocket formed with the drooping lid of ectropion accumulates debris. Both defects may alter the normal sweeping movement of the lid across the cornea and alter the flow of tears.

Skull fractures

Fracture of the base of the skull can damage or sever the optic nerve with sudden blindness and other signs of such fracture.

Degenerative

Proliferative optic neuropathy

Proliferative optic neuropathy was described in two aged horses by Saunders et al. (1972). There were no discernible visual disturbances, the lesions being detected in the fundus during the examination of 100 aged horses at an abattoir. Small, protuberant, white-gray, solitary nodules were found at the optic nerve of one eye in each of the horses, all thought to be at least 20 years old. Histologically, these nodules were composed of foamy cells, which reacted weakly with oil red O. Accumulations of these foamy cells were found at thc optic disc and also within the optic nerve. In both cases, the surrounding vasculature was tortuous. Saunders et al. (1972) differentiated this lesion from exudative optic neuritis reported in the earlier European literature. Major points of difference included sudden blindness and multiple, bilateral lesions with hemorrhage in optic neuritis, neither seen in proliferatic optic neuropathy. Saunders et al. thought that an earlier report by Gelatt et al. (1971) described essentially the same lesion. Riis and Rebhun (1990) concluded, from the study of a case of proliferative optic neuropathy in an aged pony, that the lesions were actually granular cell tumors.

Fundic pigmentation abnormalities

Matthews et al. (1990) described focal or generalized hypopigmentation or hyperpigmentation of the retinal pigment epithelium. These are common, nonspecific degenerative lesions according to the authors. They also found peripapillary choroidal degeneration, associating this with mural thickening and hyaline vascular degeneration. Eight percent of horses in Great Britain had this lesion.

Ocular and adnexal neoplasia

The common neoplasms of the eye and adnexa are squamous cell carcinoma, melanoma, and sarcoid. These tumors are described in Chapter 15, "Integument." Specific features for the eyes and adnexa are given below.

Squamous cell carcinoma

There are a number of studies on the incidence and biological behavior of squamous cell carcinoma. Twelve of 94 skin tumors in the Onderstepoort collection were squamous cell carcinomas ("acanthomas") of the conjunctiva or orbital region (Jackson 1936). Schwink (1987) discussed factors influencing morbidity in 43 cases. She found that draft horses that lacked pigmentation around the eye were more likely to have tumors. She calculated an incidence of 1:35.6 (1 horse in 35.6 will develop the tumor) for draft horses; 1:117.4 for ponies; and 1:1188.7 for a variety of light horses including Appaloosas, Arabians, Thoroughbreds, Standardbred, and American Saddlebred horses. The mean age was 9.9 years with no sex predisposition. The common sites included the membrana nictatans (37.5%), cornea or limbus (12.5%), conjunctiva (12.5%), and eyelid (12.5%).

Dugan et al. (1991) made similar observations in 147 horses, presenting data similar to that of Schwink. They also found multiple tumors in 26% of their cases.

King et al. (1991) studied 43 cases of squamous cell carcinoma in Florida horses. A majority were light breeds: 32% Appaloosa, 18% Thoroughbred, and 14% Quarter horse. Appaloosa horses, which lack periocular pigmentation, were overrepresented since only 3.5% of the hospital population were this breed. The average age was 11.8 years, slightly older than reported by Schwink.

All investigators noted that the neoplasm is locally aggressive, metastasis occurring in roughly 6%–10%. Solar radiation has an obvious role in the pathogenesis of the neoplasm, but this has not been explicitly investigated.

These tumors are of variable gross appearance depending on site, duration, and rate of growth. Neoplasms on the conjunctiva, nictatans, and limbus appear tan-white or gray. The surface is generally irregular with a tendency to papillomatoid irregular projecting masses. The surface is easily traumatized and ulcerated. In warm areas the tumors can be infested with arthropod or habronema larvae.

Microscopically, these are typical squamous cell carcinomas, with cords of poorly to well-differentiated squamous cells infiltrating adnexa and sclera. Keratinization is variably present and even absent in more aggressive lesions, a general characteristic of squamous cell carcinoma in horses.

Medulloepithelioma

Medulloepitheliomas have been described in the ciliary body (Saunders and Rubin 1975; Riis et al. 1990). In one case, the mass arose from the ciliary body at the ora serrata (Riis et al. 1990). It occupied approximately one-half of the posterior chamber and displaced the lens. Microscopically, it was composed of pleomorphic, stratified columnar cells arranged in rows or occasional rosettes. Most cells had moderate amounts of eosinophilic cytoplasm. Mitotic figures were rare.

Hemangiomas and hemangiosarcoma

Hemangiomas and hemangiosarcomas are rare in the eyes and adnexa. Bolton et al. (1990) reported three cases in Thoroughbreds from 7 to 22 years old. Two of the lesions were aggressive, requiring enucleation. The lesion was characterized by endothelium-lined vascular channels.

Intraocular melanoma

Six cases of intraocular melanoma were reported by Barnett and Platt (1990) who also reviewed 12 cases in the literature, most being in gray horses. This site is uncommon, intraocular melanoma being considerably less common than the cutaneous form. In this series, all arose from the iris. The horses were 6–16 years old. All tumors had sharply defined borders and were composed of a mixed population of polygonal and spindle-shaped cells containing variable amounts of melanin.

Retrobulbar melanoma

Sweeney and Beech (1983) found a retrobulbar melanoma causing exophthalmos in a 16-year-old gray horse. In one of our cases of intraocular melanoma, a portion of the mass extended through the sclera into the overlying conjunctiva with cords of pigmented neoplastic cells following the blood vessels.

Adnexal lymphosarcoma

Uveal tract melanomas

Uveal tract melanomas have been reported in horses (Moulton 1978) but are uncommon.

Milne (1986) reported a malignant melanoma of the thoracic inlet, which produced **Horner's syndrome** in an 8-year-old gray pony. The case is described with the nervous system.

Membrana nictitans

Glaze et al. (1990) reported a case of adnexal lymphosarcoma arising in the membrana nictitans. We have seen other cases of ocular involvement with lymphosarcoma, probably metastatic.

Optic disc

A very rare astrocytoma of the optic disc was reported by Gelatt et al. (1971). During routine fundoscopic examination of a 15-year-old Quarter horse mare, a small, fleshy mass was protruding from the edge of the optic disc. At postmortem the mass protruded into the vitreous from the optic disc. Histologically, it arose from the optic fiber layer of the disc and was composed of well-differentiated, loosely arranged astrocytes. While there were a few bizarre nuclei, most were typically spherical.

Vestre et al. (1982) identified a fleshy mass on the edge of the optic disc in a 15-year-old American Saddlebred gelding. The mass was grossly similar to the optic disc astrocytoma of Gelatt et al. Histologically, there was a proliferating mass of large, vacuolated cells adherent to the edges of the optic disc. The mass was diagnosed as a benign **xanthoma**. The description is not unlike that of the proliferative optic neuropathy discussed earlier.

Diseases of the ear

Many of the conditions affecting the skin also affect the external ear. Most are discussed with the skin (see Chapter 15, "Integument"). Auditory structures, especially in the middle and inner ear, deteriorate rapidly after death, and postmortem changes may obscure some subtle lesions.

Inflammatory

Otitis

Otitis externa, media, and interna have all been described [Cohrs in *Joest* (1969)]. They are uncommon although we have seen several ataxic horses at postmortem with purulent otitis media.

Ceruminous otitis externa

Horses can have a variant of ceruminous otitis externa, a condition in which the external ear canal is plugged with desquamated epidermal cells and/or cerumen. The plugs are hard and gray-white. Cohrs in *Joest* (1969) reported a case of bilateral ceruminous otitis externa in a 15-year-old half blood with hearing problems.

Ear ticks

Infestation of the external ear canal with ear ticks *Otobius megnini* or *Dermacentor nitens* may cause focal alopecia or ataxia and neurological signs (McMullan 1982). Bacterial infection or irritation and self-inflicted trauma can induce ceruminous gland proliferation and hyperplasia of the epidermis of the ear canal (Soulsby 1965).

Congenital and developmental

Aplasia of the external ear

Aplasia of the external ear (anotie) is rare. The middle and inner ear are normal. Atresia of the external ear canal has not been reported in the horse.

Hypoplasia of the external ear

Hypoplasia (mikrotie) may involve only the external ear, but is usually found together with malformation of the middle and inner ear [Rzaczynski (1718) cited in *Joest* (1969)]. The defect may accompany other malformations of the head.

Traumatic and mechanical

Trauma with hemorrhage may damage any part of the ear. This is seen most often with fracture of the skull. Cohrs cited in *Joest* (1969) mentions that "birth trauma" regularly is associated with hemorrhage in the middle and inner ear.

Mummification

Mummification of the external ear has been reported with ergot poisoning and purpura hemorrhagica.

Degenerative

Primary isolated peripheral cochlear degeneration

Primary isolated peripheral cochlear degeneration was described by Kolmer (1907). He found that 50% of the horses he examined had loss of the organ of Corti, ganglion spirale, and nerve fibers. This was confirmed by Cohrs (1923, 1928) cited in *Joest* (1969). No clinical abnormalities were detected. Odberg (1978) found loss of high-frequency hearing in some older horses, and this may be related to the changes reported by Kolmer and by Cohrs.

There are no gross lesions. Histological changes were found in the organ of Corti. The vestibular apparatus, utriculus, sacculus, semicircular canals were histologically normal. In histological preparations the sacculus may be obliterated with the free lateral wall applied to the medial wall. Nerves and other components of the auditory apparatus are normal, suggesting this is a postmortem change or artifact.

The degenerative changes in the organ of Corti are usually bilateral and of variable severity. Lesions are found primarily in middle and basal windings, mostly affecting the first half of the basal winding to the middle of the second winding. The beginning of the basal winding is often, but not always, spared. The scala vestibuli and tympani are normal. Reissner's membrane can, as postmortem change or artifact, fall off the tympanic wall. The limbus spiralis, basilar membrane, the tympanic covering, Reissner's membrane, and the spiral ligament are unchanged.

The organ of Corti is atrophied, as are the nerve fibers and ganglion cells. The neuroepithelium is replaced by a single layer of squamous epithelium. There may be no or few ganglion cells. The space normally occupied by nerve fibers and ganglion cells is replaced by loose connective tissue. There may be different degrees of degeneration. For example, outer hair cells can disappear first, followed by inner hair cells. The pillar cells gradually collapse. No inflammatory reaction was seen with these degenerative changes. There were no changes in the acoustic nerve nuclei in the medulla.

This condition is generally seen in horses over 5 years and increases in frequency with age. No breed, sex, or haircoat correlations were reported. Cohrs hypothesized that the first changes were seen in ganglion cells, with the degeneration of the organ of Corti as a result. There have been no recent studies of this condition and the etiology is unknown. It may be compared with the loss of high-frequency tones in aging humans.

Neoplasia

Papillary acanthoma

Papillary acanthoma (hyperplastic dermatitis) has been seen on the inner surface of the external ear in older horses. It is a flat or wartlike growth of varying size and shape, usually pigment free but, if pigmented, black. Histologically, it begins as proliferation particularly of stratum spinosum, with stratum corneum and cylindricum little changed. It is known at this stage as acanthoid wart. Later, papillary development occurs and the lesion is classified as papillary acanthoma.

Squamous cell carcinomas are rarely seen. So-called teratomas, tumors of mixed origin, do occur (ear tooth), but are rarely seen in light horses. Aural plaques are discussed with the skin (see Chapter 15, "Integument").

CHAPTER 6

Locomotor System, General

Muscle

Fibers

It has been long recognized that skeletal muscle contains fibers with differing morphology (Robertson 1910; Trautmann and Fiebiger 1952). With histological methods, **pale** and **red fibers** have been distinguished. The latter are more granular, smaller in diameter, more abundantly supplied with blood vessels, and more clearly striated longitudinally than the pale fibers in which cross striations are more pronounced. The pale fibers—anaerobic, fast-twitch fibers—contract more rapidly but fatigue sooner than the red fibers. Histochemical methods have permitted more precise classification. The pale fiber of traditional histology is the type II fiber, rich in glycogen, and the red fiber is the type I fiber, rich in oxidative enzymes and myoglobin (Hulland 1985). Further subclassifications have been made, but their functional and/or pathological significance are not clear. An approach to such understanding is the study of glycogen-depletion patterns of the different muscle fiber types in muscles of trotting horses (Lindholm et al. 1974a). It has often been shown, however, that fiber types, cross-sectional areas, and capillarity vary considerably from one part of a muscle to another. While it seems evident that these variations are related to function and may have pathological relevance, neither can be securely approached with present knowledge.

Rigor mortis

Rigor mortis begins, on average, within 2 to 3 hours after death and proceeds from fore to rear: heart–diaphragm–cranial and cervical muscles–fore leg–rear leg. Rigor wanes in the same order, usually beginning 12–24 hours after death. Rigor may begin earlier if there has been heavy, muscular work just prior to death, in cases of tetanus, strychnine poisoning, and with drowning. Ziegler (1969) mentions cataleptic rigor; that is, rigor occurring so soon after death that it appears to overlap live muscular contraction. It is said to occur in horses dying while working very hard at speed.

The normal pH of 7.4 of muscle drops quickly after death, reaching 7.0 or less in a matter of an hour or 2. Similar drop in pH occurs in other tissues as well. Tendon and connective tissue pH drops at about the same rate as muscle pH.

Ziegler (1969) says that rigor occurs in the dead fetus in utero, but we have not observed this in the horse. Zeitzschmann and Krölling (1955) mention massive necrosis of muscle fibers in fetal sheep, cat, and rat as a normal feature of skeletal muscle development. This has been seen in horse fetuses as well, but not studied in detail. The term, *necrosis*, is probably unfortunate since the cell death is a feature of normal development and, so, a form of *apoptosis* (Kerr 1987).

At present the classification of diseases of skeletal and cardiac muscle of the horse is problematic. In the absence of well-defined causes the classification must be largely clinical and pathological and, in both instances, muscle disease is distressingly stereotyped. We consider exertional, nutritional, allergic, and infectious. The incidence of the several forms of muscular disease has been given by Freestone and Carlson (1991) for 67 cases. They found over 75% related to exercise, about 10% infectious, 6% allergic, and about 4% nutritional.

Exertional myopathy

There are several conditions to be considered in this category. The clinical signs and pathological findings are similar in all. It is generally true that well-fed animals appear to be more susceptible, a point considered below.

Exertional myopathy (racetrack disease, *rennpferdkrankheit*) was described as early as 1890 (Hutyra and Marek 1920). Clinical signs begin after heavy, fast work or, less often, during work: pain, difficult breathing, fever, and heavy sweating. As well as firm consistency of the muscles of the back, neck, and legs, there are spasms and muscular fasciculations. The loin and croup muscles are more often and more severely affected. There may be no defecation and anuria. Myoglobinuria is uncommon. After a few days the major signs abate, leaving muscular irritability, spasm, weakness, and stumbling. Usually, recovery occurs in less than 3 weeks.

Recumbency myopathy

This characteristically occurs after a prolonged period of recumbency, whether for surgery or because of weakness, colic, and so forth. The animal is in pain, with a stilted, halting gait. There may be excessive sweating. Affected muscles are usually firm or hard and painful on palpation. The muscles on the down side are usually, but not invariably, more severely involved. There may be dyspnea, anuria, and/or absence of defecation. The signs may gradually abate and the animal recover. Myoglobinuria can occur and is a poor prognostic sign.

Restraint myopathy

This differs little from the above except that it follows entrapment, whether or not recumbent. Formerly, physical restraint in the absence of sedation could be followed by the clinical signs described above. Horses trapped in fences or down and struggling in confined boxes or vehicles can be affected.

Tying-up myopathy

This modern term certainly applies to the racetrack disease described above. We consider them the same. Hammel and Raker (1972) and McEwen and Hulland (1986), among others, have noted that females are more often affected. It has also been reported that epizootics can occur in horses racing in heavy, muddy going as well as in hunters working, for example, in crusted, deep snow (Hammel and Raker). Wintzer and Glasnap (1973) described a myopathy apparently localized to the croup region in trotters, 19 of 20 being females. It is not clear that this is a different entity.

Paralytic myopathy

Paralytic myopathy (azoturia, Monday morning disease) was recognized in antiquity, Apsyrtos (Leclainche 1936), and rediscovered at least by 1813 [Gohier cited by Cadeac (1899a)]. Clinically, at least, it is an exaggeration of tying-up myopathy. It typically affected, and affects, the heavy draft horse or well-muscled individuals of other breeds. It occurred most frequently in animals on full feed and work given a period of rest without reduction of feed intake, followed by a return to work (Carlström 1931/32). Cadeac (1899a) emphasized the higher frequency during cold weather or with changes of weather. The clinical signs are those of exertional myopathy with the addition of significant myoglobinuria in most cases. Rupture of the psoas muscles may occur (Ziegler 1969). A similar condition was seen in draft oxen under similar conditions (Burson 1912), suggesting, perhaps, predisposition of herbivora (see "Nutritional myopathy," below). The large quantities of myoglobin released during degeneration of skeletal muscle appear as myoglobinuria and may cause myoglobinuric nephrosis with tubular necrosis and eventual acute renal failure (Hadlow 1962).

While the precise pathogenesis of exertional myopathy remains unclear, certain observations are made. Carlström showed that there was an accumulation of glycogen in the skeletal muscle during the rest period and suggested that release of that glycogen with conversion to lactic acid was the immediate cause of the necrosis of muscle. With the onset of work glycogen is broken down by glycolysis with the accumulation of large amounts of lactic acid. There is too much lactic acid produced simply because there is too much glycogen immediately available, the glycolysis being enhanced by the adrenalin released in response to work stimulus. The predisposition of nervous, excitable animals, including females, can be thus rationalized.

It appears that high-carbohydrate feeding is a factor in excess glycogen accumulation in muscles. Herbivorous animals, on natural diets, obtain most of their glucose by hepatic gluconeogenesis from the fatty acids produced by cellulose digestion. High levels of soluble carbohydrate in the diet entail more glucose absorption, as such, with storage in muscle. While such readily available glucose would be "burned off" for energy in the working animal, it would be stored as glycogen in the resting animal. The basic pathogenesis of exertional myopathies, then, may be sought in the unusual, if not absolutely abnormal, amounts of readily available glucose provided to a metabolic system designed to operate with glucose provided largely, if not entirely, by gluconeogenesis. van den Hoven et al. (1986) have suggested that "loosely coupled" mitochondria may be a factor. This appears to mean insufficient adenosine 5′-triphosphate (ATP) production leading to a defect in oxidative phosphorylation, all the result of metabolic defects or inadequate supplies of essential nutrients. This observation is not incompatible with the Carlström hypothesis.

There is an obvious vascular component in the exertional myopathies. The anaerobic conversion of glycogen to lactate will not damage muscle if the lactate is removed expeditiously for metabolism by the liver. Inadequate perfusion or, at least, perfusion inadequate for the amount of lactic acid being produced, is relevant. This implies, as well, that elevated levels of lactate do not have to be present in the blood even with significant muscle damage.

"Rheumatic" myopathy

This has been described as a distinct clinical entity (Hutyra and Marek 1920; Cohrs 1961). It is said to be induced by chilling with recovery in about a week. The clinical signs are essentially those of exertional myopathy. Hosie et al. (1986) and Whitwell et al. (1988) described acute myopathy in horses at pasture in Scotland and England, noting that similar cases were known in Ireland, Canada, and Wales. Onset was associated with unusual and severe, wintry conditions. Cases have been seen in horses, acclimated to hot, humid summer weather, taken into air conditioned clinics for some hours and, then, returned outdoors. An association of azoturia with low temperature and chilling was emphasized by Cadeac (1899a).

Thumps and spasms of the diaphragm

There are numerous reports in the old literature of spasmodic contractions of the diaphragm in fatigued horses during hot weather (Friedberger and Fröhner 1895; Cadeac 1896). There are reports of this condition associated with tonic spasm of the facial and masseter muscles and clonic spasms of the temporal muscles. Nighbert (1900/01), from a large experience, reported that this occurred more often in animals, at rest and/or pasture for a more or less lengthy period, that were suddenly put to vigorous or extended work. Recovery usually occurred within a few up to 24 hours. In the modern era this is seen most commonly in Standardbred horses trained for long periods in hot, humid weather. No pathological studies have been reported.

Paralysis of the diaphragm

Only rare cases of paralysis of the diaphragm have been reported. Laulanie (1886) cited by Cadeac (1896) established the diagnosis in a live horse by simultaneous measurement of flank and chest movements. At postmortem the phrenic nerves were normal grossly and histologically, while the diaphragmatic muscles showed hyaline and granular degeneration.

Exertional syndrome

A specific exertional syndrome has been seen in **stallions**. The horses were in paddocks adjacent to a breeding shed during hot spring weather. They were not breeding that day but could see mares coming and going to the breeding shed all day. The horses ran themselves much of the day along the fences, sweating profusely. No untoward results were noted for about 5–7 days other than stiffness and slight depression. Then, the animals became markedly depressed and passed large quantities of myoglobinuric urine. Several died with acute uremia. At postmortem there was marked myoglobinuric nephrosis. There were scattered pale areas in a number of muscles, with minimal interstitial edema and petechiae. The histological findings are given below.

Localized exertional damage

Localized exertional damage of muscles is cited clinically but difficult to define morphologically in the absence of, at least, biopsy evidence. Isolated damage to specific muscles of the legs appears to be uncommon. Localized pain over the croup and loin are discussed (Jeffcott 1975, 1980; Wintzer 1986), but there is little or no pathological evidence for muscular disease per se.

Pathology

Gross and microscopic lesions of the muscular system are essentially identical in all forms of exertional/hypoxic myopathy, varying in pathological severity approximately in parallel with the clinical severity. Lindholm et al. (1974b) and McEwen and Hulland (1986) described the changes of tying-up, and Carlström (1931/32) and Ziegler (1969) described the quantitatively more severe changes of azoturia. McEwen and Hulland found that type II fibers, the fast-twitch, glycogen-rich, pale fibers, were preferentially affected in the tying-up syndrome. The affected muscles may be pale and/or streaked yellowish-white, with edema in the interstitial connective tissues. In all forms the muscles of the rear legs, back, and pectoral region are more often and/or severely affected.

Histologically, there is serous infiltration of the intermuscular connective tissue with dilated vessels, punctate hemorrhages, and variable degrees of degenerative change of the muscle fibers. This varies from nuclear pyknosis and fatty degeneration of single fibers to widespread swelling, granulation, hyaline degeneration, and necrosis. With time a light to moderate infiltration of mononuclear cells and regenerative activity may be seen. Vascular lesions, other than the evidence of edema and hemorrhage, have not been described.

Lindholm et al. (1974b) examined biopsies of the gluteus medius muscle in a series of Standardbred horses as tying-up developed. During the first 4 hours there was interstitial edema and focal degenerative changes in muscle fibers. An early degenerative change may be enlarged, hypercontracted fibers that show histochemical defects (van den Hoven et al. 1986). There was an increased amount of glycogen and enlarged mitochondria. During the 18–24-hour period the edema was more marked, as were the degenerative changes in the muscle fibers. There was marked depletion of glycogen and degeneration of the mitochondria. Type II fibers were preferentially affected. These findings are consistent with Carlström's observation of excessive glycogen accumulation in the muscles in paralytic myopathy.

Fatigue

Fatigue is frequently cited in this book as a causal factor in many lamenesses. While a valid and subjectively understood phenomenon, fatigue is difficult to define in specific, objective terms. Smith (1917) has provided an extensive discussion of draft and riding loads, including considerations of velocity and endurance. For purposes of discussion, fatigue may be considered as **passive** and/or **active**. Passive fatigue is taken to be diminution or loss of the ability of a structure or tissue to resist the forces applied to it. Examples include tendons and bones weakened by repetitive loading, analogous to the eventual rupture of, for example, a piece of wood, metal, rubber after repeated bending. The analogy is incomplete since biological materials repair the damage of repeated loading, and any putative fatigue failure is the result of loss of equilibrium of the damage–repair equation. Indeed, it is unclear with biological materials just what is damaged in most cases and to what extent the repair process is involved in the final failure. Shear failures of carpal bones are useful examples.

Active fatigue

Active fatigue is defined here as a function of muscular work. As muscles fatigue—whether because of exhaustion of local energy reserves, failure of replacement of such reserves, vascular insufficiency, and so on—they can do less work, exert less force, and lose phasic coordination. The latter means that any given muscle or group of muscles may not contract at the proper time or rate required by the loading experienced. Such uncoordinated muscular action may well be of greater significance in, for example, bowed tendon than passive fatigue of the superficial flexor tendon itself.

Horses are designed for moderate speeds over considerable distances with occasional bursts at maximum velocity and without external loads. Humans obviously do not use the horse according to design specifications, and specific training techniques are needed to prepare the horse for the work required. As early as 1350 BCE an Hittite training manual showed that chariot horses underwent rigorous training similar to that of Standardbred horses in the days of heat racing (so-called interval training). The animals trotted, galloped, loaded and unloaded, with rest intervals all through the day and into the night. Although the distances worked are difficult to translate into modern terms, 50 and more total miles per day were usual (Kikkuli 1977). Since scholarly research indicates that the Hittites earlier learned their horsemanship, at least in part, from the Hurrians (flourishing about 1500 BCE in the general area of the Black and Caspian Seas), it is apparent that the need for such careful and rigorous training for the life and death vicissitudes of warfare had long been known.

Nutritional myopathy

Also known as dystrophic myodegeneration, vitamin E–selenium deficiency, this has been described in several domesticated species, including the foal (Hartley and Dodd 1957; Dodd et al. 1960; Kroneman and Wensvoort 1968; Platt and Whitwell 1971; Sandersleben and Schlotke 1977). Thoroughbred, donkey, and pony foals are usually affected between birth and 7 months of age. The onset may be sudden or subtle with lethargy and a stiff, stilted gait. The more acute form usually follows exercise, foals going down and dying within a matter of hours. In Thoroughbred foals there are extensive muscular changes, including degeneration of the myocardium. Myoglobinuria is not infrequent. Less severe cases may recover with treatment. Skeletal muscle degeneration is present in donkey and pony foals, but may only be detected histologically.

Affected muscles are paler than normal and/or streaked with white lines and flecks. Histologically, there is an essentially noninflammatory myodegeneration with swelling of muscle fibers, loss of striations, hyalinization, fragmentation, and necrosis. Evidence of regeneration may be seen in longstanding cases. Lesions are usually not seen in the heart though fine-droplet fatty degeneration was noted by Sandersleben and Schlotke (1977).

Necrosis of fatty tissues was a prominent feature of the disease in ponies and donkeys and less prominent in Thoroughbred foals in the Platt and Whitwell series, but was a major feature in the Thoroughbred foals reported by Dodd et al. (1960). Sandersleben and Schlotke did not mention this lesion in their 46 cases, and the breeds were not given. The lesions appeared as indurated plaques in the subcutaneous tissues of the dorsum and sides in depressed, inappetant, feverish foals. At postmortem both subcutaneous and internal fat were involved, with the characteristic necrotizing and inflammatory lesions of yellow fat disease (Jubb et al. 1985). Platt and Whitwell found fibrinoid necrosis of capsular and medullary arterioles of the adrenal gland with associated focal necrosis and calcification in the zona fasciculata. Dodd et al. found foci of necrosis in the adrenal in one case. Fatty change may be found in the liver and kidney, and vascular lesions similar to those in the adrenal may be present in the kidney.

Apart from the foal, vitamin E—selenium deficiency in horses is not well defined. Degeneration and atrophy of the maxillary muscles of adult horses has long been known though of infrequent occurrence (Cohrs 1961). **Enzootic myoglobinuria**, long described in the European literature, appears, in fact, to be nutritional myopathy (Hutyra and Marek 1920).

The clinical signs of nutritional myopathy in the adult horse differ somewhat from those of exertional myopathy. The onset can be rapid in both cases, but with nutritional myopathy there is rarely pain, firm spasm, or fasciculation of the muscles. The muscles of mastication are more often affected in nutritional myopathy, and the disease usually has a longer course than exertional myopathy.

The loin, croup, and psoas muscles are involved, sometimes the muscles of the chest and legs. In foals the masticatory, pharyngeal, and laryngeal muscles are more often involved than in adults. Steatosis has not been reported in adult horses.

Histologically there is degeneration with swelling, hyalinization, fragmentation, and fatty degeneration as well as regenerative changes in longer-standing cases. Zschokke, cited by Ziegler (1969), found edematous infiltration of the intermuscular connective tissue and mild leucocyte infiltration in early cases. Bleeding may occur in the interstitial tissues, particularly of the psoas muscles and quadriceps femoris. In severe cases there may be similar changes in heart muscle, and there may be myoglobinuria.

The major differences between exertional and nutritional myopathy appear to be more involvement of the muscles of the head, longer course, and myocardial lesions in the latter. As well, arteriolar vascular lesions have been described in nutritional myopathy but not in exertional myopathy. These vascular lesions are characterized by hyaline degeneration of the media of small arterioles as reported in other species. While such vascular changes have not been described in the exertional myopathies, they are seen occasionally in purpura hemorrhagica.

In any given case it may not be clear whether the primary problem is exertional or nutritional or both. The cases described by Owen et al. (1977) as examples of nutritional myopathy are indicative. While the histological changes strongly support the contention that they were dealing with nutritional myodegeneration, the histories and clinical signs were an interesting mixture of nutritional and exertional, specifically that form of the latter called postcolic azoturia.

Vitamin E–selenium deficiency is a recognized entity in the young of a number of domesticated species, including the foal, but suggested as an entity in the adult animal, primarily in the horse. It may be that marginal vitamin E–selenium levels can be tolerated reasonably well in less athletic animals, for example, cattle, sheep, swine, but become limiting in working horses. In an earlier day a condition very like exertional/nutritional myopathy of horses occurred in draft oxen, except that the muscles of the pectoral limb were preferentially affected (Hutyra and Marek 1920). Hadlow (1962) reviewed cases of clinical disease and death in young cattle and sheep following exertion (driving, shipping), which were apparently related to vitamin E–selenium deficiency.

It is probable that the exertional myopathies are multifactorial: marginal vitamin E–selenium levels, fatiguing exercise, and, perhaps, glycogen levels, as suggested by Jubb and Kennedy (1970). Other factors such as ambient temperature may play a role. There would appear to be no sharp line of distinction among exertional, nutritional, and rheumatic myopathy in the horse, any given case being variably multifactorial.

Allergic myopathy

We use this term with the reservation that the pathogenesis of **purpura hemorrhagica** is undefined. Degenerative changes in the muscles are but a component of a more widespread vascular disorder. The condition is also considered with the hemolymphatic system.

Biggers and Ingram (1948) have provided a unique historical review of the disease, apparently first definitively described and given the name, purpura hemorrhagica, by Field in 1843.

There are hemorrhages in the skin and mucosae and bloody edema of subcutaneous and submucosal tissues. The mucosa of the nose, pharynx, and larynx are preferentially affected. The more distal portions of the respiratory tract are less often involved. There may be hemorrhages in the mucosa, muscularis, and serosa of the stomach and small intestine, less often more distal portions of the intestinal tract. The earliest clinical sign is petechiation of the nasal mucosa followed by urticarial plaques in the skin and/or more generalized edema of the subcutaneous tissues. Yellowish edema fluid with punctate hemorrhages infiltrates the intermuscular connective tissue. The muscles undergo parenchymatous and fatty degeneration and are gray-brown or yellowish brown and softened with streaks of punctate hemorrhage (King 1949). Inflammatory cell infiltration may occur later in the course of the disease. In an occasional case there is hyalin or fibrinoid degeneration of the media of small muscular arteries/arterioles, but this is exceptional.

A morphological variant of purpura hemorrhagica, consistent with the Henoch-Schöenlein form of the disease in the human, was described by Gunson and Rooney (1977).

Bacterial myositis

Chronic purulent myositis

This was a purulent, interstitial myositis, seen especially in the ventral part of the sternocleidomastoideus muscle of draft horses. It was a chronic, fibrosing process laced through with foci of purulent exudate. The initial lesion was believed to be a wound (harness, collar) infection with extension into the muscle. Usually called botryomycosis in the older literature, it probably was a mixed infection with staphylococcus and streptococcus. The former may have been fortuitous since the common pus-forming wound infection of horses is caused by *Streptococcus zooepidemicus*. The condition is seen infrequently since the decline of the working draft horse.

Corynebacterium pseudotuberculosis has been reported as a cause of subcutaneous abscesses, particularly of the pectoral region (50%) (Miers and Ley 1980). For the role of this organism in acute and chronic lymphangitis, see Chapter 15, "Integument." The abscesses can involve the underlying muscle, but are more localized, in general, than in the interstitial myositis described above. The condition seems to be prevalent in California and adjoining areas. The mode of infection is not certainly known. The number of cases peaks in October and November, normally a dry period in that area. The incidence varies from year to year, apparently being highest after winters of high rainfall. Transmission by biting insects is suspected, but not established.

Sarcosporidia spp. have been reported as a cause of myositis in horses in Europe (Schebitz and Hartwigk 1950; Freudenberg 1956; Cohrs 1961). The muscles had multiple foci of gray-white, firm fibrous tissue. Histologically, there was replacement of muscle tissue by fibrous tissue with masses of eosinophils and other mononuclear cells surrounding necrotic, caseous cores of debris. Degenerating sarcosporidial forms could be seen in the involved areas. It was believed that dead, and not living, sarcosporidia elicited the inflammatory reaction. The condition is rare in Europe; only about a dozen cases have been reported. The Halle clinic encountered three cases in 70 years. Sarcocystis infestation of muscle, in the absence of disease, is common both in Europe and North America, up to 90% infestation having been found at slaughter in horses in Europe.

We have seen two cases, over about 30 years, consistent with the German descriptions, but can add little to the question of etiology. It was our impression that the granulomatous lesions in the muscle were of parasitic origin, resembling the lesions produced in the liver and pancreas by the migration of *S. edentatus* larvae and in the pancreas by *S. equinus* larvae. As pointed out by Hadlow (1962) in an excellent review of muscular disease, sarcosporidia have not been unequivocally shown to be the cause of this disease. The same is true of the role of sarcosporidia in segmental encephalitis/myelitis. In both cases pathogenicity may be a function of abnormal species infesting the horse and eliciting inflammatory reactions not usual with adapted species. While entirely speculative, there may be common ground to be found among eosinophilic dermatitis, myositis, enteritis, and collagenolytic eosinophilic granuloma of the skin and arytenoid.

Myotonia

Myotonia congenita has been recorded in three horses (Hammel and Raker 1972): a Thoroughbred, a Welsh pony, and an Appaloosa. The cause and possible hereditary factors are not known. Of the 3 cases, 2 improved with age, while the Appaloosa became worse. The affected muscles, specifically those of the rear quarters, appeared overdeveloped with prolonged after-contraction and difficulty relaxing.

Ries (1913) reported a similar or identical condition in an unspecified number of horses of unspecified breed. The condition was progressive, with an insidious onset around 6 months of age. Some cases were followed to 3 years of age. The muscles of the croup and shoulder were primarily and symmetrically affected, appearing hypertrophic and hard when stimulated and atrophic once delayed relaxation occurred. Ries noted that Günther (1859, 1866) (no reference given) had seen similar cases in Mecklenberg and Hannover where they were known as "eisballen" (ice balls, presumably because of the hypertrophic appearing, hard muscle).

Histologically, in the Hammel and Raker cases, the muscle fibers were about twice normal size. The largest myofibers, invariably occurring in groups, had irregular contours with deep, membrane-lined clefts, and central nuclei. The perimysial connective tissue was normally distributed, but increased in amount.

Hyperkalemic periodic paralysis

This condition has been reported in Quarter horses (Spier 1992). It appears to be hereditary and analogous to a similar autosomal dominant condition in humans. Animals of all ages are affected, particularly males between 2 and 4 years. It is characterized by intermittent episodes of muscular tremor, fasciculation, weakness, collapse, and hyperkalemia. Consistent histopathological changes have not been reported.

Miscellaneous

Hypertrophy of the *mm. sternothyroidei, omohyoidei, and sternohyoidei* up to 3–4 times normal size may be seen in long-standing cases of cribbing and windsucking [Pader (1893) cited by Ziegler (1969); Fröhner (1905)].

Dimples may be found in the skin over the brachiocephalicus muscle, the shoulder, and the biceps femoris and semitendinosus muscles. These have been called *lanzenstichen* (lance stabs) and *prophet's thumb mark*, colorful if inaccurate names. Cohrs (1961) attributed them to muscle rupture and healing, but histological study shows no evidence of scarring or other damage. They appear to be congenital or hereditary, more often seen in Thoroughbreds and Arabians, with the histogenesis unknown.

Neoplasia

Benign

There are a few reports of leiomyoma and rhabdomyoma (myoma) in horses, but we have seen no cases (Ziegler 1969). Hemangiomatous masses varying from pea- to hen-egg size may be found in the interstitial connective tissue of superficial muscles, as well as in the intermuscular fascia and overlying skin. These lesions appear to be the same as those described in the skin and other organs and are, apparently, a congenital **hemangiomatosis** (Julien 1912; Cohrs 1961; Ziegler 1969). The histological picture varies from benign tangles of normal blood vessels to cavernous hemangiomas or hemangiosarcomas to undefinable admixtures.

Malignant

Several cases of "round cell sarcoma" were compiled by Ziegler (1969). No bona fide case of rhabdomyosarcoma has been reported, and we have seen no tumors other than hemangiomatosis.

Bone

Nutritional bone disease

Nutritional secondary hyperparathyroidism

This is an ancient disease of the horse, reported in virtually all parts of the world under a variety of descriptive names. Krook and Lowe (1964) and Krook (1969) have provided a definitive discussion of the pathology and pathogenesis. Some early references are in Leblanc et al. (1902).

The disease is an imbalance of calcium and phosphorus in the diet, phosphorus being present in excess. With the resulting hyperphosphatemia, hypocalcemia develops, and the parathyroid glands undergo hyperplasia. Increased parathormone removes calcium from bone in order to renormalize the calcium/phosphorus balance in the circulation.

Removal of calcium from bones causes characteristic clinical and pathological changes. Bone is removed by osteolysis with replacement by fibrous connective tissue; thus, the terms, *osteodystrophia fibrosa, osteitis fibrosa*. This process may, and in the cranial skeleton usually does, lead to an increase in volume of the affected structures; thus, the common term, *big head.*

The sites of predilection are, in decreasing order: cancellous bone of the skull, cancellous bone of the ribs and metaphyses of long bones, other cancellous bone, outer circumferential lamellae of long bones, Haversian systems of compact bone, and interstitial lamellae of compact bone (Krook 1969). Since the earliest clinical sign is intermittent lameness, before enlargement of the maxilla and mandible, the resorption of bone is probably progressing in the subchondral cancellous bone and outer circumferential layers earlier than the above predilection sequence indicates. The *lamina dura dentis,* the rim of compact bone around the roots of the teeth, is removed early in the disease, already noted by Leblanc et al. (1902).

The removal of the outer circumferential lamellae in the pathogenesis of splints is discussed there. Marconi cited by Leblanc et al. (1902) was apparently the first to recognize nutritional secondary hyperparathyroidism as the cause of ligamentous avulsions and fractures in older horses. Many were avulsions of the distal sesamoid ligaments from the sesamoid bones, occurring before evidence of involvement of the bones of the head. Removal of cancellous bone weakens the subchondral support of the articular cartilage of any joint, leading to collapse, erosion, and ulceration of the cartilage.

Osteitis fibrosa is the only condition in the horse causing subchondral bone failure as a primary factor in the pathogenesis of articular cartilage damage.

The parathyroid glands may be enlarged and more easily found than usual. The normal preponderance of dark chief cells is shifted to light chief and water clear cells, morphological evidence of increased parathormone production. One must be aware of the larger and lighter parenchymal cell characteristic of the normal equine parathyroid.

The morphological pattern in any given case will depend upon the age of the animal, degree of mineral imbalance, and duration. Lesions develop more rapidly in young animals as would be expected.

While calcium/phosphorus imbalance is the immediate cause of the disease, it is not always clear why such an imbalance has developed. Under controlled feeding conditions it is invariably the human choice of feedstuffs. At pasture, however, other factors may cause imbalance. Walthall and McKenzie (1976) described the disease in pastured horses in Queensland, suggesting that oxalates in the grasses rendered calcium insoluble and unavailable for absorption. There are other reports, cited by Walthall and McKenzie, of the disease in southeast Asia where oxalate-containing grasses are dominant pasture species.

Blaney et al. (1981) have shown that high levels of oxalate in pasturage can reduce calcium absorption in grazing horses, so that nutritional secondary hyperparathyroidism develops. They concluded that nutritional secondary hyperparathyroidism may occur in horses grazed solely on pastures in which calcium to oxalate ratios are less than 0.5, with such ratios occurring in grasses with more than 0.5% total oxalate. Their work was done in the Far East where, as noted, certain indigenous grasses accumulate significant quantities of oxalate. There have been no reports of oxalate-induced hyperparathyroidism in North America and Europe.

The possible role of heavy phosphate fertilization of pastures in producing the condition is discussed with splints (see Splints in Chapter 7 "Fore Leg").

Calcium deficiency

Low-calcium diets, per se, without calcium/phosphorus imbalance, reduce the size and density of skeletal tissue in the growing horse (Thompson 1986). The probable role of such a deficient diet in an "outbreak" of condylar fractures of Mc3 is discussed in Chapter 7. There are no pathological changes, other than quantitative bone loss, in young animals on a calcium-deficient diet.

Atrophy

Simple loss of bone substance, cancellous and cortical, is bone atrophy seen, for example, with severe lameness, postnatal contracture, and paralysis. Bone atrophy can be recognized radiographically and develops more rapidly and overtly in young animals. The gross appearance is obvious, and there are no specific histological changes. Bone atrophy is caused by disuse, of whatever cause, and is to be distinguished from osteitis fibrosa and osteomyelitis. **Osteoporosis** is undefined in the horse. Bona fide **rickets** and **osteomalacia** have not been reported.

Hypertrophic osteopathy

This has been seen in horses with tuberculosis or tumors in the lungs (Wirth and Pommer 1931; Obel 1969; Jubb and Kennedy 1985a). Guoth (1940) reported a case without intrathoracic disease. The disease was already known in the horse in 1902, Leblanc et al. We have seen one case in a 2-year-old Thoroughbred filly with granular cell myoblastoma of the lung. Most cases of this tumor in the lungs of horses have, however, not been associated with hypertrophic osteopathy. The lesions of the bones are as in other species, and the pathogenesis is unknown. The low frequency of tumors and tuberculosis in horses no doubt accounts for the low incidence.

Multiple cartilaginous exostoses

This has been reported in several species, including the horse. In foals and horses up to about 5 years of age, symmetrical or asymmetrical cartilaginous exostoses appear on the ribs, tibia, radius, tuber calcis, metatarsus, metacarpus, scapula, and dorsal spines of the vertebrae. Disorderly cartilaginous masses form on the metaphyseal cortex near epiphyseal plates (Dämmrich 1985) and undergo endochondral ossification. This is an hereditary condition compatible with a single dominant autosomal gene (Leone et al. 1987).

Fractures

Bones break according to mechanical principles. While predisposing factors such as nutrition and genetically determined conformation are important, the final pathway of bone failure, fracture, is stereotyped. The frequency of fractures in the population may be suggested by the data of Verhaar (1965). In the Netherlands, he found long bone fractures in about 0.3% of horses and ponies, with a somewhat higher frequency in younger animals. In the Prussian army, during peacetime, late 1800s, there were 3473 fractures among 280,000 horses presented for veterinary care, about 1.2%. The frequency (percentages) for different bones was (Fröhner 1905):

tibia	18
pelvis	16
proximal phalanx	13
radius	8
cervical vertebrae	8
metacarpus	7
lumbar vertebrae	3
thoracic vertebrae	2.5
humerus	2.5
olecranon	2.5
rib, femur, phalanges, occipital bone	2.0
scapula, frontal bone, maxilla, mandible	1.0

Fractures are variously classified, usually on orthopaedic and/or radiographic criteria (Stachak 1991). Here, the classification is based on the forces causing the fractures with attention to the modifying factors of pathological (predisposed) fracture and fatigue.

Most fractures of long bones are single event. There is either an increase of total force or a misapplication of force by misstep or trauma. These fractures are caused by forces generated by muscles and by the misplacement of the foot on the ground rather than by external trauma as such. This was well understood by Fröhner (1905). Most "small bone" fractures, on the other hand, are related to repetitive trauma (fatigue) and predisposing pathological changes in, for example, articular cartilage. Such fractures occur in the carpal bones and the dorsal lip of the proximal phalanx, among others. A given bone may suffer either type of failure. The proximal phalanx, for example, is subject to pathological shear fractures of the dorsal lip as well as to single-event, long-bone, "screwdriver," failure. Bone that one might be reluctant to call long—thoracic vertebrae—nevertheless fails as a single event.

The basis for analysis of single-event, long-bone fracture is the approximation that bone is a solid material, which fails in a brittle manner (Alms 1961). While bone is clearly not completely solid and has complex elastic-plastic behavior, it obeys the rules of brittle fracture mechanics.

Bone is subject to compression, tension, and shear. Many of the fractures can be simulated with sticks of chalk, appropriate force being applied by hand.

Tension

Simple tension causes transverse fracture, at right angles, to the tensile force. In an ideal material the fracture is a straight, flat plane, but the imperfections of real materials preclude such smooth fracture planes. Simple tensile failure does not occur in the live horse.

Compression

Compression of a column of material causes *vertical shear* failure. The axial compressive force is resolvable into two component forces: a normal force resisting failure and the shear force causing failure. There is a second type of shear, parallel to the loading force, but it does not seem to be an important factor in fracture of horse bones.

Vertical shear failure, alone, is only seen as bucked shin, but is a feature of many combined loading and pathologically predisposed fractures.

Bending

When a piece of material—bone or chalk—is bent, the convex side is in tension and the concave side in compression. Tension and compression are greatest at the outer edge and decrease to zero at the neutral axis. If the bending of a brittle material progresses to failure, it does so in tension along the characteristic transverse plane. The initial crack reduces the cross-sectional area, tensile failure occurs in the next deeper layer, and so on across the bone.

Pure bending failure is rare in the horse. It might be expected with a sufficiently large external force delivered to a bone neither bearing weight nor compressed by muscular action, that is, to a bone not under axial compression.

Bending and axial compression

This failure does occur, specifically with some fractures of the third metacarpal and metatarsal bones, the radius, and the thoracic vertebrae. The bone is bent and subjected to axial compression at the same time. If the forces are sufficient, tensile failure begins on the convex side of the bent bone. As the fracture plane progresses across the bone, the cross-section area is reduced, and the axial compressive force together with the compressive force of bending causes vertical shear failure to complete the fracture.

The relative size of the transverse and oblique

components of the fracture depends upon the magnitude of the tensile and compressive forces. This fracture in humans and small animals often has an intact soft tissue hinge on the side of the bone under compression when failure occurred. The large forces and displacements of equine fractures almost invariably destroy the hinge.

Torsion

If a brittle column is twisted in opposite directions, failure occurs in a plane about 45° to the long axis. In this plane, the disruptive effects of tension and shear are greatest. Such pure oblique failure has not been seen, but may be demonstrated with chalk.

Torsion, bending, and axial compression

This combination loading is the common cause of failure of the humerus, tibia, femur, metacarpal and metatarsal three, and the phalanges. The initial failure begins on the convex side of the bent bone and progresses in an about 45° plane in each direction until the upper and lower ends of the fracture plane lie in a vertical line—one above the other on a proximodistal line—on the compressed side of the bone. The fracture is, then, completed by a vertical crack joining the two ends of the spiral crack. A soft tissue hinge is rarely preserved.

Consideration of the topography of the fracture planes enables determination of the probable position of the leg at the time of failure. The analysis may be complicated by the presence of secondary fractures, but careful rebuilding of the macerated bone often permits determination of the primary and secondary fracture planes.

An example of such analysis is fracture of the humerus in horses galloping at a moderate pace. The fracture topography usually suggests that the affected leg was abducted at the time of failure: spiral-tensile-shear failure on the medial surface with the vertical fracture line on the lateral surface of the bone. In a number of cases, film or videotape of the accident confirmed the postmortem analysis.

Fractures of the epiphyseal plate

These occur infrequently in young foals with the epiphyseal plate as the *locus minoris resistentia*. The distal epiphyseal plate of the third metacarpal or metatarsal bone is usually involved. The fracture is simple bending failure with the transverse fracture plane on the tensile side and the shear failure on the compression side. Silbersiepe et al. (1986) mentioned that partial or complete epiphyseal fractures of the proximal femoral epiphyseal plate were seen in Cold blood foals, particularly well-grown, well-fed animals.

Fracture of the pelvis

These are not uncommon, but may go unrecognized other than as a severe lameness that gradually resolves. Silbersiepe et al. (1956) reported that 20% of all fractures seen in the Berlin clinic were of the pelvis:

1. outer angle of tuber coxae
2. fracture of whole tuber coxae
3. fracture of shaft. This may go with no. 2.
4. pubis—commonest pelvic fracture. May be seen together with:

4a. fracture of the shaft of the ilium. May also involve the acetabulum.

5. fracture of the ischium
6. fracture of the tuber sacrale

Jeffcott (1982) reviewed 50 pelvic fractures in 41 horses in England over an 8-year-period with essentially the same topography. There were more fractures in younger horses and a tendency for more fractures in males than females. Little and Hilbert (1987) reviewed 19 cases of fracture of the pelvis over a 10-year period. They found a higher frequency in young horses, females, and American Saddlebreds. Rutkowski and Richardson (1989) reviewed 100 cases. They found no breed predisposition, but did find twice as many cases in fillies as in colts.

Fracture of the outer angle of the tuber coxae occurs in so-called gluteal tendonitis (see Chapter 8, "Rear Leg"). Fracture of the tuber sacrale may occur with severe luxation of the sacroiliac joint. It may also be broken when the rear legs are snapped down to open the pelvic cavity during the postmortem examination.

Fracture of the skull

Fracture of the skull is not uncommon. Depending upon the blow or kick, running into fences and posts, a variety of forms may be seen. Often the animal rears or falls over backward with the force delivered to the occiput. The blow rostrally against the occiput causes the fracture to begin as tensile failure near or at the ventral, basilar, junction of the occipital and sphenoid bones. The fracture propagates dorsocaudally, bilaterally, opening the external ear canals and finishing dorsally near or at the junction of the occipital and parietal bones.

The animal is usually recumbent and remains

so until destroyed. Blood in the external ear canal, often detectable only by swab, is virtually pathognomonic. This fracture was described at least as early as 1845 by Cartwright cited by Smith (1976).

Fatigue failure of bone

Fatigue is considered in the specific sense of failure of a material as a result of repeated loading. Such failure is not well understood in inanimate materials and is more difficult to assess in biological materials, which are damaged and repaired simultaneously. Many tend to ascribe to fatigue, often under the incorrect rubric "stress," almost any biological material failure not otherwise explained.

During training and racing, the carpal bones, for example, are subjected to repeated **impulse** (impulse is force multiplied by time of action, $Im = F \times T$). If abnormal shearing forces are repeated sufficiently, the articular cartilage is damaged, its energy-absorbing capacity reduced, and even normal forces will be transmitted without attenuation to the subchondral bone. This additional force, for which the bony tissue is not prepared, can cause damage. The damaged bone repairs, laying down new bone—sclerosis. The process of damage–repair–damage is intermittent, damage occurring during exercise and repair during nonexercise periods, in general.

The following has been proposed (Rooney 1969). The repeated episodes of damage and repair cause an increase in the number of cement lines in the bone (Weinmann and Sicher 1955). These lines are fiber-free areas of cement substance laid down on free surfaces when bone ceases growth. They are included unchanged within the bone when growth resumes. In the case of intermittent damage and repair leading to sclerosis, there is an increased amount of bone and number of cement lines.

In general, the mineral component of bone resists compression and the collagen component resists tension, and the two share in resisting shear. Fatigue failure may be initiated by shearing the collagen-free cement lines. That is, the cement lines are more susceptible to failure in shear, being composed of mineral only while the bone tissue, composed of mineral and collagen, is resistant to shear. Once the cement lines fail, multiple stress raisers are present and macroscopic fracture occurs. This hypothesis has been partially confirmed (Carter and Hayes 1977; Katz 1980).

Other factors may, of course, be contributory. Shear strength of bone depends upon hydrodynamic as well as structural factors. Sclerosis will increase the amount of bone, but decrease vascular perfusion. Since the shear strength of bone is decreased as fluid decreases, sclerotic bone tends to fail in shear.

Aging

More fractures, in general, are seen in younger animals, presumably because of greater natural activity as well as more use of younger animals by humans. On the other hand, those fractures seen in older animals are often more comminuted and shattered than in younger animals. In the horse, failure stress and bone ash increase up to 4–7 years of age and decline thereafter, as in other species (El Shorafa et al. 1979). Bynum et al. (1971) showed that moduli of elasticity, failure strength, and rupture strength increased and then decreased with increasing age. Old bone, therefore, is not as strong as young bone and breaks more easily and with more shattering and comminution. It is to be noted that this does not require specific pathological change, such as the senile osteoporosis of humans, but, simply, aging itself. Senile osteoporosis has not been defined in the horse. Bone atrophy, as noted elsewhere, does occur with disuse, for example, fracture or contracture, in horses of any age and is not to be confused with the specific osteoporosis of the aging human. Fröhner (1905) recognized that the bone of older horses was more brittle than that of younger horses. He attributed the increased brittleness to senile atrophy, but such atrophy has not been defined morphologically, and we have seen no evidence for it. Indeed, it is probable that the increased brittleness of old-age fracture is to be attributed to the loss of collagen strength with age.

Osteochondrosis

Osteochondrosis has been defined in the horse since the 1960s, but it has been present, otherwise called arthrosis or chronic infectious arthritis, in horses for much longer. Cadeac (1909), for example, showed osteochondrosis of the medial ridge of the talus (his Fig. 102), although not identifying it as such. He cites earlier authors on chondro-osseous bodies in a number of joints, and some of these probably originated as osteochondrosis. Jeffcott (1991) has provided a review of the literature from 1972 to 1991. Dämmrich (1985) did an excellent review of the pathology of osteochondrosis.

One can, in retrospect, consider that patellar luxation and hypoplasia of the lateral ridge of the femoral trochlea was associated with osteochondrosis rather than osteoarthritis (Williams 1897/98). Osteochondrosis of the distal tibia, nonmarginal osteochondrosis of the medial condyle of the femur, and nonmarginal osteochondrosis of the medial ridge of the talus, for example, have not been found in the older literature, with the exception of Cadeac (1909) as indicated.

Either the lesions were not looked for, were misinterpreted, or did not occur with sufficient frequency to attract attention. Since the horse population of earlier days comprised largely heavy draft animals and half bloods, it might be that the modern light horse is more prone to osteochondrosis. While that cannot be established, the evidence suggests that osteochondrosis is less common today in draft animals, ponies, and grade animals than in, for example, Thoroughbreds and Standardbreds. In one study, for example, osteochondrosis was found in the medial ridge of the talus in about 25% of the Thoroughbred autopsy population, while it was present in only 5% of the grade, mixed-breed horses (Rezabek and Rooney 1992).

About 20%–30% of the Thoroughbred and Standardbred autopsy population have osteochondrosis in at least one site. Clinical recognition is about 10%–15% of the population examined. The discrepancy is largely the result of the small size and purely cartilaginous nature of many of the lesions. The frequency, in any given foal crop on any given farm, varies from zero to 30%, averaging about 10% to 15% over a period of years. This variability makes the selection of controls for experimental studies difficult, and it is hardly appropriate to use low or zero-incidence animals such as ponies or Arabians as controls for high-incidence Thoroughbreds and Standardbreds. Although the data is limited, there is a strong suggestion of predisposition of the left rear leg for osteochondrosis of the lateral ridge of the femoral trochlea and the medial ridge of the talus. No explanation has been offered. There is a 2:1 or 3:1 male predisposition, at least for osteochondrosis of the cervical vertebrae, sagittal ridge of the distal end of the tibia, and the medial ridge of the talus.

Arabian horses and ponies are only slightly, if at all, affected. Zeller et al. (1978) had never seen a case of osteochondrosis of the distal end of the tibia in the pony. We have not seen osteochondrosis in any site in a limited number of pony breeds and Arabians at postmortem. It is, perhaps, unnecessary to note that osteochondrosis is not limited to horses and humans; it has been seen, for example, in rabbits, rats, dogs, swine, and poultry.

Prenatal osteochondrosis

Osteochondrosis is defined as delay in endochondral ossification, that is, a delay in the conversion of cartilage to bone. In the context of prenatal development, this means that the cartilage model of a bone has properly formed, but the conversion of that model to bone is delayed. This occurs, in the horse, primarily in small bones such as the carpal, tarsal, and sesamoid bones. Prenatal delay of ossification presents in three ways:

1. At birth, the bone comprises more cartilage and less ossified tissue than normal. This is to be distinguished from hypoplasia in which the cartilage model of the bone is smaller than normal. There are two forms. In the first, there is more cartilage than normal, but there is a definite zone of endochondral ossification, capillaries being present only in the hypertrophic cartilage. In the second form, delay apparently occurring earlier, there is no clear zone of endochondral ossification. Larger blood vessels are still present in the cartilage, not having retreated from the cartilage as they normally do.

There are three possible outcomes: (a) endochondral ossification proceeds and no abnormality occurs—this would not be recognized; (b) the bone is deformed, compressed by postnatal loading, and the involved leg has an angular deformity; or (c) the compression is great enough to crush the bone (Rooney 1969).

2. The delay appears as secondary ossification centers. Such centers have been recognized in the proximal sesamoid bones and the distal sesamoid (navicular) bone. In the former, there are two ossification centers, one for the body and one for the apex. In the latter, two or three centers may be present.

In a large series of Thoroughbred foals followed from birth to a year of age, such secondary ossification centers in the proximal sesamoid bones were seen in the fore legs of 10%, either unilaterally or bilaterally. The rear legs were not examined. They appeared radiographically during the first 2 months of life and returned to normal in about 2 weeks (Thompson and Rooney 1992). It appears that a transverse fold or line of somewhat thinned cartilage remains throughout life as a marker of this event. The thinned line of cartilage is apparent grossly, but the bone is normal. There is no evidence of predisposition for fracture. Although these secondary centers appear after birth, they may already be present, potentially or in fact, before birth and not seen radiographically until there is sufficient ossification.

Ellis (1979) described what he considered to be fractures of proximal sesamoid bones in young foals. While some of his cases may have been true fractures, some were probably examples of secondary ossification centers, particularly in view of the absence of lameness. Stashak (1987) mentions bipartite proximal sesamoid bones in young horses, leaving the question of fracture or secondary ossification unaddressed.

As many as three ossification centers have been observed in the navicular bone at postmortem with the cartilage "marker" lines in the hyaline cartilage, only, of the dorsal surface. Parenthetically, both aplasia and hypoplasia of the navicular have been seen radiographically and at postmortem.

A secondary ossification center may either be a true congenital variant or give that appearance as a result of delayed ossification. In the congenital form the cartilage model is invaded by two separate sets of blood vessels, so that ossification begins in two distinct parts of the cartilage model. When interruption or delay of endochondral ossification occurs, there is a single center, and the cartilage continues to grow. With the resumption of ossification, a fold remains in the cartilage, giving the appearance of a secondary ossification center. It is not possible, once ossification has been completed, to know which process occurred. We tentatively suggest that a fold of cartilage indicates resumption of ossification of a delayed single center, while a thinned line of cartilage is the marker for two ossification centers.

Crushing of the small bones of the tarsus, less commonly the carpus, has been seen in a number of Thoroughbred and Quarter horse foals within the first few months of life. Ossification of these bones should be nearly completed at birth. Rooney (1969) described crushing of the central and third tarsal bones of the hock with islands of cartilage present in the crushed bones as evidence of delayed ossification. The delay was caused by hypothyroidism, hypothyroid goiter, caused by excess iodine intake by the pregnant mares (Baker and Lindsey 1968). Hypothyroidism causes delay in the conversion of cartilage to bone (Looser 1929). (See Chapter 4, "Endocrine System.")

Since the first reports, a number of additional cases of crushing of the central and third tarsal bones has been seen and others reported (Dewes 1982). In most cases there was no history of excess iodine intake and, in some, the lesion was unilateral. Obviously, then, the delay of ossification can occur in the absence of a known cause, such as hypothyroidism, leaving only the generalization: congenital and/or genetic defect.

Dewes's six cases were premature foals or twins. With the premature foal weight-bearing could begin before the appropriate amount of ossification of the tarsal bones had occurred. Similarly, twins are smaller than normal, development delayed, and the ossification of the tarsal bones incomplete at birth.

Krook and Maylin (1989) discuss prenatal delay of ossification as osteochondrosis. They hold that it is caused by excess dietary calcium, an hypothesis that requires more than purely morphological evidence.

3. A variation, particularly of the category described in 1, above, is encountered with some regularity in radiographs of young horses and at postmortem. Rather than an overall delay of ossification, focal areas of delay are found. Indeed, in some cases this is not delay at all, but normal variation in the rate of conversion of the cartilage model to bone. Endochondral ossification does not proceed at an even pace over the whole of any given articular cartilage. Some areas ossify more rapidly than others, as discussed with the histogenesis of osteochondrosis of the cervical vertebral articular facets (Rooney 1969). The topography and chronology of endochondral ossification of articular cartilage for most joints has not been studied, and it is not always possible to know when an area of thicker cartilage is normal or delayed.

Postnatal osteochondrosis

Postnatal osteochondrosis affects either the articular cartilage or the epiphyseal plate or both—and only while those cartilages are undergoing endochondral ossification. While that is obvious for the epiphyseal plate, it is somewhat less obvious for the articular cartilage. Endochondral ossification of the articular cartilage continues for a time after birth, while the end of the bone is growing in size and acquiring adult form. As already indicated, the time of cessation of growth and ossification varies from area to area for any given articular cartilage.

The postnatal osteochondroses of the horse may be classified:

Localized:
Marginal articular
Nonmarginal articular
Epiphyseal
Generalized: zinc/copper

Localized osteochondrosis

The basic premise is that the final common pathological pathway involves delay in endochondral ossification, followed by necrosis of the cartilage close to the chondro–osseous junction, with the healing process providing the final form of the lesion (Fig. 6.1). A differentiating feature of postnatal as opposed to prenatal osteochondrosis, then, is the occurrence of necrosis in the former.

Arthrosis may occur in joints with lesions of osteochondrosis, complicating the pathological picture. Osteochondrosis is characterized by one or more lesions *only* in the convex articular surface, while arthrosis and arthritis are characterized by involvement of both joint surfaces with erosion, ulceration, marginal osteophyte production, and fibrosis of the joint capsule. In fact, secondary arthrosis is not at all common in joints with osteochondrosis. It does occur in the cervical intervertebral joints and in more severe cases of osteochondrosis of the lateral ridge of the femoral trochlea. Secondary arthrosis is uncommon in other sites. Subchondral cystic defects, per se, do not establish

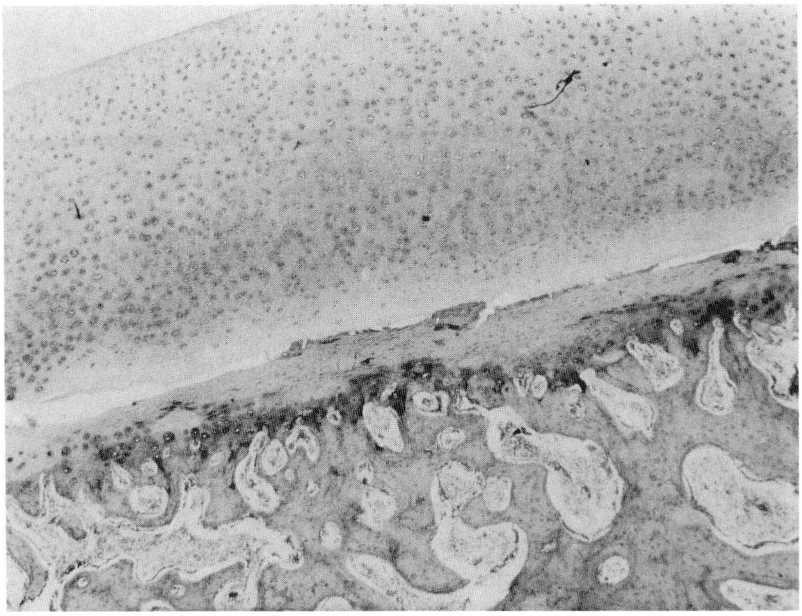

6.1. Low power, H & E of early osteochondrosis. There is necrosis and loss of chondrocytes in the inner third of the articular cartilage. Necrotic debris can be seen in the space, and reparative cloning of chondrocytes is apparent at *lower left* in the cartilage still in continuity with bone.

a diagnosis of osteochondrosis since these occur with arthrosis and arthritis as well (Trotter et al. 1982). Usually, then, arthrosis and osteochondrosis are immediately differentiated by the fact that the former always affects both joint surfaces, while the latter only affects the convex joint surface.

Osteochondrosis can only develop while articular and epiphyseal cartilage are growing. In Thoroughbred and Standardbred foals most lesions of articular osteochondrosis appear during the 3rd to 6th postnatal months. Lesions may appear earlier in foals with fracture of a paired limb or marked angular or other congenital deformity of the legs. Osteochondrosis of the epiphyseal plate, for example, is routinely found in the lateral part of the distal radial epiphyseal plate in foals with lateral deviation of the leg. This contrasts with the usual medial site, nearing 1 year of age, in fast-growing foals. No lesions have been seen in the fetus that predispose to postnatal osteochondrosis.

Known causes of delay of endochondral ossification include hypothyroidism, excess estradiol, and increased pressure on areas of endochondral ossification (Trueta and Trias 1961). There are delays of ossification of the small bones of the tarsus and carpus for which a cause is not known but a genetic basis suspected. While nutrition is frequently suggested, the only definable nutritional factor is excessive rate of gain causing increased pressure on the ossifying bones. No specific nutritional deficiency or excess has been identified.

Excessive zinc intake is certainly associated with generalized osteochondrosis, as discussed below, but has not been implicated in localized osteochondrosis. Experimental studies have indicated that excessive calcium or protein intake is not related, while excessive phosphorus and energy may be related (Jeffcott 1991). Excess energy may operate through weight gain, while excess phosphorus should manifest as osteitis fibrosa. Since lesions of osteitis fibrosa have not been seen or reported in early, developing cases of osteochondrosis, the relationship is obscure, if true. Tetracycline is a suspected agent of delay in the foal after birth as noted below.

Marginal articular. This form is seen, for example, in the cervical intervertebral joints, the lateral ridge of the femoral trochlea, and the dorsal end of the sagittal ridge of the distal end of the tibia. The histogenesis of this form was described by Rooney (1969) in the cervical intervertebral joints. Excessive pressure on those portions of the joints last undergoing ossification led to necrosis of the cartilage near the chondro-osseous junction. The articular cartilage continued to proliferate, and the overgrown cartilage was invaded by blood vessels, forming one type of secondary ossification center. The overgrown cartilage was converted to bone giving the end-stage form of osteochondrosis dissecans (see Central nervous system—spinal cord: Cervical stenotic myelopathy in Chapter 16, "Nervous System").

Osteochondrosis of the cervical intervertebral joints is unique in that it develops on both articular surfaces. As noted by Rooney (1975) and Dämmrich (1985), localized osteochondrosis is characterized in all other sites by restriction to convex joint surfaces. The reason is an increase of force per unit area in the deeper part of convex surfaces, in contrast to the decrease of force per unit area in the deeper parts of concave surfaces. Osteochondrosis develops on both surfaces of the cervical articular cartilages because there is little difference in the curvature of the mating surfaces.

The increased pressure leading to marginal osteochondrosis of the cervical articular facets is thought to be mechanical, involving the length of the neck and weight of the head (Rooney 1969). As with many osteochondroses, males are affected more often than females (Dämmrich 1985), a fact compatible with the mechanical hypothesis. The mechanical hypothesis is also compatible with genetic factors operating through the conformation of the animal.

Marginal osteochondrosis of the lateral ridge of the femoral trochlea has a similar histogenesis, the abnormal pressure being exerted on the lateral ridge by the misplaced patella.

Osteochondrosis of the dorsal end of the sagittal ridge of the distal end of the tibia is common and usually bilateral. It is the only osteochondrosis of the horse that is the result of osteochondral fracture. Routine postmortem examination of the tarsocrural joint of foals has provided examples of the early osteochondral fractures with a hinge at the dorsal end of the shear fracture line. These fractures are probably caused by rapid flexion of the joint during protraction of the leg and are more common, as the mechanics would suggest, with straight leg conformation.

Nonmarginal articular. This form is seen in the medial condyle of the distal end of the femur and the medial ridge of the trochlea of the talus (see Chapter 8, "Rear Leg"). It is less common in any of the three bones of the phalanx, the distal end of Mc3, and one of the small tarsal or carpal bones (Fig. 6.2).

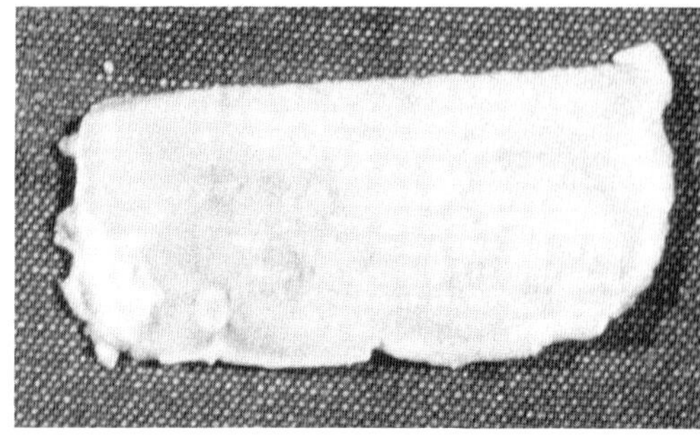

6.2. Nonmarginal osteochondrosis of the radial carpal bone. The lesion extends into the subchondral bone and would, in principle, appear on radiographs.

The histogenesis is similar to that of marginal osteochondrosis (Fig. 6.3). Pressure on the cartilage leads to overgrowth of the cartilage; that is, the cartilage continues to grow, but is not converted to bone because the epiphyseal circulation is compromised by pressure. When the critical diffusion thickness is reached, necrosis occurs in that portion of cartilage at the end of the nutrient pathways, that is, the inner third. If the necrosis is not severe, the core is sloughed and, with sealing of the chondro–osseous junction, a groove or pit is left as the final form of the lesion. With more marked necrosis, sloughing of the core opens the subchondral area to the joint surface. Synovial fluid can, then, enter the subchondral bone and induce a so-called *subchondral cyst,* its cavity filled with a mucoid, Wharton's jellylike material and surrounded by sclerotic bone. This lesion is no different than that found when ulceration caused by arthrosis or arthritis opens the subchondral area to synovial fluid.

During healing of such a lesion, the cartilage will proliferate and the matrix flow, so that the channel from joint surface to subchondral bone may be occluded. Careful serial sectioning will always reveal the presence of a patent or previously patent, now occluded, channel.

The overgrowth of cartilage characteristic of marginal osteochondrosis is not seen with the nonmarginal form since the growing cartilage cannot escape the pressure that induced the lesion. Overgrowth is characteristic of osteochondrosis of the cervical articulations and of the osteochondral fracture of the distal tibia. While it may be apparent in some lesions of the lateral trochlear ridge of the stifle, so much cartilage may be sheared off secondarily, at this site, that overgrowth cannot be appreciated.

Nonmarginal osteochondrosis of the medial femoral condyle is of specific interest. It is commoner in the straight leg of the Thoroughbred than in the, on average, more angulated leg of the Standardbred. With less angulation, the axial compression force through the medial femoral condyle is greater. It is of more than passing interest that the medial femoral condyle is the commonest site of nonmarginal osteochondrosis in the quintessential straight-legged animal: the human.

Osteochondrosis of the epiphyseal plate. This was described pathologically by Rooney in 1963 although it had been recognized clinically much earlier (Fig. 6.4). The medial part of the distal epiphyseal plates of Mc3 and the radius are most commonly affected nearing the time for normal closure of those plates. The pathogenesis of this "epiphysitis" is that of nonmarginal osteochondrosis,

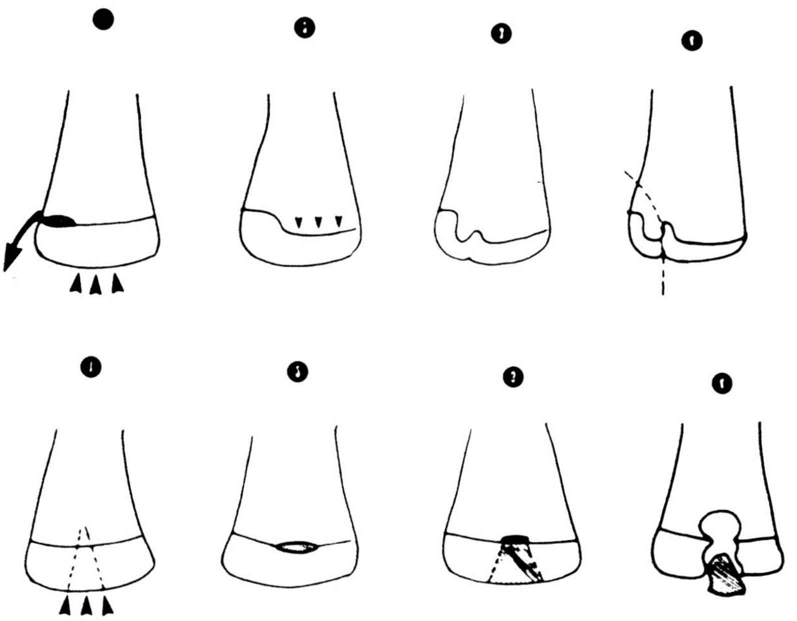

6.3. Diagrams of the development of marginal (*above*), and nonmarginal osteochondrosis (*left to right*).

pressure compromising the metaphyseal circulation and causing delay or cessation of endochondral ossification. The cartilage of the epiphyseal plate continues to grow and, eventually, undergoes necrosis (Fig. 6.5).

Since the lesion characteristically develops near the time of epiphyseal plate closure, healing is usually uneventful (Rooney 1963, 1969). The metaphyseal circulation is protected to some extent from the effects of pressure by numerous vascular anastomoses across the epiphyseal plates (Rooney 1969) (Fig. 6.6). When these anastomoses close, as harbingers of epiphyseal plate closure, the metaphyseal circulation loses its safety factor, and osteochondrosis of the epiphyseal plate occurs.

Osteochondrosis of the epiphyseal plate is frequently associated, as one might expect, with osteochondrosis of the related convex joint surface. Usually there is no evidence of osteochondrosis of the concave joint surface or its related epiphyseal plate. There can be lesions in the plate associated with the concave joint surface when the lesions in the plate with the convex joint surface are particularly marked. The clearest examples are in foals rendered three-legged lame by a fracture or radial paralysis of the paired leg. Evidence for increased pressure is the sclerosis of metaphysis and epiphysis accompanying the damage to the epiphyseal cartilage (Fig. 6.7).

To answer the question raised by Brown and MacCallum (1976) in their study of crossbred Quarter horse, Belgian, and Percheron foals, many

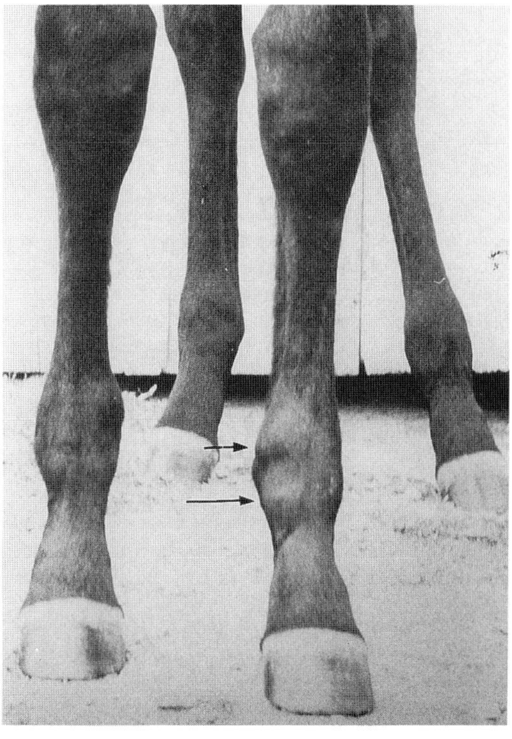

6.4. Epiphyseal compression, distal region of third metacarpal (Mc3) and proximal region of proximal phalanx (*arrows*).

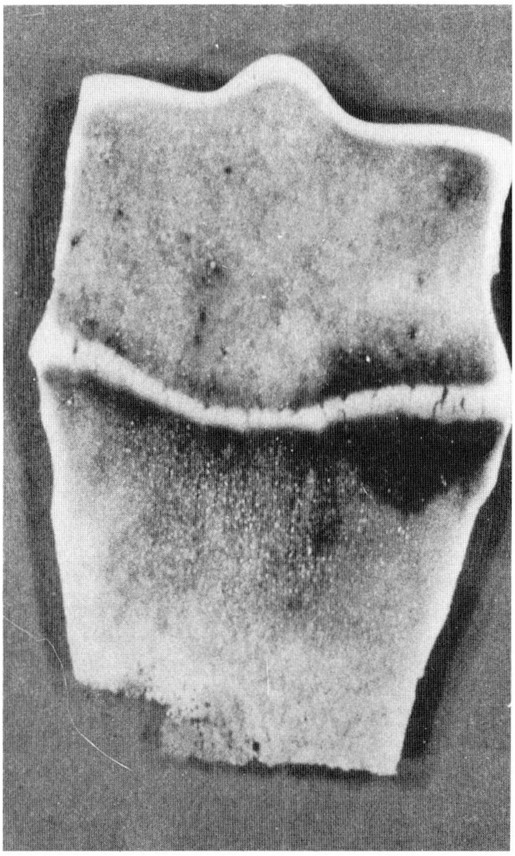

6.5. Early lesion of epiphyseal compression. The vessels crossing the epiphyseal plate are apparent. There is hyperemia in the subchondral bone of the articular cartilage, on the epiphyseal side of the epiphyseal plate, and as a pressure wedge or cone on the metaphyseal side of the epiphyseal plate. This was a three-legged lame foal.

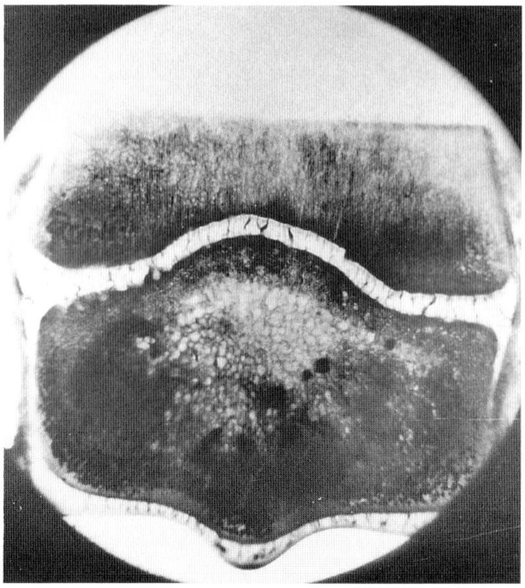

6.6. Cleared, india ink-injected, slab of the distal end of the third metacarpal (Mc3) showing the numerous blood vessels crossing the epiphyseal plate.

Thoroughbred, Standardbred, and Quarter horse foals will have osteochondrosis of the epiphyseal plates of the fore legs at postmortem in the absence of clinical evidence of disease. There is a gray area between normal closure of the plate and closure occurring with variably greater than normal compression loading, both usually occurring at the same time.

There is anecdotal evidence that a higher frequency of postnatal osteochondrosis of whatever type may be occurring in foals given tetracycline. No experimental or pathological studies have been done. Tetracycline's known action of slowing bone growth may cause an iatrogenic postnatal osteochondrosis. While it is certainly true that osteochondrosis long preceded the discovery of tetracycline, attention should be directed to the possible untoward skeletal effects of this antibiotic or any other bone-seeking drug, both in the pregnant mare and the growing foal.

Generalized osteochondrosis

This condition has been known for many years in central Kentucky and has been reported from other areas of the United States and Europe. While largely a disease of the individual foal, epizootics have occurred.

The onset is sudden with marked swelling of multiple joints and debilitating pain. The initial clinical signs suggest septicemia with joint-ill, but there is little or no febrile response or other evidence of septicemia.

At postmortem virtually every joint is affected, including those of the vertebral column. The articular cartilage is lifted from the subchondral bone in variable-sized sheets, and large pieces of cartilage may be free in the joint. Even normal appearing cartilage can often be readily peeled away from the underlying bone. Both convex and concave joint surfaces are affected, the former somewhat more severely.

Histologically, there is necrosis of the articular cartilage near the chondro-osseous junction. The pathological process is identical in nature and location to that seen in the early stages of marginal

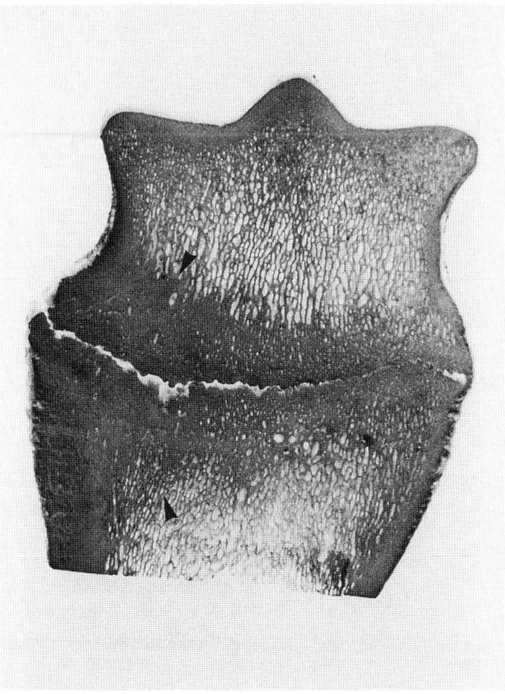

6.7. A transilluminated ground section of distal third metacarpal (Mc3) with epiphyseal compression. The *arrowheads* indicate the sclerosis in epiphysis and metaphysis that accompanies increased pressure and loss of stability of the damaged epiphyseal plate.

and nonmarginal, localized osteochondroses. There is, at most, a mild inflammatory reaction in the synovial membrane.

With time there is rapid regeneration of cartilage from the joint margins and from islands of cartilage immediately adjacent to the subchondral bone. Regeneration may succeed in re-covering the denuded joints, but the normal topography of the joint surface is not re-covered.

With regeneration, the foals may, eventually, appear to be sound but will probably never withstand heavy training. Many are destroyed because of severe crippling early in the course of the disease or as a result of cervical stenotic neuropathy following osteochondrosis of the cervical articular facets.

The cause is now certainly known to be excessive intake of zinc, the main source being paint on white plank fences. Outbreaks have occurred when foals had access to newly painted fences. The individual case is probably the foal that develops an appetite for flaking white paint on fence panels. When animals ingest either flakes or gain access to newly applied paint and become intoxicated, excessive quantities of zinc are found by chemical analysis of the liver. In retrospect sporadic cases, in central Kentucky, have always been on white fence farms and not on black fence (creosote/asphalt paint) farms.

It has been suggested that copper deficiency, whether mediated by zinc or self-standing, is the immediate cause of the necrosis of the cartilage (Bridges et al. 1984; Bridges and Harris 1988; Bridges and Moffitt 1990). All of our cases have had high levels of zinc in the liver with normal levels of copper. Bridges and Moffitt produced the disease by feeding high levels of zinc and demonstrated hypocupremia. Bridges and Harris apparently produced generalized osteochondrosis in four foals on a low-copper, milk-replacer diet, though high levels of zinc were found in the livers. While these results suggest that copper and copper–zinc interaction are important factors in generalized osteochondrosis, there is no hard evidence that they play any role in the localized osteochondroses. Normal copper levels in the fetus and foal are higher than those in the adult horse: about 300 ppm dry matter in the former and about 30 ppm in the latter.

Cohrs (1961) indicated that identical lesions in the joints may be caused by selenium poisoning, but refers to Hupka (1955) to the effect that environmental zinc and lead were responsible. Hupka identified the condition in foals in the vicinity of foundries and reproduced it in two foals by feeding dust collected around the foundries. Some spontaneous cases became roarers as well (lead neuropathy). He believed that lead was primarily responsible, with zinc also involved. Gunson et al. (1982) and Eamens et al. (1984) reported similar findings with environmental pollution by zinc.

CHAPTER 7

Fore Leg

General

Lameness has been a major concern of horsemen and veterinarians for centuries. Pathologists, however, have shown little interest, most of the pathological descriptions in the literature being those of clinicians, or worse. For that reason and personal interest, the discussion here of the lesions of lameness is extensive. Matters of a biomechanical nature, including predisposing conformation, the role of different types of work, and so on, are touched upon but cannot be given the attention they deserve (Rooney 1969).

Probably nowhere in equine pathology is the interaction of genetic and environmental factors so apparent or so important as in the pathogenesis of lameness. Pathology, epidemiology, and genetics offer, together, a rich, intellectually rewarding, and financially destitute opportunity for the study of lameness and breakdown (Mohammed et al. 1991).

A number of conditions have become uncommon as the use of horses has changed. They are included for historical interest, and because they are part of the complex continuum of damage to the locomotor system. The outward manifestations of many conditions—spavin, curb, splints, and ringbone—were known to ancient Greek veterinarians and no doubt to the horsemen of the steppes and mid-East soon after domestication of the horse.

Statistics

The major sites of lameness in Prussian military horses in the late 1800s (Bartke 1900) may be compared to those of Thoroughbred racehorses in 1980 (Jeffcott et al. 1982) (see Table 7-1).

The Prussian cavalry and artillery horses were subjected to heavy loads for protracted periods, leading to hock, pastern, and tendon (check ligament of deep flexor) damage, while the Thoroughbred racehorse specializes in carpal and hoof problems of all types. The fetlock joint is damaged in all horses subjected to the loads imposed by people.

For the embryological development of the fore and rear legs, see Carlens (1927) and Sack (1991).

Shoulder

The head of the humerus presents, as a normal feature, a variably obvious **craniocaudal groove** in its lateral aspect. This groove is not present in the newborn foal, gradually developing during the first year of life. It may represent slow, limited wearing by the lateral edge of the glenoid.

The **glenoid** cavity of the scapula is normally

Table 7-1. Comparison of lameness in Prussian military horses in the late 1800s with that in Thoroughbred racehorses in 1980

	Prussian[a]	English TB[b]
Joints	2	1
Bones	3	2
Muscle	4	3
Tendons	1	4
Joint and Hoof		
Hock	1	5
Fetlock	2	2
Pastern	3	6
Shoulder area	4	NR
Hoof	5	1
Croup area	6	4
Carpus	7	3

Sources: [a]Bartke 1900.
[b]Jeffcott et al 1982.

Note: Rankings are used for most common (1) to least common (7) since the data cannot be compared one to one. NR = no report.

even and smooth at birth. Some time after birth, the central cartilage softens and partially disappears, leaving either a variable size bony crater covered by synovial membrane or an irregular cleft of folded cartilage. This feature is routine in the glenoid beyond 3–6 months of age. While not typical, this may be a **synovial fossa**. Carlens (1927) apparently accepted it as a synovial fossa. Cadeac (1909) shows such an area in the glenoid, but misinterpreted it as pathological erosion. Indeed, he misinterpreted synovial fossae in all locations as pathological, as did Percivall (1834) and not a few writers since.

There are reports of osteochondrosis of the laterocaudal part of the head of the humerus and the glenoid of the scapula (Schebitz 1968; Meagher et al. 1973; Schmidt et al. 1975; Mason 1977). We have not seen this osteochondrosis in over 10,000 postmortem examinations. The few postmortem cases in the literature had lesions of both the humeral head and the glenoid, suggesting arthrosis or chronic infectious arthritis rather than osteochondrosis. As noted elsewhere (see Chapter 6, "Locomotor System, General"), localized osteochondrosis is characterized by restriction to convex joint surfaces. The laterocaudal part of the head of the humerus ossifies somewhat later than the rest of the head of the humerus, and this could be mistaken for osteochondrosis radiographically.

Chronic infectious arthritis of the shoulder, as well as other joints, causes severe lameness in yearling horses. The chronic arthritis, with severe loss and distortion of joint cartilage and architecture, follows acute infectious joint disease early in life, with lameness appearing at the time the animal is broken for training. (**Arthritis** is for joint disease caused by infectious agents; **arthrosis** means degenerative or traumatic, noninfectious disease.)

Bicipital bursitis

This condition, well known in earlier times, is now uncommon. The acute clinical signs are characteristic: near refusal to move the leg forward but ability to move it backward, fixing of the leg to prevent movement and pain, reluctance to bear weight, marked lifting of the head, and stumbling when moving. Similar, though less pronounced, signs are present in chronic cases.

Dollar (1920) wrote, "a chronic bursitis (which may be bilateral) is produced in tramway and omnibus horses by half-falls or slipping in rapid driving." The same observation was made by Cadeac (1907). It occurred in those farm horses working in the furrow during spring plowing, that is, slipping. Slipping or falling, so that the leg slips backward with the shoulder flexing and the elbow extending, causes a sudden increase of tension in the biceps brachii tendon, tearing tendon fibers. Inflammation with swelling and pain follows.

Our few postmortem cases were long standing. There was chronic proliferative synovitis, excess synovial fluid, and moderate disorganization and scarring of the surface of the biceps tendon. Acute, purulent synovitis has been seen following diagnostic injection and in foals with septicemia. In one chronic case, in an old horse, the biceps tendon and bursal wall had metaplastic calcification and ossification.

Infraspinatus bursitis

As with bicipital bursitis, this condition is uncommon in the modern era. There is supporting leg lameness, the leg bearing weight but abducted to avoid pressure on the painful infraspinatus bursa and tendon (Dollar 1920). No reports of the postmortem findings have been found, and we have seen no cases.

Fractures

Scapula

Fractures of the scapula are uncommon and usually in young horses as the result of falls and collisions. The supraglenoid tubercle (*tuber scapulae*) may be fractured at or near the epiphyseal plate. The scapula may fracture through the neck, more often in older horses. In both cases the mechanism is simple bending failure.

Humerus

Fractures of the humerus are always mixed: bending, axial compression, and torsion. The position of the leg when the fracture occurred can often be deduced by reconstruction and study of the fracture planes. Frequently there is compression of the lateral aspect and tension of the medial aspect of the humerus as the leg impacts the ground in a markedly abducted position. There is no predisposition by sex or leg, though the fracture is more common in young Thoroughbred racehorses, usually occurring while the animal is galloping at less than full speed.

Various reports have suggested that incomplete, "stress" fractures of the humerus are predisposing for overt fractures. The evidence is unconvincing. The term, *stress fracture*, is undefined jargon in veterinary pathology.

Olecranon process

Fractures of the olecranon process of the ulna take two forms. In the foal the fracture is usually through the epiphyseal plate, while it is through the body of the olecranon process in the older horse. In both cases there is simple bending failure as a result of powerful triceps muscular contraction, often as the animal is trying to stop falling to that side.

Elbow

This joint is virtually immune from pathological changes with the exception of the purulent synovitis of foal septicemia and scoring or wear lines (see below). The synovial fossae of the humeroradial and humeroulnar joints are variably sized from one leg to the other and from horse to horse, as are the fossae found in the functionally comparable tarsocrural joint (Fig. 7.1).

Synovial fossae

The function of synovial fossae is not known. They are not present at birth, but appear within the first few months of life. Mehlfeld et al. (1984) have suggested a nutrient function. It is more probable that they serve a lubricating function in large joints (Krölling and Grau 1960; Rooney 1969). Modes (1938), however, did not believe they served as synovial fluid reservoirs. He described the development of the fossae as progressive thinning of the cartilage with disappearance of the calcified cartilage. Once the cartilage had completely atrophied, it was replaced by fibrous synovial membrane with remnants of degenerate cartilaginous material. He believed lack of pressure to be the reason for development of the fossae. Schulz (1914/15) discussed synovial fossae, but offered no suggestions about function.

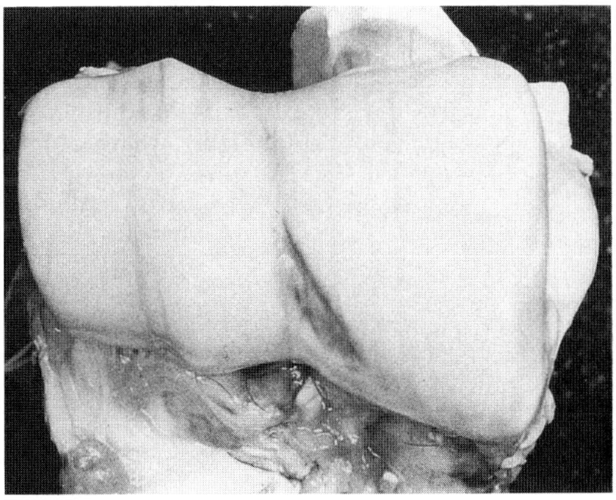

7.1. Distal end of humerus with a synovial fossa and scoring or wear lines.

Hygroma

This acute/chronic bursitis of the bursa between the skin and olecranon process is usually known as **shoe boil**. There is inflammation of the wall of the bursa with accumulation of excessive amounts of synovial fluid. The condition tends to be chronic and persistent. It is generally believed to be caused by irritation by the shoe when the horse is lying down. Goubeaud (1899/90) observed that the condition was commoner in horses kept in straight stalls, rarely being seen in animals at pasture or in loose boxes, whether shod or unshod. He proposed that the elbow striking the packed dirt or the plank floor of the straight stall as the horse was rising initiated the inflammatory process.

The elbow and tarsocrural joints are functionally similar (Schnappgelenke) and characterized by a snapping action in osteoligamentous preparations that is not seen in undissected specimens or the live animal (Rooney 1990a). The phenomenon has been recognized at least since the 1800s [references in Updike (1984); and Rooney (1990a)].

Wear lines

A common, clinically silent, lesion of the elbow is scoring or wear lines in the articular cartilage (Fig. 7.1). As in the tarsocrural joint these scoring lines are usually present in the absence of other lesions. Histologically, they are simply grooves in otherwise normal cartilage. While the grooves may become deeper with time, they are eventually self-limiting and not a cause of clinical lameness. There appear to be two pathogenetic pathways for scoring lines:

1. They appear in one elbow joint when there is significant lameness in the same or, more often, another leg. This can only be appreciated early in training or work when the animal first experiences a significant, painful lameness. Older horses, veterans of many lamenesses, will usually have scoring lines in both elbows.

Young horses with ataxia, such as cervical stenotic myelopathy, will routinely have bilateral scoring of the tarsocrural joints, less often the humeroradial joints. This suggests that irregular, intermittent impulse loading of the joints as a result of pain or ataxia is directly related to the genesis of the scoring lines. The precise mechanism cannot be further specified, although turbulent synovial fluid has been suggested as the eroding agent (Rooney 1969).

2. Scoring lines appear in the carpus, intratarsal joints, intervertebral joints, and fetlock joint once a focal erosive arthrosis has occurred in the joint. Turbulent synovial fluid, arising in the eroded areas, has, again, been suggested as the cause of these scoring lines (Rooney 1969).

Aging of articular cartilage

Young articular cartilage in all joints, and including fibrocartilage, is white with a slightly bluish cast. In the young foal the blue color is more apparent since the limiting bone plate has not formed and cut off the color of the bluish subchondral bone marrow. With age the cartilage becomes whiter, shading towards a gray, opaque color. These gross changes are not reflected in histological changes of the cartilage. Yellow, yellow-brown discoloration is pathological, though it may appear so late in life that clinical effects are trivial. This discoloration is accompanied by variable loss of matrix metachromasia, loss of chondrocytes, and reparative cloning of chondrocytes. These remarks apply to all articular cartilage.

Fore arm

Normal ulna

The entire ulna is present in the early fetus, 4–6 weeks (Carlens 1927), but soon reduces to the proximal olecranon process and the distal lateral malleolus of the radius. Often, particularly in younger animals, the shaft of the ulna remains as a distinct fibrous band with areas of bone or cartilage. The fusion of the distal end of the ulna, as the lateral malleolus, to the radius is completed early, but the line of fusion remains as a distinct white band not to be mistaken for a healed fracture. Persistence of the complete ulna has been seen as a recessive defect in Shetland ponies (see Chapter 4, "Endocrine System").

Fractures

Fractures of the olecranon process have been discussed. Clinical texts indicate that fractures of the radius are not uncommon, but no frequency data is available. We have seen few at postmortem and those either in foals or in horses undergoing difficult recovery from anesthesia. In foals most fractures have been simple bending failures near midshaft often with a history, and evidence at postmortem, of having been kicked. Radial fractures in older horses have been of mixed type with a pronounced torsional component. Reconstruction showed that the leg was too far forward when load was suddenly applied, as when a horse is trying to stand before complete recovery from anesthesia.

Carpus

Arthrosis

Traumatic arthrosis of the dorsal aspect of the distal, articular cartilage of the radius and the opposed dorsal aspects of the articular cartilage of the radial carpal bone (RC) and the third carpal bone (C3) are among the commonest lesions of racing Thoroughbred and Standardbred horses. Such lesions are uncommon in horses that do not race, whatever the breed. Cadeac (1909) said that cavalry horses, steeplechasers, racehorses, and hackney coach horses were more commonly affected. It is clear that carpal arthrosis is a high-speed lesion. Virtually every Thoroughbred that has trained and raced has lesions of the carpus. The frequency in Standardbred racehorses is lower but still significant. Lesions may appear earlier in the left carpus, but the frequency at postmortem is essentially equal, left and right, whatever the direction of the race course turns (Wyburn and Goulden 1974). Most reviews of lesion frequency have been radiographic and, therefore, reflect the incidence of reparative osteophytes rather than arthrosis per se.

Of the two sites, RC/C3 is, by far, the more common (Figs. 7.2 and 7.3). The lesions first appear in the articular cartilage of the dorsal margin of RC/C3 as fraying and erosion of the articular cartilage. This progresses to deeper erosion and ulceration. As the lesions progress, scoring lines may appear in the otherwise uninvolved cartilage, and osteophytes develop on the joint margins. Pannuslike growths of granulation tissue can extend

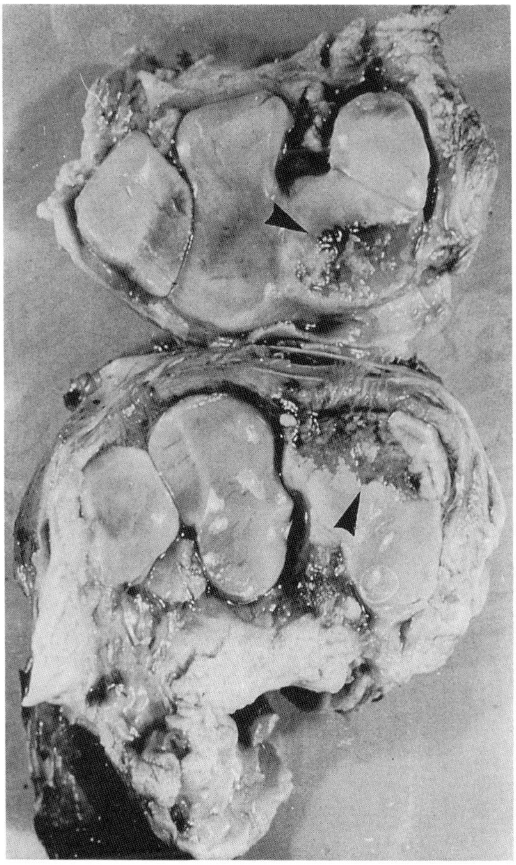

7.2. Proximal and distal row of carpal bones with erosion/ulceration of the distal face of radial carpal bone three (RC3) (*arrowheads*), and the mirror lesion on the proximal surface of the third carpal bone (C3).

from the thickened synovial membrane unto the eroded articular cartilage (Fig. 7.3).

Before intraarticular steroids were introduced, the lesions shown here were the largest seen. An animal with such lesions did not race. Since the advent of intraarticular steroid injection, the size and severity of the lesions has increased (Fig. 7.4). Indeed, with repeated use of steroids there may be complete disintegration of the carpus with RC, C3, and other small carpal bones virtually reduced to bone dust and powder. Such catastrophic failures were rare before steroids.

As the cartilage damage proceeds, the underlying subchondral bone undergoes progressive sclerosis. *Sclerosis* is a term to be used in relation to pathological processes. Subchondral bone becomes *denser* with increasing age and weight, training, and other hard work, this normal process being the response of bone to increased loading. Even though the mechanism for increasing bone per unit volume may be the same in both instances, sclerosis should be reserved for increasing density in relation to pathological, and not normal, factors.

Fractures

Chip

Chip fractures, so-called, of the dorsal lip of RC and/or C3 are not uncommon and virtually always pathological. That is, they occur as the result of loss of articular cartilage and the decreasing shear strength associated with subchondral sclerosis. Shear failure occurs, then, with even normal compressive loads. Osteophytes may be, and often are, mistaken for shear fractures on radiographs.

The lesion of the distal end of the radius, lateral aspect, is unique among arthroses of the horse in that a mirror image lesion is not usually present on the opposing surface of the intermediate carpal bone. This lesion rarely is as severe as the RC/C3 lesion. Periarticular osteophytes usually are present. In keeping with the pathological findings, the lameness associated with this lesion is generally less severe than with the RC/C3 lesion.

Mechanical arguments and anecdotal experience indicate that the radial lesion is associated with over-on-the-knee and the RC/C3 lesion with back-on-the-knee conformation. These describe the static or standing appearance of the fore leg, lateral view. Conformational defects such as this have long been associated with lameness, and mechanical arguments have defined that relationship. It is also true that the leg can assume positions, dynamically, which are equivalent to these static defects. With fatigue of the flexor muscles, for example, the carpus can dorsiflex too much, the dynamic equivalent of static back-on-the-knee conformation (Rooney 1969).

The arthrosis is caused by shearing forces, which are the result of desynchronization of the movements of the small carpal bones caused, in turn, by the static and dynamic conformational factors discussed above and in Rooney (1969).

Congenital and/or genetic factors apart from overall conformation may be present. Hypoplasia of one or more carpal bones may be unrecognized in the live animal. One Thoroughbred stallion went out of racing because of carpal arthrosis and sired many foals with frank hypoplasia of the carpal bones (Fig. 7.5).

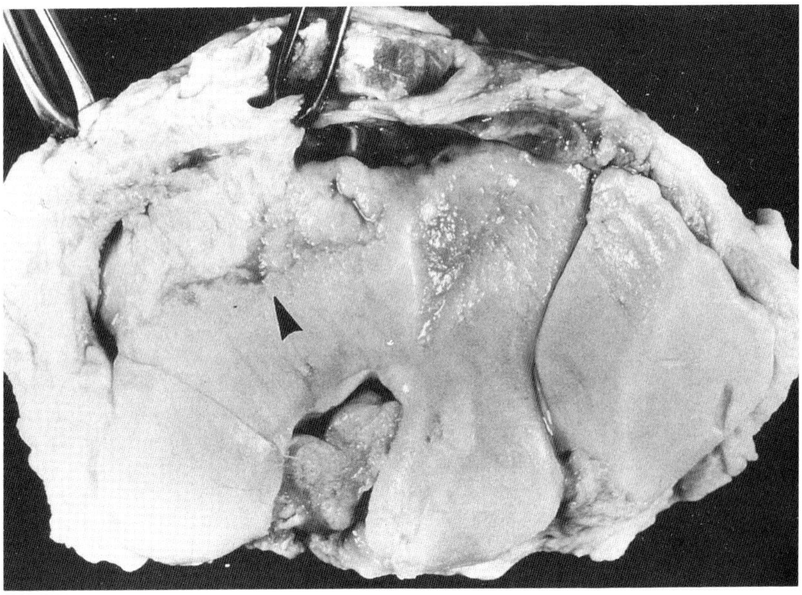

7.3. Ulcerative arthrosis of the proximal surface of third carpal bone (C3) (*arrowhead*). The forceps hold the joint capsule showing "pannus" extending from capsule to the damaged joint surface.

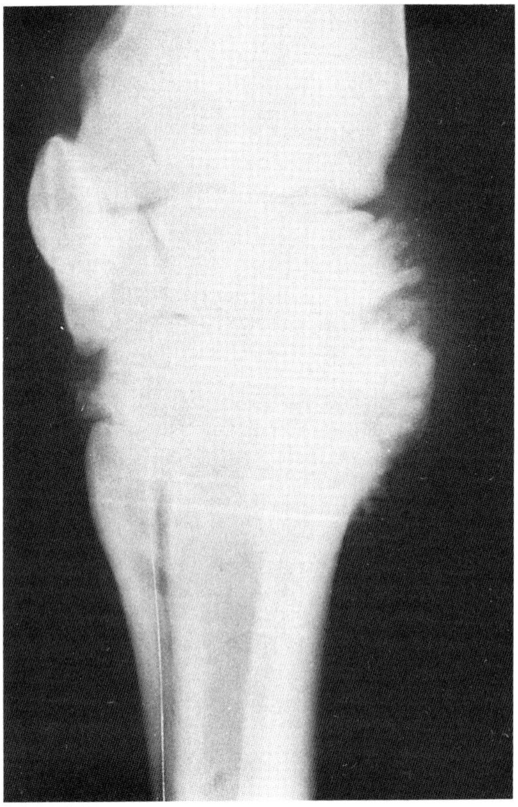

7.4. Radiograph of carpus subjected to multiple injections of steroids. Characteristic explosion of osteophytes accompanying massive articular cartilage destruction.

Third carpal

Although most fractures of the third carpal bone are pathological, following upon arthrosis, single-event shear fractures, particularly of C3, do occur (Fig. 7.6). Referred to as slab fractures, these are, in fact, shear failures caused by compression force. The pathogenesis is essentially the same as for chip fracture. That is, if cartilage damage is done by misapplication of force to RC and C3, then a sufficiently large force, misapplied in the same manner, will cause failure of both cartilage and bone: fracture. True pathological or single-event fractures of the dorsal aspect of the radial carpal bone have not been seen. They are frequently described in the clinical literature, but pathological examination indicates that the bony masses seen on radiographs are, in fact, osteophytes.

Third metacarpal

A shear fracture of the proximal, dorsomedial aspect of the third metacarpal (Mc3) bone is seen infrequently and usually in Standardbred racehorses. Most of these animals become sound, and only a few healed lesions have been seen at postmortem. Ross and Martin (1992) described seven cases in a large clinic over a 12-year period, a low frequency consistent with our postmortem experience.

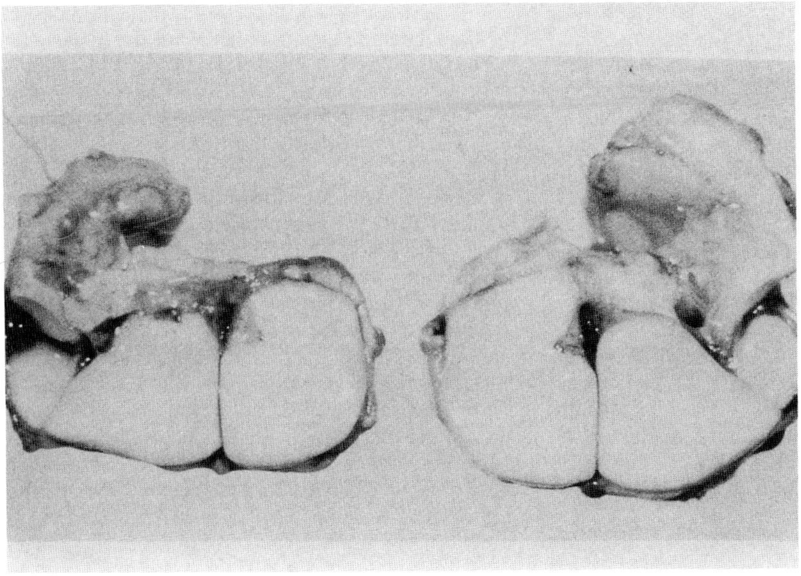

7.5. Proximal rows of carpal bones from a foal. The set on the *left* is hypoplastic.

Accessory carpal bone

This fracture may be more common in jumping horses. Wyburn and Goulden (1974) found only 4 racing Thoroughbreds among 55 cases. It is simple bending failure with the transverse component, tensile failure, beginning on the lateral side and finishing with a very small oblique, compression, failure on the medial side.

The pathogenesis appears to be asynchronous contraction of the two muscles inserted on the accessory carpal bone (Rooney 1969). Fatigue—inadequate force of contraction—or delay of contraction of the ulnaris lateralis muscle would predispose to fracture caused by the contraction of the flexor carpi ulnaris muscle. This can be simulated with a simple model.

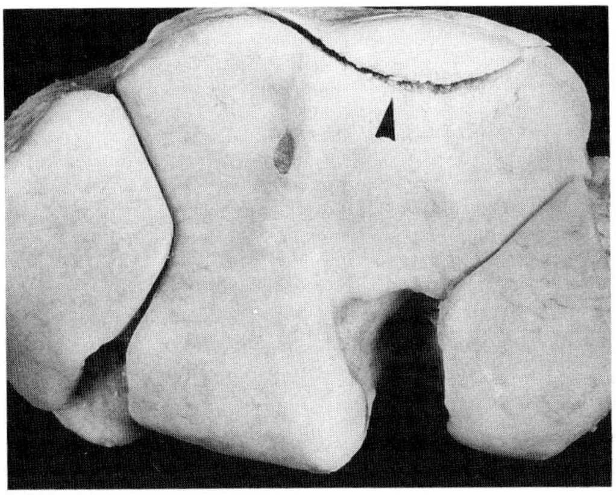

7.6. Macerated specimen of single-event fracture (*arrowhead*) of the third carpal bone (C3).

Fourth intermediate carpal

These are uncommon shear failures as a result of asynchronous force application (Auer et al. 1986).

Miscellaneous

Osteochondrosis is uncommon in the carpus. Only one or two cases of nonmarginal osteochondrosis of the third carpal bone have been seen. The carpometacarpal joint is rarely the site of lesions other than the purulent synovitis of foal septicemia. Synovitis of the carpal synovial sheath has been described under the sobriquet, **carpal tunnel syndrome** (Mackay-Smith et al. 1972). This is not, however, a self-standing entity as in the human. The synovitis is either aseptic and secondary to fracture of the accessory carpal bone or purulent in foal septicemias or following diagnostic injection.

Metacarpus

Bucked shin

This common affliction of the young racehorse, primarily Thoroughbred, was hardly described before the modern era. Guoth (1927) recognized the condition in racehorses, noting that it had long been known. He described the periosteal new bone formation, relating it to the remodeling of the third metacarpal bone during the earlier stages of training for racing. He did not recognize the characteristic fracture of the dorsal cortex of Mc3. Bogdaschew (1937) described the remodeling of Mc3 with thickening of the dorsomedial cortex. He found this thickening to be greater in work, draft, horses than in galloping horses. He found no differences among the breeds he examined, other than between heavy and light horses.

It is now generally recognized that bucked shin is a shear fracture of the dorsal cortex of Mc3 (Fig. 7.7). Multiple microfracturing has been proposed as a lesion, but without morphological evidence. The evidence is that bucked shin is a single, shear fracture of the dorsal cortex with periosteal and endosteal new bone formation as part of the healing process.

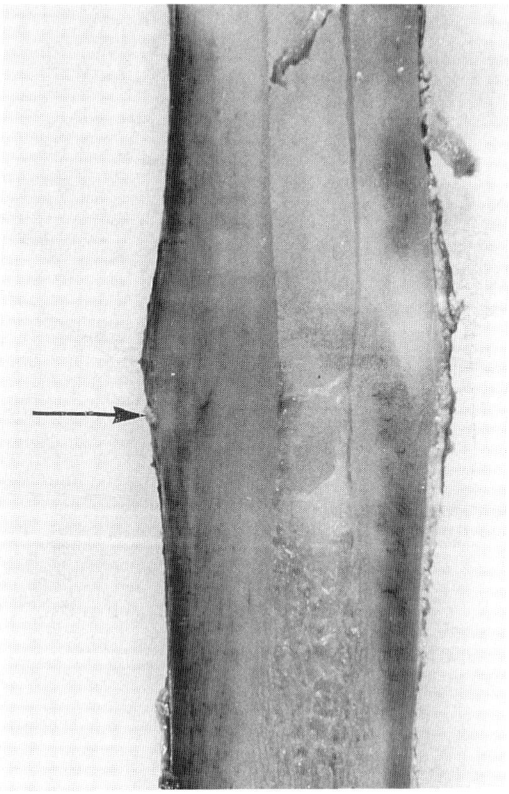

7.7. Sagittal section of the third metacarpal bone (Mc3) of a horse that "bucked the shin" about 30 days previously. The *arrow* indicates new periosteal bone formation, callus. The almost closed, oblique fracture line is present as a *dark line* in the cortex.

The fracture occurs on either the dorsomedial or dorsolateral aspect of Mc3, does not propagate all the way through the dorsal cortex, and extends proximally at about a 30°/60° angle to the long axis of the bone. In some cases (see below) the fracture may run out proximally to form a so-called **saucer fracture**.

Healing is rapid with simple shear failure, the fracture line barely perceptible grossly at about 30 days, when healing, histologically, is effectively completed. New bone forms on the periosteal surface in the vicinity of the initial failure and is gradually remodeled and removed after the fracture heals. New bone formation occurs on the endosteal surface as well (Devas 1961). While difficult to see on clinical radiographs, it is apparent in the postmortem specimen.

There appear to be two topographical forms of bucked shin (Norwood 1978; Haynes 1980). The first, and more common, occurs on the dorsomedial aspect of the middle third of Mc3. In the few cases available for study, this type appears to occur in, or at least in close association with, remodeling areas of Mc3. The third metacarpal is essentially circular in cross section before race training begins. As training progresses Mc3 remodels to a more oval cross section with new bone laid down on the dorsomedial aspect of the bone. This new bone is laid down, initially, as a latticework, which gradually fills in, forming mature osteonic bone. The shear fracture occurs in the newly formed latticework bone.

The second type of shear fracture occurs in the dorsolateral cortex in bone that is not remodeling. This type is more often associated with nonunion and/or saucer fracture and, on average, occurs after remodeling of the dorsomedial surface has been completed, that is, in somewhat older horses (Haynes 1980).

The pathogenesis of bucked shin fracture is unclear. It is obviously a lesion of the young racehorse and is usually seen in older horses only if they have worked strictly on grass before being subjected to American-style dirt tracks. That is, Mc3 remodels, as described above, on dirt tracks but much less so on turf. The grass horse, when subjected to the dirt track, undergoes Mc3 remodeling at whatever age. Jeffcott et al. (1982) found that about 9% of lamenesses were bucked (sore) shins in England on grass courses, while the frequency approximated 70% in American horses training and racing largely on dirt tracks (Norwood 1978; Haynes 1980).

The topography of the fracture, at a theoretical angle of 45°, actual angle of 30°/60°, to the long axis of Mc3, indicates shear failure, and shear is the failure mode for compression. It is apparent, therefore, that too much bending of Mc3 with the dorsal surface in compression is the final pathway for bucked shin. One mechanism for that is the sudden stop after the foot "skis" through the cushion to impact on the hard base of a dirt track. Toe grabs or other friction-increasing devices on the bearing surface of the shoe will exaggerate the sudden deceleration and large, impulse forces.

Fractures

Condylar

Fractures of the distal end of Mc3 and the third metatarsal (Mt3) are among the commoner fractures of high speed horses (Fig. 7.8). One study found 64% of cannon bone fractures to be of this type (Alexander and Rooney 1972). Among 25 cases in Thoroughbred racehorses, 9 and 8 affected the left and right Mc3, respectively, and 2 and 5 the left and right Mt3, respectively.

In order to understand the pathogenesis of these fractures, we first briefly review the normal movements under load. As the body weight is applied to the leg, the fetlock joint dorsiflexes and translates distally because of coffin joint rotation. Because of the cam construction of the several joint surfaces, this dorsiflexion is accompanied by a spinning of Mc3–Mt3 and the proximal phalanx around their long axes from medial to lateral.

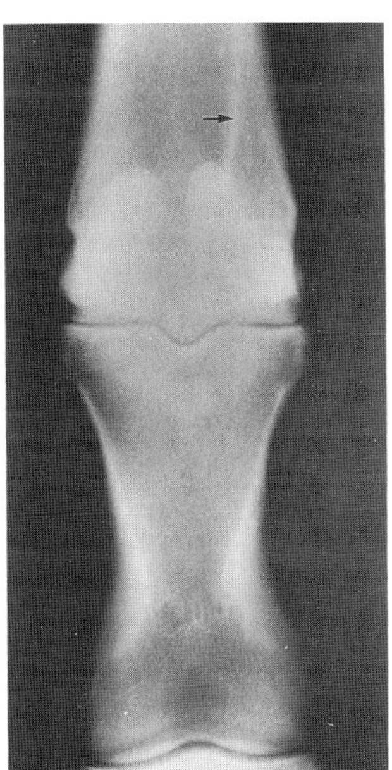

7.8. Nearly healed condylar fracture of the third metacarpal (Mc3) indicated by *arrow*.

Toward the end of support, vertical force on the leg decreasing, the spinning movement is in the opposite direction, from lateral to medial. The angular displacement of this spinning movement at the fetlock is about 7°–10°. The joints, then, are moving in three dimensions, and these movements must be precisely synchronized at high rates of acceleration.

The necessary mechanical conditions for fracture of Mc3 are that the proximal phalanx remains stationary, or nearly so, with the fetlock in the fully dorsiflexed position, while Mc3 makes the lateral to medial spinning movement. Fracture will occur as the moving lateral condyle of Mc3 strikes the stationary lateral aspect of the proximal end of the proximal phalanx. Such an out-of-phase, asynchronous movement would be expected near the end of the support phase when the fetlock dorsal angle should be increasing. These fractures almost always are completed by the formation of a slab on the lateral aspect of Mc3.

Condylar fracture of Mt3 occurs because the lateral to medial rotation of Mt3 is out of phase, ahead of, the lateral to medial rotation of the proximal phalanx. Unlike the Mc3 fracture, the Mt3 failure occurs while both bones are spinning, but the proximal phalanx is spinning later than Mt3. These fractures, in contrast to those of Mc3, often do not form a slab, the fracture progressing a variable distance proximally in Mt3. This is singularly dangerous since complete, secondary, failure of Mt3 may occur.

The basic pathogenesis is that elevation of the pastern during the second half of the support phase is completely (Mc3) or partially (Mt3) delayed. The exact cause of such delay can vary from case to case. Some relevant causes are: foot slipping on the surface, fatigue of the flexor muscles, breakover delayed by excessive length of toe, and too-sharp turning with overloading of the inside leg.

While out-of-phase movements provide the final common pathological pathway, predisposing factors may be present. A case study makes the point. A farm that raised and raced its own horses had Mc3 condylar fractures in four 2 year olds in the same year. The animals were racing in three different parts of the country when the fractures occurred. The feeding program of the farm was reviewed for the period before these animals left the farm and went into training. The program had been changed during that period, and retrospective nutritional analysis indicated that the calcium–phosphorus intake had been considerably below the recommended level for growing horses. The feeding program was corrected, and there has been no further untoward incidence of fractures of Mc3 (Thompson 1989). Although no material was available for pathological study, osteitis fibrosa would not be expected; rather, probably an inadequate amount of bone is because of calcium deficiency (see Bone in Chapter 6, "Locomotor System, General").

Other

Most fractures of Mc3, Mt3 in foals are midshaft with severe comminution and contamination. Reconstruction indicates simple bending failure, in many instances with the history of a kick or a mare stepping on a recumbent foal. Fracture of the distal epiphyseal plate has been seen at postmortem, but is not common. Both the midshaft and epiphyseal plate fractures are characterized by transverse, tensile failure with a shear component.

Shear failure of the proximal, dorsal aspect of Mc3 may be seen in racehorses with multiple fracture/collapse of the carpus after long-term intraarticular steroid administration. This is similar to, but more catastrophic than, the dorsomedial fracture already described.

A number of reports have appeared on "lesions" predisposing to fractures of the third metacarpal bone as well as other bones: endarteritis (obliterans) of older animals, normal increased density of cancellous bone in trained animals, normal Renaut bodies in peripheral nerves, and so on. The reports are trivial and not cited.

Tendon

Tearing, general

Lesions of tendons and ligaments are, primarily, disruption and tearing of collagen bundles and fibers. While one may argue whether such tearing is purely mechanical or occurs following ischemic necrosis, the fact remains that lesions with pain and lameness are characterized by loss of continuity of tendon fibers and consequent inflammation. Tearing of tendons has long been known, at least to Xenophon, circa 390 BCE (Dakyns 1897).

There are two ways in which tendons can tear:

1. The tendon may be stretched beyond its functional limit, that is, the tensile force generated in the tendon is greater than the maximum stress of the tendon. *Stress* is used here, and throughout, as defined in mechanics: the force within a structure resisting deformation of that structure by an externally applied force. Stress, then, is a material property of the structure, in this case, the tendon. Such overstretching of a tendon is uncommon.
2. The tendon may be torn as a result of sudden changes of direction of application of the external force: vector changes, third-order acceleration. These vector changes may be associated with the generation of impulse, as well. *Impulse* is force measured over a specific period of time and is change of momentum. This will be considered in more detail later. A homely example may be given. Try to tear apart a piece of rope by pulling on each end. If unsuccessful, snap and jerk the piece of rope until it tears apart. Sudden vector changes of acceleration have been employed, as well as large forces applied over brief periods of time. The case will be made that superficial flexor tendon tearing, check ligament tearing, and thoroughpin, for example, are caused by such vector/impulse mechanisms.

Compromised blood supply

The role of compromised blood supply may be addressed. It is certainly the case that either mechanism of tendon tearing, exceeding the strength of the tendon or abnormal vector/impulse behavior, will damage small vessels (lymphatic, venous, arteriolar, and capillary) as well as tendinous, interstitial collagenous, and elastic fibers. While it may be postulated that vascular failure precedes collagenous failure, the point is moot. To propose that mechanical factors are unimportant and that some unspecified "occlusion" or other vascular malfeasance causes primary ischemic necrosis cannot be countenanced until and unless such malfeasance is demonstrated. The situation is not unlike that of the proposed vascular origin of navicular disease in the absence of valid morphological or functional evidence.

Stay apparatus

The tendons of the stay apparatus of the fore leg are the most frequently injured. The primary pathogenesis is to be sought in genetically modulated, environmentally induced trauma.

Onchocerca reticulata

Onchocerca reticulata have been suggested as causative and/or predisposing factors, but there is no evidence that these worms are common in horse tendons, at least in North America, or that they predispose an infested tendon to tearing (Cohrs 1961). *O. reticulata* is, or was, common in Europe. Of 43 horses, donkeys, and mules examined the parasite was found, primarily in the interosseus, in 35 (Pader 1901/02). The parasite was first identified by Hermann and Blisweis in Vienna in 1840, cited by Pader (1901). Even with heavy infestations there was little or no tissue reaction.

Exposure to pressure and shear

Tendon surfaces exposed to shear and pressure, such as the biceps brachii and that portion of the deep flexor in contact with the navicular, are composed of a thick, pleated mass of collagen fibers, rather than the parallel fibers of the purely tensile parts of the tendon. Drahn (1922) observed that the cells in these areas were not typical tendon cells but were ovoid and surrounded by a capsule, like cartilage cells. In fact these are cartilage cells, and the tendon surfaces exposed to pressure and shear are fibrocartilage.

Studies in species other than the horse have shown that training increases the resistance of tendons to applied loads because of the increase of tensile properties and mass (Woo et al. 1970).

Biomechanical aging

Frischbier (1928) investigated the biomechanical aging of some tendons of the fore leg of horses in vitro. The common and lateral digital extensors and the superficial flexor lost both strength and elasticity with increasing age, while the deep digital flexor did not change significantly. The interosseus was not examined. The decreases were approximately exponential, resembling the curves for stress relaxation of equine tendons in vitro (Rooney 1991a). Since stress relaxation appears to be a function of breakdown of collagen cross-links, aging change may have a similar basis. There is no explanation for the apparent lack of aging of the deep flexor tendon. The tendons of Cold bloods had a lower elastic limit and a higher elongation limit than the tendons of half bloods at all ages. Riemersma and Schamhardt (1985) found no age effects in their series, but their animals were 4–8 years old, while those of Frischbier ranged from 6 to over 20 years.

Mechanical behavior

Frischbier (1928) also noted that the flexor tendons behaved as hard springs (Thompson and Stewart 1986), elongation decreasing with increasing load, while the extensor tendons behaved more nearly as soft springs, elongation increasing with increasing load. The hard spring behavior is considered to be characteristic of tendons (Viidik 1966).

The common and lateral extensor tendons were tested in vitro by Thompson et al. (1992), and the behavior of the extensor tendons and the extensor branches of the interosseus were shown to be dependent upon the direction of movement of the fetlock and coffin joints: hard spring during dorsiflexion of the fetlock/palmar flexion of the coffin and so-called **constant-load** (Wahl (1963) during palmar flexion of the fetlock and coffin. It was apparent in these studies, as well as in unreported studies, that there are differences in cross-sectional area, density, and stress–strain behavior of the flexor tendons of the left and right fore legs of the same horse. No clinical or pathological correlations have yet been made, and these observations suggest further study.

The passive function of the flexor tendons and the interosseus were investigated experimentally by Lishman (1908) cited by Smith (1917) and Forssell (1914/15). A review of the passive function of tendons is given by Dimery et al. (1986) and Alexander (1990).

Fracture of medial splint bone, Mc2

Tearing of the deep flexor check ligament

Avulsion fracture of the proximal m. interosseus

These three conditions will be considered together, even though they may not appear to be clinically or pathologically related.

The pathology is understood by consideration of pathogenesis. All three conditions usually occur in horses that pull loads. In the modern era the Standardbred racehorse and contest pulling horses are at risk. The evidence of earlier times was that pulled check ligaments were by far the commonest lesions of the fore leg (Siedamgrotsky 1891). In the modern era tearing of the superficial flexor tendon takes pride of place. Silbersiepe et al. (1986) indicated that check ligament strain was commonest in draft horses, 75% having such a lesion. Ziegler (1969) quotes figures from 1909 that 70% of all tendon tears were of the deep flexor check ligament, 8%–9% in the superficial flexor tendon, and 18% in a branch of the suspensory ligament. While similar data are not available today, autopsy experience shows just the reverse for check and superficial flexor tearing, reflecting the preponderance of draft animals in the old population and the preponderance of light horses in the modern population. Standardbred horses are prone to both superficial flexor tearing, related to speed, and check ligament tearing, related to pulling loads. Draft horses used in pulling contests are prone to check ligament tearing.

The basic pathogenesis of these conditions is the carpus buckled, incompletely dorsiflexed, at the moment of impact of the foot with the ground. Stability analysis shows that the buckled position of the carpus is unstable; the specific physical events will be given below. At any velocity beyond a slow walk, a leg protracts fully forward and then retracts, through the air, before impacting with the ground. The velocity of retraction equals the velocity of the body, so that horizontal velocities and accelerations are canceled at the moment of impact (Rooney 1969).

Fracture of the splint bone, Mc2

The carpus completes dorsiflexion after impact of the foot and before the coffin joint rotates significantly. In this case the snapping of the carpus acts through the deep fascia to fracture Mc2, the medial splint bone. The fracture may occur anywhere from the middle to distal third of the bone (Fig. 7.9). The mechanical reasoning is given elsewhere (Rooney 1969) (see Chapter 10, "Stability and Lameness"). Silbersiepe et al. (1986) stated that splint bone fractures are 10 times more common in the fore legs than the rear legs; 88% of the fractures were of Mc2. Standardbreds and Thoroughbreds were most frequently affected. In our experience Standardbreds are more often affected.

Not all fractures of the splint bones are in the distal portion or of the medial splint bone. These fractures are usually attributable to external trauma:

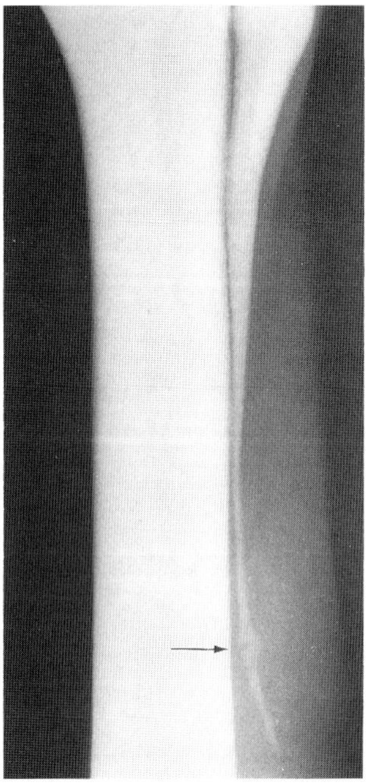

7.9. Fracture of the distal end of the second metacarpal (Mc2) (*arrow*) with callus.

interference. It is assumed that the normal epiphyseal plate at the distal end of the splint bone is not mistaken for a fracture. This epiphyseal plate closes between 12 and 18 months in Cold bloods, variably earlier in light horses.

Tearing of the deep flexor check ligament (accessory lig, *NAV* 1983)

The carpus completes its dorsiflexion as the coffin joint is rotating significantly. This causes a snapping, abnormal acceleration of the deep flexor check ligament, with tearing of that ligament in its middle third.

Schifferli (1908) reported that the tissue reaction to tearing of the check ligament of the deep flexor was less localized than in other tendons because of "less differentiation" of the tissues of the inferior check. The fibers of the check were thicker and grosser than in the deep flexor tendon, and less tightly organized, with more interstitial ground substance containing connective tissue cell elements with unusually well-stained nuclei (chondroid tissue). When repair begins after a tear, the fibers and ground substance become basophilic and even hyaline. Cartilage and bone formation may be more frequent in the repair of check ligament tears than in other tendons. We confirm Schifferli's observations, but have seen too few repaired check ligaments to evaluate the frequency of chondrogenesis and osteogenesis.

Avulsion fracture of the proximal m. interosseus

The normal nuclei of the tendon fibers of the *m. interosseus* are, on average, larger and more nearly spherical or ovoid than those of the other digital tendons. They are more basophilic, more numerous, and often in chains. Variably obvious basophilic, granular cytoplasm may be apparent (Krölling and Grau 1960). These appear to be *chondroid cells* like those seen in the intersesamoidean ligament and, often, in the interosseous ligaments between the second/fourth and third metacarpal bones, as well as in the superficial and deep flexor tendons (Webbon 1978a,b). While a formal study has not been done, chondroid cellular tissue appears to be more common in the interosseus than in the other sites and is present in the interosseus of the newborn foal.

Despite statements to the contrary, skeletal muscle is always present in two nearly parallel columns in the proximal third of the interosseus (Szakall 1899) (Fig. 7.10). It has been proposed that this muscle assists in damping vibration of the

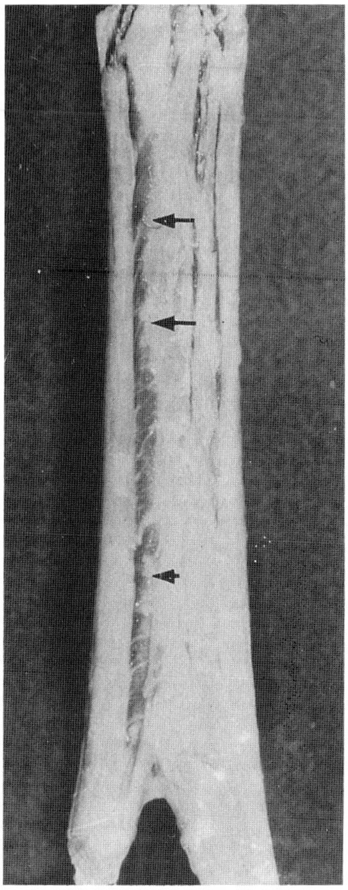

7.10. The muscle of the interosseous medius (*arrows*).

interosseus (Rooney 1973a,b,c). Occasionally, degeneration and dystrophic calcification of the muscle tissue has been found histologically, but there were no relevant clinical histories.

Avulsion of the interosseus

Avulsion fracture of proximopalmar Mc3 has only been recognized in recent years (Bramlage et al. 1980). It is probable that the so-called "blind splint" was (and is) such an unrecognized fracture. There is no such thing as a blind splint.

The carpus is dorsiflexed and not yet snapping into dorsiflexion as the coffin joint rotates significantly. This concentrates the force in the interosseus to its proximal attachment to the proximal end of Mc3, causing avulsion fracture of that attachment. Normally, the force in the proximal end of the interosseus is distributed to the attachments on the palmar surface of the carpus as well as to those on Mc3 (Fig. 7.11).

The reason for palmar flexion of the carpus at impact is to be sought in the individual case: fatigue—delay of protraction and/or retraction caused by hobbles or the force on the collar under draft. That such palmar flexion occurs in animals under heavy draft can be verified in the photographs of Muybridge (1957), for example. One would, also, expect palmar flexion of the carpus in jumping horses, particularly with heavier riders, higher jumps, and fatigue.

Proximal suspensory desmitis

Proximal palmar cortical fracture

These conditions have been described in the clinical literature (Dyson 1990), but no pathologic observations have been reported, and we have seen no examples. The evidence is not convincing.

Bowed tendon

This is tearing of the superficial flexor tendon in its middle third with the tear beginning on the palmar aspect of the tendon. It is an ancient affliction of the horse [Xenophon cited by Morgan (1962) and Leclainche (1936)]. The clinical terms, *high* and *low bow*, are pathologically meaningless. The tendon tears in its middle third and the external swelling is a function of the severity of the tear and the resulting volume of blood, tissue fluid, and inflammatory exudate. A small amount of fluid will not tend to migrate distally: the external appearance of high bow. A large amount of fluid will migrate distally: the external appearance of low bow.

Histologically, or with moderate magnification, there are, in the acute case, many torn tendon fibers with hemorrhage. Most fibers are torn across, tensile failure, while some may be torn obliquely. Overall, in all but the most severe cases, the tear has a generally sawtooth pattern (Alexander 1909). A number of clinical writers say that tendons and ligaments can be "strained" or "sprained" without tearing of the tendon or ligament. The diagnosis of strain or sprain is incoherent in the absence of tearing and disruption of tissue. Such opinions, not based on pathological observation, are reminiscent of the malign misinformation that bowed tendons were, in fact, only tearing of the tissue around the superficial flexor tendon [Coleman cited by Smith (1976)]. Dick (1869) cited by Smith (1976) dissected tendon "sprains" and knew they were torn tendons. Forssell, Siedamgrotsky, and other continental writers also recognized that the tendon was torn.

The misinformation purveyed by the pathologically ignorant Coleman persisted well into the mid-1900s and, indeed, persists even today.

Healing of the torn superficial flexor tendon is that of any collagenous structure. Granulation tissue forms, gradually replacing the hemorrhage and degenerate, necrotic debris. Histological examination of tendons at intervals after initial damage shows that the process of healing by granulation goes on for at least 9 months and perhaps longer than 15 months in a given case (Silver et al. 1983).

Microscopic sections show areas of normal tendon fibers interlaced with granulation tissue at all stages of maturation as well as multiple areas of hemorrhage. Ziegler (1969) stated that the scar tissue never becomes true tendon, the fibers being shorter and the new tissue more cellular than normal tendon. Williams et al. (1980) have shown that the granulation tissue is Types III, IV, and V collagen, rather than the Type I collagen of the original tendon bundles. These collagen types derive from the peritendinous and endotendinous connective tissue and, probably, blood vessels. The scar tissue is primarily Type III collagen, an elastic collagen characteristic of blood vessels and less stiff and strong than Type I collagen. Twenty percent to 30% of the total collagen, after repair, consisted of Type III collagen. The repair cells are more basophilic than normal fibroblasts, and Williams et al. (1980) believed them to be myofibroblasts, cells perhaps concerned with contraction of healing wounds (Cheville 1983). The suggestion, then, is that the scar tissue formed after tearing of the tendon is more elastic, less strong, derived from blood vessels, and of myofibroblast type. No replacement of the original, Type I, tendon fibers apparently occurs.

The newly formed fibers are laid down at random in the damaged tendon as already observed by Alexander in 1909. Those fibers in line with the tensile force, or nearly so, mature, while those not so aligned are torn by normal fluctuations of tensile load as the animal moves, lies down, and arises. This process continues until, eventually, there are sufficient fibers in nearly appropriate tensile alignment. At that time the tendon is healed, usually with more fibrous tissue present than in the original, undamaged tendon (hamhock bow). During the long course of healing, chondroid, cartilaginous, and, eventually, bony tissue may form. While it appears that injection of steroids into tendons will almost always be followed by ossification, such ossification can occur during noniatrogenic healing. Krüger (1938) found 15 cases of calcification or ossification of tendons of the legs among 224 cases examined in the presteroid era. Gurlt (1831) cited by Alexander (1909) found ossification in tendons as did Tombs (1841) cited by Smith (1976). As already noted, Schifferli indicated cartilage and bone formation to be more common in repair of the check ligament of the deep flexor.

Widespread dystrophic calcification of tendons, ligaments, and arteries is seen in horses given large quantities of vitamin D and in horses ingesting day-blooming jasmine (*Cestrum diurnum*), which contains an active vitamin D-like substance (Krook et al. 1975). Discrete areas of calcification in tendons may be the end stage of *O. reticulata* infestation (Cohrs 1961).

Attention has been given, as already noted, to the putative role of the vascular supply in superficial flexor tearing. The most provocative evidence for a significant vascular role in bowed tendon was that the superficial flexor tendon is essentially avascular in its middle part, and that the primary failure occurred in this area (Strömberg 1971). Three facts refute that view: (1) If the central part of the tendon is avascular, why would hemorrhage occur? (2) Histological sections of the superficial flexor tendon show as many vessels in the central as in the peripheral area. (3) If one injects india ink with a fine needle just under the peritendon and makes cross sections, it is apparent that the india ink moves along the tendon, following the fiber bundles and gradually spiraling in to the center of the tendon (Rooney 1973b). Tearing on the palmar aspect of the tendon, then, will result in hemorrhage in that immediate area with blood dissecting proximally and distally toward the central part of the tendon. This is readily explained by the spiraling course of the tendon fibers (Forssell 1915; Evans and Barbenel 1975), the ink moving in the looser connective tissue among those fibers.

It has been suggested that the centers of tendons are devoid of blood flow when the tendons experience large tensile forces. It is difficult to understand why, if that be the case, the superficial flexor is more frequently damaged than other tendons.

The cause of bowed tendon appears multifactorial. Certain facts will be adduced:

1. Bowed tendon occurs in racing horses in late training or early racing (Rooney and Genovese 1981).
2. Bowed tendon shows a distinct increase in frequency in racing horses in hot and/or humid weather.

In both cases fatigue, as a result of too much speed for the level of training in no. 1, and as a result of heat and humidity in no. 2, seems evident. Numerous older authors have noted a lower frequency of tearing of tendons when horses were adequately trained and not pushed too hard. Edwards (1923) considered high-speed work, fatigue, and lack of fitness as important predisposing factors. Smith (1917) made similar observations. Although not demonstrated in horses, there is evidence that tendons in general become stronger with exercise (Woo et al. 1980). Inadequate training, then, could be a predisposing factor, in this sense, in any given case.

3. It is a general rule that excessive tensile force in a tendinous structure will cause failure at or near a tendo-osseous junction. This, together with calculations showing that the fetlock joint would dehisce before the tensile strength of the superficial flexor could be exceeded, strongly indicates that too much tensile force, simply overstretching the tendon, is not a sufficient explanation.

It is proposed that superficial flexor tendon tearing occurs in the same manner as tearing of the deep flexor check ligament, by snapping—abnormal acceleration. An example illustrates. The foot is on the surface with the vertical force increasing as the coffin and fetlock joints close, tensile force increasing in all components of the stay apparatus. Before reaching midsupport, the surface breaks away ("cups out"). The angular displacement of the joints is suddenly reversed—the pastern reverses upward instead of continuing a smooth course downward. The superficial flexor tendon, and the other members of the stay apparatus, experience a sudden decrease of tensile force. The surface now holds once more, the foot reaches the hard base of the racetrack for example. The direction of movement is reversed once more, with the tensile force in the tendons suddenly increasing again. These sudden and abnormal accelerations—vector changes—are analogous to the cracking of a whip. The change of slope of the ground reaction vertical force curve shown by Dow et al. (1991), when a horse tore the superficial flexor tendon, is compatible with these observations. That is, the slope of a force curve is, in effect, a derivative of the acceleration, mass being constant, so that the slope is a measure of abnormal, third-order acceleration. These observations provide a subtle and unique example of the gait-lesion-gait principle (see Chapter 10, "Stability and Lameness").

Fatigue, however induced, would predispose to abnormal accelerations of the tendon by reducing or, in the extreme case, eliminating muscular tensioning force.

Clinical experience indicates that a predisposing, conformational, factor is the upright pastern. This is justified, mechanically, by the fact that, during loading, the pastern moves through a greater angular distance, in the same time, than the more sloping pastern. This, of course, entails greater angular acceleration of the coffin and fetlock joints and, so, greater linear acceleration in the tendon. The tensile force in the tendon is a function of that acceleration, and, so, the predisposition for bowing of the horse with upright pasterns. Fröhner (1905) and Alexander (1909) recognized that the long toe, low heel, that is, upright pastern, was predisposing for tearing of the superficial flexor tendon.

Splints

Jordanus Ruffus (1250) gave splints the name *supraos.* Dollar (1920):

> . . . a bony enlargement developed between the large and small metacarpal bones, generally on the inner side, less commonly on the outer side of the leg. . . . The real disease, i.e., the condition causing lameness, is an osteoperiostitis associated with formation of enlargement. Two periods can, therefore, be distinguished: the first that of inflammation; the second that of complete development, in which the inflammation is absent. During the first, lameness is therefore very general, but disappears during the second.

The inflammatory stage is often called *green splint* and the completed stage is called *cold splint* (Fig. 7.11).

> The process usually starts in the periosteum or in the interosseous ligament, which fixes the internal small splint bone to the cannon bone. Irritation of the bone and deep layers of periosteum causes a productive osteoperiostitis, and the process of splint formation is completed by ossification of the newly formed material. . . . The splint itself generally assumes an elongated form lying parallel with the small splint bone. When the inflammatory process has subsided, and the formation of the splint is complete, pain and lameness generally disappear, though the splint itself remains as a blemish (Dollar 1920).

In the early stages there is disruption of the interosseous ligament with avulsion from either or both the cannon and splint bone. In cases of longer duration, inflammation largely absent, the normally white interosseous ligament consists of bundles of collagen fibers interspersed with areas of brownish, translucent chondroid tissue (Fig. 7.12). When

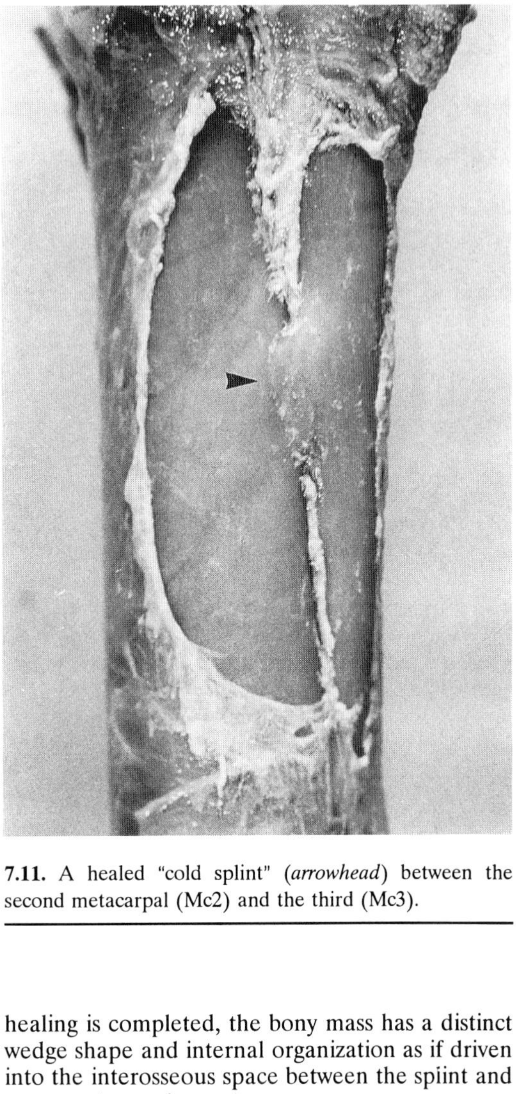

7.11. A healed "cold splint" (*arrowhead*) between the second metacarpal (Mc2) and the third (Mc3).

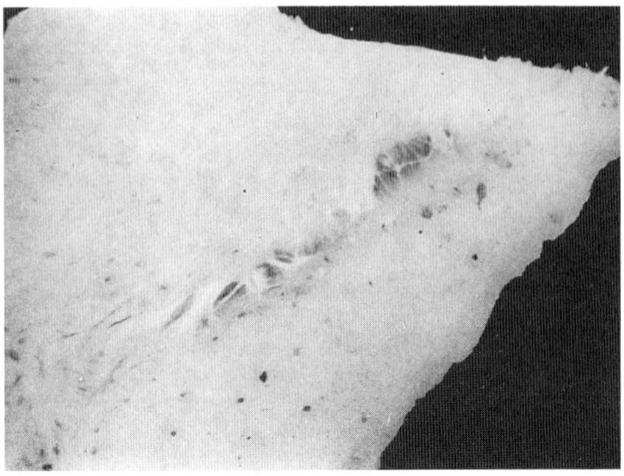

7.12. Cross section of the second and third metacarpal (Mc2 and Mc3) showing the chondroid metaplasia (*translucent gray* in photograph; translucent brown in fresh state) in the interosseous ligament.

healing is completed, the bony mass has a distinct wedge shape and internal organization as if driven into the interosseous space between the spiint and cannon bone in order to prevent movement (Rooney and Prickett 1966).

The translucent, brownish chondroid may be found in the interosseous ligament of Mc3/Mc2 of many young horses without evidence of inflammation or new bone formation. Chondroid tissue apparently is intermediate between collagenous and cartilaginous tissue. There appears to be no work specifically on the function of chondroid tissue. Its presence in collagenous structures that undergo considerable loading and movement, either from the start such as the *m. interosseus* or as a functional adaptation, suggests that it is an adaptation to movement and load (Krölling and Grau 1960).

As discussed by Rooney and Prickett (1966), if the head of Mc2 articulates with the third carpal bone, as it usually does, the loading of Mc2 by C3 involves both a linear, distal displacement and a mediopalmar displacement of Mc2. This displacement in two directions simultaneously appears to predispose the medial interosseous ligament to tearing. Mc4 is loaded by C4 only and moves only distally in a nearly linear manner. Fröhner (1905) reported Prussian army data that 80%–90% of all splints of the fore leg were medial.

Splints are rare in the rear leg and occur because of tearing/avulsion of the interosseous ligament between Mt3 and Mt4, on the lateral side of the leg. The articular loading patterns are the reverse of those given for the fore leg, so that Mt4 experiences two directional movement, while Mt2 moves in one direction only. Among 784 splints in Prussian army horses only 38 were in the rear legs (Bartke 1900).

The final common pathway for splints, therefore, involves both the amount of load (scalar) and the direction(s) of load application (vector). In a study of nutritional secondary hyperparathyroidism, Krook and Lowe (1964) showed that the outer layer of cortical bone is removed first under the influence of parathyroid hormone. This could be a predisposing factor in individuals as well as in groups of young horses. Several outbreaks of splints have been seen in yearlings on newly and heavily phosphate-fertilized pasturage with presumed imbalance of calcium and phosphorus. The outbreaks ceased when the animals were moved to normal pasture. The case is not proven since pathological studies could not be done, but is suggestive.

Fetlock

The word, *fetlock*, probably derives from *fetter* and *lock* from the practice of hobbling horses to prevent straying. Lesions of the fetlock are more common than in any other joint no matter the work to which the horse is set, and pain arising from the fetlock is one of the commonest causes of complete or partial loss of usc, particularly in young horses.

The fetlock joint is, in fact, two joints: the metacarpophalangeal and the metacarposesamoidean. There is an obliquely oriented transverse ridge that separates the two joint surfaces. In fact, all joints of the digit act as two joints in one: the distal end of the proximal phalanx articulating with the middle phalanx, and the proximal fibrocartilage of the middle phalanx and the distal end of the middle phalanx articulating with the distal phalanx and the navicular bone.

Immediately palmar to the transverse ridge, in the angles of this ridge with the sagittal ridge, the articular cartilage is often, though not invariably, thinner, with the bluish-violet color of the underlying bone marrow showing through. Recent clinical literature seems to have uncritically accepted these areas as synovial fossae. Since synovial fossae, by definition, are not covered by cartilage but by a fibrous synovial membrane, these areas are not synovial fossae.

There are six lesions of the fetlock and/or its immediate environs:

1. dorsal arthrosis (osselet);
2. transverse arthrosis (gullwing);
3. sesamoiditis;
4. fracture of sesamoids,
   (a) apical and
   (b) basal;
5. total/partial dehiscence; and
6. osteochondrosis.

Aging changes occur in the digital arteries and are discussed with the cardiovascular system (see Chapter 1). Even with apparent total obliteration of one digital artery, collateral circulation is sufficient to prevent lesions or lameness. Supperer (1953) described infestation of the walls of the digital arteries of both the fore and rear legs by a specific parasite, *Eleaphora böhmi.* The infestation, while striking and inducing a localized inflammatory reaction, did not compromise the vascular perfusion of the digit. This parasite has only been reported from Europe, specifically Austria, in about 6% of the animals examined, and has not been found in central Kentucky, at least, despite careful search [Lyons E (1992), personal communication].

Dorsal arthrosis

Together with transverse arthrosis, this is the commonest lesion and is seen, to some degree, in all four fetlock joints of virtually every horse under the loads of people.

The fully developed, classic lesion is arthrosis of the dorsal aspect of the articular cartilage of the proximal phalanx with mirror image arthrosis on the dorsal, proximal articular cartilage of the distal end of Mc3 and Mt3 (Figs. 7.13, 7.14, and 7.15). The arthrosis is characterized by erosion and ulceration of cartilage, reparative granulation tissue developing from the subchondral spaces of ulcerated areas, periarticular osteophyte development, and inflammation and fibrosis of the adjacent joint capsule and the *synovial flap.* This bilobed flap is formed by the synovial membrane and hangs down into the dorsal pouch of the fetlock joint. As the arthrosis progresses the flap may either disappear or, less frequently, become considerably enlarged and thickened by scar tissue containing numbers of hemosiderophages. This has been called **villonodular synovitis** (Nickels et al. 1976). Veenendaal and Moffatt (1980) examined similar masses and

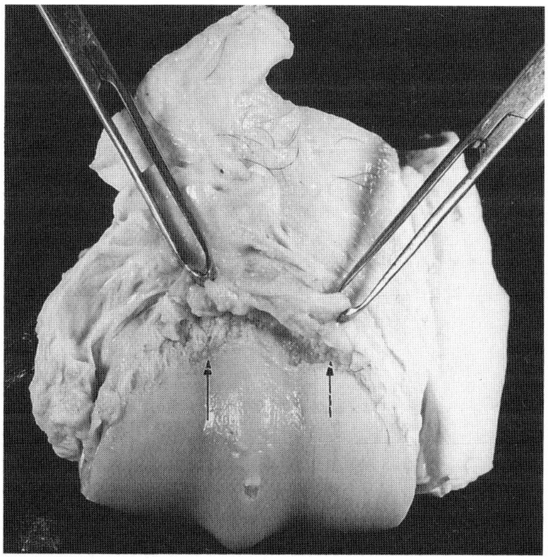

7.13. Metacarpophalangeal joint, distal end of the third metacarpal (Mc3). The characteristic erosion/ulceration (*arrows*) of the dorsal limits of the articular surface of so-called "osselet." Scoring lines are also present. The defect in the sagittal ridge is an artifact.

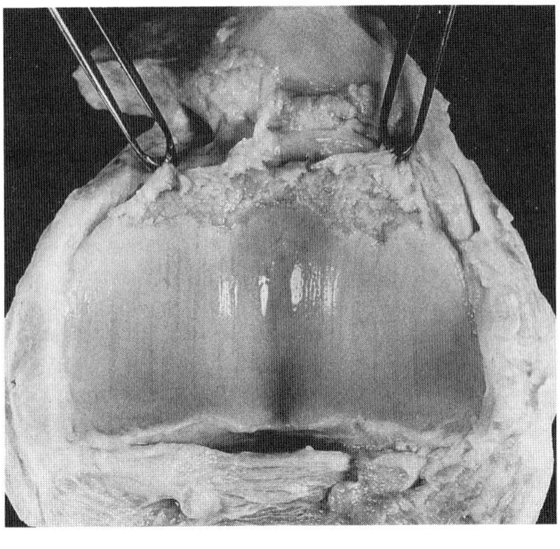

7.14. Metacarpophalangeal joint, proximal end of proximal phalanx. Mirror lesions for Figure 7.13 on the dorsal lip of the proximal phalanx. Pannus extends from joint capsule to the ulcerated cartilage, and scoring lines are present.

thought them inconsistent with the human lesion of villonodular synovitis. As Richardson (1991) has correctly pointed out, it is a reparative process, part of chronic arthrosis, and not a self-standing entity.

Subchondral lytic defects do occur but are uncommon. In fact, it may be taken as a rule that the subchondral lytic defects of arthrosis are rare with strictly marginal arthroses, and more common

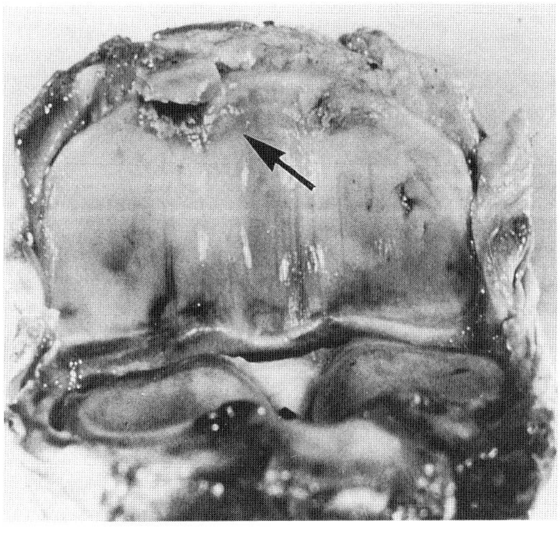

7.15. Proximal end of the proximal phalanx with a pathological, shear fracture (*arrow*) of the dorsomedial edge.

when the arthrosis involves areas away from the margin.

Wear lines, scoring of the articular cartilage, are common in the developed and developing case of dorsal and transverse fetlock arthrosis. It has been suggested (Rooney 1969) that they are the result of turbulence of the synovial fluid induced by erosion and ulceration of the articular cartilage.

The process begins with degeneration of the articular cartilage of the dorsomedial lip of the proximal phalanx and the mirror image area of the articular cartilage of Mc/Mt3. This proceeds rapidly to erosion with inflammation of the adjacent synovial tissues, giving rise to the hot, painful enlargement characteristic of so-called "green osselet." This enlargement is, in part, the result of inflammatory fluid accumulation in the synovial membrane itself and, in part, the result of the increased production of synovial fluid by the membrane. Increased production of synovial fluid is a characteristic of the inflammatory process of articular tissues.

As the dorsomedial lesion progresses, an identical lesion usually develops in the dorsolateral articular cartilage. The dorsomedial lesion always appears first and is always larger than the lateral lesion when, as is usually the case, both are present. It is a general rule of equine joints that lesions appear first medially because of the "spinning" of the component bones around their long axes as the joints move, that is, three-dimensional joint movement. This, in turn, is related to the larger size of the medial parts of joints, entailing greater acceleration and, so, forces on those parts of the joint surfaces and margins. This is discussed in Rooney (1969). The three-dimensional nature of equine joint movement was described at least as early as 1919 (Stoss 1923).

Restitution to normal does not occur. As the lesions progress, the erosions increase in area and may penetrate to the subchondral bone (ulceration). Periarticular osteophytes develop, at least roughly parallel with the articular cartilage changes. When ulceration occurs, granulation tissue is induced in the subchondral marrow spaces and grows into the deeper portions of the ulcerated areas. With time this granulation tissue ages to scar tissue and may undergo fibrocartilaginous transformation.

The inflamed synovial membrane may adhere to the eroded areas, forming a pannuslike mass. This is demonstrated by careful traction, tensing the tendrils of synovial membrane stretching over to the damaged articular cartilage. It appears that the synovial membrane proliferates as part of its reaction to cartilage damage and adheres to the fibrin and/or matrix bared in the eroding cartilage.

The usual terms, *acute* and *chronic*, applied to

arthrosis, can be misleading. The acute inflammatory reaction is certainly present, but the lesions do not become chronic, so much as they persist. Healing and new damage go on intermittently or simultaneously, so that there is a cycle of incomplete repair, ongoing damage. In retired horses one eventually sees a quiescent joint, permanently scarred and without ongoing, active destruction of articular cartilage.

The periarticular osteophytes and pathological fractures undoubtedly gave rise to the term, *osselet* (little bone). Periarticular osteophytes may appear as separate pieces of ossified tissue on radiographs, though they are always continuous with the bone of origin. Pathological shear fractures are not uncommon, particularly of the more severely affected dorsomedial lip of the proximal phalanx. As discussed with carpal arthrosis, such fractures occur in the sclerotic bone underlying eroded, ulcerated articular cartilage. Sclerotic bone is drier than normal bone, and drier bone has a lower shear strength. Even normal compressive force delivered to the area during dorsiflexion of the fetlock joint can, then, cause shear failure (Fig. 7.15).

The pathogenesis of all forms of fetlock joint damage (with the exception of osteochondrosis) is qualitatively similar and will be discussed at the end of this section.

There is, normally, a small synovial bursa between the deep face of the common extensor tendon and the fetlock joint capsule (Sisson and Grossman 1953). This may undergo soft, painless enlargement (Wintzer 1986). It is not associated with lameness and not to be mistaken for dorsal arthrosis.

Transverse arthrosis

While osselet arthrosis has long been recognized, transverse or gullwing arthrosis has not been clinically defined. The immediate clinical differentiation of osselet and gullwing arthrosis is the visible swelling caused by inflammation and increase of synovial fluid on the dorsal aspect of the fetlock in the former case and on the palmar/plantar aspect in the latter. In this latter location the increase of synovial fluid has often been called *windpuffs* or *windgalls.*

The lesions and histogenesis of dorsal fetlock arthrosis pertain, in general, to transverse arthrosis as well. Erosive lesions appear along the transverse ridges on the medial and lateral condyles of the articular surface of Mc3/Mt3 (Fig. 7.16). The earliest lesions are just behind the ridge, on the articular surface for the proximal sesamoids. The ridge itself is quickly involved, but the erosions do not extend forward to the articular surface for the proximal phalanx. Thus it is that only the synovial membrane of the metacarposesamoidean joint reacts to the damage, with the increase of synovial fluid apparent on the palmar/plantar aspect of the fetlock joint. The erosive lesion on the medial side is always larger than on the lateral, but it appears that both are always present, and probably of simultaneous onset. In contrast to dorsal arthrosis, there are often attached shreds and flaps of cartilage, some of which eventually become transient cartilaginous free bodies. They are transient because they adhere to the synovial membrane and are removed.

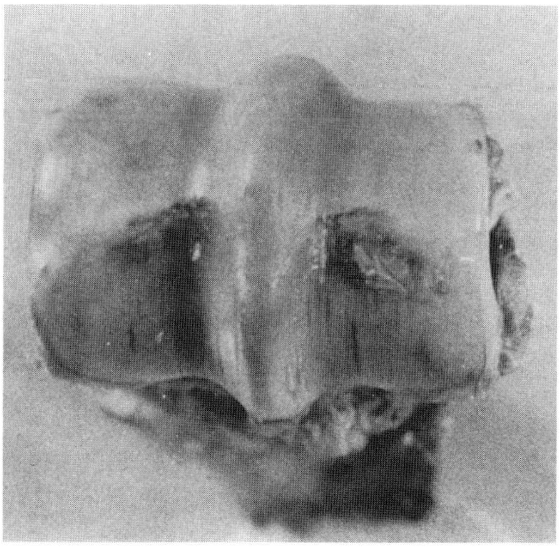

7.16. Distal end of the third metacarpal (Mc3) with gullwing arthrosis localized along the transverse, gullwing, ridge that separates the sesamoid and phalangeal articular surfaces of Mc3. Scoring lines are also present.

The mirror image lesions are in the articular cartilage of the basal border of the proximal sesamoid bones. While the damage on the transverse ridges is obvious, these basilar lesions are narrow and easily overlooked. As they progress, osteophytes develop in the periarticular tissues adjacent to these basilar erosions. These may be detectable radiographically and, incorrectly, considered to be either chip fractures or "calcification" in avulsed distal sesamoidean ligaments. (See "Sesamoiditis," below.) These osteophytes are also to be distinguished from the condition described next.

Petersson and Ryden (1982) reported 57 cases of so-called avulsion fracture of the proximal, plantar or palmar, border of the proximal phalanx, that is, in the area just considered. No pathological description was given. These lesions were seen primarily on the medial side of the rear legs of Standardbred racehorses. Nilsson et al. (1973) and

Sandgren (1988) also described these "ossicles." Barclay et al. (1987) preferred the term *osteochondral fragmentation* as did Houttu (1991). Hardy et al. (1987) found four cases, radiographically, among 71 young horses without lameness. They believed them to be osteochondrosis dissecans. Gröndahl (1992) examined 753 yearling Standardbreds radiographically and found this change in 11.8%, more often on the lateral aspect of the rear legs.

We have seen a number of examples at postmortem in both the fore and rear legs of horses of several breeds with most in the rear fetlocks of Standardbreds. In all cases they were bilateral, discrete, mature bony masses in the space between the basal border of the sesamoid and the proximal border of the proximal phalanx. The histological picture was unremarkable: normal mature bone. They lay between the synovial membrane and the short sesamoidean ligaments with no obvious origin from those ligaments. There was no history of lameness in these horses and no evidence of tearing, avulsion, fracture, or other pathological change. While the cause is unknown, it is our impression that they are benign, not related to fracture or trauma, and probably congenital.

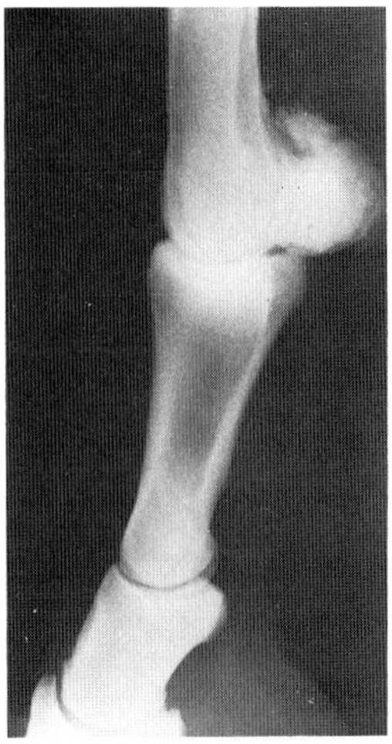

7.17. Radiograph of severe sesamoiditis, avulsion of ligamentous and tendinous tissue with osteophyte proliferation.

Sesamoiditis

This is a variably extensive and severe avulsion of the tendoligamentous attachments of the proximal sesamoid bones. The *m. interosseus* inserts proximally into the proximal sesamoid bones, while the straight, oblique, short, and cruciate sesamoidean ligaments arise from the distal borders and the intersesamoidean ligament (palmar ligament, *NAV* 1983) from the axial borders. Functionally, one may consider the interosseus and the sesamoidean ligaments as a continuous passive fibroelastic supporting system. The proximal sesamoid bones are intercalated into this system in an area of high compressive loading since fibroelastic tissue has very little compressive strength. The sesamoids are analogous to the patella in the quadriceps tendon, again, an area of high compressive loading.

The lesion is tearing and avulsion of the tendoligamentous insertions in the proximal sesamoid bones (Fig. 7.17). Acute inflammation is followed by repair: formation of granulation tissue and new bone in the torn, damaged areas. The repair process is that described for the pathogenesis of splints. The lesions of the intersesamoidean ligament described by Berge (see below), we consider a component of sesamoiditis. The pathogenesis is certainly overstretching and avulsion of the intersesamoidean and other ligaments as the sesamoid bones move too far with excessive dorsiflexion of the fetlock joint. The pathogenesis, then, is similar to that of basal fracture of the sesamoid. With sesamoiditis the avulsion of ligaments is caused by moderate and repeated overdorsiflexion of the fetlock, while basal fracture is caused by marked dynamic overdorsiflexion and impulse loading as a single event.

Arthroses of the fetlock joint permit eventual return to reasonably sound work (working sound). It is well known that sesamoiditis usually does not permit return to performance, pasture soundness being the best result. While there is no ready explanation, it may be observed that in the case of splint or nonarticular ringbone, for example, working soundness is possible once bony ankylosis has occurred. In the case of sesamoiditis ankylosis does not and cannot occur. Chronic or enduring pain, then, seems to be a characteristic of tendoligamentous avulsive processes unless movement is completely obviated.

Sesamoid, other

Wisner et al. (1991) reported osteomyelitis largely localized to the axial border of the proximal sesamoids, with involvement of the adjacent intersesamoidean ligament (palmar/plantar ligaments, *NAV* 1983). Five of their 7 cases were in the rear leg.

Berge (1933) described lesions of the intersesamoidean ligament primarily in the rear legs of heavy draft horses. He cited a report by Matisz that such lesions were 4 times as common in the fore legs and suggested that population could account for the difference. Less severe changes were tearing and fibrillation of the fibers of the plantar surface of the ligament with hemorrhagic discoloration of the adjacent tissues. More marked lesions were larger, focal defects often with granulation tissue. In some cases he found foci of discoloration within the ligament in the absence of changes on the plantar surface. Most often these lesions were immediately adjacent to the axial border of the sesamoid bones and associated with focal areas of necrosis and/or granulation tissue in the sesamoid bones. No reports of this entity, as such, have been found in the more recent literature (but see below), and we have not seen such lesions except in association with sesamoiditis. Indeed, in our opinion, this is part of the lesion complex of sesamoiditis. Berge shows one case that clearly was sesamoiditis.

While the osseous and ligamentous changes reported by Wisner et al. and Berge are certainly pathological, translucent, dark brown discoloration of the intersesamoidean ligament, per se, is not necessarily a pathological change. Székely (1930), cited by Berge, found 25% to 36% of animals with such areas in the interior of the intersesamoidean ligament and assumed it to be pathological change. Hertsch and Becker (1986) reported that the axial borders of the sesamoids of 28.5% of slaughter horses showed radiographic irregularities. The fore legs were affected twice as often as the rear legs. They also indicated that the intersesamoidean ligament was discolored brownish or black. Histological examination was apparently not done.

The intersesamoidean ligament is a fibrocartilage in which **chondroid metaplasia** appears grossly as translucent dark brown foci (Zeitzschmann et al. 1943). Such foci are routinely found in the intersesamoidean ligament of many horses without evidence of lameness (Rooney 1970; *NAV* 1983). In the absence of other changes, chondroid metaplasia is not pathological. Alexander (1909) found chondroid tissue (which he called cartilage) in both normal and damaged superficial flexor tendons. Beckmann (1936) found chondroid metaplasia in 73 of 180 intersesamoidean ligaments.

Fractures of the proximal sesamoid bones

Fractures of the proximal sesamoid bones are almost unique to the racing horse. Apical fractures are commonest in the rear leg of racing Standardbreds (Fig. 7.18), while basal fractures are more often seen in the fore leg of the racing Thoroughbred (Fig. 7.19). Another racing breed, the Quarter horse, perhaps has a lower incidence of such fractures for reasons suggested below. Sesamoid fractures also occur in jumpers but are rare in work horses (Wirstad 1963).

The proximal sesamoid bones, as the distal sesamoid and the small bones of the carpus and tarsus, are primarily composed of cancellous bone

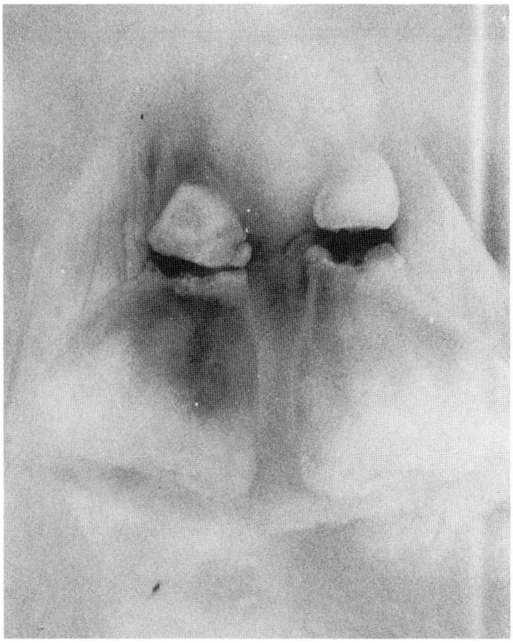

7.18. Unusual example of bilateral apical fractures of proximal sesamoid bones of left rear leg of a Standardbred horse. The specimen has been partially cleared in oil of wintergreen.

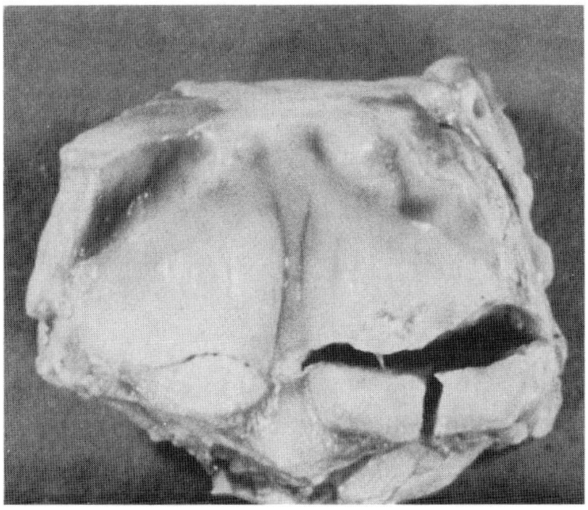

7.19. Bilateral basal fractures of the proximal sesamoid bones of a Thoroughbred racehorse. The medial fracture is more proximal than the lateral and has a secondary "T" failure.

within a compact bony shell. The orientation of the cancellous trabeculae parallels that of the principal forces applied to those bones. In the case of the proximal sesamoids, both large tensile (suspensory apparatus) and compressive forces (distal end of Mc-Mt3) are experienced, and the trabeculae reflect those forces. With age and work, the trabeculae in all of these bones become thicker and denser: work hypertrophy and/or hyperplasia. Such increases in density should not be termed *sclerosis*, implying pathological change.

Two ossification centers may occur in the proximal sesamoids. There is a larger center for the base and body and a smaller center for the apex as discussed with osteochondrosis, below.

Basal fracture

Basal fracture of the sesamoid bones is the most frequent lesion of "breakdown" in the Thoroughbred racehorse—fracture, occurring in about 50% of such catastrophic failures. While a variety of contributory factors have been suggested, it appears that impulse overloading of the leg is the basic event.

Osteochondrosis of the sesamoids has been reported as a predisposing factor by Krook and Maylin (1989), but not confirmed by us or others. Wirstad (1963) found no sex difference in Thoroughbreds though the numbers were small. The frequency of proximal sesamoid fracture in Thoroughbreds is greater on the American-style racetrack with short, inadequately banked turns than on race courses with fewer, wider turns, such as those in England, Ireland, and France. Many sesamoid fractures occur in or near the turns. The low frequency of sesamoid fractures in Quarter horses is probably related to the fact that these horses race almost entirely on the straight.

The topography of the fracture line (see "Fractures," above) is transverse, approximately at right angles, to the long axis of the bone and, so, the result of tensile failure. Tensile failure, in this case, can be the result of either: bending induced primarily by the compressive force from Mc/Mt3, or pure tension exerted by the suspensory system. Since the fracture lines are purely transverse, it is apparent that tensile force predominates, but compressive force is not unimportant as will be seen. The fracture is usually near the base but may be nearer the middle of the bone.

The pathogenesis is overdorsiflexion of the fetlock joint, so that the sesamoids are pulled over the transverse ridge on the distal end of Mc3. As the sesamoids move over the ridge there is concentration of compressive force on the basilar part of the sesamoid, and fracture occurs. This resolves the question implicitly raised above concerning the relative importance of compressive and tensile forces in the pathogenesis of such fractures. As the sesamoid moves over the ridge, the tensile force of the suspensory system increases. The compressive force is concentrated, acting momentarily through the ridge only. This observation was made by Wirstad (1962), rediscovered by Rooney (1969) and Stede et al. (1977). At this instant the concentration of force causes a significant momentary increase in the tensile component of the bending force, which, added to the considerable tensile force in the suspensory system, causes transverse failure of the bone. Immediately after failure begins, the tensile forces exerted by the suspensory system predominate and, so, the bone fails with the topography of pure tensile failure. In more direct terms, once the bone breaks, the tensile pull of the suspensory system pulls the broken pieces apart before any compressive/shear effect can occur.

The medial sesamoid will be at greatest risk because of the spinning movement of the fetlock joint pulling it over the transverse ridge before the lateral sesamoid bone. Once any bone is broken, and energy still remains in the area, secondary fracturing can and frequently does occur. The so-called T fracture of the sesamoid is an example. Once the major transverse failure has occurred, the small perpendicular failure can readily be accomplished by the tensile force of the extensor branches of the suspensory and the metacarposesamoidean collateral ligaments.

Apical fracture

This fracture is largely confined to the Standardbred racehorse, affecting the lateral sesamoid bone of the left rear leg (Spurlock and Gabel 1983). Wirstad believed females were predisposed, in a report in 1962, but said that males were more often affected in a 1963 report. Both reports may be statistical aberrations. We have seen no sex differences.

It appears that the concentration of compressive force, causing bending tensile force to be added to suspensory system tensile force, occurs when the compressive force peaks before the sesamoids have cleared the "shelf" formed by the proximal plantar limit of the metatarsosesamoidean joint surface. The lateral sesamoid is fractured more often than the medial because it is taller than the medial sesamoid and, so, last clears the shelf as the fetlock rotates. There may be apical fracture of the lateral sesamoid alone—most common—or of both the lateral and medial sesamoids, but never of the medial alone. It has been suggested that too slow *retraction* of the left rear leg in counterclockwise turns causes the delay of fetlock movement, delay in clearing the shelf, and, so, apical fracture (Rooney 1969).

Total/partial dehiscence

Catastrophic failure of the fetlock occurs most commonly in the galloping racehorse (Berge 1933; Rooney 1982). Usually this failure is the result of basal fractures of both sesamoids, with multiple secondary fractures and tendoligamentous avulsion from the shattered sesamoid bones. One may argue primary avulsion followed by fracture and vice versa. Since sesamoid fractures occur alone and with avulsion, while massive avulsion only occurs in the presence of fracture, fracture would seem to be the primary event.

Under North American racing conditions a breakdown occurs in about 2% of all races run, affecting about 0.2% of all horses that race. The left fore leg (counterclockwise racing) is most commonly involved. Sesamoid fractures, alone or as a component of breakdown, are more frequent during the hotter months of the year (fatigue) and are distinctly a function of racing around turns.

Osteochondrosis of the distal Mc3, Mt3

There are reports (Yovich et al. 1986) of localized osteochondrosis of the dorsal part of the sagittal ridge of Mc3 and Mt3. We have only seen lesions of this ridge in cases of generalized osteochondrosis or with joint infection, active or chronic. The latter lesion, in the healing phase, can resemble osteochondrosis. While the lesions described by Yovich et al. may, indeed, be localized osteochondrosis, we are inclined to believe them examples of healing-phase infectious arthritis.

Pastern

Osteophytosis (ringbone)

Ringbone is a catchall term subsuming several specific entities of the digit. Hell in *Bayer-Fröhner* (1900) indicates that ringbone was known to ancient Greek veterinarians. The process observed clinically and radiographically is osteophytosis—reparative new bone formation. The underlying pathological process leading to such reparative new bone formation is either arthrosis of the pastern joint or tendoligamentous avulsions. The word, *pastern*, derives from the Latin for pasture, implying tethering a horse by the pastern while grazing.

There are four conditions to be considered: cab horse disease, articular ringbone, nonarticular ringbone (leist), and pyramidal disease. The terminology is historical and descriptive.

Cab horse disease

This is a mass of new bone on the proximal end, dorsolateral aspect, of the proximal phalanx of the fore leg, approximately in the area of attachment of the tendon of *m. extensor lateralis.* Hickman (1964) called this cab horse disease since it was seen in horses working at fast pace on paved streets. We have only seen the condition, in massive form, in a few old Thoroughbred horses not known, and unlikely, to have worked as carriage horses. Wintzer (1986) described a similar, if not identical, condition in trotters under the name, **periostitis ossificans**. The pathogenesis is unclear. Since the lesion appears in the area of insertion of the lateral extensor tendon, it is tempting to consider avulsion of this insertion under conditions similar to those described for pyramidal disease, that is, sudden palmar flexion of the fetlock as the foot leaves the ground at the end of support. Fatigue or uncoordinated muscular activity could leave the tendon operating in a purely passive manner on the check ligament at the carpus (Zietzschmann et al. 1943; Rooney 1986), so that avulsion because of dynamic overstretching of the tendon occurs.

Arthrosis (articular ringbone)

This is the usual cause of so-called high ringbone in light horses but is uncommon, at least in Thoroughbred and Standardbred racing horses (Figs. 7.20 and 7.21). Despite earlier speculations about pathogenesis (Rooney 1969) the pathogenesis of virtually all cases in light horses must be based on the observations of early writers (Percivall 1834; Dadd 1854), and the paradigmatic work of Haakenstad (1955) with Norwegian Döle horses. The early writers specifically incriminated the short, upright pastern as predisposing for ringbone though the distinction between articular and nonarticular was not clearly made.

Haakenstad found that certain lines of Döle horses regularly developed pastern arthrosis by 3 to 4 years of age. By careful examination and detailed anatomical measurements before the onset of clinical disease, he found that there was hypoplasia of the sagittal ridge of the proximal end of the middle phalanx. As discussed elsewhere (Rooney 1969), the proximal phalanx spins around its long

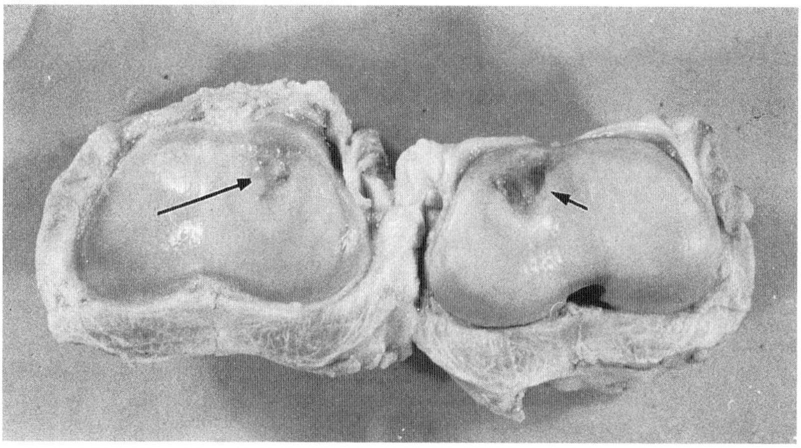

7.20. Middle interphalangeal joint (pastern joint). There is ulceration (*arrows*) of the dorsomedial part of the distal end of the proximal phalanx and a mirror lesion on the dorsomedial part of the middle phalanx.

axis on the middle phalanx articular surface, that spinning displacement being limited, in part, by the ridge as well as the straight distal sesamoidean ligament and the superficial and deep flexor tendons (see Chapter 10, "Stability and Lameness"). With hypoplasia of the ridge, the spinning movement goes too far, and there is a concentration of force on the dorsomedial aspects of the opposing joint surfaces. It is in this area that erosion and ulceration of the cartilage first appears. The usual repair process of joints supervenes, osteophytes forming first in the area immediately adjacent to the damaged cartilage.

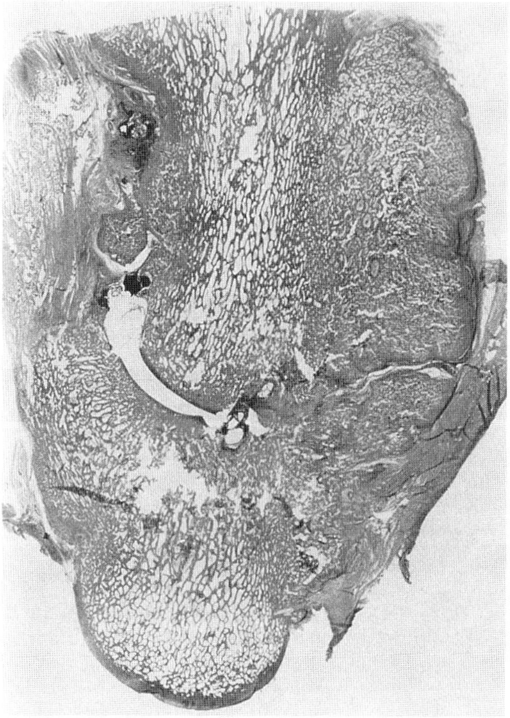

7.21. Sagittal section of well-developed pastern arthrosis with periarticular osteophytes (ringbone) and ankylosis.

Since learning of Haakenstad's work, we have attempted to determine if hypoplasia was the underlying defect in sporadic cases of pastern arthrosis encountered at postmortem. Despite the fact that the majority of cases were well developed and of long duration, it appears that most did, indeed, have hypoplasia of the sagittal ridge as the primary defect. In some the hypoplasia was sufficiently marked that ulcerative lesions were present in the palmar/plantar lateral portion of the joint as well as in the dorsomedial portion, evidence of even greater "over-spinning" of the joint. In all cases only one joint was involved in a given horse. The hypoplasia is certainly congenital and probably hereditary; it is certainly hereditary in the Döle horses.

Tearing of the straight sesamoidean ligament

Pastern arthrosis occurs in the absence of hypoplasia and in concert with extensive scar tissue in the straight sesamoidean ligament. The pathogenesis in these cases, all polo ponies, was, first, tearing of the straight sesamoidean ligament. With weakening of this ligament, part of the restraint of the spinning movement is lost and too much spinning would lead to force concentration and cartilage damage by the same final pathway as sagittal ridge hypoplasia. Stashak (1987) has a classic radiograph (his Fig. 8.101) of coexisting damage of the straight distal sesamoidean ligament and pastern arthrosis. Although all our cases were in polo ponies, such tearing of the straight sesamoidean ligament might be expected in other horses doing similar work, such as cutting and rodeo work.

Periarticular ringbone (*lysst*)

The Norwegian word, *lysst,* (German: *leist*) is included because Haakenstad (1955) provided significant clarification for the pathogenesis of these lesions. He showed that certain lines of Döle horses tend to have larger, boxier proximal pastern bones and that osteophytosis of ligamentous insertions around the pastern joint was more frequent in such animals (Figs. 7.22 and 7.23).

This may be interpreted as follows. The osteophytes of nonarticular ringbone are the later stages of the repair process of ligamentous avulsion from bone. The mechanics of spinning and rotating structures involves *moments of inertia,* that is, resistance to such movements. The larger the structure the greater the moment of inertia and the greater resistance to movement. This leads to delays eventuating in out-of-phase movement of the proximal phalanx relative to the middle phalanx, so that snapping, abnormal acceleration occurs.

Even with normally constructed phalanges, fatigue and rough farm terrain would predispose to irregular impact of the hoof with the surface. Such irregular impacts, the pastern joint not "locked" in the close-packed position (Rooney 1969), can cause snapping of the pastern joint into dorsiflexion or palmar/plantar flexion with avulsion of the ligaments around the joint. The joint cartilages are not injured under these circumstances so long as the sagittal ridge and tendoligamentous restraints are normal.

A particular form of nonarticular osteophyte formation was described by Siedamgrotsky (1891). Following healing and shortening of a torn deep flexor check ligament, the pastern was more upright and, so, the pastern joint liable to buckling or snapping into palmar flexion. Such snapping can

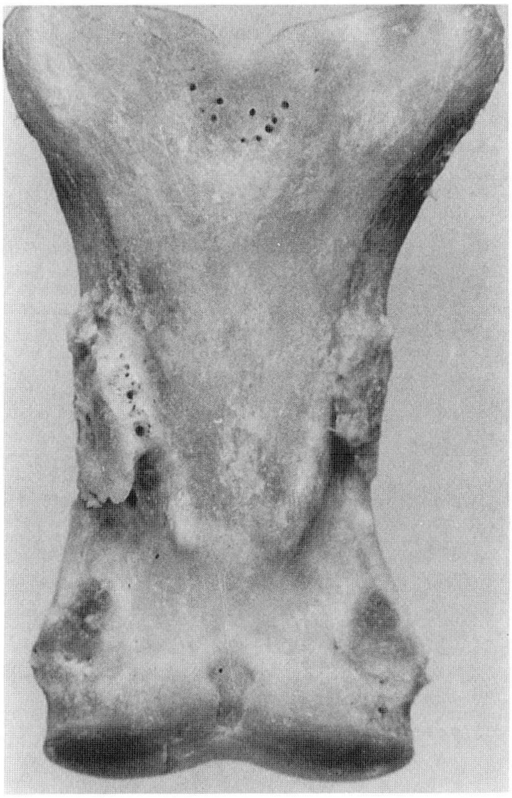

7.22. Palmar aspect, proximal phalanx with osteophytes in ligamentous insertion, as described by Haakenstad (1955).

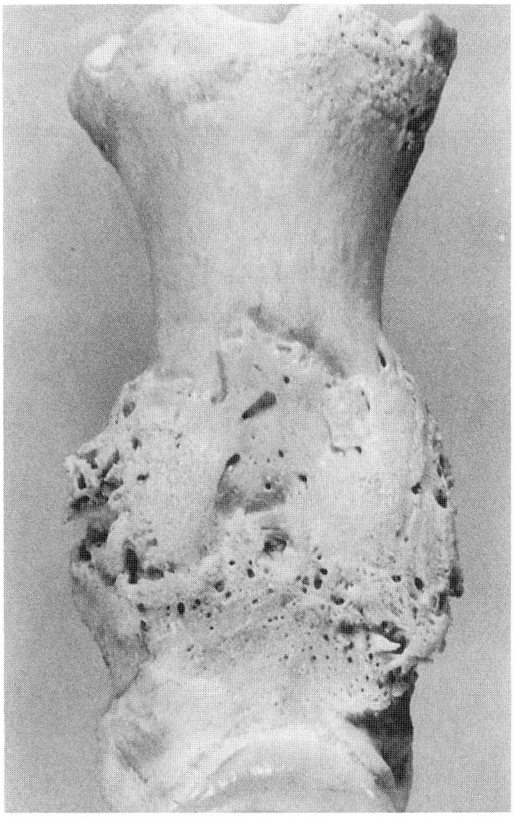

7.23. Macerated specimen of periarticular osteophytes and ankylosed middle interphalangeal joint, "high ringbone."

avulse the attachments of the distal digital annular ligament (Zietzschmann et al. 1943; *Lig. anulare digiti*, *NAV* 1983) on the lateral borders of the proximal phalanx with osteophytic healing. Siedamgrotsky saw this lesion, together with overall thickening of the distal digital annular ligament, primarily in heavy work horses (Fig. 7.24). Similar, though less obvious, osteophytosis may occasionally be seen in light horses with short, upright pasterns. It may occur together with osteophytosis of the attachments of the suspensory ligament of the navicular bone (*collateral sesamoid ligament*, *NAV* 1983), in young horses with postnatal contracture.

Insertion desmopathy

Hertsch et al. (1982), Huskamp and Nowak (1988), and Tóth (1989) have described so-called insertion desmopathy in the navicular area: osteophytes in the insertions of the collateral sesamoid ligaments, the navicular/distal phalanx ligament (*Lig. sesamoideum distale impar*), and the ligaments between the navicular bone and the cartilage of the foot (*Lig. chondrosesamoideum med. et lat.*). Tóth (1989) found such osteophytes in 247 of 296 navicular bones examined at slaughter.

While osteophyte formation is clear evidence of avulsion and repair, the clinical significance is unclear in the absence of any clinical history for these animals. We have seen osteophytes in these sites in older Thoroughbred and Standardbred horses, but much less frequently than reported by Tóth in what were, we assume, Cold blood and Warm blood horses.

Extensor process avulsion (pyramidal disease)

The extensor (pyramidal) process of the distal phalanx is the site of insertion of the common digital extensor tendon of the fore leg and the combined long and lateral digital extensor tendon of the rear leg.

Osteophytosis of the extensor process is low ringbone or **pyramidal disease**. Articular and nonarticular osteophytes around the pastern joint are usually called high ringbone, but the use of the terms, *high* and *low*, is not clearly defined. The osteophytes are the result of avulsion of the tendinous insertion on the extensor process, the joint cartilage not being affected.

It has been shown (Rooney 1986) that the extensor tendon is tightly bound to the deep fascia on the dorsal aspect of the pastern both in the fore and rear legs. It appears that avulsion occurs after the foot leaves the ground, sudden tensile force developing in this passive tendinous system as the coffin joint palmar/plantar flexes. This might be expected in animals with large, heavy feet and/or feet modified by the addition of heavy shoes, pads, or other gaiting devices. Carriage horses, draft horses, and gaited horses are at risk. An example is the Paso Fino horse, which characteristically works with a very fast, trappy "slow gait." Pyramidal disease is common in such horses and related to the acceleration of the foot as it lifts off the surface.

This condition has been described as a fracture of the extensor process (Frank 1935; Scott et al.

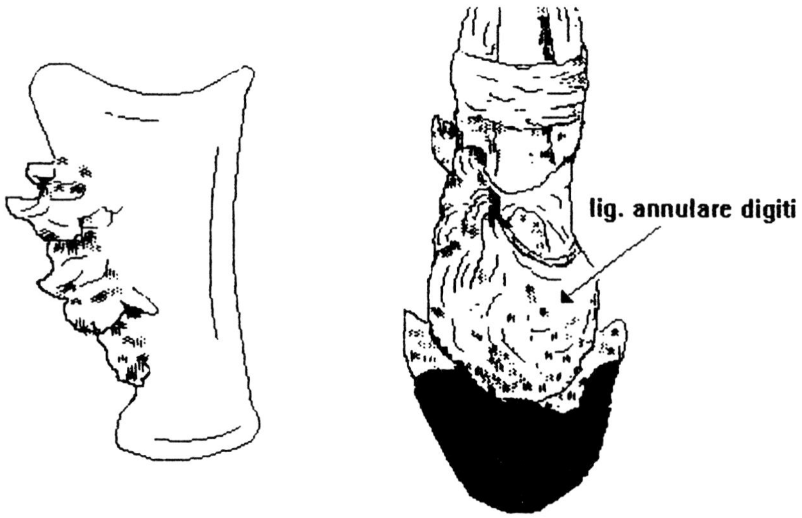

7.24. Drawing of the scarred and irregularly thickened ligamentum anulare digiti and of the associated osteophytes on the proximal phalanx, after Siedamgrotsky (1891).

1979). There is a fine line of distinction, perhaps, between avulsion and avulsion fracture, the former a pulling out of the bone and the latter a pulling out with some pieces of bone. The pathogenesis is the same, whatever the name.

Fracture of phalanges

Proximal

Pathological fractures of the dorsal lip, proximal end of the proximal phalanx were discussed with lesions of the fetlock joint, above.

Fractures of the proximal phalanx—*screwdriver, split pastern*—occur most frequently in Thoroughbred horses that train and race on turf and in horses used for rodeo, cow pony, and similar work. The fracture is caused by a combination of torsion, bending, and axial compression (Figs. 7.24 and 7.25).

During the second half of support, as the pastern is elevating—the fetlock moving from dorsiflexed to palmarflexed—the proximal phalanx is spinning around its long axis from lateral to medial. The dorsal surface of the phalanx is under tension and the palmar surface under compression. If this spinning movement suddenly accelerates, the ridge on Mc3 acts as a wedge, prying off the fracture slab of the proximal phalanx. The spiral component of the fracture is on the dorsolateral aspect of the bone, that part under tension. The vertical component is on the palmar aspect since that part is in compression. A sudden backward slipping of the foot on the surface, for example, on wet grass or on ice, can provide the sudden acceleration.

While the fracture described is classic, a few have been seen with the spiral component on the

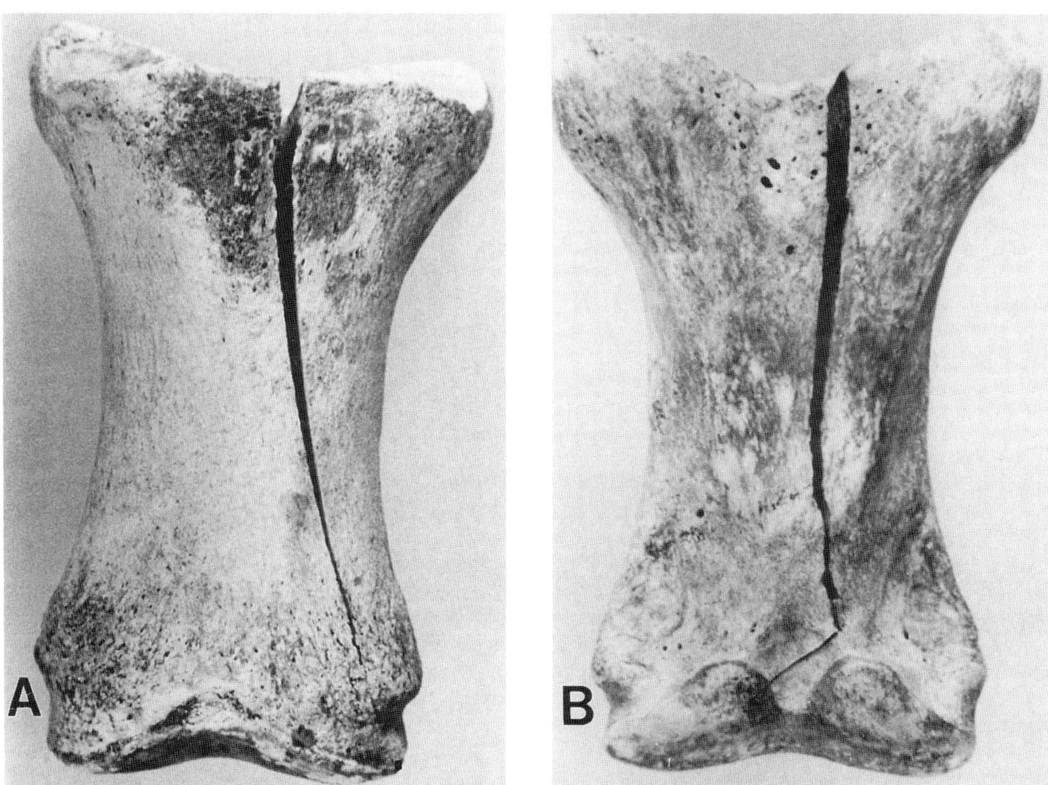

7.25. Incomplete fracture ("screwdriver") of the proximal phalanx, dorsal view (*A*) and palmar aspects (*B*): the curved, tensile/torsion, fracture line on the dorsal and the vertical, compression, fracture line on the palmar surface, respectively.

palmar surface and the vertical component on the dorsal surface, the exact opposite. Fortunately, in those few cases, the fracture occurred, and was heard, as the foot slipped forward on a smooth concrete surface. A case of this type in a racehorse was described and illustrated by Miller (1901).

Secondary fractures of the proximal phalanx often occur after the initial failure, particularly in older horses. They take the variety of forms shown in surgical texts.

Middle

Fractures of the middle phalanx may be most common in western performance horses (barrel racing, cutting) (Turner 1982). Very few have been available for pathological study. Torsional forces appear to predominate. The general principles of fracture pathogenesis are applied to the pathogenesis of a given case, though extensive secondary fracturing can make the analysis difficult (Fig. 7.26).

Distal

Fractures of the distal phalanx are not uncommon, particularly in the fore leg, and are of two types: so-called sagittal fracture and fracture of the palmar processes (angles). Yovich et al. (1982) reported these fractures in 1.1% of their clinical population. Scott et al. (1979) reviewed 65 cases, 47% in Standardbred racehorses. Weaver (1969) reported nine cases and cited Pires (1949) to the effect that 0.32% of lamenesses of the foot were such fractures. Weaver suggested that they represented 2% of all cases of lameness. Most occur in racing horses.

Sagittal fractures almost invariably extend into the joint cartilage and are nearly at a 45° angle, lateral or medial, to the axial midline (Fig. 7.27). They are, then, shear failures as a result of excessive compression, probably the result of concentration of force (increased force per unit area) as by stepping on a stone or a hard ridge on the surface

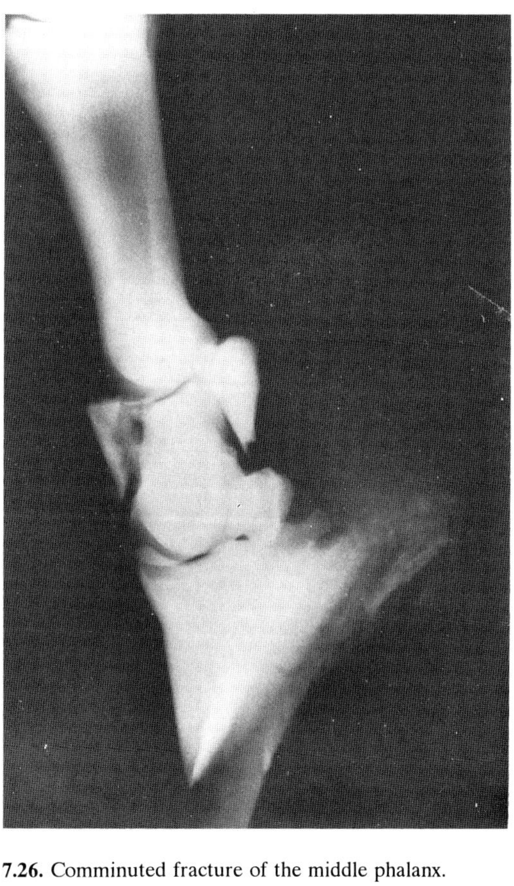

7.26. Comminuted fracture of the middle phalanx.

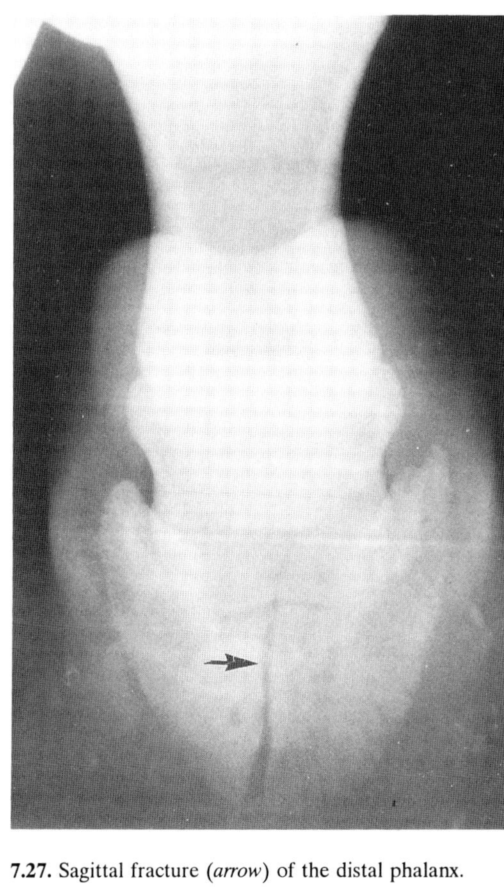

7.27. Sagittal fracture (*arrow*) of the distal phalanx.

or as a result of uneven impact of the hoof with the surface. In 47 of 53 cases of this type (Scott et al. 1979) the fracture line ran from the lateral half of the distal phalanx to the articular surface of the left fore foot, or from the medial half to the articular surface of the right fore. This is consistent with the impact of the foot with the surface in counterclockwise turns, force being concentrated on the lateral aspect of the left fore at impact and on the medial aspect of the right fore at impact.

Fracture of the palmar process appears to be simple bending failure, again as a result of concentration of force on the quarter or heel by uneven impact of the foot with the surface (Fig. 7.28). Scott et al. (1979) found 8 of these among 65 cases. With either fracture, predisposing factors may be present. A painful lesion of the foot, for example, corn or abscess, may cause the horse to change the impact position of the foot and, so, provide the necessary concentration of force.

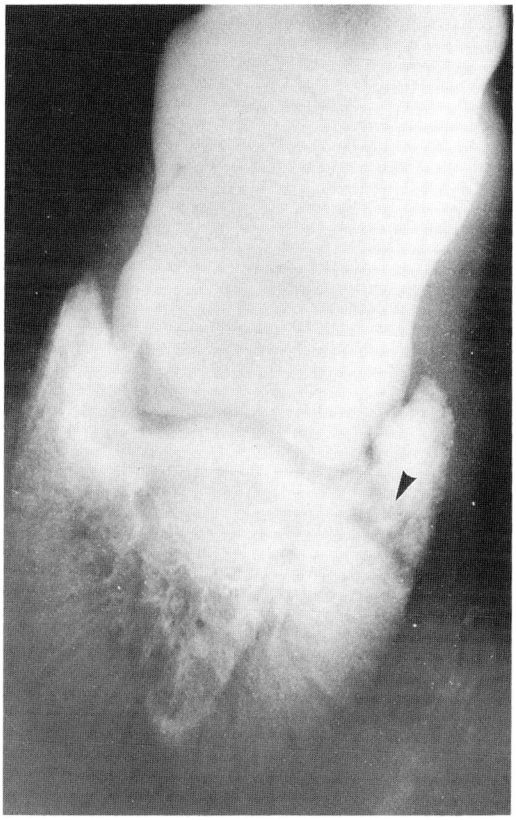

7.28. Fracture (*arrowhead*) of the palmar process. Callus is evident.

Digit

Adequate routine examination of the foot is hampered by the difficulty of removing the hoof wall without damaging underlying structures. Some considerations are given with autopsy method (see Chapter 19). The mechanics of the foot are of obvious and basic importance in the understanding of disease processes of the foot. Despite the passage of years, the description of the hoof "mechanism" collated by Smith (1917) can hardly be improved upon.

Navicular disease

The causes and pathogenesis of navicular disease remain in dispute. It has been recognized as a specific entity at least since Turner (1816) cited by Smith (1976). Smith, in fact, makes a strong case that Moorcroft was familiar with the condition in 1794 and had examined afflicted horses at postmortem no later than 1800. Navicular disease is defined here as primary pathological changes in the fibrocartilage of the navicular bone and the deep flexor tendon within the confines of the navicular bursa (Fig. 7.29).

The fibrocartilage of the flexor surface of the navicular bone contains blood vessels during fetal life (Fig. 7.30). These vessels degenerate and disappear before or within a few weeks after birth (Delius 1982). Occasionally, one or more segments of such vessels remain as brownish, translucent foci in the cartilage. Histologically, they are discrete, homogeneous, and eosinophilic (Figs. 7.31 and 7.32). They are similar, if not identical, to the "blood cysts" that occasionally occur in the heart valves (Cohrs 1961). These foci, apparently, disappear with age since they are never seen beyond the first few months of life (Rooney 1985). There is no evidence that they predispose to articular cartilage damage.

A synovial fossalike formation is often present in the sagittal ridge of the flexor surface in its middle third (Westhues 1938; Delius 1982). It is a variably deep transverse depression but may take more rounded form or be doubled. The base is covered by a thin layer of cartilage. It occurs in about 20%–30% of navicular bones (Delius 1982). In a given horse fossae may be present in one, two, three, or all four navicular bones. The fossa is of no pathological significance, but is incorporated into the erosions and ulcerations of navicular disease. If a synovial fossa, it is unusual in having an intact cartilaginous base.

The following observations are based on the

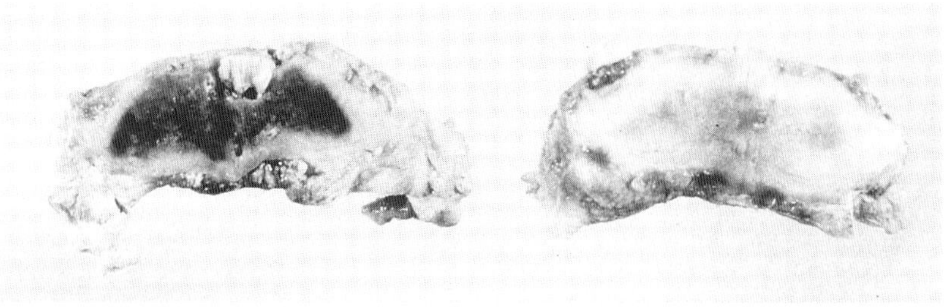

7.29. Navicular disease. The lesions of the *right* specimen are of characteristic location and less advanced than those on the *left*.

postmortem examination of over 10,000 horses, always including gross and, often, histological examination.

The palmar/plantar fibrocartilage of the navicular bone is white in the young horse, becoming gray to gray-tan with age. The surface of the deep flexor tendon, subject to both shear and compression loading, is modified as already described and reiterated here. The parallel tendon fibers are replaced by a thick, pleated mass of fibers with fibroblasts replaced by chondrocytes—fibrocartilage.

In many older horses a tannish-yellow, translucent change appears in certain areas of the cartilage, specifically the distal and proximal ridges of the palmar surface of the navicular. This is characterized microscopically by eosinophilia and fraying of the superficial surface of the fibrocartilage with depletion and cloning of chondrocytes. Mirror image changes occur in the fibrocartilaginous surface of the deep flexor tendon. These aging changes occur in the absence of any *pathological* changes in the underlying subchondral bone. They occur in the rear legs as well as the fore, but are never as marked as in the fore legs. Many have suggested that changes occur in the subchondral bone before, and are predisposing for, the changes in the fibrocartilage (Smith 1886; Oxspring 1935; Ammann 1987). Dick cited by Smith, on the other hand, believed the cartilaginous changes to be primary, which is our experience.

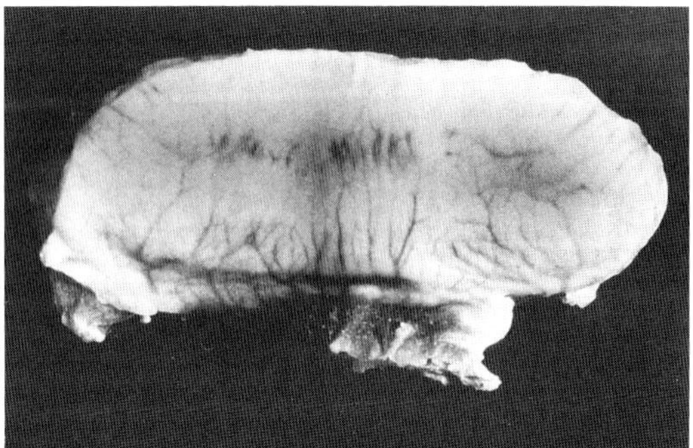

7.30. Normal blood vessels in the fibrocartilage of the prenatal and immediate postnatal navicular.

The subchondral bone in the young horse is cancellous and becomes denser, more bone per unit volume, with age and work. This is comparable to the increase in density that occurs in other small bones and subchondral bone in all sites with age and work. The pathological evidence is that erosive, ulcerative damage of the navicular fibrocartilage and the corresponding surface of the deep flexor tendon occurs with and without changes in the subchondral bone. Pathological changes of the subchondral bone, reaction of the subchondral bone to the influx of synovial fluid through ulcerated fibrocartilage, has not been seen in the absence of fibrocartilage damage and, indeed, frank ulceration of that fibrocartilage. Increased density of the subchondral and cancellous bone is not pathological; it is, as already noted, the response to increased loading with age and work. Fibrocartilage damage, on the other hand, is seen in the absence of such changes in the subchondral bone. The process is no different than classic descriptions of arthrosis of any joint (Collins 1950). Focal subchondral sclerosis and "cyst" formation follow on ulceration of the overlying cartilage with intrusion of synovial fluid into the subchondral marrow.

The so-called vascular channels, **sesamoid canals** (Hertsch et al. 1982), of the distal border of the navicular bone are, in fact, outcroppings of the coffin joint cavity, lined with synovial membrane, which carries microscopic vessels to that membrane and into the navicular bone. The shape and number of these pouches is variable between horses and among legs in the same horse (Hertsch 1981). There is no evidence that the shape or number of these pouches is correlated with the occurrence of pathological change either within the navicular bone or in the navicular fibrocartilage (Delius 1982).

Wintzer and Dämmrich (1971) described distal widening of the flexor articular surface of the navicular, together with shortening of the distal navicular ligament (*Lig. sesamoideum distale impar*) and exostoses in the insertions of the ligament and the deep flexor tendon. The widening of the navicular flexor surface is real and not uncommon in

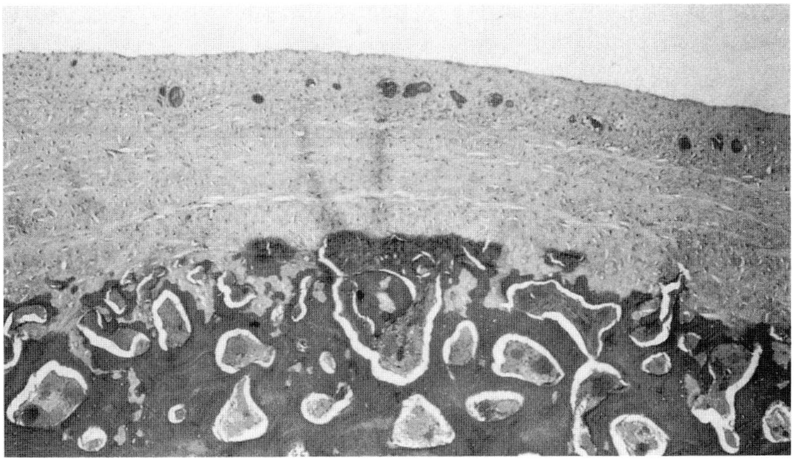

7.31. Low power of vascular "rests" in the fibrocartilage of the navicular.

older horses, appearing to be an adaptive remodeling rather than a pathological change. We have not seen the exostoses and the illustrations are unconvincing.

While it is not certain that these aging changes are early changes of navicular disease, we believe that to be the case, navicular disease being, at least in part, an accelerated aging process. The aging changes are most frequent on the distal ridge of the navicular surface, followed by the proximal ridge. All cases of early, frank erosion of the fibrocartilage found at postmortem have been in the same areas. As the erosive lesions proceed to ulceration and confluence, the process is always most severe on and between these two ridges near the center of the palmar articular surface.

By far the greatest majority of horses with obvious lesions had been used for jumping or had worked on hard surfaces for prolonged periods (carriage, police). Most were over 5 years of age. An exception is made for many Quarter horses, which develop lesions earlier if used for the types of work described. Thoroughbred and Standardbred racehorses rarely have significant lesions of the navicular unless used for jumping or hard-road work after retirement from racing. It is of course

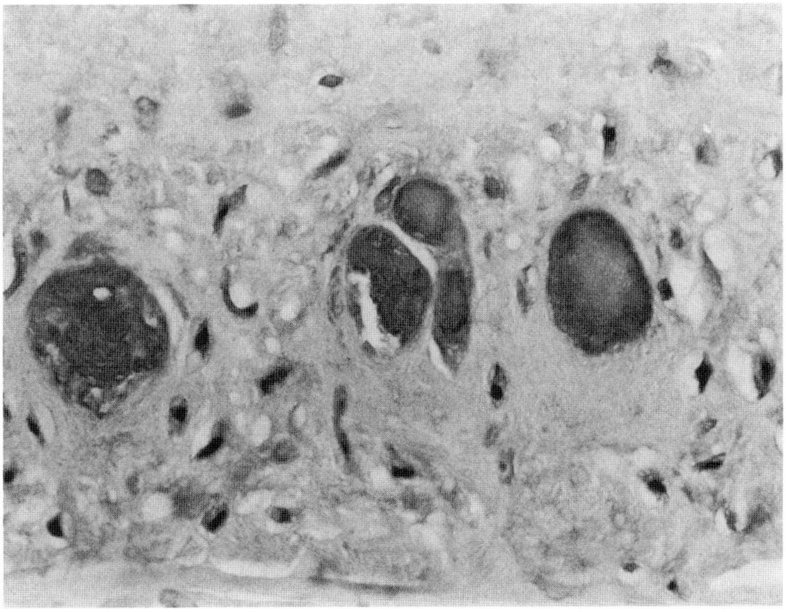

7.32. Higher power of Figure 7.31. Homogenous, eosinophilic masses in the lumina of segmentally occluded vessels.

possible, though unanswerable, that navicular disease would be more frequent in racehorses if their careers were prolonged and comparable in duration to the careers of carriage, police, and jumping horses.

Navicular disease is a significant clinical problem in Warm blood and draft horses. Navicular disease of the rear feet is rare although minor degrees of aging change are seen. We have seen navicular disease of all four feet in a few Hackney ponies and in horses that have worked for considerable periods on the hard surface of a treadmill.

Lowe (1976) examined the epidemiology of 5900 clinically diagnosed cases of navicular disease among 89,000 admissions to veterinary hospitals. He recognized the problem of accurate clinical diagnosis of the disease, showing that among eight clinicians at one clinic the rate of diagnosis of navicular disease varied from 3.1% to 18.1%. The diagnosis was commonest in the 7- to 14-year age group. Overall the frequency of navicular disease was 5%–6%, while in the 7- to 14-year group it was 12%. Geldings were more often affected, followed by mares and stallions. Quarter horses and Thoroughbreds were at greater risk than other breeds, with Quarter horses somewhat more at risk than Thoroughbreds. Arabian horses and ponies had significantly low risk. No conclusions could be drawn about the relative importance of intrinsic breed factors versus characteristic work for breeds. Ackermann et al. (1977) reviewed 74 cases. They found geldings at greatest risk, followed by stallions, and females. Quarter horses were at greater risk than other breeds.

Löhrer (1981) examined the clinical records of 8340 horses in the Swiss cavalry, of which 23.5% developed navicular disease and 13.4% were destroyed because of the disease. He attributed this frequency to the hard work of the cavalry horse. Hannoverian horses were more affected than the Swedish horse, Polish horse, French horse, Irish horse, and Holsteiner. The Swedish horse was much more frequently affected than the French or Polish. The highest risk was for horses 6–11 years of age. Virtually no new cases were seen after 12 years. The frequency of navicular disease decreased during the 15-year study period, particularly amongst the Hannoverians. This was attributed to more careful selection of breeding stock. The Irish hunter was least affected. In the whole population females were significantly more affected than geldings, in contrast to the findings of others. Within individual breeds, no significant differences in sex incidence were found.

Stornetta (1988) examined the clinical frequency of navicular disease between the offspring of two stallions of the Franches-Montagnes breed and a control group of varying lineage unrelated to the two stallions. One stallion had navicular disease, and the other was sound. Although the numbers were small, 67 animals, Stornetta believed there was clear evidence for an hereditary predisposition to navicular disease in this breed. Mey et al. (1967) reached similar conclusions in a study of Dutch saddle horses. Salis-Schindler (1967) examined the frequency of navicular disease among the descendants of five half blood Swedish stallions of Hannoverian origin. He considered that the disease was not directly transmitted, but that there was an hereditary predisposition and that the use of the horse was the primary factor.

The evidence suggests a multifactorial etiology, involving genetic (conformation) and environmental factors. A mechanical pathogenesis for this disease has been proposed and tested in vitro (Thompson et al. 1991). In brief, it was shown that out-of-phase rotations of the coffin and fetlock joints would cause an abnormal increase of tensile force in the deep flexor tendon. Increased tensile force means increased normal force (force perpendicular to the navicular fibrocartilage surface) and, so, increased friction of the surfaces of the tendon and the navicular fibrocartilage. The insidious onset of navicular disease is consistent with repetitive damage by this mechanism. Additional evidence for the role of friction is that, in reasonably early cases, the frayed and torn fibrocartilage is stripped from distal to proximal as would be the case if the increase of friction occurred as the foot rotated from toe to heel on the ground. This observation was made by Smith, as well, in 1917.

The specific event causing the out-of-phase rotation is hoof impact with the ground toe first, rather than flat foot or heel first as is normal. Toe-first impact occurs routinely when a horse lands from a jump, with fatigue at the walk, and when pulling heavy loads (Muybridge 1957). As Smith wrote in 1917, "In heavy draught-work on the level it may sometimes be noticed that the toes of the fore-feet are the first to make contact with the ground. This is due to the animal being unable to extend his shoulders properly owing to the load." It should be noted that the rear feet, also, tend to land toe first when under heavy draft (see below).

Repetitive toe-first impact is a feature of large body–small foot (absolute or relative). That is, the amount of energy generated in the small foot by the large body/load is too great for immediate storage and dissipation by the small foot. The foot, therefore, "bounces" or rocks back and forth heel-toe, toe-heel causing repeated impulses of tension and normal force on the navicular-deep flexor interface. This effect can be exaggerated by hard surfaces of low resilience. Indeed, enough work on hard surfaces, as carriage, police, or treadmill horses, can induce navicular damage in quite normal horses with only moderate loads.

It is reasonable to ask why navicular disease is much less common in the rear feet. Given the hypothesis, the explanation is that the action of the rear digit is different from the fore. That is, in the fore leg rotation of both fetlock and coffin joints occurs immediately and together at impact as the load comes unto the leg. The out-of-phase rotations can, then, occur as described. In the rear leg, however, the coffin joint rotates immediately after impact and nearly completes its rotation before the fetlock begins to rotate (Rooney 1969). Toe-first impact can occur and be corrected before the fetlock begins to rotate and generate significant tension in the deep flexor tendon.

The toe-first impact is an example of the gait–lesion–gait principle (Rooney 1969), which states that the gait anomaly that causes a lesion is the gait anomaly produced by the established lesion. Navicular disease is the paradigmatic case.

Leuthold (1975) saw three horses with "fracture" (avulsion) of the extensor process of the distal phalanx, which subsequently developed navicular disease. The common extensor, inserting on the extensor process, is in part responsible for proper positioning of the foot for impact. If it is not able to do so, as in these cases, toe-first impact could be expected.

Other considerations are:

1. The body, mass, of the horse being too large relative to the size of foot—a genetic factor. The size of the foot relates to the ability of the digit to resist impulse loading and dissipate energy. The smaller the foot, the less "material" to absorb energy and bouncing occurs as noted above. With extreme imbalance of load and foot size, instability and impulse forces are generated sufficient to cause navicular disease or fracture without toe-first, vibratory loading.
2. The load (body plus rider/draft) being too large relative to size of foot. [This is the environmental case of that described in no. 1.]
3. Hard surfaces causing high impulse loading and contributing to nos. 1 and/or 2, above.
4. The stability aspects of navicular disease are considered in the chapter on stability (see Chapter 10, "Stability and Lameness").

Many have attempted to incriminate vascular lesions of various sorts in navicular disease (Nemeth 1974; Colles and Hickman 1977; Fricker et al. 1982). The changes described are artifactual, normal, or questionable. Experimental occlusion of vessels to the navicular did not produce the lesions of navicular disease, and there is no unequivocal evidence for a primary role for ischemia in navicular disease.

Fracture of navicular bone

This is uncommon, usually affecting bones severely damaged by navicular disease, or as the result of osteomyelitis following puncture wounds of the sole. The exception to the rule is the heavy-bodied, small-footed Quarter horse. In these animals the force applied to the navicular bone by the deep flexor tendon can, apparently, be of such magnitude, and of impulse type, that single-event fracture occurs even in the absence of predisposing disease. In a sense such fractures represent the extreme case of navicular disease. The fracture plane is nearly parallel to the long axis of the digit and to one side of the median sagittal ridge (Fig. 7.33). In three cases (Vaughn 1961) a sufficient

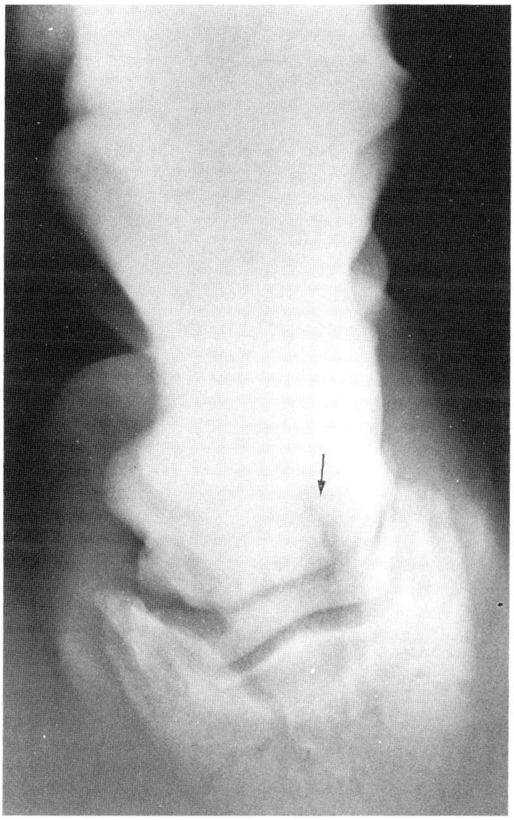

7.33. Fracture (*arrow*) of navicular bone.

period was allowed for healing to occur by fibrous nonunion, but the animals remained lame.

While no incidence data is available, the navicular bone not uncommonly ossifies from two or three centers, rather than the normal single center. The evidence for this is a neatly linear proximodistal fold (or two such folds) only in the dorsal, hyaline articular cartilage. There may be an infolding or thickening of bone in relation to this cartilage fold, which can be seen radiographically and, so, mistaken for fracture. We have seen a few cases of hypoplasia and complete aplasia of the navicular bone.

Avulsion of the collateral ligament of navicular

Osteophytes may appear on the medial and lateral ends of the navicular bone, in the attachments of the collateral ligament of the navicular bone (formerly, the suspensory ligament of the navicular bone) (Fig. 7.34). This occurs most often in horses with upright pastern conformation, including young horses undergoing postnatal contracture (Norberg 1967). These avulsion and repair osteophytes are to be differentiated from the arthrosis and repair osteophytes of advanced navicular disease.

The pathogenesis is found in avulsion of the collateral ligaments from the ends of the navicular bone as a result of the snapping into palmar flexion ("knuckling") of the pastern joint in the horse with an upright and, so, unstable, pastern.

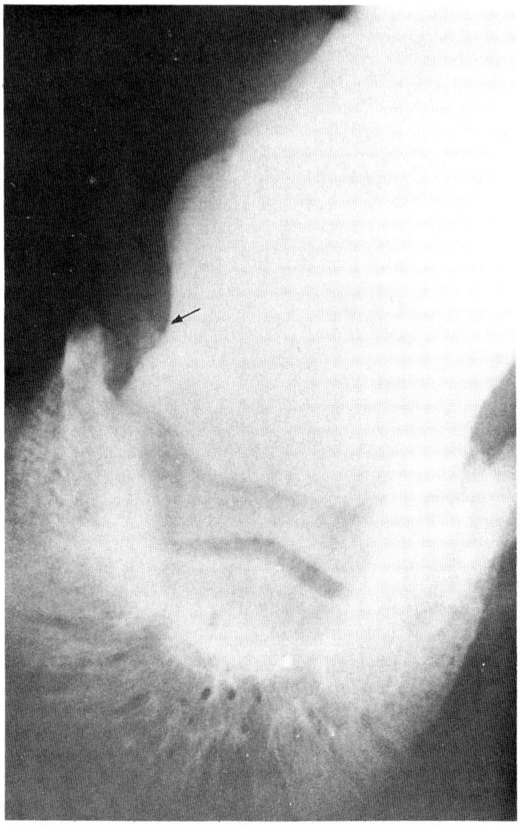

7.34. Osteophytes (*arrow*) on the abaxial borders of the navicular bone. They may be present here with navicular disease, but are also present with avulsion of the collateral ligament of the navicular bone with upright pastern conformation.

Ossification of cartilages of the hoof

Ossification of the lateral and medial cartilages of the hoof—**sidebone**—was a disease of the heavy horse with a somewhat lower frequency in the light horse (Fig. 7.35). The frequency of the condition in the modern light horse is not known and may be less than in former times.

The function of the cartilages of the hoof has not been defined. They are predominantly fibrocartilage with an admixture of elastic fibers (Schuster 1941). The following observations may be made. At the faster gaits, the impact of the foot is heel-quarter-toe. At the walk the usual impact is nearly or absolutely flat footed. With heel-quarter-toe impact the foot is flat on the ground in no more than 0.01 seconds, given a total support time of about 0.1 seconds. There is, then, only a brief time when the heels and quarters are supporting weight alone, that is, without significant assistance of the distal phalanx.

The heels, quarters, cartilages, and digital cushion serve as impact shock absorbers. The task for that first 0.01 second is to store and dissipate *energy* and not to deal with the large linear forces that rapidly grow to peak at midsupport. Once midsupport is reached the major forces in the leg are largely dealt with by distal phalanx and its attachments to the hoof wall at the toe and quarters. The palmar structures—cartilages, digital cushion, and flexible hoof wall—have stored energy, which will be regained as the load comes off the leg during the second half of support.

These observations are consistent with those of Smith (1917), Heusser (1928), Akerblom (1930), and Schuster (1941). While the medial and lateral fibrocartilages are a component of this elastic, energy-storing mechanism, there is still no clear reason why they are cartilage rather than, for example, fatty collagenous pads like the digital cushion. It has been suggested that, in addition to

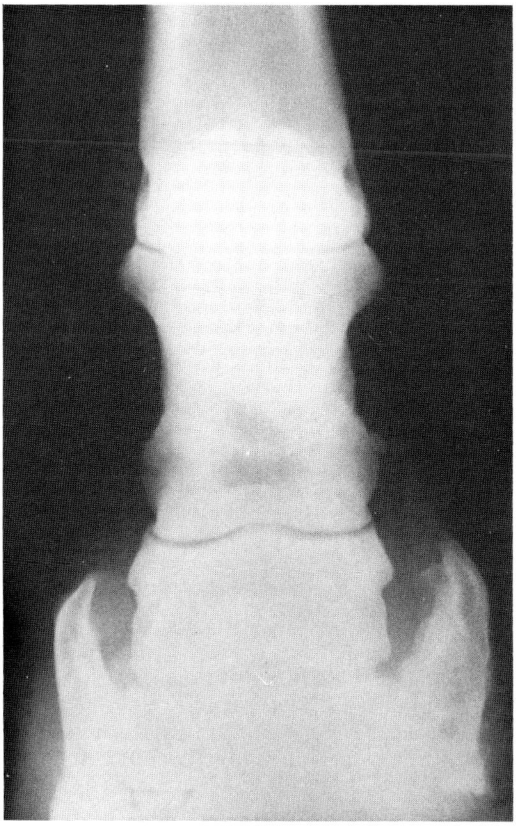

7.35. Well-developed bilateral ossification of the cartilages of the distal phalanx, "sidebone." There is also new bone formation on the distal end of the proximal phalanx, probable nonarticular ringbone.

their elastic-energy function, the cartilages provide a somewhat rigid support and pathway for the movement of blood in the extensive axial and abaxial venous plexuses of the digit (Rooney 1969). Heusser (1928) suggested that the hoof wall and cartilage separate during loading of the foot, blood flowing into the vessels in the space so formed. As the foot unloads, the cartilage and hoof wall come together again and, so, press the blood upward.

The cartilages of the distal phalanx ossify slowly with age at the chondro-osseous junction. Premature ossification occurs in this same area, rarely as foci some distance from this junction. The process of ossification is normal, the pathogenesis only being apparent in early cases where there is granulation tissue in and involving the laminae and corium between the hoof wall and the cartilage. This granulation tissue invades the cartilage, and the capillaries induce ossification. The arteries and veins that normally traverse the cartilage do not induce ossification, but capillaries invariably induce ossification when in proximity to cartilage.

Tearing and disruption of laminae and corium, with granulation tissue formation, should, in the early stages, be associated with pain localizable to the quarters of the foot. This is one form of the **sheared heels** described by Moyer and Anderson (1975) and Moyer (1979). The reasons for such damage have been suggested by the elegant observations of Dollar (1920), reiterated by Volkmann (1936). Dollar noted that heavy horses working on hard ground (carriage and draft horses in cities) commonly developed sidebone in the lateral cartilage of the left fore leg. Horses are generally trained to turn to the left (near side). Turning to the left, the horse tends to place the foot on the ground under the body with the outside wall of the hoof impacting with the ground first (functional base, narrow).

This accords with anecdotal evidence that the base-narrow conformation predisposes to lateral sidebone while the base-wide, toed-out conformation predisposes to medial sidebone. The general case may be made that uneven impact of the foot with the ground, concentrating force on one side or the other, causes tearing/bruising of the soft tissues between the hoof wall and the lateral cartilage. Bilateral sidebone may be sequential: pain of a developing lateral sidebone leading to preferential medial wall impact and subsequent medial sidebone and vice versa. Akerblom (1930) observed that there was less movement of the hoof wall at the quarter when the related cartilage was ossified.

Persistently contracted hooves are associated with the development of sidebone. Narrow feet are liable to uneven impact. If contracture of the foot begins after sidebone begins, a *circulous vitiosus* is established. Improper, unbalanced trimming of the hoof is also associated with eventual development of sidebone. The medial or lateral hoof wall is cut too short or left too long with preferential impact on the longer wall concentrating force and damaging the soft tissue supporting structures (Solleysel 1711).

Heusser (1928) felt that the initial lesion was tearing of the several ligamentous and tendinous attachments to the axial surfaces of the cartilages as the hoof rotated off the ground at the end of support. The strain in these ligaments at this time was thought to be greater in draft horses than light horses, explaining the higher frequency of the condition in those animals. Since our experience with heavy horses is limited, we cannot disagree with Heusser. It is possible, even probable, that tearing of tissue on either the inside or outside of the cartilages could lead to the pathogenesis suggested above. Using a maceration technique, Heusser clearly demonstrated insertions of the deep flexor tendon on the cartilages of the hoof, as well as on the distal phalanx (see Chapter 19, "Autopsy Method").

Pedal osteitis

This condition is poorly defined and only discussed in the clinical literature. Lameness is localized in the foot without evidence of sidebone, navicular disease, corn, and so forth. Radiographs suggest osteolysis and/or osteophytosis of the edges of the distal phalanx either at the toe or quarters and heels. When the toe is involved the condition is, properly, **road founder**, which is discussed with laminitis (see next section). Involvement of the quarters and heels is problematic and often a diagnosis of desperation and inadequate radiographic technique. No unequivocal example of pedal osteitis, other than road founder, has been seen at postmortem.

Other lesions of the foot

As pointed out by Dyson (1991) and well known to equine veterinarians, there are many horses with pain in the foot for which causes are not found. The foot is difficult to examine satisfactorily at postmortem, and few horses with foot lameness are presented, or identified when presented, for postmortem. As a result our knowledge of these occult causes is limited. Experience indicates, however, that the laminar lesions described above for the early stages of sidebone and road founder are not defined clinically, but can be found by careful postmortem dissection. Early cases of true navicular disease and avulsion of the suspensory ligament of the navicular bone, also, can be missed clinically, but are definable at postmortem.

A so-called **synovitis of the coffin joint** with increased amounts of synovial fluid and elevated pressure has apparently been observed, but no pathological descriptions have been found, and we have not seen a case at postmortem.

Laminitis

This is an ancient disease of the domesticated horse, as old, no doubt, as domestication itself [Aristotle 330 BCE and Xenophon 445 BCE: Darmstaedter et al. (1908) and Leclainche (1936)]. The care exercised by Hittite horsemen in providing feed and water after work suggests that they may have been aware of the relationship to laminitis as early as 1350 BCE (Kikkuli 1977).

In a compilation of claims paid by insurers of horses, laminitis ranked 10th, approximately 4% of all losses.

Laminitis is a common complication of many conditions, largely related to the association of horse and human. These include ingestion of large quantities of water after a period of deprivation, placental retention and metritis, sepsis, colic and intestinal ischemia, grain overload, endotoxemia, hepatic steatosis, excessive concussion, and corticosteroid administration (Hood et al. 1979; Moore et al. 1991a,b). Horses eating hoary alyssum, *Berteroa incana,* and black walnut, *Juglans nigra,* may develop acute laminitis (Galey et al. 1990; Geor et al. 1992). It is well known that walnut shavings or sawdust should not be used as stall bedding because of the high frequency of laminitis.

Laminitis is more common in stallions than mares or geldings, according to Dorn et al. (1975). Amoss et al. (1979) showed increased levels of adrenal-derived testosterone in mares and geldings with experimental laminitis. Mares develop laminitis most commonly between 4 and 7 years, while stallions develop it later, between 7 and 10 years of age (Garner et al. 1978). The disease is 4 times more common in ponies than in horses in the experience of Garner et al. (1980), but is frequently more severe in the horse (Dorn et al. 1975; Garner 1980). Some seasonal variation in the incidence in ponies was noted in one study (Peremans et al. 1991).

The work of Amoss et al. (1979) has not been confirmed. The frequency data reported is to be taken cautiously. In our experience the significant correlations are to be found with environmental and management factors and not with sex or age. Although anecdotal, pony laminitis is more frequent with the arrival of spring grass, so long as one is considering the Shetland pony. This breed by far outstrips other ponies in the frequency of laminitis, largely mechanical, as discussed below.

Obel (1948) developed a classification of the clinical disease. Horses with Obel grade 1 laminitis shift feet frequently when standing. When trotted, they have shortened stride. Obel grade 2 horses move at the walk and trot but with stabbing, shortened stride. Obel grade 3 horses move reluctantly and resist attempts to lift the affected or contralateral feet. The most severe grade, Obel grade 4, is characterized by marked reluctance or absolute refusal to move, including going down.

Systemic clinical signs are also seen in horses with spontaneous and experimental—carbohydrate overload with cornstarch and methyl cellulose—laminitis. Parry (1984) found the mean systemic systolic/diastolic pressure in two horses with acute laminitis to be 206/146 mm Hg coccygeal, uncorrected value, significantly higher than normal mean pressures of 112/77 mm Hg. Garner (1975) and Amoss et al. (1988) considered this a response to intense pain. The pathophysiologic basis of the hypertension, increased cardiac output, increased left ventricular ejection rate and heart rate, and delayed decrease in plasma volume, was studied in carbohydrate-induced acute laminitis by Garner et al. (1977). No further studies have been found, and the role of hypertension in laminitis is unclear.

A decrease in plasma volume, serum sodium, potassium, and chloride levels has been observed in carbohydrate-induced acute laminitis. The electrolyte abnormalities were thought to be caused by activation of the renin–angiotensin–aldosterone system (Hood et al. 1979; Clarke et al. 1982). Increased levels of plasma renin and serum catecholamines, which could exert pressor effects on vasculature, have been found in horses with experimental laminitis (Amoss et al. 1988). Increased packed cell volume has been observed in spontaneous and experimental cases (Coffman and Garner 1972). The role of any of these changes in the pathogenesis of the disease is unclear and problematic.

Two basic forms of the clinical disease may be defined pathologically.

Mechanical

Mechanical laminitis—road founder—is tearing of the corial tissues between the distal phalanx and the hoof wall. The lesion is most severe at the toe, extending a variable distance around toward the quarters (Fig. 7.36). Histologically, there is disruption of collagen fibers with hemorrhage and edema in the acute stage, followed by granulation tissue and fibrosis.

The condition was seen primarily in carriage horses: animals with heavy bodies, relatively light legs, and long toes for high "action." In the modern era the incidence is not known, at least in part, because of lack of differential recognition of the clinical signs.

Mechanical laminitis is not uncommon in Shetland ponies in nonindigenous areas in the spring of the year. These animals put on weight very rapidly with the flush of new grass. As well, the hoof of the Shetland, well adapted genetically to the harsh wearing conditions of the islands, is not worn down on less abrasive grass pastures. These circumstances—rapid increase of weight and inadequate wearing—lead to an overly long toe, around the tip of which a greater weight of animal must be rotated at the end of support. With slight modification the pathogenesis applies to the heavy carriage horse, as well: long toe for high action, hard surfaces, and long periods of work.

Vascular

This is the common, generally recognized, form of laminitis. The clinical signs are well known. Variations of the basic clinical pattern are given various names, such as "sinker," by clinicians and farriers. There variations are largely related to the rapidity of displacement of the distal phalanx, in turn related to the extent and severity of the laminar necrosis and the weight of the animal (Figs. 7.37 and 7.38).

There are three circumstances leading to vascular laminitis. The classic and most frequent form is in horses ingesting too much water and/or

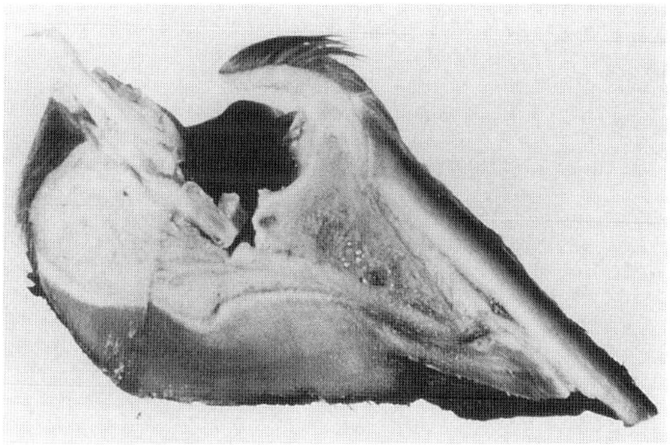

7.36. Road founder or pony-type laminitis with tearing of the laminae and corium near the toe. Note the length of the toe as compared to Figure 7.37.

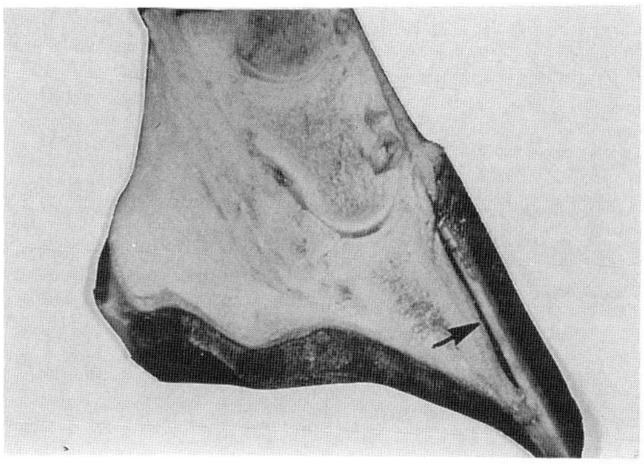

7.37. Acute, classic laminitis. The laminae of the wall at the toe are destroyed (*arrow*) and replaced by a lake of free blood.

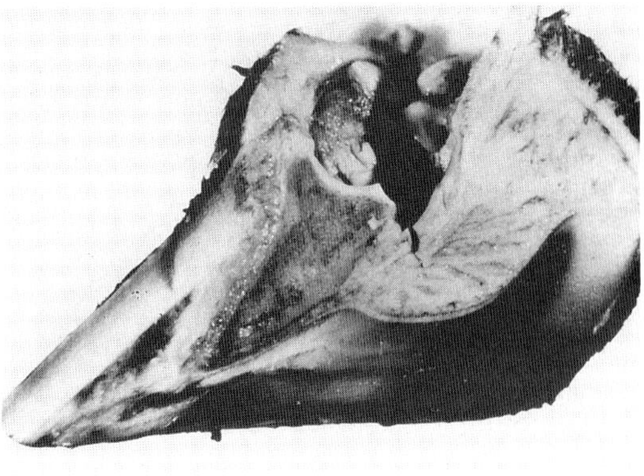

7.38. Laminitis of some duration with rotation of the distal phalanx and granulation tissue formation in the gap.

feed after an enforced fast, prolonged work in inclement weather, improper long distance shipping, and so on. The second is the postparturient mare with laminitis, almost invariably associated with retained placenta. The third form, static vascular laminitis, occurs in horses which are three-legged lame, confined to small standings, and, so, unable to move about at will.

The pathology is the same in all three cases. If the postmortem is done during the acute phase and before rotation of the distal phalanx begins, the laminar/corial area is intensely congested with loss of tissue substance and frank hemorrhage (Fig. 7.37). With or without rotation, granulation tissue gradually fills the necrotic area. Without rotation, healing and reorganization progresses apace and a near normal foot is regained. With rotation the granulation tissue fills the larger space, eventually becoming a mass of scar tissue (Fig. 7.38). Some degree of regeneration and reorganization of the germinal epithelium does take place, so that the foot resumes nearly normal growth even though the displacement may cause distortion of the foot.

Histologically, the earliest changes in spontaneous cases have been vascular dilatation, hemorrhage, and edema in the corium, accompanied by ischemic necrosis of the germinal epithelium of the hoof wall. The epithelial cells are swollen with pale staining cytoplasm and karyorrhectic and karyolytic nuclear degeneration. Vacuolation of cells, frank necrosis, and disruption of the epithelial architecture quickly follows. These changes are nonspecific, suggesting only anoxia. Obel (1948) described the process clearly, though his interpretation of cause has not been substantiated. Cohrs (1941a) suggested that the fibrinoid swelling and necrosis of the corium that accompany the epithelial changes were evidence for an allergic process, but that is problematic.

There are no qualitative pathological differences among the three types of vascular laminitis. The usual form involves all feet, although the fore feet are more severely affected because of the greater static load. Postparturient laminitis is characterized by its severity, rapid course, and clinically evident involvement of all four feet. In both cases the rapidity of rotation of the distal phalanx, or almost straight distal displacement of the phalanx, is related to the extent and severity of the necrosis and disruption of the soft tissues between the hoof wall and the phalanx, and to the weight of the animal.

Static

Static vascular laminitis characteristically involves only the one supporting fore foot. Clinicians at Colorado State University found that allowing free movement of the three-legged animal in a paddock effectively prevented such laminitis. Such cases have only been seen at postmortem some time after onset, with no pathological differences from classic laminitis. Failure of adequate venous return from the foot with subsequent stagnant anoxia would appear to be the pathogenesis.

Transport

European veterinarians have long recognized a transport laminitis in horses shipped for considerable distances without adequate rest periods. The clinical signs are those of classic, vascular laminitis but are usually mild and disappear with exercise. Stagnant anoxia would appear to be the pathogenesis here, as well, clearly related to long periods of confined transport.

While the multiple causes and precise pathogenesis of classic vascular laminitis remain undefined, the evidence indicates inadequate capillary blood flow as the immediate cause of the ischemia.

Physiological and anatomical studies (Hood et al. 1978; Pollitt and Molyneux 1990) indicate that shunting by arteriovenous anastomoses in the papillae and laminae are probably involved. Nickel (1941) had already indicated a role for the arteriovenous anastomoses in laminitis. Obel (1948) showed that changes occurred in the epithelium of the chestnut as well as in the laminae of the hoof with acute laminitis.

Rooney (1984) pointed out that arteriovenous anastomoses of the glomus type are as common adjacent to the dermoepidermal junction of the chestnut as they are in the papillae and laminae of the hoof [Hyrtl (1864) cited by Clara (1956); and Pollitt and Molyneux (1990)] (Fig. 7.39).

In the dermal papillae of the distal end of the laminae, the periople, coronary band, sole, and

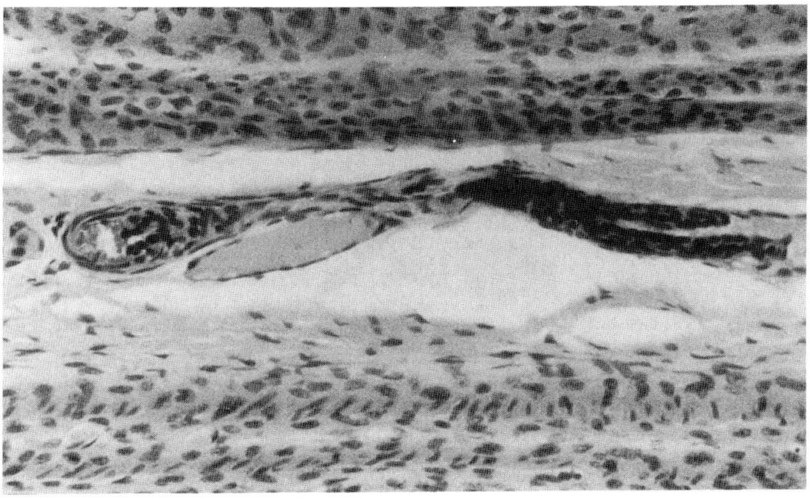

7.39. High power view of glomustype arteriovenous anastomosis in the corium of the hoof. The arterial vessel is to the *left* and the opening of the arteriovenous anastomoses into the vein is to the *right*.

frog, there are numerous glomus-type arteriovenous anastomoses. In addition, at the tip of each papilla of the distal ends of the laminae, there is a direct, nonglomus, arteriolar–venular shunt (Schummer 1949, 1951). Schummer may have only examined the papillae at the distal end of the laminae, and it is not known if such shunts are present in papillae of the other parts of the foot as well. Apparently, Pollitt and Molyneux (1990) did not identify this shunt in their preparations. They did, however, recognize direct arteriolar–venular shunts, apparently of this nature, in the laminae (Pollitt and Molyneux 1987). It may be speculated that this shunt, occurring after the arteriole has given off the capillary network, serves as an overflow pathway for blood that has not entered the capillaries (Clara 1956; Schummer 1949, 1951). There are, then, two arteriovenous anastomotic systems: the glomus type seen in both papillae and laminae and the direct shunts in the tips of the papillae. The former are, undoubtedly, under neurohormonal control (Pollitt and Molyneux 1987b), while the latter may act passively as indicated.

Pathogenesis

Anatomical and physiological studies of the digital microcirculation have attempted to unify hypotheses regarding the pathogenesis of laminitis. Digital blood flow measurement studies by Robinson et al. (1976) and scintigraphic radiography by Trout et al. (1990) showed increased blood flow in the feet of laminitic horses and ponies. Angiographic studies by Coffman and Garner (1972) and radiolabeled albumin studies by Hood et al. (1978), however, showed regionally decreased laminar circulation. These apparently contradictory observations can be reconciled by models of vascular shunting through arteriovenous anastomoses as proposed by Robinson et al. (1976) and Hood et al. (1978). Increased capillary pressure, the result of high venous vascular resistance, was believed to cause increased transmural movement of fluid, leading to buildup of interstitial edema fluid in horses with early experimental laminitis (Allen et al. 1990).

These flow and perfusion studies must be cautiously interpreted since different techniques were employed in a variety of equids, anesthetized and unanesthetized.

The role of neurohumoral mediators and vasoactive peptides in the pathogenesis of laminitis has been studied. Akerblom (1934) proposed that histamine released during intestinal dysfunction could cause laminitis, and Garner (1980) proposed a similar role for coliform endotoxin. While experimental infusion of either mediator may produce some of the systemic signs associated with laminitis, they do not cause laminitis (see below).

Robinson et al. (1975a,b), using isolated limb circulation techniques in anesthetized ponies, found that the circulation of the limb was not autoregulated. Local administration of acetylcholine, histamine, and prostaglandins E_1 and E_2 decreased prevenous vascular resistance, while serotonin and epinephrine caused prevenous vasoconstriction and decreased the diameter of veins. Vasodilators such as acepromazine and isoxsuprine were shown to be effective in vitro antagonists to norepinephrine. Such compounds have been useful in treating clinical cases of laminitis (Baxter et al. 1989).

Robinson et al. (1975) did not measure the effects of these mediators on the laminar microcirculation, but speculated that the overall effects of venous constricting agents like serotonin and epinephrine would favor the development of edema. Several investigators, studying black walnut laminitis, found that aqueous extracts of the material potentiated vasoactive effects of catecholamines (Galey et al. 1989, 1990). These vasoactive mediator effects could be antagonized by α- and β-adrenergic receptor blockers and with nonspecific calcium channel blockers such as nifedipine (Galey et al. 1989). Studies of the action of dopamine on isolated digital vessels indicated that it might induce vasoconstriction, an effect not completely mediated by action on α-adrenergic receptors (Baxter et al. 1991). Recently, Wilcke et al. (1993) proposed that certain chemical mediators of inflammation stimulate laminar microvascular endothelial cells, which in turn secrete prostanoids, endothelin, and endothelium-derived relaxing factor. These endothelium-derived mediators may, then, initiate a sequence of vascular changes leading to acute laminitis.

It has been suggested that microvascular pooling of blood or alterations in clotting are factors in the development of laminar ischemia and degeneration. Obel (1948) saw thrombosed laminar vessels in some horses with stage 3 laminitis. Hood et al. (1979) proposed that consumptive coagulopathies were a factor in the development of carbohydrate overload laminitis, but platelet numbers, activated partial thromboplastin time, and fibrin split products were roughly similar in nine horses that did and did not develop laminitis.

Johnstone and Blackwell (1984) described a case of colic with laminitis in a postpartum 5-year-old Belgian mare with a coincident consumptive coagulopathy. In a definitive study of coagulation and fibrinolysis in carbohydrate-induced laminitis, Prasse et al. (1990) were unable to find significant changes in platelet counts, mean platelet volume, prothrombin, and activated partial thromboplastin times, or concentrations of antithrombin III, fibrinogen, plasminogen, α_2-antiplasmin, protein C, thromboxane B_2, or fibrinogen degradation products. Belknap and Moore (1989) found no beneficial effect of heparin treatment in a retrospective study of 71 horses with a variety of intestinal disorders. Thus, there is no experimental and little clinical evidence to suggest that either disseminated intravascular coagulation or an imbalance in coagulation and fibrinolysis plays a role in the development of laminitis. Indeed, the significance of intravascular coagulation as other than an accompanying and secondary disorder in any disease of the horse is highly problematic.

The association of grain or carbohydrate overload and laminitis suggested a role for endotoxin. Attempts to induce laminitis with single injections of endotoxin have been unsuccessful (Sprouse et al. 1987). Clinical signs of Obel grade 1 laminitis (weight shifting lameness) were induced by 24-hour infusion of endotoxin (Duncan et al. 1985). Thirty minute infusion of endotoxin in an isolated, perfused limb preparation increased total vascular resistance and decreased digital blood flow (Hunt et al. 1990). Precapillary resistance was increased, but postcapillary resistance did not change significantly (Hunt et al. 1990).

Sprouse et al. (1987) considered thrombocytopenia, hypovolemia, and limb hypothermia, sometimes seen in laminitis, to be characteristic of endotoxemia. They measured endotoxin in horses with carbohydrate-induced laminitis and found a convincing correlation between increased plasma endotoxin levels and Obel grade 3, reluctance to move, laminitis. They proposed that some cases of laminitis were caused by localized Swartzmann reactions in which complexes of endotoxin and antibody lodged in small vessels and elicited inflammatory reactions. Favorable therapeutic responses to heparin and α-adrenergic blocking agents like phenoxybenzamine seemed to support this hypothesis. Sprouse et al. (1987) noted that equids are exquisitely sensitive to endotoxin and may already have antibodies that would facilitate an immune-mediated vasculopathy.

Despite these arguments, there is no solid evidence that endotoxin plays a primary role in laminitis or any other disease of the horse. The measurement of endotoxin levels in the blood is inexact at best. Favorable clinical responses to drugs are always highly subjective in the absence of controlled clinical trials. Such trials are rare to nonexistent in equine medicine.

The possibility of antigen–antibody immune complexes lodging in the laminar vessels and causing laminitis was proposed by Stanek et al. (1984). They studied circulating levels of immune complexes in the serum of 14 horses with early or healing laminitis. Statistically significant elevations were found. There has, however, been no demonstration of the deposition of such complexes in the laminar vessels, a necessary prerequisite to further study of the significance of immune complexes in laminitis.

Obel (1948) proposed that the primary defect in laminitis was death of keratinocytes and a failure of keratinocytes to differentiate. Larson (1956) studied the production and maturation of keratin in the hoof and found keratinocytes failed to incorporate the critical sulfur-containing amino acid cystine during acute phases of laminitis. Sulfur is essential for the formation of keratin and differentiation of the laminar epithelium (Budras et al. 1989). Ekfalck et al. (1991) reviewed investigations bearing on the hypothesis that the primary cause of laminitis was death of laminar cells. They proposed that multiple factors, including vasospasm and ischemia, binding of endotoxins, injudicious use of corticosteroids, and deficiency of sulfur-containing amino acids, were all predisposing.

Several investigators have proposed that abnormal placement of epidermal growth factor receptors causes inappropriate laminar epithelial cell proliferation and failure of keratinocyte differentiation (Grosenbaugh et al. 1988, 1990, 1991). Kameya (1980) and Kameya et al. (1980) proposed that the hyperplasia of laminar epithelial cells, which is so prominent in healing laminitis, was caused by abnormal maturation and cell differentiation.

While these studies are of interest, there is no convincing evidence that the changes are other than those secondary to a primary ischemic event followed by healing.

The following elements of pathogenesis are suggested. During normal movement some portion of the increased flow of blood to the digit is shunted by the arteriovenous anastomoses directly from the arteries to the enormous valveless venous plexus of the foot [Storch (1893) cited by Smith (1917); Zietzschmann (1943); and Krölling and Grau (1960)]. This may serve as a shock-absorbing and heat-removal system (Smith 1917). The pumping of blood out of the venous plexus as load is applied to the foot was clearly described by Smith (1917). In classic laminitis the shunting occurs before there is an increase of blood flow, so that the capillary bed is underperfused and anoxic. Thus, the pathway for classic vascular laminitis may be entirely normal, the disease occurring when the timing of the events of that pathway is inappropriate. The responsible agent(s) may, then, be normal vasoactive factors, which act at an inappropriate time on the arteriovenous anastomoses.

It has long been recognized that "high nerving," bilateral neurectomy of the digital nerves at the fetlock, eventually and almost invariably leads to necrosis of the epithelium with sloughing of the hoof. This may be thought of as a *slow laminitis*, with the derangement of the nerve supply to the digital vessels, specifically the arteriovenous anastomoses, leading to long-term inadequate capillary perfusion and chronic ischemia.

All the evidence indicates that laminitis, in all its manifestations, with the possible exception of the postparturient, is a disease of domestication. The classic form of vascular laminitis is certainly related to feeding practices. While laminitis does follow severe colic, renal disease, severe necrotizing processes, walnut shavings bedding, and so on, experiments with carbohydrate overload (Akerblom 1934; Teeter 1969) clearly show that derangements of the digestive process by unnatural feeding and watering are of singular importance.

Hoof

Despite the oft noted importance of the foot and, specifically, the horny hoof wall, sole, and frog, there is little information available on the pathology of these structures. Even with sufficient interest, routine pathological examination of this technically intransigent tissue is difficult.

Heymering (1990) provided an extensive historical bibliography on the hoof and farriery. Verschooten et al. (1989) conducted extensive studies on hoof shape, form, and growth in half blood horses. The rate of hoof growth decreased with age and during the winter. There was increased growth in the spring. Increased work and hard, uneven surfaces increased the rate of growth. Xenophon (390 BCE) stressed the favorable effect of cobblestones in stables on hoof growth and toughness—this at a time when horseshoes were unknown. Later writers also reported the same benefits for paved stable flooring (de Gray 1639). The hoof of the foal grows rapidly, nearly reaching adult size by 10 months of age. Morgan (1962) suggested that the word *frog*, at least in Xenophon, derived from swallow, the frog resembling the tail of that bird.

The origins of the nailed shoe, like the origin of the stirrup and domestication itself, is unknown. It is certain that the nailed shoe was unknown to the Greeks, Romans, and earlier peoples. During Greek and Roman times some form of shoe, probably leather, was strapped to the feet of asses to protect them as they carried loads. The evidence suggests that nailed shoes appeared around 800–900 CE (White 1978). It has been suggested that the Celtic Druids were the first farriers and kept the secret to themselves, and secret, in many ways, it remains.

Normal structure

Nickel (1938, 1939, 1949) did elegant studies of the structure of the cornified structures of the foot. The hoof wall, frog, bulbs of the heels, and sole are composed of **horn tubules** of distinctive structure in a mesh of equally distinctively structured **interstitial horn**. His work is summarized here for eventual use in pathological studies of the hoof. Bolliger (1991) added information including histochemical studies of normal horn.

The hoof wall comprises the outer perioplic layer, which extends distally from the coronary band to end about two-thirds of the way to the distal border. Inside the periople is the **stratum medium**, comprising the bulk of the hoof wall, with an innermost **stratum lamellatum**, the laminar horn. The stratum medium, at the toe, presents an outer, dark, pigmented zone and an inner, unpigmented zone. At the toe the outer zone is 2 1/2 times as wide (section parallel to the bearing surface) as the inner zone. Toward and into the dorsal part of the quarter the two zones are of equal width. In the quarter itself the inner zone is 1 1/2 times the width of the outer zone. In the heels and bars the outer zone disappears altogether, the stratum medium comprising the entire inner zone.

The individual horn tubules are made up of layers or lamellae of cornified cell cords surrounding a medulla, not unlike hair. The medulla contains dying or dead cell masses and may be empty, particularly near the distal border, the bearing surface. The tonofibrils of each layer of the horn tubules are specifically oriented, providing an overall structure elegantly oriented for stress in all directions.

Although composed of variably oriented layers, the horn tubules have a predominant orientation of layers (tonofibrils). In the toe region the inner zone is composed of tubules with predominantly steep spirals, while the tubules of the outer zone are predominantly flat spirals. Moving from the toe region to the quarter the steep spiral tubules are replaced by flat spiral tubules, so that the stratum medium of the quarters, heels, and bars is composed entirely of flat spiral tubules. As well, the periople, frog, and sole are entirely composed of predominantly flat spiral tubules. Tubules with steep spirals, then, are mainly found in the inner zone of the hoof wall in the toe region.

Considering these steep spiral tubules as elastic springs, they are preloaded in order to deal with compression loading, while the flat spirals are preloaded to deal, primarily, with tensile forces. This explanation is compatible with, though not exactly that of, Nickel. In effect, as the body weight pushes the distal phalanx distad, a bending force is exerted on the hoof wall through the corium and the laminae, so that the inner zone is under compression and the outer parts of the hoof wall are in tension. The steep spiral, compression tubules disappear in the quarters and are not present in the heels, bars, frog, and sole, suggesting that these portions of the hoof capsule are primarily adapted for tensile rather than compressive loading.

One may, also, note that the linear forces to which the hoof wall is normally subjected are always parallel to the horn tubules.

The **interstitial horn** of the toe, quarters, heels, and bars forms an interlacing meshwork in which the tubules are embedded. As a generalization, the interstitial horn is oriented, in three dimensions, at about a 45° angle to the horn tubules. The tubules are oriented to restrict the compression and tension caused by normal bending of the hoof wall while the interstitial horn resists shear.

It is well known that there is considerable variation in the quality of horn, for example, hardness, tendency to cracking, as well as the shape and form of the hoof: underrun heels, narrow, flat-footed, and so forth. It is equally well known that many of these characteristics, are, at least congenital, usually hereditary, and predispose to bruising, cracking, thrush, and so on. Even a casual comparison of the hooves of feral horses, subject to natural selection, with domesticated horses makes the case. The feral hoof is well formed, if not fitting the usual conception of that term, evenly worn, and very hard. Smith (1917) noted that the horn of the unshod hoof was much harder than that of the shod hoof, so hard, "as to resist the entry of a nail." Despite this knowledge, there has been little morphological study. Hamori (1983) discusses the question of the inheritance of hoof characteristics in domestic horses and states, based on a considerable experience, ". . . the genetically determined constitutional characteristics of the hoof are more important than daily cleaning and maintenance."

Sebaceous-type glands are present in the depth and walls of the cleft of the frog, producing a fatty secretion [Mettam (1896) cited by Smith (1917); and Trautmann and Fiebiger (1952)]. In the donkey the glands are scattered throughout the frog (Trautmann and Fiebiger).

Cracks

Cracks of the hoof wall occur at the toe, quarter, and heel and begin at the bearing surface or the coronary band.

The orientation of the horn tubules provides sufficient explanation for the orientation of the cracks. Examination of a limited number of bearing-surface cracks at postmortem, as well as breaking pieces of the hoof wall in vitro, shows that failure occurs in the interstitial horn and, so, is failure in shear. This observation permits at least a preliminary consideration of the pathogenesis of cracks that begin at the bearing surface. As indicated in Figure 7.40, during loading the frontal section of the hoof experiences a circumferential tensile force, analogous to hoop tension (Fairman and Cutshall 1953). The wall is bent, causing vertical compression, with the hoop tension at right angles tending to pull the horn tubules apart, and failure occurring by shearing of the interstitial horn. The well-known relationship of dry horn and cracking is related to the decrease of shear strength with drying. The hoop stress, that is, the resistance to the hoop tension caused by loading, is increased by the presence of the shoe nailed to the foot. The nailed portion of the wall, then, moves less than the

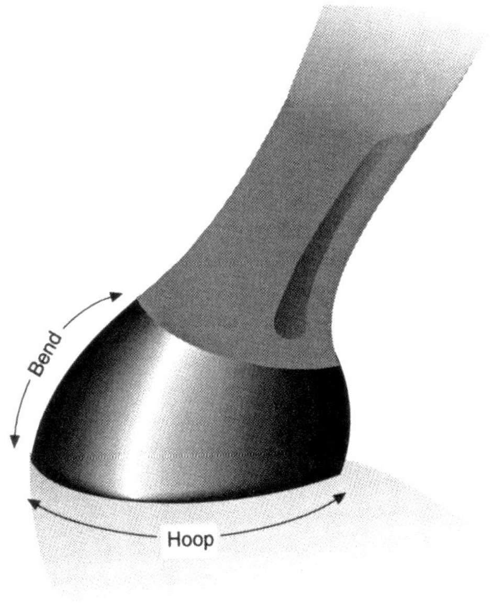

7.40. Schematic indicating the bending and hoop or circumferential forces on the hoof as it is loaded.

unnailed part, and quarter cracks typically occur at this junction of small and large movement. While the final common pathway for cracks involves shear failure of the interstitial horn, the quality of the horn, state of hydration, uneven impact with the ground, hoof trimming, contracted hoof, and other factors in the individual case are predisposing. One may note, specifically, the high frequency of quarter cracks in Standardbred racing horses that are reshod frequently (nail hole stress raisers) and race on hard surfaces (large impulse forces).

Pathogenetic pathways for cracks beginning at the coronary band are problematic in the absence of pathological information. It is certainly the case that wounds and severe bruising of the coronary band can cause at least temporary failure of formation of horn with the appearance of a crack. Once such a defect begins, the forces within the hoof wall assure separation and distal progression.

Percivall (1834) said that quarter cracks were more common in the forefeet and toe cracks in the rear feet. He further said that toe cracks were almost always in heavy draft horses working on hard surfaces, that is, in the city. Toe cracks of the rear feet may be related either to toe-first impact of the foot with the ground when horses are under draft, or concentration of force at the toe as the foot is breaking over. The latter may be preferable since the front feet usually impact toe first under heavy draft as well. Toe cracks are not uncommon in younger animals with contracture of the deep flexor tendon, the force, thereby, concentrated at the toe. They are also seen with chronic laminitis, the connective tissue supporting structures of the wall lost or weakened.

Thrush

Thrush is a superficial infection beginning in the frog and frog sulci and characterized by fetid, gray-black exudate. The horn is soft, macerated, or brittle with a characteristic odor. If untreated it spreads by undermining adjacent normal horn. Kochi (1947) reported that 30%–50% of horses in Switzerland develop thrush and that it was twice as common in the rear feet. He described the histopathology in detail. There is marked thickening of the stratum spinosum and stratum germinativum with loss of stratum corneum. The cells of the stratum spinosum and germinativum undergo vacuolation with necrobiotic nuclear changes and vacuolated spaces between the cells. There is marked increase in mitotic activity in the stratum germinativum. The interstitial horn is lost before the tubular horn. There are large numbers of cocci, diplococci, and small rods in the detritus. The corium is not markedly affected, unlike canker, but there are small hemorrhages, edema, and hyalinization of collagenous tissue. Kochi measured the width of the feet of affected and unaffected horses, confirming that narrower feet are predisposed with wet conditions and inadequate exercise.

Percivall (1834) said that the word, *thrush*, came from the French, frush, in turn from Latin, furca: or fork, referring to the shape of the frog. Frush, however, is given as a Middle English word in *Webster's* (1964).

Canker

Canker (pododermatitis chronica verrucosa) was commonest in the rear feet of draft horses and is still seen more often in those animals. It is described as a chronic, proliferative dermatitis, beginning in the caudal part of the cleft of the frog and gradually expanding to the sole and wall. A greasy, cheesy mass with a foul odor is adherent to filamentous or cauliflowerlike epithelial proliferations (Wintzer 1986). There is marked hyperplasia of both the epithelium and the connective tissue of the papillae of the corium (Hutyra and Marek 1920). The epithelium does not keratinize, but simply degenerates to a necrotic mass, which covers the hyperplastic papillary bodies.

Burgi (1910) gave a detailed histological description of this condition in the sole, frog, and wall of the hoof. The early lesion was characterized by proliferation of the corium and epithelium, particularly of the secondary laminae in the hoof wall, with continuing production of horn. With progression the proliferation continued, but there was no transition to stratum corneum; no horn produced. The fully developed lesion was characterized by absence of horn and marked thickness of the epithelium. In cases involving the hoof wall the primary laminae were up to 900-μm thick, while the secondary laminae were up to 300 μm. In the corium the connective tissue cell nuclei were enlarged and the collagen swollen. There was infiltration of lymphoid cells and a few neutrophils. The exuberant growth of the multilayered epithelium, with numerous mitotic figures, formed feathery, villous, and cauliflowerlike proliferations from which the preexisting horn sloughed away. The epithelial cells were enlarged, often with vacuolated cytoplasm and fluid-filled spaces between the cells. The undermining of the sole or frog was the result of the sloughing of horny tissue away from the underlying epithelium.

Westhues (1937) and Brunemann (1941) described canker as a primary acanthosis and parakeratosis, noting that the changes in the corium were secondary and that the interstitial horn was more resistant than the tubular horn.

These descriptions, with that of Hutyra and Marek (1920), suggest that canker could be a true papillomatosis with proliferation of both epidermis and papillary connective tissue. Secondary infection would account for the necrotic, odoriferous gross lesion. This was suggested by Dadd in 1854.

Burgi indicated that many unsuccessful attempts had been made to transmit the disease by contact, inoculation of material into wounds in the hoof, and intravenously. He examined cases of **grease,** chronic verrucous dermatitis involving the skin of the pastern, and believed the lesions to be identical to those of canker. However, he found only 4 cases of simultaneous disease among 45 cases studied. Schäper and Weischer (1938), among others, have provided evidence for a complex hereditary basis for the condition.

Chronic progressive dermatitis

Chronic progressive dermatitis (pododermatitis chronica progressiva) was described by Björck and Nilsson (1971), and Wintzer (1986) has seen cases. The sole is primarily affected, beginning near the white line as opposed to the similar lesion of thrush. The fore feet of Standardbred horses were particularly affected. The histological findings were similar to those of thrush. The cells of the stratum corneum were swollen and vacuolated with intercellular fluid accumulation. The stratum germinativum was hyperplastic, forming unkeratinized secondary papillae. The cause is not known, and it has apparently not been recognized other than in Scandinavia and Germany.

Keratoma

Keratoma is a discrete mass of firm horn within the hoof wall. It causes lameness and forms a ridgelike, vertical deformation of the wall. The mass is composed of disoriented, hyperplastic epithelial cells. The older literature suggests keratoma is the product of a chronic inflammatory reaction. Our few cases have been of long standing, without evidence of chronic inflammation or other cause. (See Chapter 15, "Integument").

Other causes of lameness of the foot

Localized infection of the foot is not uncommon, including abscesses of the sole and **gravel.** The latter is a purulent infection near or in the white line, which migrates proximally to open at the coronary band. While purulent processes typically migrate distally by gravity, the pumping action of the foot moves the infection proximally—as it moves venous blood proximally. Abscess and gravel often occur as recurrent sequelae of chronic laminitis. **Seedy toe** is undefined pathologically. There is apparent maceration and separation of the tissues forming the junction of the sole and hoof wall, which predisposes to infection, gravel. It is seen as a sequela of laminitis as well as in improperly worn or trimmed hooves.

Reddish or brownish **discoloration of the white line** is seen, particularly in the freshly trimmed foot. The discoloration is caused by hemoglobin pigment apparently derived from hemorrhages in the adjacent soft tissues. The condition does not seem to be related to lameness, but no systematic studies have been done.

Geyer (1992) and Zenker (1992) studied a clearly **hereditary degeneration of the horn** in Lippizan horses. Grossly, there is breaking up of the distal part of the hoof wall, seedy toe, degeneration of the horn of the white line. While the pathogenesis is not worked out, there appears to be a defect in keratinocyte formation at the coronary band leading to disorganization of tubular horn and microfracturing of the hoof wall. Approaching the bearing border the microfracturing becomes macrofracturing, with the breaking up described. Supplementation with biotin appeared to ameliorate but not prevent the condition.

Nerving

Some forms of neurectomy are legal or illegal depending upon breed use and rules. Fewer cases of illegal nerving come for pathological confirmation than in the past. When approached, the pathologist should strongly advise detailed clinical study for anesthesia of suspected areas before agreeing to the postmortem study. That can be very difficult, particularly if there is heavy scarring because of poor technique and/or repeated interventions.

Careful dissection with multiple, defined sectioning is necessary and, at the end of the day, one is still left with a purely morphological probability. The mere presence of scar tissue in the subcutis at the fetlock does not establish nerving. Since loss of sensation is the issue, the careful and detailed examination of several clinicians can be of greater value than the probabilities of morphology.

CHAPTER 8

Rear Leg

Specific diagnosis of lameness of the rear legs has always presented difficulties, largely because lameness-inducing lesions of the rear leg are bilateral and occur simultaneously, or nearly so, in several sites. This is specifically the case with spavin and lesions of the croup area. While pathology cannot completely resolve the clinical difficulties, it can help define the problems.

Conditions to be considered are abscess of the external iliac lymph nodes, sacroiliac arthrosis, sacroiliac luxation, gluteal syndrome ("tendonitis"), fracture of the tuber coxae, trochanteric bursitis, arthritis, luxation of the coxofemoral joint, and fractures of the femur. Neurogenic atrophy of the gluteus medius is discussed with peripheral nerves and thrombosis of the aortic–iliac vessels with the vascular system.

Abscess of external iliac lymph nodes

Unilateral abscessation of the iliac lymph nodes is not common and is usually found in horses debilitated by chronic disease and/or age (Webb 1882). The organism, in our experience, has always been *R. equi*, although other organisms may be present. The abscess can reach considerable size and be palpable per rectum. The splenic lymph nodes may abscess under similar circumstances, although it is unusual for abscesses to be present in both sites. The reason for the localization, in either case, is not known. There may be lameness, but often the only clinical sign is nonspecific cachexia.

Sacroiliac arthrosis

This condition was defined by Rooney (1977). A characteristic clinical finding is delay of protraction of the affected rear leg, leading to "hiking," a jerky protraction of the leg. The leg appears to remain on the ground, in support, too long. It is more frequent in, but by no means restricted to, Standardbred horses. In the early stages, the abnormal gait is apparent in the inside leg as the animal is going around a turn at the trot or pace. In fact, the condition is bilateral and, with progression, the hiking gait may be seen on the straight as well as in turns. The specific leg showing clinical signs may vary from day to day. Careful examination may reveal hypersensitivity and/or localized sweating over the middle gluteal between the tuber sacrale and the tuber coxae, presumably the result of referred pain. The evaluation of hypersensitivity in horses is highly subjective, however. The long-standing case may have localized atrophy of the middle gluteal muscle.

Postmortem examination of horses with these clinical signs, and in horses with a prior history of such signs, reveals bilateral lesions of the sacroiliac joints. The method of examination of these joints is given in Chapter 19, "Autopsy Method."

The sacroiliac joint surfaces are irregular in shape from horse to horse and from side to side in the same horse (Jeffcott et al. 1985; Dalin and Jeffcott 1986). The sacral surface is hyaline cartilage while the iliac surface is a mixture of hyaline and fibrocartilage. The significant gross lesions are focal areas of translucent brownish or yellowish-brown discoloration of the cartilage, most clearly seen on the sacral part of the joint (Fig. 8.1). Erosion and ulceration are difficult to appreciate, but can often be seen with moderate magnification and as the surfaces are drying. Osteophyte proliferation occurs around the margins of the joint surfaces. This can be difficult to define, given the normally irregular joint margins. In long-standing cases, usually older horses no longer showing clinical signs, there may be fibrous ankylosis. There have been only rare examples of bony ankylosis. Early lesions may be difficult to detect when postmortem imbibition of blood has occurred, histological examination being necessary.

The histological appearance is that of any arthrosis; that is, there is fraying and loss of the superficial layers of cartilage, loss and cloning of chondrocytes, and decreased metachromatic staining of the ground substance. Full thickness loss of cartilage occasions fibrous ankylosis.

Dalin and Jeffcott (1986) reported these same

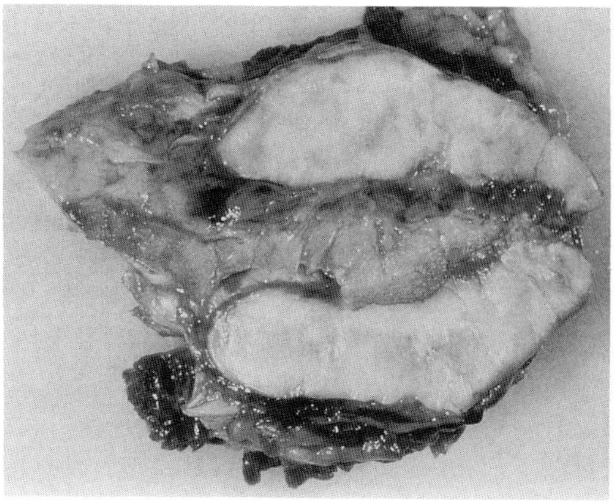

8.1. Yellow and brownish translucent discoloration of the sacral part of the sacroiliac joint: sacroiliac arthrosis.

changes, attributing them to aging. It is certainly the case that these lesions occur with aging, but occur earlier in horses that work at the trot or pace as compared to the gallop, as was pointed out by Rooney (1977). This is to the point that aging changes in joints are, in fact, pathological, and that the time of onset and rate of development are significant factors in determining clinical significance.

The pathogenesis of sacroiliac arthrosis has been described (Rooney 1981). In brief, the moments (turning forces) generated at the sacroiliac joints, by horses negotiating improperly banked turns at the racing trot and pace, cause excessive movement of those joints and, so, arthrosis. Since horses, over a lifetime, walk and trot more than they gallop, gradual damage to these joints by such movement should and does occur. Reiterating, clinical signs occur when the rate of aging change increases, as at racing speeds on improperly banked turns.

Sacroiliac luxation

This was described by Cadeac (1907), Velling (1926), and Rooney et al. (1969). It is commoner in horses that jump and is usually unilateral, though an occasional horse may luxate the opposite side at a later time. Most animals recover, but do not return to their original jumping form. The onset of lameness is acute, followed quickly by dorsal displacement of the tuber sacrale on the affected side. In the earlier stages the displaced tuber sacrale may be seen moving up and down as the horse walks, but soon becomes fixed. The displaced and fixed tuber sacrale is often called a "hunter bump" (Fig. 8.2). Normal prominence of the sacrum in horses with sloping croups has this name as well (Robertson 1910).

In the usual case there is tearing and avulsion of the ligaments on the cranial aspect of the sacroiliac joint. These ligaments are not well described in anatomical texts. The dorsal ligaments, which are well described, are not affected. The torn ligaments heal in a longer state, the joint remaining permanently in the luxated position (Fig. 8.3). In rare, severe cases, the joint may completely luxate, with fracture of the ilium below the tuber sacrale, mentioned also by Cadeac (1907). In such cases, the animal goes down and is unable or unwilling to rise. As the sacroiliac joints are deliberately luxated during the postmortem examination, an identical fracture or fractures may be produced, particularly in older animals.

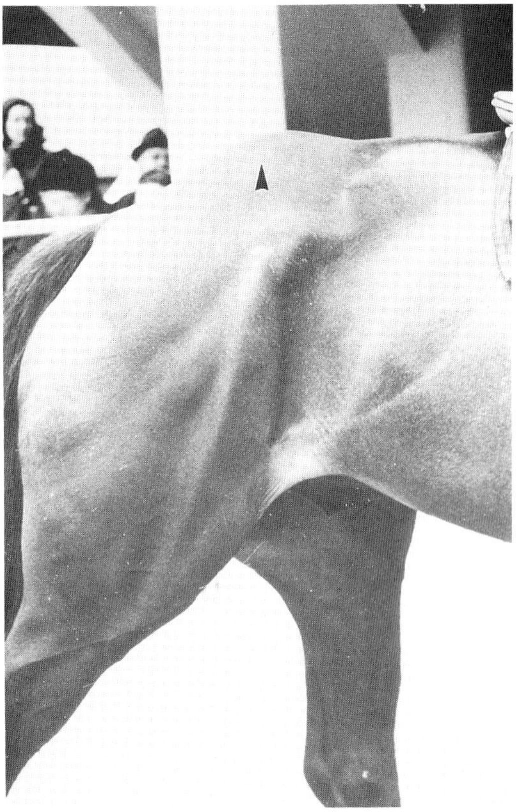

8.2. Sacroiliac luxation (*arrowhead*) in a champion jumper.

Velling (1926) described a number of cases of sacroiliac luxation in the late 1800s and early 1900s. Some of these seemed to be tearing of the dorsal sacroiliac ligaments, specifically the *lig. sacrotuberale latum,* so that the caudal end of the sacrum was tipped dorsally. Some followed severe dystocia. We have only seen luxation associated with tearing of the ventral ligaments.

The pathogenesis of sacroiliac luxation involves out-of-phase, wrong way, rotation of the rear leg around the iliac half of the joint and the vertebral column around the sacral half (Rooney et al. 1969). Such movements occur with fatigue and slipping, primarily in jumpers.

Fracture of tuber coxae

Fracture of the tuber coxae (gluteal syndrome) presents clinical signs qualitatively identical to sacroiliac arthrosis, but, on average, more severe.

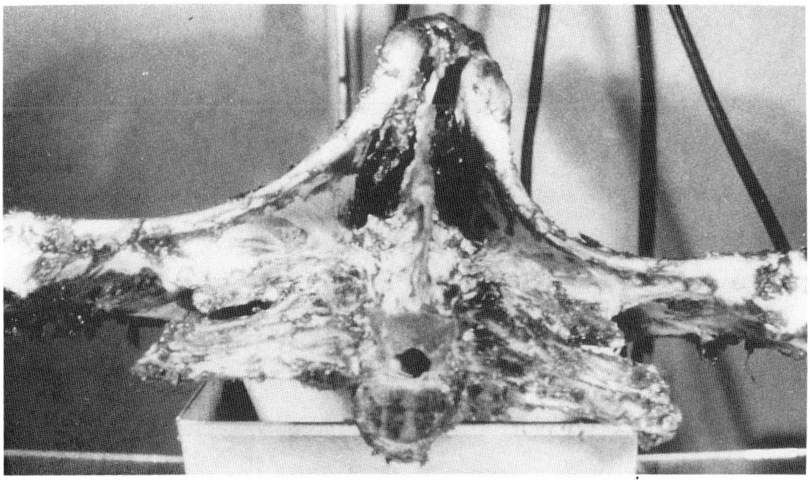

8.3. Sacroiliac luxation. Cranial view with luxation of the horse's right side, the ligaments being elongated and, so, more visible.

The clinical frequency, apparently not trivial, is somewhat greater in Standardbred than Thoroughbred horses, with no information available about other breeds. Only one case has been seen at postmortem. Given the site of the lesion, routine postmortem examination has undoubtedly missed others.

In the one case, a fracture of the tuber coxae was found on the clinically affected side. The fracture was impacted and had formed a nonunion pseudoarthrosis. Its presence was not suspected on clinical examination. It is of interest that this fracture did not behave in the classic manner of a "dropped hip." This may be explained by consideration of the pelvic fractures reported by Silbersiepe et al. (1986). There are two types of fracture of the tuber coxae. The complete type will displace distally, the dropped hip. The incomplete type, involving only the angle of the tuber coxae, does not drop and is the type discussed here. Pelvic fractures are discussed with fractures.

An important clinical point is that any lesion, whether arthrosis of the sacroiliac joint, fracture of the tuber coxae, or any other lesion in this area will produce qualitatively identical clinical signs.

Trochanteric bursitis

This condition, extensively described in the older clinical literature, does not appear to have been described pathologically. The few cases we have seen at postmortem have been iatrogenic—purulent bursitis following diagnostic injection. For several years the trochanteric bursa and the tendon of the *m. gluteus accessorius* were routinely examined in most horses coming to postmortem (approximately 400 light horses) without evidence of acute, chronic, or healed lesions. While a reasonable case (Rooney 1969) can be made for the pathogenesis of an aseptic trochanteric bursitis, it must remain speculative in the absence of morphological evidence for such an entity.

Coxofemoral joint

This joint is rarely the site of significant lesions. Acute infectious arthritis occurs in septicemic foals, in common with many other joints. Osteochondrosis is seen only in the generalized form. A few longstanding cases of dorsocranial luxation of the head of the femur have been seen in straight-legged Shetland ponies. The round ligament and accessory ligament were, of course, ruptured. In all cases a false, fibrous joint had been formed between the head of the femur and the shaft of the ileum. No cause was apparent in these chronic cases. Malark et al. (1992) reported 17 cases of coxofemoral luxation over a 15-year period primarily in ponies and Miniature horses with onset related to trauma.

The anatomical studies of Preuss et al. (1972) have shown that the accessory ligaments are, in fact, the tendons of insertion of the rectus abdominus muscles with large components of the external abdominal obliques and the tunica flava abdominis. This is discussed with rupture of the prepubic tendon.

Chronic arthritis, the sequelae of prior acute infectious arthritis, is seen. While the acute damage is done in early life, presumably during streptococcal septicemia, clinical signs often do not appear until the animal is broken for training at about a year of age. This appears to be the explanation for the case reported by Jögi and Norberg (1962). Characteristically, there is loss of cartilage on both joint surfaces, eburnation, subchondral cystlike areas, marginal osteophyte formation, and marked fibrosis of the joint capsule.

Wirstad (1948) and Haakenstad (1953, 1969) reported an apparently hereditary malformation of the hip joint of Norwegian Döle horses. The clinical signs generally did not appear until about 8–12 years. Haakenstad believed the basic malformation to be wider than normal joint space with a flattened, shallow acetabulum and flattened femoral head, usually bilateral. Secondary arthrotic changes developed, including erosion of cartilage, eburnation, osteophyte formation, and loss of the round and accessory ligaments. Luxation and subluxation followed loss of the ligaments.

Silbersiepe et al. (1986) reported that fractures of the proximal epiphyseal plate of the femur occurred in draft horse foals, particularly large, well-grown animals. Lienaux and Zwanenpoete (1910) said such fractures were frequent in Belgian foals and described the clinical features. Hunt et al. (1990a) reported 25 cases in foals over an 18-year period, a very low incidence. We have seen only a few cases in light horse foals. Fractures of the femoral shaft are uncommon: combined compression, bending, and torsion and almost invariably comminuted (Fig. 8.4).

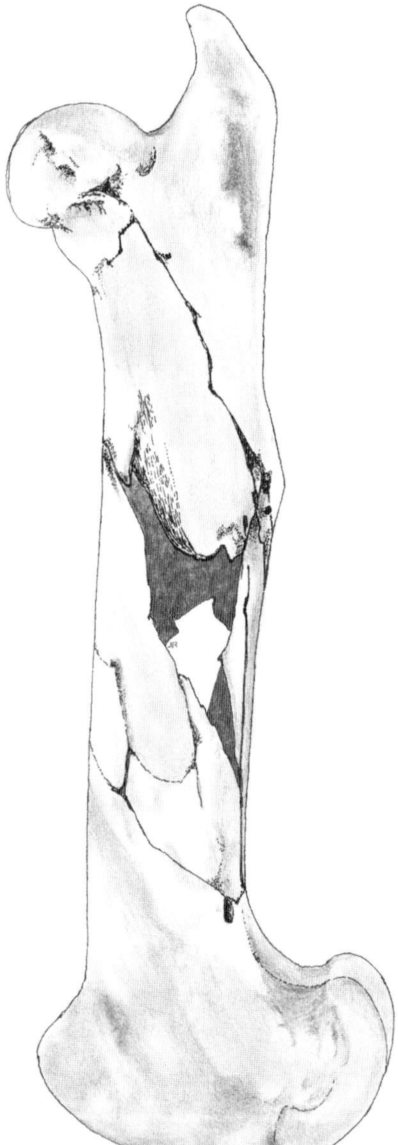

8.4. Comminuted fracture of femur, reconstructed as far as possible.

Stifle

The stifle comprises the femoropatellar and the femorotibial joints. It is a large, complex joint often indicted, but seldom convicted, as a site of lameness. At least one reason for the low frequency of stifle lesions is the fact that the stifle, like the coxofemoral, scapulohumeral, humeroradial, and tarsocrural joints moves less while loaded than the more distal limb joints.

The origin of the word, stifle, is unclear, perhaps referring to the apparent role of the patella in restraining—stifling—movement of the joint. The first determination of the coefficient of friction of an animal joint was made on the stifle in vitro and was $\mu = 0.02$.

The conditions to be considered are arthrosis, upward fixation of the patella, lateral luxation of the patella, cruciate ligament avulsion, femoropatellar osteochondrosis, and femorotibial osteochondrosis. Purulent synovitis is discussed with diseases of foals.

Arthrosis

With the exception of purulent gonitis of foals or iatrogenic gonitis in older horses, arthrosis is rare in the stifle of the modern light horse. Silbersiepe et al. (1986) and Wintzer (1985) mention arthrosis, apparently of the medial femorotibial joint, in heavy horses in draft work. Cadeac (1909) described this arthrosis of the medial femorotibial joint in heavy horses, specifically noting that it was more common in such horses than in riding horses. We have seen no example in our few heavy horse postmortems.

Upward fixation of patella

There are no lesions associated with this condition. It is an inadvertently recurring normal action of the rear leg. The condition was well known in antiquity [Apsyrtos cited by Leclainche (1936)].

As the stifle is extended, caudal angle increased, the movement of the tibia on the femoral condyles is both extension and a spinning or curving movement from medial to lateral. This may be demonstrated on the osteoligamentous preparation: the femur is held stationary and a moderate straight upward pull is exerted on the patella, simulating the quadriceps femoris. The tibia moves from the flexed to the extended position. The patella rides proximally along the ridges of the femoral trochlea. As the tibia approaches and passes about 143°–145° caudal angle, the medial to lateral curving path suddenly curves back from lateral to medial. The patella follows and, with the final lateral to medial turn, hooks over the proximal end of the medial ridge of the femoral trochlea. This is the normal mechanism of "locking the stifle."

Normally, extension of the joint to 143°–145° does not take place while the animal is moving. If it does, inadvertent locking may occur, particularly in horses and ponies with very straight hind leg conformation. Cadeac (1909) noted that the condition was common in Breton horses, noted for their straight hind legs. In such animals the joint is closer to 140° than the 135° of the normal standing position. Inadvertent hooking of the patella is more apt to occur in such individuals.

Inadvertent locking is seen, in less severe form, in young horses in the earlier stages of training before muscle tone has fully developed. Such muscular "weakness" predisposes to overextension and, so, inadvertent locking of the stifle (Cadeac 1909). The clinical signs of sacroiliac arthrosis, specifically hiking, are often, and incorrectly, said to be those of inadvertent upward displacement of the patella.

Lateral luxation of patella

The underlying lesion is variably severe hypoplasia of the lateral ridge of the femoral trochlea with partial luxation of the patella (Figs. 8.5 and 8.6). In the partially luxated position the patella provides the pressure necessary for the development of osteochondrosis. This osteochondrosis tends to localize in the middle third of the lateral ridge (see "Osteochondrosis of femoropatellar," below).

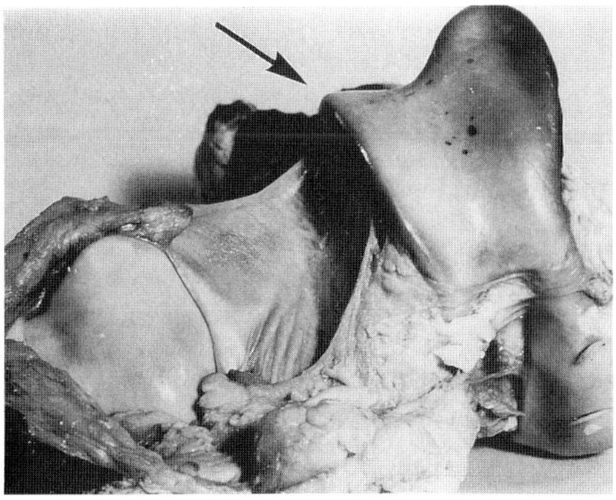

8.5. Normal femoral trochlea, with *arrow* indicating lateral ridge of the trochlea.

Rathor (1967) described hereditary patellar luxation in Shetland ponies in the Netherlands. The hereditary nature of the condition was also suggested by the work of Nilsson (1947) with Ardennes breed draft horses in Sweden. Strömberg (1976) presented photographs of osteochondrosis of the lateral ridge of the femoral trochlea with hypoplasia also present. Pfeiffer (1935), Berge (1936), and Peters (1935) described the condition in German Cold bloods, most often in the left stifle, though both right and bilateral cases were seen. One of Berge's cases is illustrated in Cohrs (1961). The animals were foals and young horses up to 2 1/2 years of age when often subtle clinical signs of

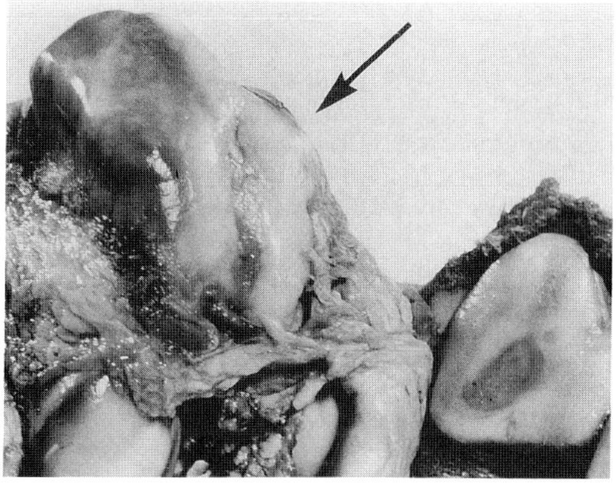

8.6. Hypoplasia of the lateral ridge of the femoral trochlea (*arrow*) with osteochondrosis following.

lateral luxation of the patella were noted. These authors described lesions of the lateral ridge of the femoral trochlea, which they considered to be arthrosis, but which were probably a mixture of arthrosis and osteochondrosis.

Leuthold (1943) described lateral luxation of the patella with flattening of the lateral ridge of the femoral trochlea. Rooney et al. (1971) described 2 bilateral cases, 1 Standardbred and 1 Morgan foal. Hypoplasia of the lateral ridge was present and, in retrospect, osteochondrosis of the lateral ridge. Williams (1897/98) described a bilateral case in a bred trotting filly and illustrated the hypoplasia of the lateral ridges. Noirjean (1945) reported a 1%–1.5% frequency of the condition in the Franches-Montagnes, a small, about 13 hands, mixed-use animal of Swiss origin. The history and characteristics of the breed are summarized by Stornetta (1988). Thirty-four cases of varying severity were seen: in the left leg, 21 cases; in the right leg, 6 cases; in both legs, 7 cases.

Silbersiepe et al. (1986) noted that luxation of the patella could be minimal and difficult to detect. He suspected that osteochondrosis was the pathological process, rather than arthrosis. Priester et al. (1970) found 60 cases (19 in ponies) of patellar luxation in an assemblage of academic veterinary clinic populations, a 23 per 10,000 rate (0.2%), probably somewhat less than the true frequency. Perhaps the earliest case is that of Bènard in 1828, cited by Lanzillotti-Buonsanti in *Bayer-Fröhner* (1900). Pritchard saw the condition in 1849 in England cited by Smith (1976).

The pathogenesis includes an hereditary, primary hypoplasia of the lateral ridge of the femoral trochlea, which allows displacement of the patella. The displaced patella entails misplaced compressive forces on both the patella and the lateral ridge, resulting in osteochondrosis of the marginal type. This form of osteochondrosis is largely restricted to the middle third of the lateral ridge and the patella.

The predilection for the left rear leg is striking and unexplained. This left-sided predilection is also seen with nonmarginal osteochondrosis of the talus. It is well known that horses, on average, prefer to turn to the left, indicating a preference for supporting body weight on the left legs. If this is true of usual standing as well, more weight would be carried over time on the left legs than on the right. Given the hypothesis that weight bearing is a significant component of the pathogenesis of osteochondroses, a reasonable, though speculative, case can be made for left-sided predilection.

Avulsion of cranial cruciate ligament

This is uncommon and usually seen as a shipping, pasture, or barrel racing accident. Avulsion of either or both cruciates may occur with massive damage to the stifle in shipping accidents. The few cases we have seen were killed soon after the accident, and we have no information about long-term effects. Tearing of the cranial cruciate without avulsion has been suggested on but slender evidence (Prades et al. 1989).

Osteochondrosis of femoropatellar

Osteochondrosis has been discussed as a result of lateral luxation of the patella. Osteochondrosis of this joint also occurs in the absence of luxation (Fig. 8.7). Marginal osteochondrosis of the lateral ridge may be accompanied by nonmarginal-type osteochondrosis of the medial ridge, usually with some degree of involvement of the patella. This form, occurring in the absence of hypoplasia, is more frequent in horses with a more angled rear leg conformation, that is, the smaller caudal angle of the stifle characteristic of, but not limited to, Standardbred horses. Such conformation directs more linear force into the femoropatellar joint. The marginal osteochondrosis of the lateral ridge in these joints tends to occur in the distal third of the ridge, while that associated with hypoplasia of the lateral ridge tends to be in the middle third.

In general, this osteochondrosis is less severe than that seen with hypoplasia of the lateral ridge, but may still be sufficient for debilitating lameness.

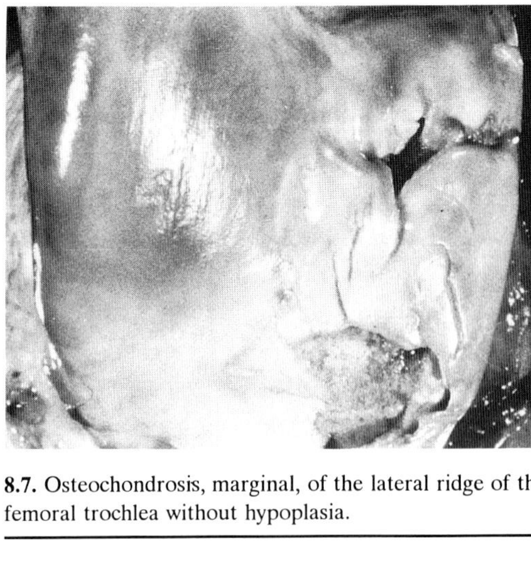

8.7. Osteochondrosis, marginal, of the lateral ridge of the femoral trochlea without hypoplasia.

Osteochondrosis of femorotibial

Nonmarginal osteochondrosis is not uncommon in the medial femoral condyle. It is usually no more than a dimple or folding of the convex articular cartilage, which extends to, but not through, the subchondral bone plate (Fig. 8.8). If it does extend into the subchondral marrow, a subchondral, lytic defect is formed (Fig. 8.9). This is a roughly spherical area filled with mucoid, mesenchymal connective tissue and surrounded by a variably thick zone of sclerotic bone (Fig. 8.10). It is morphologically identical to the subchondral defects found with ulcerative arthrosis, and, as noted elsewhere, is the reaction of subchondral bone and marrow to the presence of synovial fluid. It is often, and incorrectly, called a cyst.

This osteochondrosis is more frequent in the straight-legged (Thoroughbred-type) animal. Osteochondrosis of both the femoropatellar and femorotibial joints is rarely present in the same animal. A few cases of femorotibial nonmarginal osteochondrosis, however, have been seen together with the osteochondrosis of the lateral ridge of the femoral trochlea secondary to hypoplasia of that ridge.

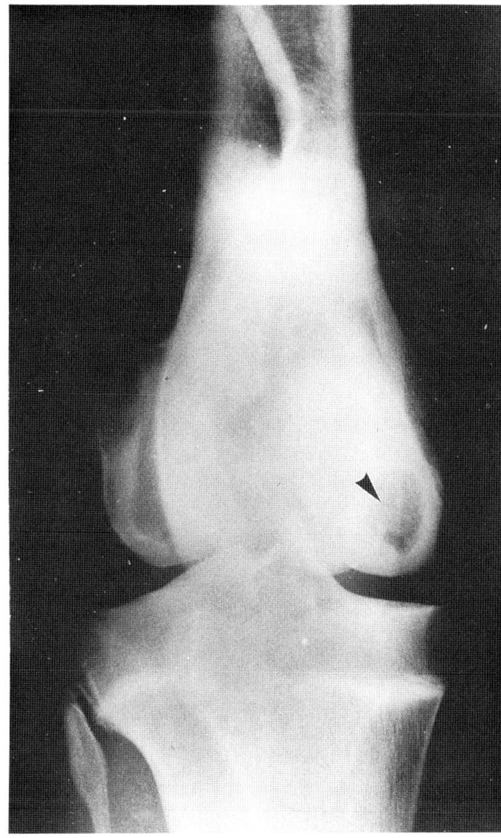

8.9. Radiograph of large subchondral defect (*arrowhead*) in medial femoral condyle.

Fibrotic myopathy

This was described by Lamy (1901/02) and Dihlmann (1922). Lamy saw one case and Dihlmann two cases of metaplastic bone formation, "osteoma," in the semitendinosus muscle. The gait was described as chickenlike, a reasonable fit to the description by Adams in 1966. The characteristic clinical picture follows tearing of the distal third of the semitendinosus muscle. It occurs most frequently in horses used for cutting and roping, but occurs as well in horses that have caught the rear foot in the halter, over a picket rope, and so forth.

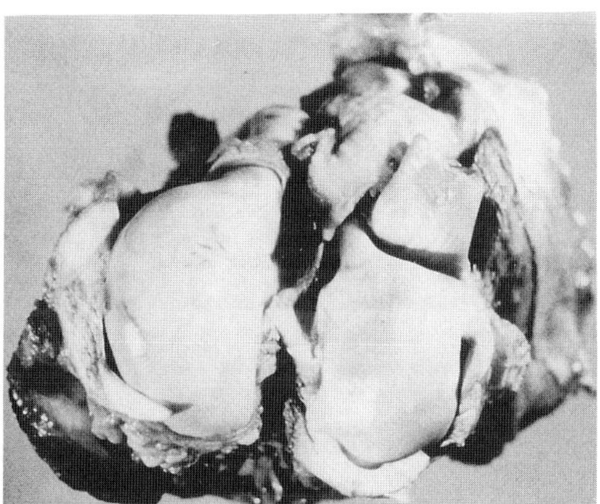

8.8. Minimal osteochondrosis, nonmarginal, of the medial condyle of the distal end of the femur. The lesion is a series of 5-6 groove infoldings of the articular cartilage that did not open into the subchondral space.

The acute lesion is tearing and dehiscence of muscle fibers with hemorrhage. Healing is by fibrosis, often with metaplastic formation of cartilage and bone. The pathogenesis involves the foot sliding forward or being held in the forward, protracted, position. The opening, extension, of the stifle generates a moment around the stifle, which is to be resisted by an opposite sense, flexion or closing, moment generated by muscle action. The biceps femoris and semimembranosus insert close to the center of rotation of the stifle and, so, generate only small resisting moments. The semi-

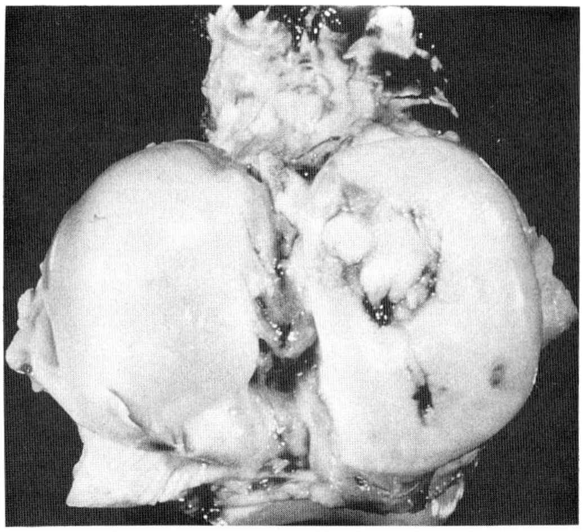

8.10. A type of gross lesion associated with Figure 8.9: one large and one smaller nonmarginal osteochondrosis.

tendinosus inserts distal to the center of rotation, generates a significant moment and, so, is the muscle/tendon torn when its moment is exceeded by the "slipping forward" moment (Rooney 1969) (Fig. 8.11a and b).

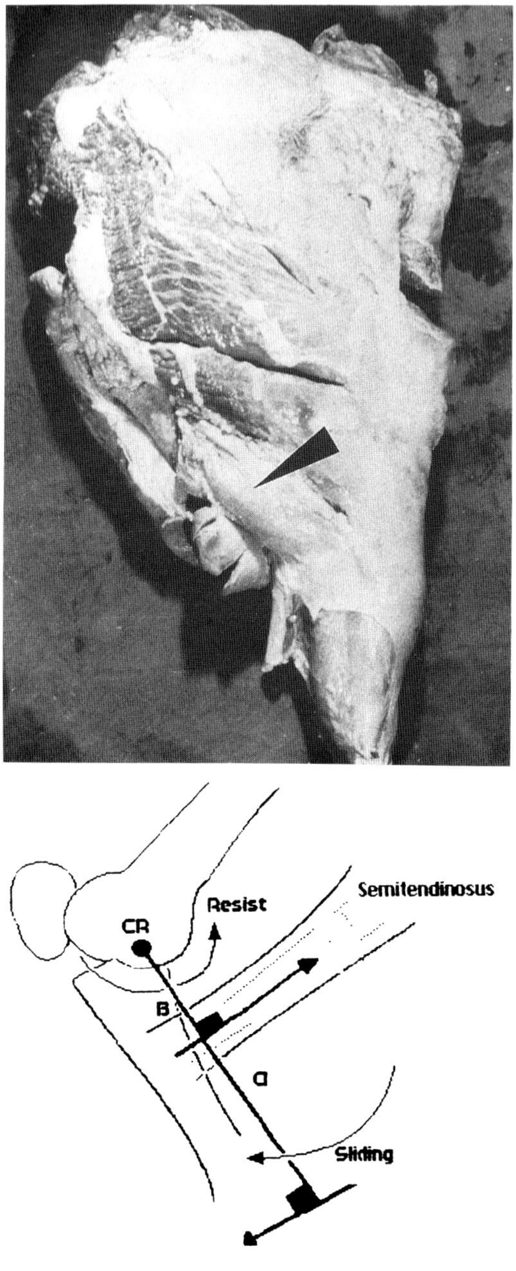

8.11. (*above*) Torn semitendinosus muscle (*arrowhead*) replaced by fibrous tissue. (*below*) Pathogenesis: the sliding force acting around center of rotation (CR), over the distance **a**, generates a moment (*sliding arrow*), opening the stifle joint. This is resisted by semitendinosus acting around CR over the distance **b** (*resist arrow*). The biceps and semimembranosus insert around the CR and, so, generate no significant moment forces around the stifle.

Fracture of tibia

This is one of the commoner fractures; invariably a compression, bending, torsion failure of the shaft (Figs. 8.12 and 8.13). Fröhner (1905) well understood these fractures, writing that they occurred as the horse fell onto the markedly flexed rear leg. They are not rare in cutting, roping horses.

Hock

The hock has long been considered a major site for lameness of the working horse, a clinical judgement supported by pathological observation. The origin of the word *hock* is unclear, perhaps from Old English or Old Norse for heel.

Tarsocrural joint

There are four lesions to be considered, all of which, if they achieve clinical significance, are characterized by effusion of synovial fluid into the

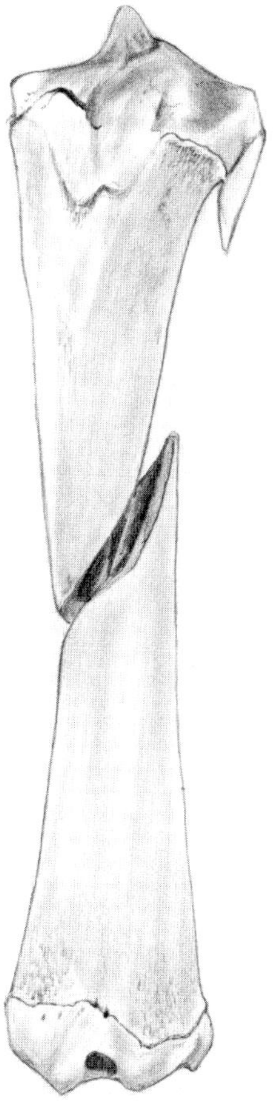

8.12. Fracture of tibia, dorsal view, spiral component.

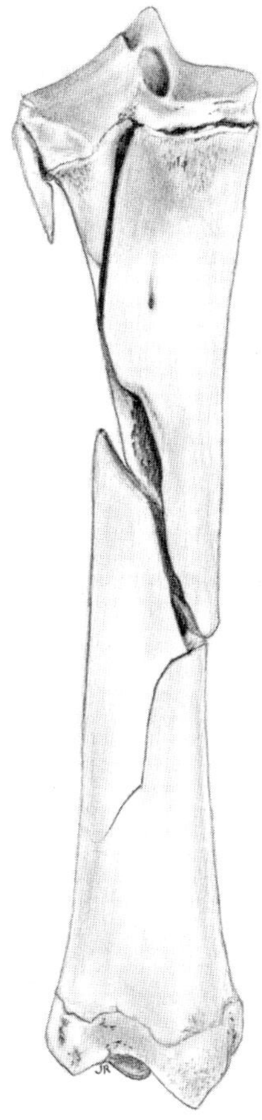

8.13. As Figure 8.12, caudal view with more vertical component.

tarsocrural joint—bog spavin. The functional anatomy of this joint is mentioned with the elbow and in the chapter on stability (see Chapter 10, "Stability and Lameness").

Osteochondrosis of distal tibia

Osteochondrosis of the dorsal end of the distal ridge of the tibia is bilateral, less often unilateral. It is a variable-sized mass of cartilage-covered bone with fibrous attachment to the parent bone (Fig. 8.14). It is not uncommon in Thoroughbred and Standardbred horses at postmortem, but is considerably less common as a cause of lameness. Schougaard et al. (1990) reported a radiographic incidence of about 12% in a group of Standardbred horses. Schebitz et al. (1975) found 14%, 53 cases among 376 horses examined for lameness and purchase.

Lesions were found in the left leg 17 times, the right 12 times, and bilateral 24 times, which accords with our experience. Zeller et al. (1978) found a radiographic incidence of 11%–12% among 1300 horses.

The postmortem incidence of this lesion is nearer 15%–20%, a number of lesions being too small to be resolved by x-ray, as is true of osteochondrosis in general. Perhaps the first report of this condition, thought at the time to be a fracture, was that of Berkeland and Haakenstad (1968).

With routine examination of this joint in foals at postmortem, the pathogenesis of the lesion becomes apparent. That is, one will see bona fide osteochondral fracture (Schebitz et al. 1975). The fracture is that of a "hinged door," with the hinge at the dorsal edge (Fig. 8.15). Since an attachment remains, blood vessels can invade the partially freed cartilage, with resulting ossification. This is the one osteochondrosis of the horse that can, with certainty, be ascribed to single-event osteochondral fracture. The fracture has been ascribed to acceleration of the leg during protraction, snapping the tarsocrural joint into flexion. The straight-leg

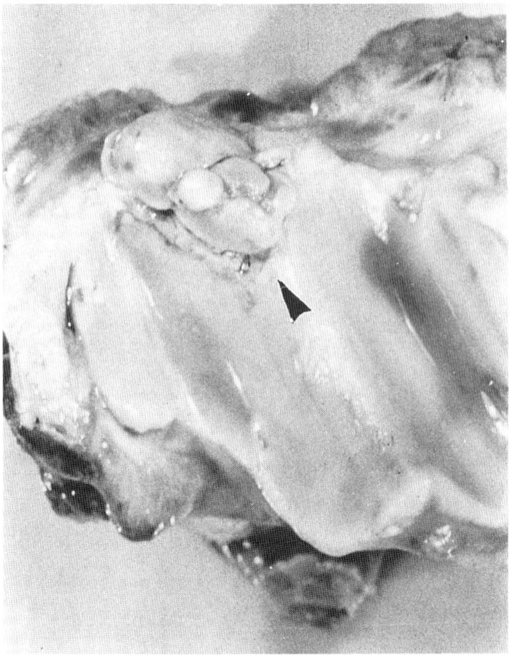

8.14. Distal end of tibia. Osteochondrosis (*arrowhead*) at the dorsal end of the sagittal ridge.

conformation is predisposing. Compressive loading applied by one bone to another over a period of time does not apply to the osteochondrosis of the intermediate ridge of the tibia, but one can say that

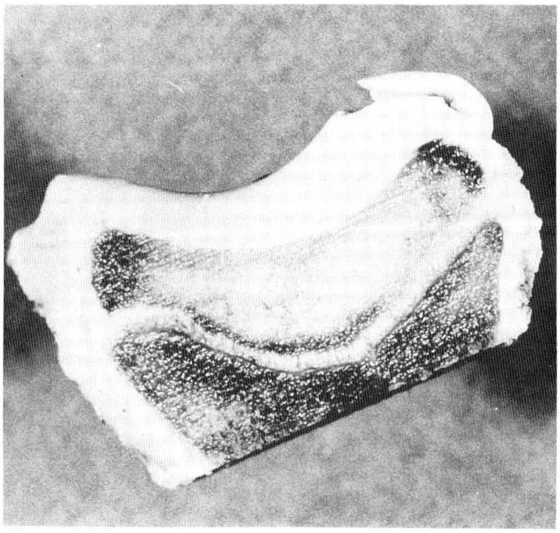

8.15. Slab of distal end of tibia of a foal with a recent osteochondral fracture of the sagittal ridge destined to become osteochondrosis like Figure 8.14.

fracture is the result of such loading as an *impulse,* a force delivered in a finite, brief, period of time.

Schougaard et al. (1990) believed they found a genetic predisposition to this condition in Standardbreds. Their numbers are small but suggestive. Such a genetic predisposition would be in keeping with the apparent conformational predisposition. Zeller et al. (1978) found the condition more often in trotting and Thoroughbred horses. There was about equal frequency of left, right, and bilateral involvement, and there were about twice as many males as females, as appears to be true of many osteochondroses.

Nonmarginal osteochondrosis of trochlea of talus

These lesions appear on either the lateral or medial ridges of the trochlea (Fig. 8.16). Our postmortem experience and that of Dämmrich (1985) are that the medial ridge is by far the more common site. The clinical literature, however, indicates that the lateral ridge is more common (McIlwraith et al. 1991). Rezabek and Rooney (1992) recorded the frequency and location of these lesions in 100 autopsies. The lesion was found in 30% of the animals examined and was in the middle third of the medial ridge in all cases. Three times as many males as females were affected, and Thoroughbreds were overrepresented. The lesion was present in the left leg about 50% of the time,

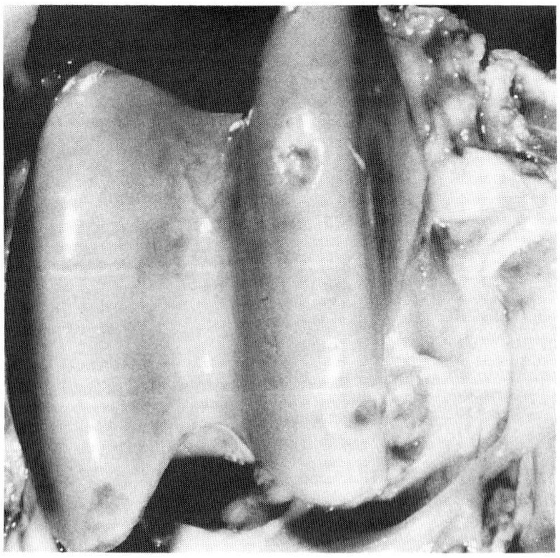

8.16. Nonmarginal osteochondrosis of the medial ridge of the talus. The apparent defect at the lower end of the ridge is an artifact, though this is where the synovial fossa described in the text would be found.

the right leg 25%, and bilateral 25%. This agrees with the overrepresentation of the left rear leg for osteochondrosis at other sites.

The lesion usually appears as a dimple in the articular cartilage, in the middle third of the medial ridge, and extending almost to or to the subchondral plate. Larger lesions extend into the subchondral bone, inducing a subchondral defect, which can be seen radiographically. Cadeac (1909) showed such a lesion (his Fig. 102).

The cause of osteochondrosis of the talus is not clear. The following observations may be made. The earliest lesion seen (Fig. 8.17), in a 4-month foal, was characterized by degeneration of cartilage in an area of thickened cartilage. In the degenerate area and other areas there was persistence of blood vessels within the cartilage. One may propose that endochondral ossification had been slowed in this particular area. Thus, the cartilage was thicker than surrounding cartilage, and the blood vessels, which should have retreated from the cartilage by this time, were still present. The blood vessels, then, were indicators of delayed ossification. With such delay in ossification, the cartilage was thicker than it should be when postnatal weight bearing began. Even normal weight bearing, then, could be associated with further compromise of the circulatory-dependent process of endochondral ossification and lead to osteochondrosis by the mechanism already described. The cause for the localized delay of ossification in utero is, of course, not addressed by this hypothesis.

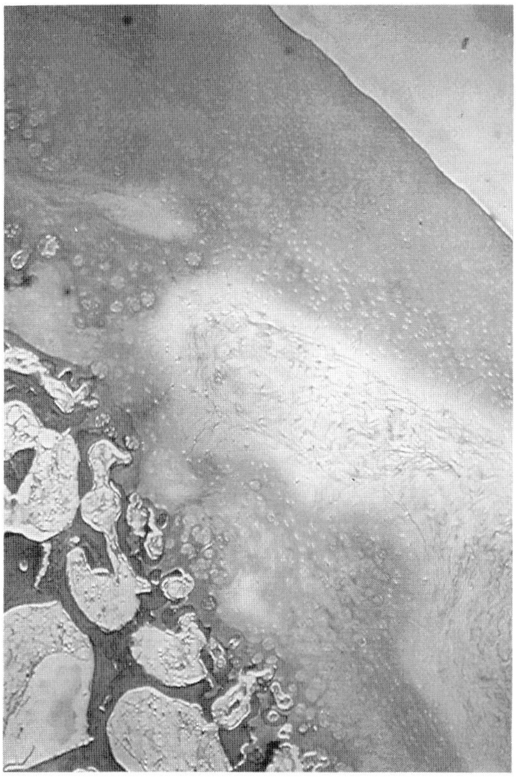

8.17. Moderate power, H & E of an early, developing osteochondrosis of the medial ridge of the talus. See the text.

A second, less common, defect in the cartilage of the talus appears in the distal third of the medial ridge. It is craterlike, more nearly resembling a synovial fossa than osteochondrosis (Sippel 1942). Rezabek and Rooney (1992) found this in about 10% of their horses.

Osteochondrosis of malleoli of tibia

There is reference in the surgical literature (McIlwraith et al. 1991) to osteochondrosis of the dorsal part of the medial malleolus of the tibia. Dämmrich (1985) mentions dissecans lesions of thickened cartilage, or "impression" fractures, of the medial, less often the lateral, malleoli. We have not encountered examples in either site.

Nonmarginal osteochondrosis of central and third tarsal bones

Dimple or groove defects typical of osteochondrosis may be present in the articular cartilage of either of these two bones, some with a subchondral defect large enough to be seen radiographically. Most have been found incidentally at postmortem. In several cases in yearlings with obscure, persisting lameness of a rear leg, they were the only lesions found. There is no evidence here, as with most osteochondroses, of progression to arthrosis.

Arthrosis of dorsal articular grooves of tibia

In many cases of bog spavin, with or without osteochondrosis, erosive lesions are present at the dorsal margin of the medial and lateral articular grooves of the distal end of the tibia (Rooney 1973c). The lesions are always small, somewhat larger medially than laterally, and do not progress to larger and/or deeply ulcerative lesions. It is reasonable to assume, though without proof, that these erosions are sufficient to induce an inflammatory reaction, including an increase of synovial fluid. The cause of the erosions appears to be the same as that of osteochondrosis of the distal tibia (indeed, they often coexist): acceleration of the hock during dorsiflexion. As already noted this pathogenesis is associated with the straight-hock conformation, a predisposition with regard to bog spavin already known to Percivall (1834).

Scoring or **wear lines** of the talus, as noted with the elbow, are common in ataxic young horses. They are uncommon with the arthrosis just discussed or with any of the osteochondroses of the tarsocrural joint. Marked scoring may be seen in old horses, which presumably began to score the cartilage earlier in life.

Bog spavin

Increased amounts of synovial fluid in the tarsocrural joint can accompany any lesions of that joint. Increased production of synovial fluid is a component of the inflammatory reaction of synovial structures. It is not at all clear, however, why there is variation in the amount of fluid quite apart from the size or severity of the lesion(s). As well, there is no explanation for the common occurrence of bog spavin in overfed, underexercised young horses, such as yearlings being prepared for sales. Turning such animals out to pasture, providing exercise, will quickly alleviate the condition in virtually all cases. The pathogenesis is univestigated and unknown.

Spavin

This is the commonest and most important cause of lameness of the rear leg. The origin of the word, spavin, was thought to be old high German, *sparwari,* sparrow hawk (Martin 1900/01). The name apparently referred to the jerky gait of the spavined horse, resembling the normal leg movements of the sparrow hawk (Martin 1900/01). That is attractive and the more so since Jordanus Rufus knew the condition as *sparvanus* in 1250, the medieval Latin word for sparrow hawk, so that both the English, *spavin*, and German, *spat*, may derive from medieval Latin (Fig. 8.18).

Spavin is virtually inevitable in horses that carry or pull heavy weights for long periods (draft horses), pull lesser weights at higher velocities (Standardbred racing horses), jump, or work for long periods in a collected manner, for example, dressage, Paso Fino. The sickle-hock and cow-hock conformations are clearly predisposing, and the disease is invariably bilateral (Cadeac 1909). It is a disease of the domesticated horse. Martin (1900/01) examined many fossil horses from different parts of the world without finding evidence of the condition.

Spavin is arthrosis of the central tarsal (Tc) and third tarsal (T3) joint, and the T3 and metatarsal 3 (Mt3) joint (Fig. 8.19). The early lesion is

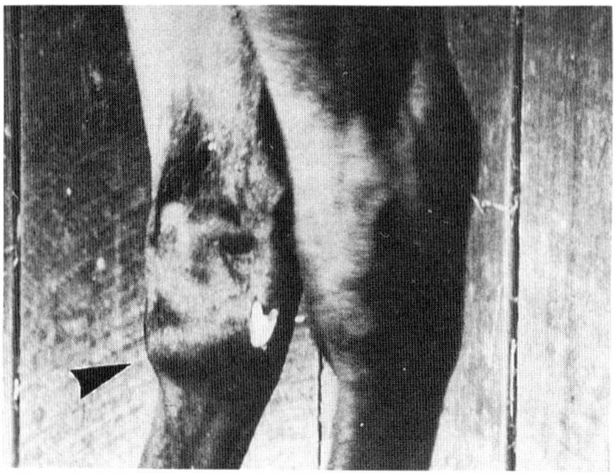

8.18. Horse with developed spavin (*arrowhead*), "bone spavin."

brownish or brownish-yellow, often translucent, discoloration of the mating articular cartilages on the dorsomedial aspect of the joint surfaces. This is followed by fraying and erosion of the articular cartilage, progressing to ulceration and fibrous and bony ankylosis (Goldberg 1918a) (Fig. 8.20). Following erosion and ulceration, periarticular new bone—osteophytes—develops on the dorsomedial aspect of the hock: bone spavin. The early stages are accompanied by acute inflammation, synovitis, with the associated pain often being referred to as **occult spavin**, since there is no obvious swelling or pain on palpation and radiographs are negative.

As discussed elsewhere (Rooney 1968, 1969) the first lesion to appear in the horse sickle-hock by conformation or working in a sickle-hock manner is in the Tc-T3 joint. The pain caused by this lesion causes a change of gait to a straight-hock dynamic conformation with the subsequent development of arthrosis in the T3-Mt3 joint. The horse that is straight-hock by heritage, specifically the Thoroughbred horse, may develop arthrosis only in the T3-Mt3 joint, but this is uncommon (Figs. 8.21 and 8.22).

Once the lesions in both sites, and in both legs, have progressed to ankylosis the animal will be working sound. The ankylosis is both intraarticular and extraarticular. Granulation tissue invades the ulcerated cartilage surfaces, fusing and gradually undergoing ossification to form intraarticular ankylosis, while the periarticular osteophytes fuse to form the extraarticular ankylosis.

It has been repeatedly suggested that there is a periarticular spavin without articular cartilage damage. Inflammation, bursitis, of the bursa under the medial tendon of insertion of the *m. tibialis cranialis* is claimed as a cause of lameness in, particularly, Standardbred horses (Lutz and Gabel 1969). Routine examination of the hock at postmor-

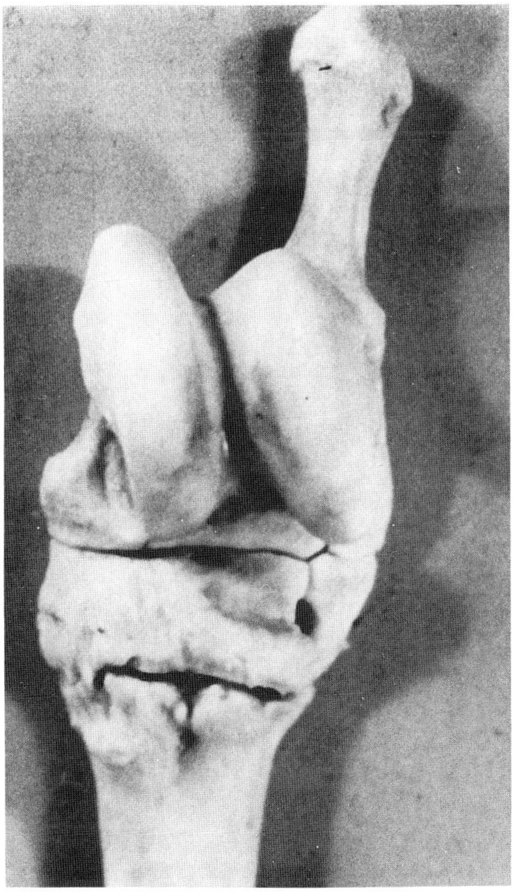

8.19. Macerated specimen of spavin with arthrosis at both sites.

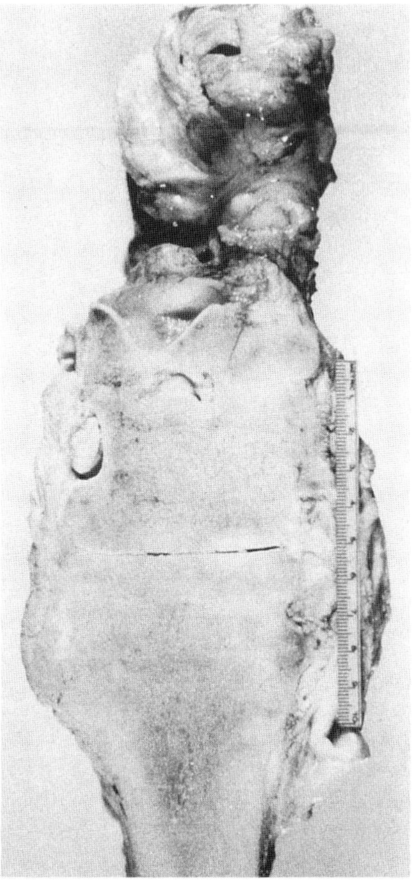

8.20. Frontal section of spavin, which is completely ankylosed at both the central tarsal, third tarsal articulation and the third tarsal, and third metatarsal articulation.

tem has never revealed either entity. This was recognized by Barrier cited by Cadeac in 1909.

The pathogenesis of spavin has been dealt with in detail elsewhere (Rooney 1969). In brief, the sickle-hock conformation entails out-of-phase movements of Tc and T3, so that shearing forces are generated in the articular surfaces, while the straight-hock entails such out-of-phase shearing of T3 and Mt3.

Rehbein

Gottlieb (1919) described enlargement of the proximal end of Mt4 as *rehbein* (deer bone). This is rarely seen in modern light horses as a congenital variant of no pathological or clinical significance.

Curb

Curb and thoroughpin are related tendoligamentous lesions, with curb more frequently or exclusively seen in the young horse in early training or work, while thoroughpin is more often seen in the mature working horse. The clinical signs are obvious, well known, and described in clinical texts. The term, curb, is probably derived from the Latin, *curvare,* by way of middle French and English, meaning curved.

The swelling, heat, and pain are caused by tearing of the fibers of the plantar part of the plantar tarsal ligament. As healing proceeds, a thickened area of scar tissue develops. Depending upon the extent of the original damage, this thickening may eventually disappear or remain for life.

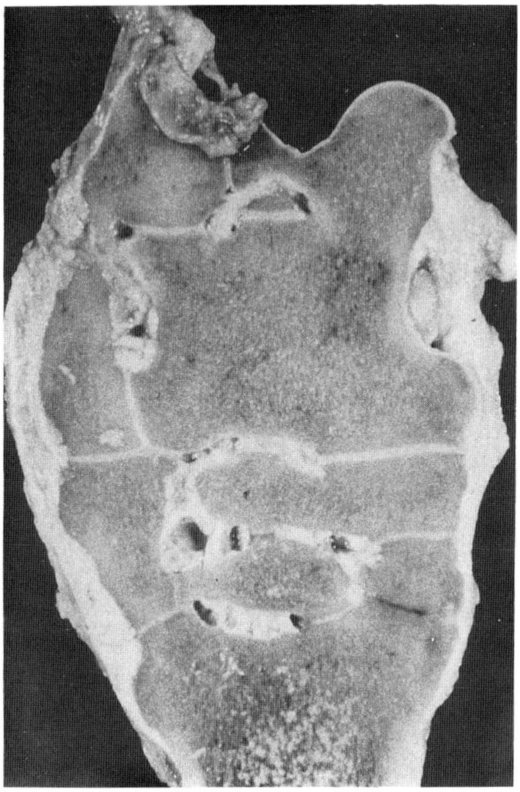

8.21. Arthrosis, spavin, of the third tarsal/third metatarsal articulation in a Thoroughbred yearling. The lesion appears as a *dark line* to the *right*, translucent brown in the fresh state.

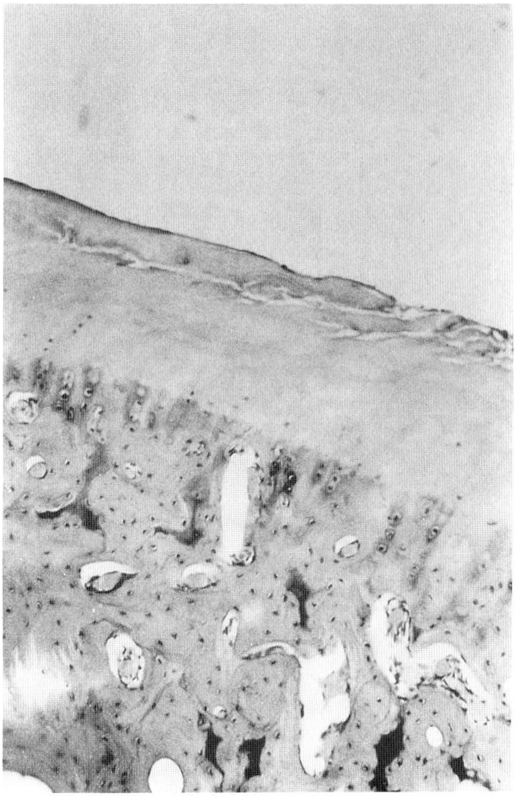

8.22. Moderate power, H & E of early arthrosis: death and disappearance of chondrocytes, cloning (*far left*), and early fraying and fibrillation.

Retearing of the ligament seems to be rare, given sufficient time for healing and the continuing maturation of the ligament.

The pathogenesis of curb is related to structural (conformational) and/or functional sickle-hock and cow-hock. Cadeac (1907) stated this clearly, noting that the predisposing sickle-hock may be either conformational or functional, as reiterated by Rooney (1969, 1981). Lawrence (1804) noted the relationship of curb and cow-hock. The proximate cause of curb is increased load, leading to a functional sickle-hock, which will be exaggerated if there is preexisting structural sickle-hock. The immature tarsal plantar ligament is the *locus minoris resistentia* (Fig. 8.23).

Thoroughpin

Thoroughpin is tearing of fibers of the deep digital flexor tendon of the rear leg within the plantar tarsal sheath, with reactive inflammation of the tendon and synovial sheath. Aseptic inflammation of synovial sheaths and joints is characterized by the usual signs of inflammation in any tissue. In the case of synovial structures, *swelling* occurs not only within the tissues as a result of inflammatory edema, but also as the result of increased production of synovial fluid.

With thoroughpin, the swelling is moderate and resolves if the amount of tendon damage is small. Often, however, the increased amount of synovial fluid will remain even after healing of the tendon with no residual evidence of the original tear. No explanation is available for the persistence of increased amounts of synovial fluid in the absence of ongoing or recurring pathological changes either in this case or in other cases, such as bog spavin. It appears that a new homeostasis, equilibrium, of production versus removal of synovial fluid is established. With this new equilibrium compatible with normal, or nearly so, function, there is no feedback to return the equilibrium to the original, undamaged state.

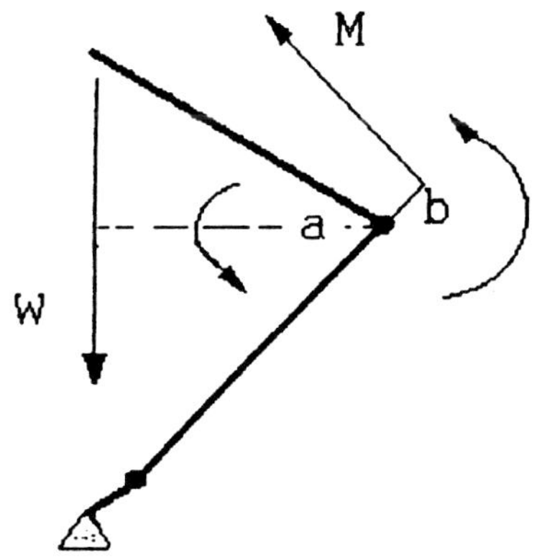

8.23. The moment forces concerned with the pathogenesis of curb and thoroughpin. See the text.

The pathogenesis of thoroughpin appears identical to that of curb. With maturation the plantar tarsal ligament becomes stronger as the cross-linking of collagen fibers is completed, and the ligament is no longer the *locus minoris resistentia.* Thoroughpin should occur more often in animals subjected to heavy loads, such as draft horses or moderate loads at higher speeds such as carriage horses. Cadeac (1907) implicated larger horses and suggested that thoroughpin (vessigon tarsien) was commoner in horses with straight, as opposed to more curved, hocks, working, therefore, in a functionally sickle-hock manner.

Luxation of superficial flexor tendon

This luxation follows rupture of the medial, less often lateral, band attaching the superficial flexor tendon to the calcaneus (Guoth 1941). The tendon is displaced to one side and, eventually, reattached by fibrous tissue in the new position. A chronic bursitis, capped hock, typically accompanies this lesion according to Ziegler (1969), but that has not been our experience. Fröhner described this in 1905, noting that it could be medial or lateral. Bilateral cases have been seen but are uncommon (Guoth 1941).

The luxation occurs, not exclusively, in jumping horses, presumably because of impulse dorsiflexion of the tarsocrural joint. There are no predisposing lesions in the torn tendinous attachments. Guoth (1941) lists improper jumping, sudden turns, sudden stop at a fast gallop, slipping of a rear foot, too heavy loads, overloading because of lameness, and trapping of a rear foot in marsh, deep mud, and so forth. All of these could cause excessive and/or sudden impulse dorsiflexion of the tarsocrural joint. Guoth believed the medial band was more frequently ruptured because it was weaker than the lateral, but gave no evidence.

Luxation/fracture of the hock

This is uncommon and usually seen in stallions (Gavard 1890; Rooney 1969; Stashak 1987; Moll et al. 1987). Characteristically, there is sudden onset of severe, non–weight-bearing pain in a stallion isolated in a paddock or, rarely, a box stall.

In several of our cases the inciting event was observed or readily reconstructed. The stallion, presumably in boredom and frustration, was kicking fiercely at the plank fence of the paddock. The foot caught on a plank, and the animal jerked it loose with single or repeated violent muscular effort. Cadeac (1907) indicated that horses attempting to free themselves after accidents entrapping the foot in equipment, tramway rails, and so forth, could luxate the hock in this manner.

Although there has been eventual recovery in a few cases, our experience, and that of Cadeac (1907), has been that the pain is persistent and severe, and the animal is usually destroyed on humane grounds. Moll et al. (1987), on the other hand, reported six cases in ponies and horses that recovered with conservative treatment.

The basic lesion is luxation/dehiscence of the proximal intertarsal joint between the talus and the central tarsal bone, with tearing/avulsion of the intraarticular ligaments. Occasional cases are seen involving only the tarsometatarsal joint (Moll et al. 1987). Fragments of bone are torn loose with the ligaments, and there may be comminuted fracturing of, particularly, the talus and central tarsal bones. The tendons of the peroneus tertius and tibialis cranialis muscles are not affected.

The pathogenesis of this condition contrasts interestingly with that of rupture of the peroneus tertius. With luxation of the hock the stifle is extending, decreasing tension, as the hock is palmar flexing, increasing tension in the peroneus tertius. The hock can, then, palmarflex sufficiently to avulse the intraarticular ligaments without developing tension sufficient to tear the peroneus tertius.

Fracture of central and third tarsal bones

So-called slab fractures, actually shear failures, of these bones are uncommon, particularly when compared to the carpus. Lindsay et al. (1982) described five cases of fracture of the third tarsal bone. Pettersson (1970) reported two cases of fracture of the central tarsal bone. Tulamo et al. (1983) reported 11 cases, suggesting they were more frequent in Standardbreds. Most cases have been seen in racehorses. Crushing fractures of these bones in foals was discussed with Osteochondrosis, above.

Fibula

The fibula, like the ulna, is complete in the early embryo, but reduces to a proximal and distal portion, the latter forming the lateral epicondyle of the distal end of the tibia. The shafts of both the fibula and ulna may be present as fibrous bands, occasionally with islands of ossification, which appear on radiographs (Zeskov 1959). The fibula and the ulna are complete in a genetic dwarfism of Shetland ponies (see Chapter 4, "Endocrine System.")

Rupture of peroneus tertius

As a clinical entity, rupture of the peroneus tertius has been long known and well described (Solleysel 1664; Fröhner 1905). It occurred in draft oxen as well as horses. No incidence figures are available, but the condition may be less frequent in the modern, light horse era.

We have not seen a case at postmortem and have found only one incomplete description in the literature (Sloan 1898/99). Clinical signs of swelling and pain are not marked, the swelling apparently being suppressed by the heavy deep fascial sheath around the muscle (Wintzer 1986). The clinical signs clearly indicate rupture. In Sloan's case there was tearing and rupture with hemorrhage, somewhere in the middle third of the tendon, as best one can discern.

The basic mechanical event is plantar flexion of the hock as the stifle is either stationary or flexing [Fröhner (1905); and Hell in *Bayer-Fröhner* (1900)]. As described by Rooney (1969) and Wentink (1978) this action is normal during the second half of support of the rear leg. An increase of stifle flexion, or hock plantar flexion, or both, increases the tension in the peroneus tertius until tearing/avulsion occurs.

The pathogenesis may develop in at least two different ways:

1. Fatigue, specifically fatigue of the protractor muscles of the rear leg, delays flexion of the hip joint (protraction of the leg), allowing the stifle to flex too much (fatigue, specifically of the quadriceps femoris muscle). This would be a "slow" pathogenesis to be expected in horses working for long periods at moderate to slow velocity, such as draft horses and endurance trail ride horses.
2. A sudden acceleration of the foot during the second half of support (slipping backward), with peak tensile force exceeding the limits of the peroneus tertius tendon. This would be expected in horses working on slippery, wet, frozen, or friable surfaces such as gravel, particularly upgrade.

The **gait–lesion–gait principle** applies (see Chapter 10, "Stability and Lameness"): the gait abnormality caused by a specific lesion is the gait abnormality that caused the lesion. The characteristic gait after rupture of the peroneus tertius is excessive plantar flexion of the hock, and the mechanical cause is the same. In general, as discussed with bowed tendon, simple overstretching of a tendon causes avulsion failure at the tendo–osseous junction. Since the tearing of the peroneus is in its middle third, sudden acceleration with snapping, as proposed for tearing of the superficial flexor tendon, would apply here as well.

Bursitis of long extensor tendon

Aseptic inflammation with variable increase of synovial fluid may occur in the subtendinous bursae of the common and lateral extensor of the fore leg or long extensor tendon of the rear leg. The bursae are normally present, though small, between the tendon and fibrous joint capsule on the dorsal surface of the fetlock. The cause is not known, but Cadeac (1907) stated that it was most common at the rear fetlock of draft horses, particularly those with short pasterns, which would include most draft horses. We have not seen this.

Flexor tendonitis/tearing

In the older clinical literature cited in Berge (1933), there is extensive consideration of aseptic lesions of the deep flexor tendon and superficial flexor tendon in their course over the plantar aspect of the fetlock joint. There was tearing of tendon fibers of the dorsal and plantar aspects of both tendons, with the deep flexor tendon more severely affected. This was accompanied by chronic inflammatory changes and increased synovial fluid in the digital sheath. The condition could be characterized as a tenosynovitis, although usually lumped as a form of "sesamoid lameness" (Gleichbeinlähme). While it did occur in the fore leg, it was apparently more common in the rear legs of heavy work horses, the pathogenesis being related to excessive tension in the deep flexor tendon as the foot rotated off the surface at the end of support. This pathogenesis may be compared with that for tearing of the check ligament of the deep flexor tendon. No reports have been found in the modern literature, though the desmitis reviewed by Verschooten and Picavet (1988) may be the same condition. We have seen no cases.

Miscellaneous

The check ligament of the deep flexor is thin in the rear leg and sometimes absent altogether. In the mule it is usually absent (Sisson and Grossman 1953). No lesions have ever been seen in the check ligament, when present, but it has been incriminated in clinical texts.

Bucked shin fracture of Mt3 has never been seen at postmortem and is certainly uncommon. Condylar fractures of Mt3 are described with the fore leg. Dorsal and transverse arthroses of the fetlock joint are seen routinely in working horses. They are as common in the rear fetlocks as in the fore, though rarely as severe. Sesamoiditis has not been seen, nor have basal fractures of the sesamoid bones. Apical fractures have been described with the fore leg. Arthrosis of the pastern joint has been discussed with the fore leg, although it is somewhat more common in the rear leg. Fractures of the phalanges and navicular bone are uncommon. Navicular disease has been seen in the rear feet together with the fore, never alone. The few cases encountered have been in Hackney ponies and in horses worked for considerable periods on the hard surface of a high-speed treadmill.

CHAPTER 9

Vertebral Column

Relatively inaccessible to clinical examination, the vertebral column is often the diagnosis of desperation for the diagnostically destitute. That applies as well to pathologists as clinical veterinarians since the vertebral column, often blamed by the latter, is rarely adequately examined by the former.

A basic reference, apart from standard anatomical texts, is Slipjer (1946). Certain relevant facts are in Rooney (1971). Jeffcott (1980) provided a clinical review of 443 cases considered to be thoracolumbar vertebral problems. Jeffcott and Dalin (1980) examined the movements of the vertebral column.

Pathological changes of the vertebral column include congenital defects, aging changes, fractures, spondylitis deformans, various ankyloses, and rare metastatic neoplasms. The osteochondrosis associated with one form of spinal ataxia, cervical stenotic myelopathy, is considered with the nervous system (see Chapter 16, "Nervous System").

Atlanto–occipital malformations

Malformations of the atlanto-occipital junction comprise varying degrees of fusion of the atlas to the skull with or without fusion of the atlas and axis. All of our cases have been in Arabian foals coming to postmortem soon after birth because of severe ataxia. The lesions are certainly congenital and perhaps hereditary.

Fracture

Thoracic

While fracture can occur, under different circumstances, in any portion of the vertebral column, the common site is thoracic vertebrae 10–14 (Zschokke in *Bayer-Fröhner* 1900) (Figs. 9.1 and 9.2). The fractures are related to lightning strike, electrical shock of other origin, tetanus, and marked uncoordinated muscle contraction, such as a young animal trying to jump a high fence and an animal cast and struggling in a horse box.

The fracture, compression and dorsiflexion bending, is caused by the dorsal vertebral musculature. If all the spinal musculature contracted simultaneously, the back would ventroflex and not dorsiflex (Rooney 1971). Since the fracture topography indicates dorsiflexion with compression failure in shear, it is apparent that electrical shock, struggling while cast, and so forth, are associated with both too-powerful and out-of-phase contractions of the vertebral muscles. That is, the *m. longissimus* (and its coactor *mm. multifidi*) and the *m. spinalis* do not contract simultaneously, and dorsiflexion occurs.

The thoracic spinal cord is usually transected or severely compressed. Rarely, fracture fragments lacerate the thoracic aorta with fatal intrathoracic hemorrhage. This is more likely with shattering of the vertebrae in older animals.

Dorsal spinal traumatic myopathy

It is of clinical importance that some animals with clear-cut clinical signs of vertebral fracture do not, in fact, have such fracture. At postmortem the vertebrae and spinal cord are intact, and there is severe tearing, disruption, and hemorrhage of the dorsal spinal muscles in the T10–14 area, dorsal spinal traumatic myopathy. The clinical histories suggest that this muscular damage is caused by the same, quantitatively less severe, mechanism as fracture. Such lesions are rare as compared to fractures, in our experience, a point of prognostic importance.

Cervical

A special case is the somersault of the jumping or steeplechase horse. While, in most cases, such somersaults cause only dismay and minor stiffness, severe disability or complete paralysis may ensue.

Somersaults entail severe ventroflexion of the neck, with tearing of ligaments and muscles on the dorsal and lateral surfaces of the cervical vertebrae. Fracture may occur with sufficiently severe falls, following the initial soft tissue failure.

Some horses recover following such accidents. One assumes that soft tissue injury was sustained and, eventually, repaired. It is an interesting and important clinical fact that such horses show ataxia of all four legs so long as there is obvious pain (splinting, guarding) of the neck. As the pain and muscular guarding gradually recede, the ataxia improves with eventual return to normal. It may be taken as a rule that severe pain causing sustained guarding of the cervical musculature will cause temporary ataxia of all four legs. Abscesses adjacent to the thoracic inlet (caudal cervical lymph nodes caused by *S. equi*, for example) may cause such splinting and ataxia. These empirical clinicopathological correlations strongly suggest that neural reflexes mediated through the neck are necessary for coordinated movement.

Bartke (1900) reported that, in Prussian army horses, 8% of fractures involved the cervical verte-

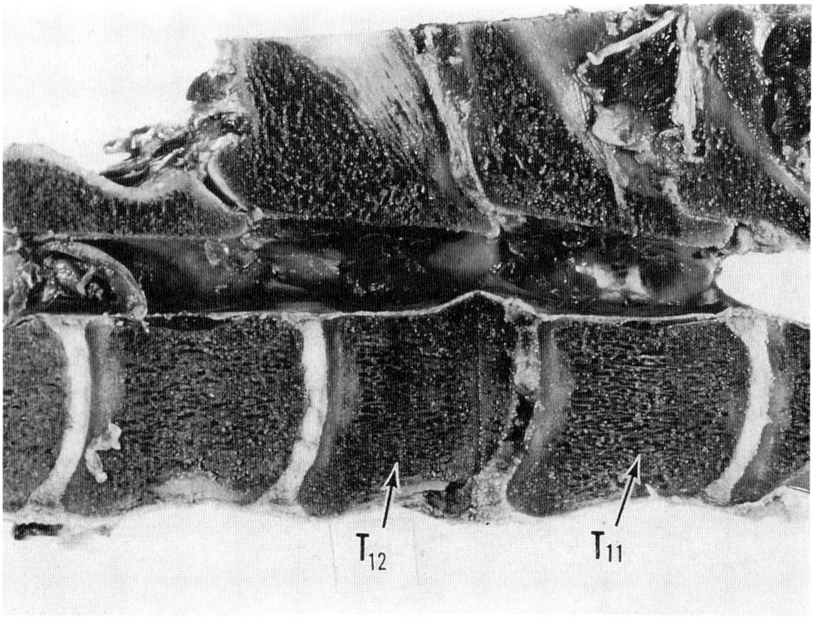

9.1. Fracture of thoracic vertebra 12 (T12). The intervertebral disk is involved and mashed bone is bulging into the vertebral canal.

brae in the following order of frequency: C3,4,2, 1,5,6, which nearly matches the order of increasing mobility of the articulations (Rooney 1969). Over 60% of these fractures involved C3 and C4. Fröhner (1905) pointed out that the ankylosis of spondylosis deformans predisposed to fracture of adjacent vertebral bodies. In recent years surgical ankylosis has been used in treating cervical stenotic myelopathy (wobbles). A number of cases of fracture of adjacent vertebral bodies have been seen following such ankylosis.

Spondylosis deformans

This is the morphological basis for many cases of so-called "cold back" in horses. The relationship between spondylosis and *sattelzwang*—cold back—was recorded by Fröhner (1905) and Vogt (1906). The lesions are most frequent in the area of the 10th through 14th thoracic vertebrae, but can involve the lumbar vertebrae as well. While no incidence figures are available, it appears that 3-day-event horses and others used for protracted periods of work with heavier riders are prone to this condition. It occurs, as well, in old broodmares as a result, presumably, of many pregnancies. It is not a significant lesion of racing Thoroughbreds and Standardbreds. In earlier times draft horses were affected, specifically smaller breeds doing heavy work (Bittner 1927). In this regard it is to be remembered that horses that pull loads are subjected to vertical forces, the forces involved in the pathogenesis of spondylosis, as well as horizontal, draft forces, and the larger the load being pulled, the larger such vertical force will be.

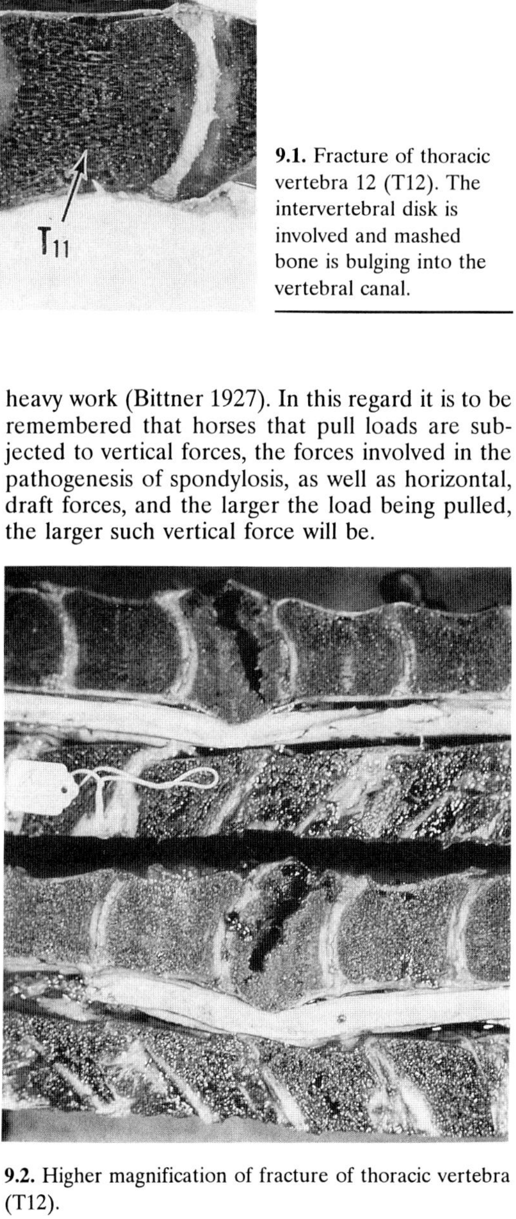

9.2. Higher magnification of fracture of thoracic vertebra (T12).

Stecher and Goss (1961) examined 245 vertebral columns from a variety of equids. In addition to variations of lumbar, sacral, and coccygeal numbers they reported a number of ankyloses of the lateral transverse joints of the lumbar region, as well as ankyloses of thoracic and lumbar vertebral bodies and intervertebral joints. These lesions were found in domesticated horses, but not in several species of nondomesticated horses and zebras. Ankyloses of the lateral transverse joints are not at all uncommon in older horses of whatever breed and may be regarded as almost normal. That is not to say, of course, that pain was not present during the active stages of ankylosis.

Stecher (1962) also reported a statistical study of the numerical variation of vertebrae in the spine of the horse, perhaps of eventual pathological interest. Robertson (1910) believed that there was a dominant inheritance of numbers of lumbar vertebrae, six vertebrae being dominant over five. He further noted that there was a tendency for the nasal bones to be convex when there were six and concave with five lumbar vertebrae, as is certainly the case with the Arabian horse.

Few cases of spondylosis have been seen at postmortem during the acute phase. A typical acute case (dying for reasons unrelated to cold back) had tearing of the annulus fibrosus of T10–11,11–12 at and around the ventral midline. There was moderate hemorrhage and fraying of collagen fibers. The tearing extended no deeper than the annulus fibrosus. The dorsal intervertebral articulations had evidently been jammed together, with fraying and erosion of the articular cartilage and hemarthrosis.

Chronic spondylosis deformans is characterized by osteophytes on the ventrolateral aspects of two or more vertebrae, usually T10–14. The osteophytes are bullus and, in advanced cases, bridge the intervertebral space as bony ankyloses (Figs. 9.3 and 9.4). The dorsal intervertebral joints may show marked destruction of articular cartilage, as well, with eventual bony ankylosis (Fig. 9.5). As a result of the dorsiflexed position of the vertebrae, the dorsal spinous processes override or impinge with formation of new bone and false joints (Vogt 1906; Roberts 1968; Townsend et al. 1986).

The pathogenesis is similar to, but obviously less severe than, thoracic vertebral fracture. Single event, or more probably repeated, dorsiflexion of the vertebral column causes overstretching and tearing of the annulus fibrosis and drives the dorsal intervertebral joints together. In the old broodmare, of course, the overloading dorsiflexion has been continuous over long periods of time. While repeated overloading may be the primary factor for dorsiflexion and tearing of the annulus fibrosus,

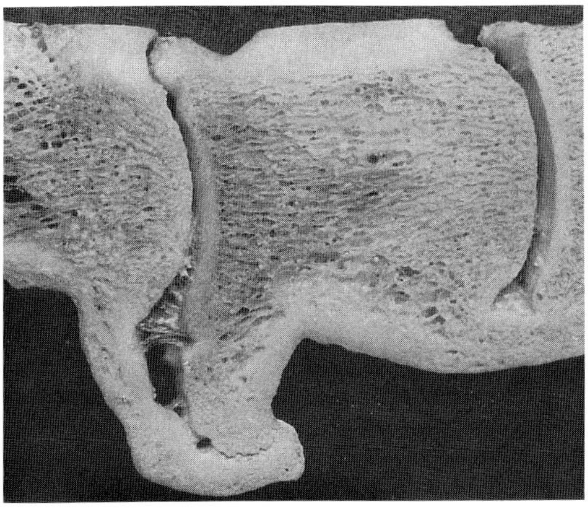

9.3. Spondylosis deformans with ankylosis.

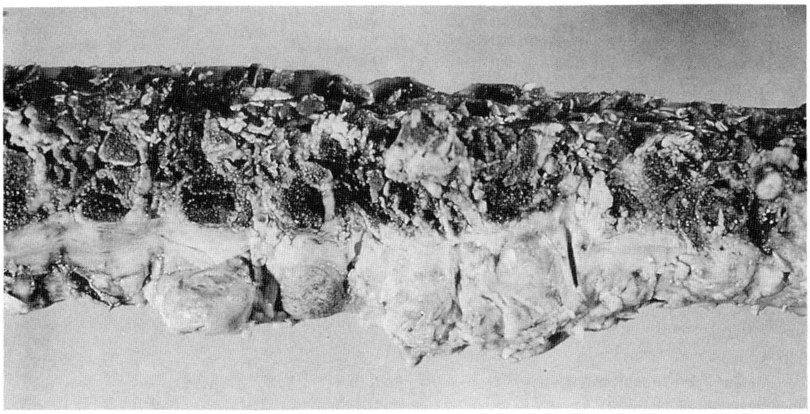

9.4. Spondylosis deformans. The dorsal spines and ribs were removed.

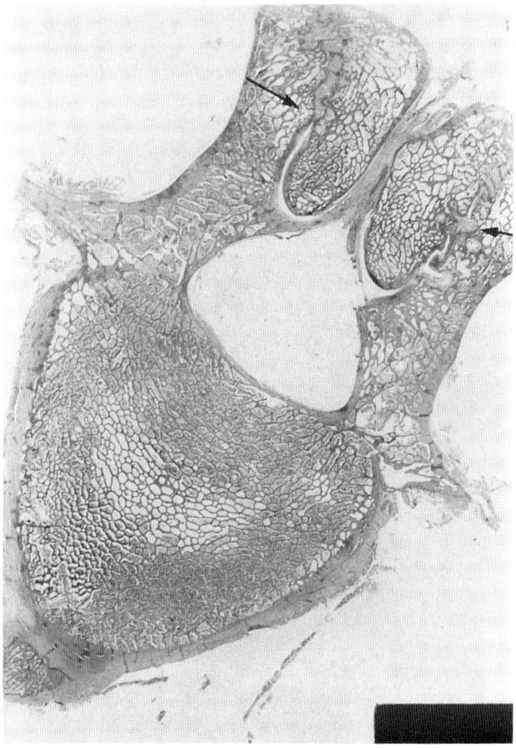

9.5. Cross section of thoracic vertebrae to show ankylosis of the intervertebral joints (*arrows*).

out-of-phase contraction of the vertebral muscles, as with fractures, may be a factor in some cases.

Vertebral disease without lesions

Clinical observation suggests a frequency of "lameness of the back" that is quite out of line with the frequency of pathological changes of the vertebral column. Two observations, one from professional riding instructors and the other experimental, support that clinical opinion and correlate with the pathogenesis of fractures and spondylosis deformans.

A typical clinical history: a young horse is broken and trained for riding by a professional trainer. It is sold for use by a rider of limited training and experience. Within a few weeks the purchaser returns with the complaint that the horse is rough-gaited, sour, resists being saddled, and is generally unsuitable for the rider—all signs of cold back. The trainer takes the horse back and, shortly, it is performing normally. Returned to the poor rider, the scenario repeats itself. It is the opinion of professional trainers that, among the many shortcomings of inexperienced riding, a most important factor is improper seat. That is, the rider does not stay in line with the center of mass of the horse; does not maintain the so-called balanced seat.

Evidence of soreness of the back is, of course, not limited to the above scenario. It is frequently diagnosed in horses in almost all types of work, and the contributing factors, such as lameness, overwork, and immaturity must be evaluated in each case.

Experiments were done with several horses using a treadmill and high-speed videography. A marker was placed at the thoracolumbar junction. The horses were moved at the walk, trot, and canter with a modest weight, about 40 kg, in saddlebags on the line of the center of mass and, again, about 20–30 cm caudal to that position. The marker traced out a smooth, sinusoidal curve with the proper loading. With improper loading, the curve was considerably rougher. Harmonic analysis showed that there was a single fundamental and very small harmonics for the normal curve, while the curve for the abnormal loading had a fundamental and a large second frequency. The variation of amplitude of the curve and the appearance of a second frequency with improper loading suggested that out-of-phase contraction of the vertebral muscles, as already described for fractures and for spondylosis deformans, could be a factor in nonlesion back problems. The vertebral column was, also, stiffer with the improper loading, which would contribute to fatigue of the vertebral musculature.

The general case is made that there is a gradient of out-of-phase contraction of vertebral muscles, from the pain and discomfort of improper riding, without lesions necessarily being present, through spondylosis deformans to fracture.

Intervertebral disks

Senile degeneration

Senile degeneration of the intervertebral disks is routine in aging horses. The lumbosacral and cervical disks are invariably involved, but only an occasional thoracolumbar disk.

The intervertebral disk of the horse and other large animals does not have a nucleus pulposus, as such. Both grossly and microscopically there is gradual grading of fibrous tissue from the thick, heavy annulus fibrosus to a looser fibrocartilaginous center with a modest amount of mucoid matrix.

With age the central part of the disk gradually yellows, becomes drier, and, eventually, disappears, leaving a space surrounded by the yellowed, frayed fibrous tissue of the annulus fibrosus (Fig. 9.6). There are invariably arthrotic changes, including scoring lines, in the vertebral articular joints, associated with such disk degeneration. Detailed chemical and morphological studies have not been done.

Clinical signs of spinal cord disease are rarely associated with senile disk degeneration. Some older animals may develop clinical signs of wobbler at ages well beyond the expected. Postmortem examination shows the osteochondrotic articular facets characteristic of cervical stenotic myelopathy, together with degeneration of the intervertebral disks of the cervical vertebrae. It appears that the increased mobility attendant upon degeneration of the disks adds to that provided by the overly large articular facets, allowing subluxation sufficient to damage the cervical spinal cord.

Hansen (1969) observed disk degeneration, apparently similar to the aging type described above, in Gotland ponies, although the degeneration occurred in young animals. There was necrosis, degeneration, and loss of the centers of the disks, and the vertebral bodies were sclerotic. The instability resulting from disk degeneration caused kyphosis, lordosis, and scoliosis. Complicating bacterial infection was seen in some cases. The animals often had marked locomotor deficits, including ataxia.

No case of degeneration and protrusion of the intervertebral disks comparable to that seen in humans and dog has been seen, probably because of the lack of a distinct nucleus pulposus. Taylor et al. (1977) claimed that fibrocartilaginous emboli causing ischemic myelopathy in a horse arose from intervertebral disk degeneration. They did not find such disk degeneration, however, and the source of the emboli in their case was, in fact, not determined. This is generally the case in humans and other animals as well, the pathogenesis of fibrocartilaginous emboli not being known (LeCouteur and Child 1989).

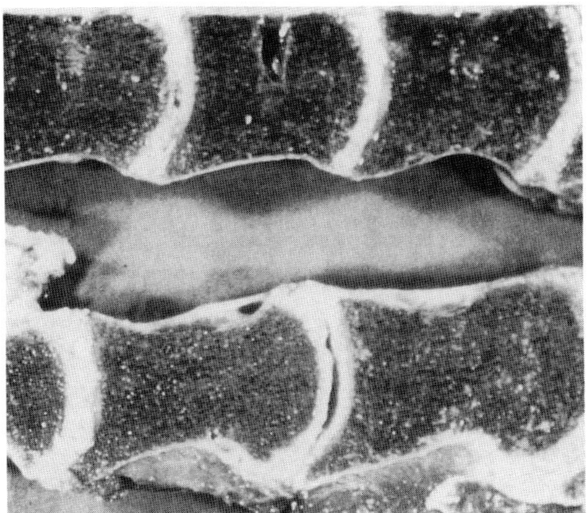

9.6. Senile degeneration of the cervical intervertebral disks. The cervical disk to the *left* is almost normal. One thoracic disk (*above*) has a small central area of tissue loss.

Foss et al. (1983) described two cases of degeneration of the intervertebral disk with dorsal bulging of the annulus fibrosus as the cause of neurological signs. Disk degeneration was confined to a single segment in each case, one a 3- and the other a 6-year-old animal, clearly not the age-related degeneration described above. The cause of the disk degeneration was not determined, but the amount of sclerosis in the vertebral bodies at least suggests osteomyelitis. Nixon et al. (1984) reported a case in an 18-year-old horse as a Hansen type II intervertebral protrusion. The report indicated that dorsal bulging of the annulus fibrosus caused the spinal cord compression, but is not convincing as a type II protrusion.

While perhaps a semantic argument, it does not appear appropriate to designate greater mobility of the intervertebral junction, with or without bulging of the dorsal annulus fibrosus, as Hansen type II disk protrusion. Pressure on the spinal cord may well result from the greater mobility, as well as the bulging, of the annulus per se. Hansen did not designate the process in the Gotland ponies as disk protrusion.

Diskospondylitis

Diskospondylitis of infection is seen occasionally in foals and rarely in adult horses (Collins et al. 1971; Adams et al. 1985). Most cases in foals have been associated with *Rhodococcus equi* and *Salmonella* sp. infections, the vertebral bodies and disks being involved by direct extension from the lung in the former and by metastasis in the latter.

Stadler et al. (1987) described a case that they considered to be Hansen type I protrusion of the C2–3 intervertebral disk. The pathological description and radiograph, however, strongly suggest that it was, in fact, diskospondylitis.

Scoliosis, lordosis, and kyphosis

Scoliosis and lordosis are congenital defects. As noted elsewhere, scoliosis is part of the syndrome of contracture of the newborn foal. The basic pathological defect with both scoliosis and lordosis is hypoplasia or aplasia of the articular facets of the intervertebral articulations, primarily of the thoracic portion of the vertebral column.

Scoliosis

With scoliosis one or more facets on one side are hypoplastic, and the vertebral column moves to the stable, scoliotic position (Rooney 1966, 1969). This occurs in utero (see Chapter 12, "Neonate"). Goubaux (1886/87) said that scoliosis could be congenital or acquired, but we have seen no acquired cases.

Lordosis

With congenital lordosis the hypoplasia/aplasia of the articular facets is bilateral at one or more thoracic vertebrae, and movement to the stable, lordotic position occurs only after birth and weight bearing (Rooney and Prickett 1967a) (Figs. 9.7, 9.8, and 9.9). In our few cases a genetic basis was probable, but could not be established.

At present variable degrees of lordosis seem to be common in certain lines of American Saddlebred horses. Conformation standards for this breed include the spread-out stance and high neck/head carriage. Taken together with the standard for high action of the forelegs, these criteria lead, mechanically, to selection for the lordotic conformation. No examples have been seen at postmortem.

Senile lordosis

Variably obvious senile lordosis occurs in aging horses in the absence of predisposing lesions. There may be arthrosis and ankylosis of the intervertebral joints and new bone formation on the articular

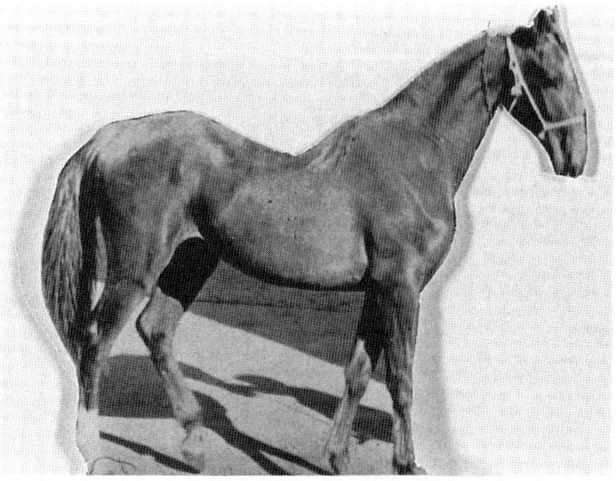

9.7. One-year-old mixed breed with congenital lordosis.

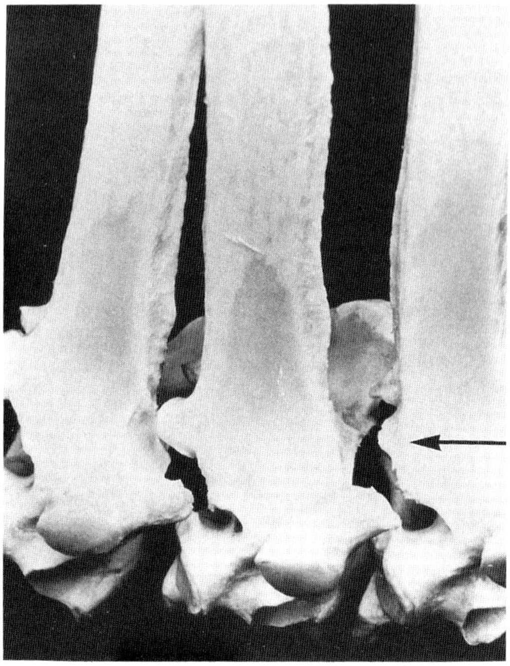

9.8. Macerated vertebrae of Figure 9.7. The *arrow* points to the hypoplastic, almost aplastic intervertebral articular processes.

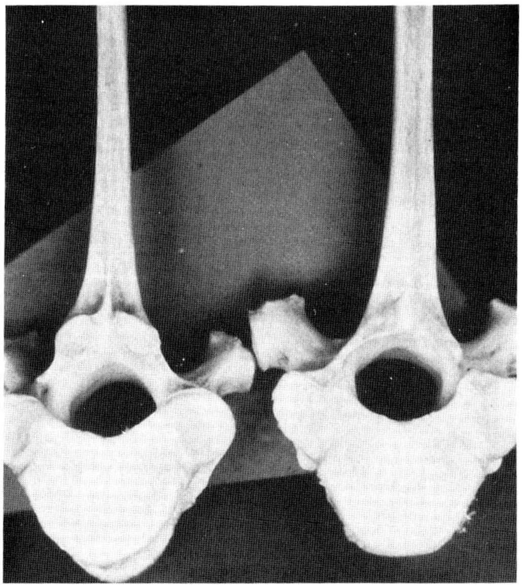

9.9. Caudal view of normal (*left*) and nearly aplastic articular processes (*right*).

processes and dorsal spines. The dorsal spines may override and form false joints (Virchow 1916). While there is some osteophyte formation on the vertebral bodes, it is less prominent than in spondylosis deformans. Goubaux (1886/87) made essentially the same observations. Senile lordosis may be considered a slowly developing spondylosis deformans, although it can occur in the absence of pathological change.

Kyphosis

Kyphosis of the lumbar region has been seen, clinically, in several yearling Thoroughbred horses. Only one has come to postmortem. There was fibrosis and osteophytosis (avulsion and repair) of the attachment of the multifidus muscle on the cranial articular processes of the first lumbar vertebra, lesions probably secondary to, rather than the cause of, the kyphosis. The condition is probably congenital, or perhaps hereditary, but adequate data is not available. Goubaux (1886/87) described kyphosis in draft horses, but his description is difficult to interpret.

Neoplasia

No case of primary neoplasia of the vertebral column has been reported. Metastasis of malignant melanoma into the dorsal spine or body of a lumbar vertebra occurs with some frequency. Clinical signs may be caused by bulging of the tumor into the spinal canal and/or as the result of pathological fracture (Dobberstein and Tamaschke 1969). Occasional cases of metastasis of melanoma to the lumbar meninges without bony involvement have been seen.

An occasional case of vascular malformation/neoplasia in or on the meninges and causing compression of the spinal cord has been seen. These are histologically identical to the vascular angiomatosis described with the skin (see Chapter 15, "Integument").

CHAPTER 10

Stability Theory and Pathogenesis of Lameness

This chapter is unusual for a textbook of pathology and may well, and probably will, be passed over on first reading. The justification is a deeper understanding of the pathogenesis of locomotor disease. The material will be unfamiliar and difficult.

Nonlinear dynamics is applied to the study of the form and normal locomotor function of the horse and to the study of the pathogenesis of lameness of horses. The resulting stability theory incorporates earlier theoretical formulations (Rooney 1969, 1989), providing necessary and sufficient conditions for a mechanical theory of the pathogenesis of lameness. From our own observations and that of many early writers, fatigue is a major initiating factor for many forms of lameness. The present analysis provides a pathway for fatigue as a cause of instability and damage. Smith (1917) has provided a classic review of the working capacity of horses for draft, carrying loads, endurance, and velocity.

Nonlinear dynamics

The concept of stability is familiar. Nonlinear mechanics objectifies that concept, posing questions of stability and instability in a coherent manner (Berge et al. 1984; Migulin et al. 1983; Moon 1987; Panovko and Gubanova 1965; Stoker 1950; Thompson and Stewart 1986).

There are two forms of stability: (1) *ordinary stability*—resistance to small variations of initial conditions, and (2) *structural stability*—resistance to small variations in the parameters of the structure itself (Berge et al. 1984). Small initial conditions must be within the vector field of the horse. As will be shown, the horse is, in general, stable in this sense. In the case of the structure itself even quite small changes in, for example, joint angles, can cause instability.

A graphical method for the solution of differential equations has been employed. Stability is examined only when the leg(s) is in support since damage to the locomotor system occurs then.

Method

The dynamics of the legs, vertebral column, and the whole horse are investigated at instants with displacements, velocities, and accelerations constant at that instant. The instantaneous figure is perturbed by initial conditions of velocity or displacement or both, and the response of the horse as trajectories—integral curves—examined. For example, if the standing horse is pushed to one side (initial conditions of displacement and velocity), the response to that push will indicate the stability status of the horse in the standing position.

The legs and vertebral column are in stick-figure form. While that may seem trivial, the stick figure is the result of the interaction of gravity and all the components of the legs and back and has great generality as an abstraction of a real body in a real world (Blum 1967; Russ 1989).

The stick figure is in a coordinate system, the *phase plane*. The vertical displacement is plotted on the horizontal axis and the first derivative plotted on the vertical axis (Fig. 10.1). Compromise centers of rotation for the fore leg and rear leg (or an individual joint) are at centers of coordinates, since it is the behavior of the trajectories in relationship to centers that determines stability. A center of rotation is a *singularity,* a point of zero displacement and velocity around which movement occurs. In the case of the whole horse there are two obvious centers, the scapulohumeral joint and the coxofemoral joint. The horizontal, *y*, axis passes through these two centers. This horizontal line is *not* parallel to the ground line. Very different results are obtained for the rear leg if *y* is parallel to the ground, as will be shown. The vector field of the horse contains singularities at each joint center as well as at a saddle point as will be seen. The phase plane is an abstract vector field. It is a rule of such a two-dimensional vector field that the trajectories cannot cross (Stoker 1950; Thompson and Stewart 1986).

The stick figure is the graphical representation of the *characteristic* of the differential equation of

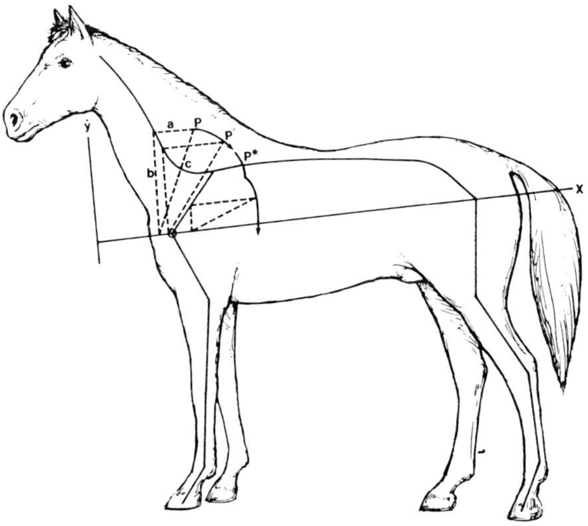

10.1. The Liénard (1928) graphical construction. See the text.

the leg. The characteristic is that portion of the differential equation containing the terms for storage and dissipation of energy in the physical system (Stoker 1950). Here, the differential equation is not written and the characteristic is the shape of the leg, which, in turn, is a function of the energetics of the leg.

The graphical characteristic is solved by finding the integral curves, the trajectories, in the phase plane. The method is that of Liénard (1928), Stoker (1950), and Migulin et al. (1983). A point is selected—an initial condition—and a line is drawn parallel to the abscissa to intersect the characteristic (Fig. 10.1). Next, a line is drawn from that intersection perpendicular to the abscissa. A third line is drawn back to the starting point. Finally, a short line is drawn in the clockwise direction perpendicular to the third line. The "head" of that short line is now a new point, and the process is repeated. The theory for the construction may be found in Stoker (1950). By convention the horse moves from right to left, facing left, so that the trajectories develop in the clockwise direction. For the "off" pair of legs the construction is carried out as if looking through the horse.

The method, as applied to the legs, is standard. For the whole horse, a nonanalytical figure, there is no a priori mathematical justification, and the construction is heuristic—the physical results justifying the means in the absence of mathematical proof.

Harmonic analysis was done on the displacement values of the stick figures, using the Fast Fourier Transform (Moon 1987), as will be discussed.

Static

In the standing position there are two singularities, the shoulder (scapulohumeral) joint and the hip (coxofemoral) joint. Trajectories arising from initial conditions near the shoulder move outward to form a *limit cycle*. With larger initial conditions the trajectory may circle before joining the limit cycle. The initial conditions may be either displacement, or velocity, or both. In all cases a limit cycle is formed (Fig. 10.2). The shoulder joint is not fixed relative to the thoracic wall as the horse is moving. Its displacement relative to the thoracic wall does not, however, change the behavior of the trajectories in the phase plane.

A displacement initial condition of the rear leg, no matter the magnitude, leads to a limit cycle centered on the hip joint (Fig. 10.3). Positive velocity initial conditions also produce trajectories that join the limit cycle. Large negative velocity initial conditions, on the other hand, give rise to large amplitude trajectories that, as will be seen,

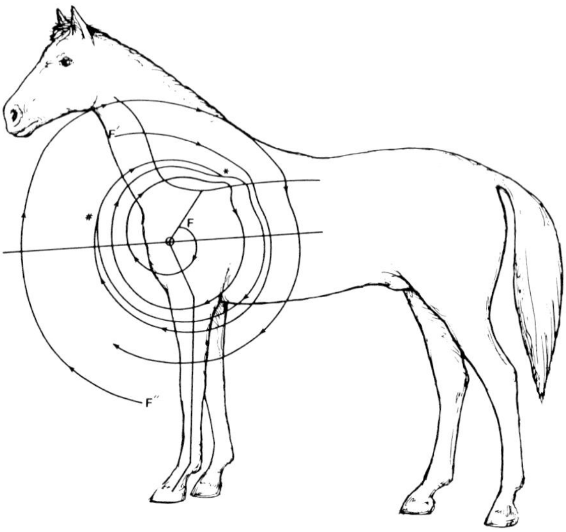

10.2. The trajectories of the fore leg. With a small initial condition at F, the trajectory spirals out to form the limit cycle at the asterisk. With a large initial condition at F′, the trajectory spirals in to join the limit cycle at the hatch. F″ is large enough that it does not reach the limit cycle as far as this construction was done.

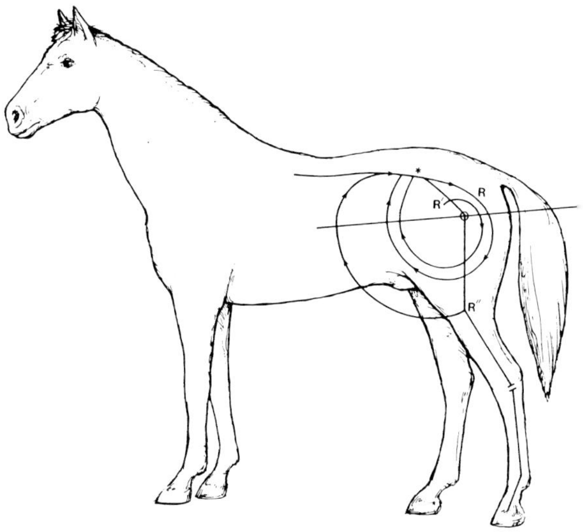

10.3. The trajectories for the rear leg. R is the limit cycle. R′ spirals out to R, while R″ spirals in, both joining the limit cycle near the asterisk.

join the limit cycle of the fore leg. Thus it is that sufficient velocity must be imparted to the rear leg to cause movement of the horse. Taking negative velocity of the leg to be opposite to the direction of velocity of the whole horse, the leg must be moving backward.

The limit cycles formed at both the fore leg and rear leg characterize *self-excited* behavior. An oscillatory system can respond to excitation in three ways. If perturbed by a brief impulse (a little push), the system oscillates and comes to rest. This is a *transient,* the frequency of which is a natural frequency of the system itself. If perturbed by a repeating, periodic force (the pistons of an internal combustion engine), there is an initial transient before the system settles down to a periodic motion, the frequency determined by the external, driving force.

In *self-excited* systems (Stoker 1950), energy supplied to the system is constant, or nearly so, such as a fan blowing. After the transient the system continues to oscillate, so long as energy is supplied, and oscillates at a natural frequency of the system. The rear legs are the principal source of energy for the movement of the horse. This energy is not continuous but is effectively so, as in pushing a swing, supplying energy as necessary to maintain (but not change) the swinging frequency.

So-called negative damping is characteristic of self-excited systems. In ordinary dissipative systems damping is positive, removing energy from the system so that it eventually comes to rest. In self-excited systems damping is dissipative—positive—in part, but the system is primarily characterized by energy being added to or generated in the system, so that it does not come to rest. In the horse, energy is passively stored in the musculotendinous system during the first half of support by stretching of the viscelastic connective tissues. Negative work by muscles contributes to this viscelastic storage mechanism (Goldspinck 1980; Rooney 1990a). During the second half of support much of the stored energy is recovered as the connective tissues shorten. This is true of other species, as well (Alexander and Bennet-Clark 1977).

In the phase-plane representation small initial condition trajectories spiral outward to a limit cycle. This is energy supplied to the system as negative damping. Large initial condition trajectories spiral in to the limit cycle. This is positive damping, dissipating energy. The limit cycle, then, is the equilibrium condition, equal amounts of energy being added to and dissipated from the system.

If the horse "locks" a rear leg by hooking the patella over the medial ridge of the femoral trochlea, the hip joint is displaced distally. The y axis joining the shoulder and hip centers is, now, parallel to the ground, or nearly so. The Liénard construction shows (Fig. 10.4) that the rear leg is now asymptotically stable. That is, the trajectories spiral in toward the hip joint. The locked rear leg is stable and the behavior of the trajectories so indicates. The transition from the asymptotically stable focus of the hip joint to limit cycling is an *Hopf bifurcation* (Berge et al. 1984), which occurs in both directions.

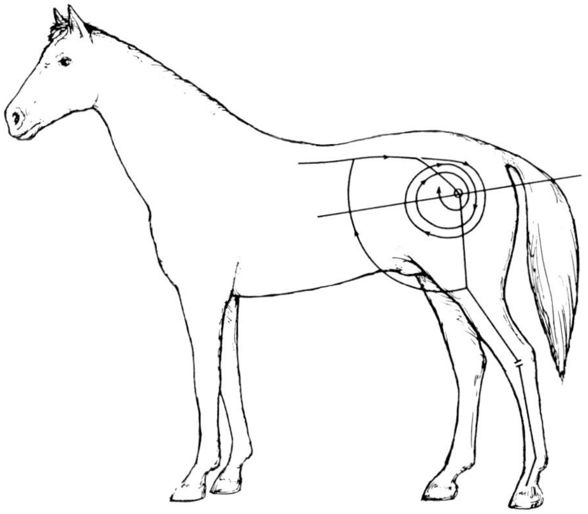

10.4. If the horse "locks" the stifle, dropping the croup down, the trajectories spiral in toward the hip joint center, a stable, noncycling condition.

Large velocity initial conditions of the rear leg, larger than appropriate for the velocity of the whole horse, are characteristic of ataxia, that is, circumduction, hypermetria. The initial condition is not small, as already defined, and there is a loss of ordinary stability.

The limit cycle of the fore leg extends to the approximate location of the center of mass of the horse. The limit cycle of the rear leg extends to the same point (Fig. 10.5). This suggests that there is a *saddle point* in this area.

If the vertebral column is perturbed (any trajectory encounters the vertebral column) (Fig. 10.6), it is apparent that the trajectories either join the limit cycle of the fore leg, or the limit cycle of the rear leg, or *bifurcate* to join both. This pertains to the standing state. During movement, trajectories arising from the fore and rear legs and the vertebral column coalesce, as will be seen. The saddle point is unstable, by definition, and small movements of the legs tend to settle around the centers of rotation of the legs themselves, rather than the saddle point; the horse does not move. In the standing

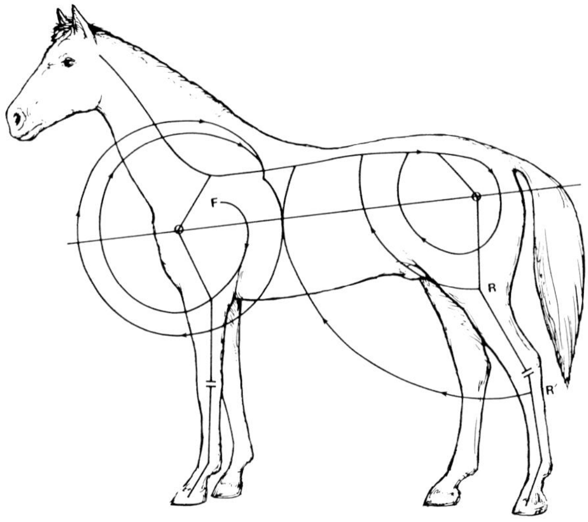

10.5. Limit cycles of fore and rear in the standing horse.

case, then, the horse is stable as the trajectories settle around the limit cycles (or asymptotic path) of the rear leg and fore leg. The stability is *ordinary*; that is, the system is resistant to small changes in initial conditions. The horse, however, is not *structurally stable*; small changes in the configurations of the legs and vertebral column can result in changes of behavior of the system. For example, the Hopf bifurcation is structurally unstable, the limit cycle changing to asymptotic and vice versa.

Physically, limit cycles imply that the standing horse is never completely stationary; there is always some oscillation. Studies with horses using high-speed videography and force plates confirm this observation (Thompson and Rooney 1992; Pratt and O'Connor 1976). If the horse could be held dead-still and then released, it would return to limit cycle oscillation. A large push causes large oscillations, which settle back into the normal limit cycle oscillation. If the initial conditions are large enough, the horse may have to move to a new position on the ground in order to regain stability, and that is movement.

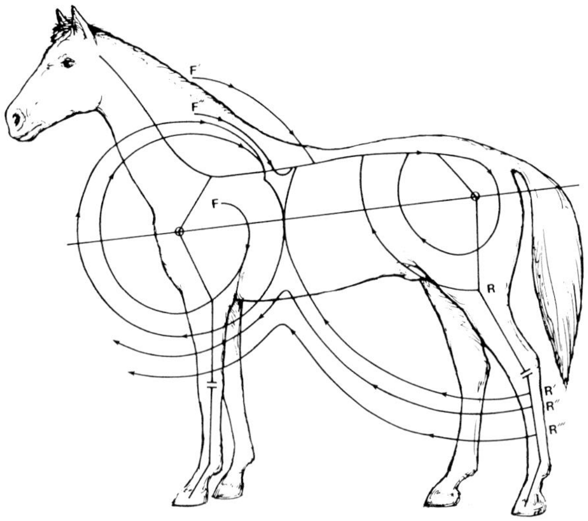

10.6. With larger initial conditions, R″,R‴, for the rear leg, the rear leg trajectories swing by saddle point to join the fore leg limit cycle. Similarly, large fore leg initial conditions intersect the vertebral column and bifurcate to stay with the fore leg or join the limit cycle of the rear leg.

Dynamic

When movement begins—the negative velocity of the rear leg is sufficiently large—the trajectory of the rear leg joins the fore leg limit cycle. The trajectories of the unstable limit cycle of horse movement behave as in Figure 10.6, involving the fore and rear legs in turn and swinging by the saddle point. A single, unstable saddle limit cycle, then, characterizes movement. This limit cycle is the result of the coalescence of the trajectories of the rear leg, fore leg, and vertebral column. The coalescence of the fore and rear legs is accomplished physically by the vertebral column and, conceptually, by the bifurcation occasioned by the vertebral column. The saddle point represents a maximum displacement, and is an unstable equilibrium point. It is reiterated that in a two-dimensional vector field (this phase plane) the trajectories cannot cross. Thus it is that a trajectory of the rear leg joins the limit cycle of the fore leg and does not cross it. The saddle point, in the phase plane, is located at $y = 180°$ and $y' = 0$ (Thompson and Stewart 1986). Integrating backwards from the saddle point, one obtains the *inset* and integrating forward from the saddle point gives the *outset* (see below) (Fig. 10.6). The saddle point is squarely on the y axis with $y' = 0$ as it should be.

The limit cycles of the fore leg and rear leg form a *separatrix,* trajectories asymptotic to the saddle point. The separatrix has an inset, a pair of trajectories approaching the saddle point, and an outset, a pair of trajectories consisting of one leaving the saddle point to form the limit cycle around the shoulder joint and the other around the hip joint. The inset and outset delimit the two periodic attractors: the fore leg and rear leg limit cycles. All trajectories within the limit cycle join the limit cycle. Trajectories originating outside the limit cycle either join that cycle or join the whole horse saddle cycle.

All trajectories of the moving horse eventually join the limit cycle of the rear leg. If the velocity of the horse increases, it is clear that a limit cycle for one velocity will be replaced by a larger amplitude limit cycle for the next, larger, velocity. Increasing velocity, then, is characterized by unstable limit cycles, increasing in velocity and amplitude in the phase plane, as velocity increases (Fig. 10.6).

In the transverse plane the fore legs and rear legs are limit cycling (Fig. 10.7).

A valuable technique for evaluating the periodic behavior of a system is harmonic analysis, a measure of the number of frequencies present (Moon 1987). In the case of the horse stick figure a single, fundamental frequency and one or two small harmonics are present, indicating periodic behavior. Harmonic analysis of the lateral or transverse outlines of the whole horse, before reduction to a stick figure, also gives a fundamental and one or two small harmonics. The harmonic analysis and the trajectories in the phase plane agree and define periodic behavior.

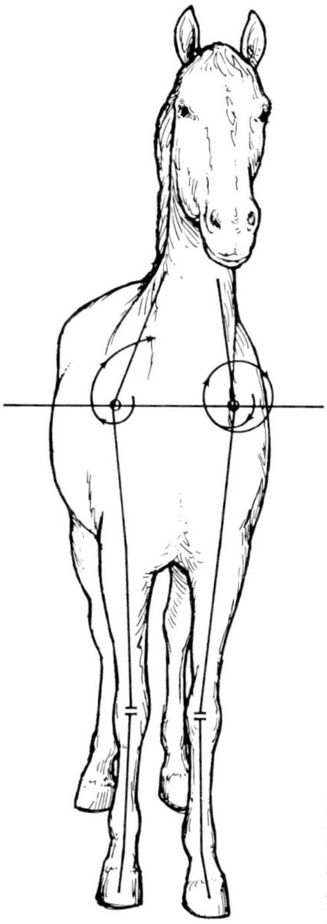

10.7. Cross section view. Limit cycles are formed at both legs; please see the text.

Individual joints

With any reasonable (small) initial condition the trajectories will join the limit cycle of the fore leg or rear leg (asymptote of rear leg if stifle is locked). While each joint will be examined as an entity, it is apparent that each joint's stability characteristic is that of the whole leg. If an individual joint becomes unstable, the whole leg remains asymptotic or limit cycling despite the instability of the individual joint.

The lumbosacral, sacroiliac, and coxofemoral joints all show limit cycle behavior given that the perturbing initial conditions are within the vector field of those joints. These joints are asymptotically stable when the hip joint is displaced distally by the locking of the stifle joint. The shoulder joint has been examined. In the usual standing position, self-excited, limit cycle behavior holds, so long as the trajectories intersect the vertebral column.

The stifle joint, like the shoulder (Fig. 10.8), displays limit cycle behavior if more proximal elements of the characteristic are intersected by the trajectory.

The elbow (humeroradial) (Fig. 10.9), and hock (tarsocrural) joints are mechanically comparable (Rooney 1969). Both of these joints are "snap joints" (*Schnappgelenke*) because of the excentric

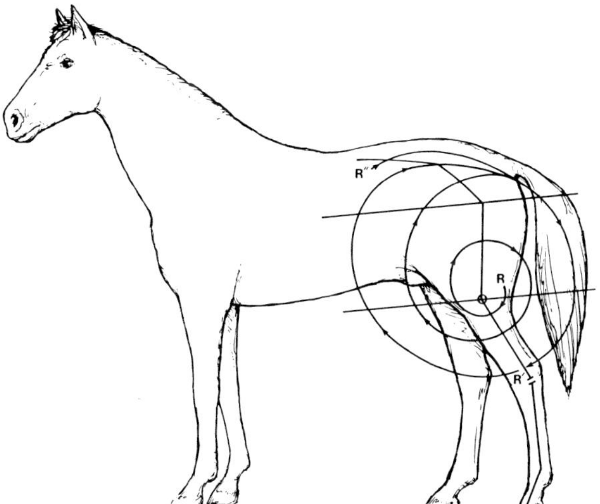

10.8. Limit cycle developed around the stifle.

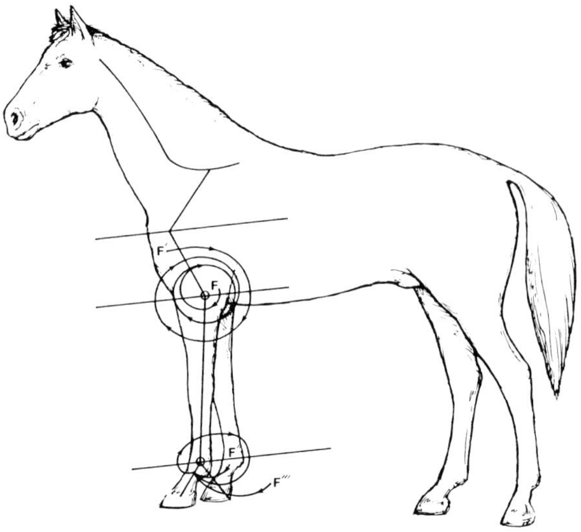

10.9. Limit cycles at elbow and fetlock.

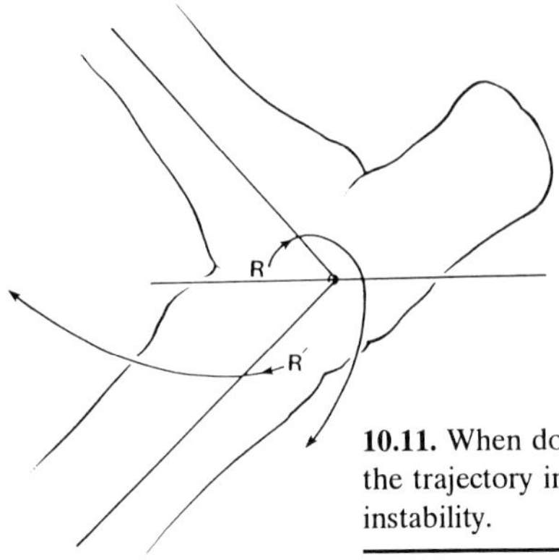

10.11. When dorsiflexed the trajectory indicates instability.

attachments of the medial and lateral collateral ligaments. Freed of all muscle and tendinous attachments, they oscillate within the range of the usual standing position. As the joint is dorsiflexed it jumps to a smaller dorsal angle. Similarly, as the joint is palmar (plantar) flexed it jumps from the midrange to the fully extended position. This latter jump is less obvious than the former, on average. The stick-figure representation of these joints shows identical behavior (Figs. 10.10–10.12). That is, the joint is limit cycling in the self-excited manner in the middle range, becomes unstable with the jump to the smaller dorsal angle, and becomes asymptotically stable with the less obvious jump to the larger dorsal angle.

This jump behavior does not occur when the dead leg is manipulated with tendons and muscles intact and has not been seen in the live horse. The nonlinear behavior engendered by the collateral ligaments is, then, smoothed to near-linear behavior by the muscles and tendons on the dorsal and palmar/plantar aspects of the elbow/hock. The tendons and muscles kinematically control the movement of the joints, and the nonlinear jump behavior does not occur. The energy optimizing aspects of the behavior of these joints is considered elsewhere in this book (Rooney 1990a).

The carpus is unstable from impact to near midsupport, limit cycling at midsupport, and stable until lift-off at the end of support. If the carpus were precisely straight, radius and metacarpal in a straight line, there would be as many limit cycles as there are initial conditions, each cycle of different amplitude. This is biologically unreasonable and the midsupport position is, in fact, a slightly over-on-the-knee alignment. This is consistent with the view that carpal arthrosis occurs during the first half of

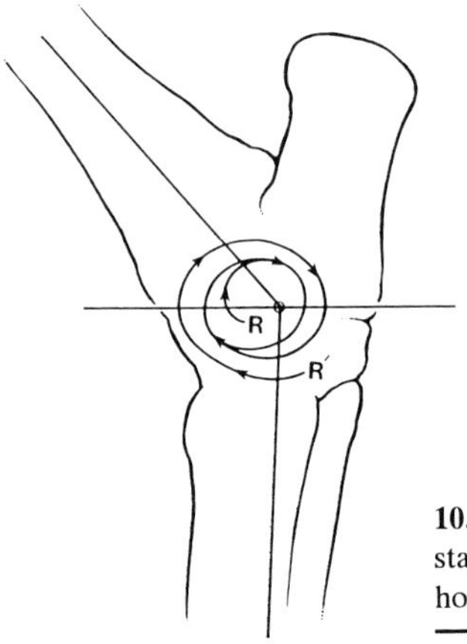

10.10. In the usual standing position the hock is limit cycling.

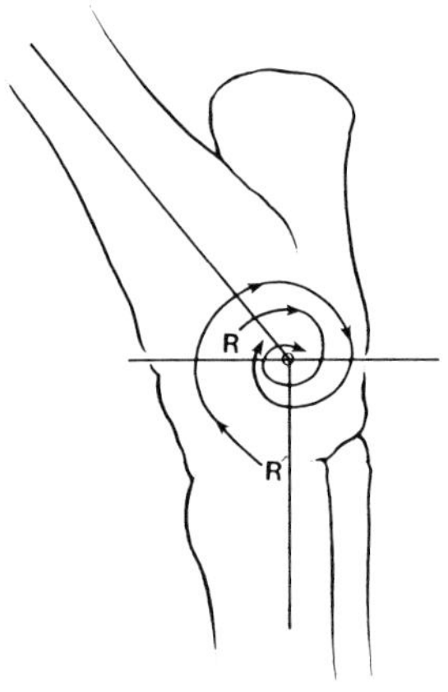

10.12. When strongly plantarflexed the trajectories spiral in toward the center, stable and noncycling.

support (Rooney 1969). The fetlock, pastern, and coffin joints are paired joints, as already noted. In all three cases (Fig. 10.9), the Liénard (1928) procedure is carried out with the proximal and both distal vectors. At the fetlock joint the dorsal aspect of the distal end of Mc3 articulates with the proximal phalanx, and the palmar (plantar) aspect articulates with the proximal sesamoid bones. The combined joints show limit cycle behavior at the usual dorsal standing angle of 140° and larger angles (Fig. 10.13).

If the proximal sesamoids are pulled over the ridge on the distal end of Mc3 (dorsal angle of the fetlock joint less than 95°), instability occurs, leading to, for example, gullwing arthrosis, sesamoiditis, and/or basal fracture of the sesamoid bones (Fig. 10.14). The analysis shows the conditions for instability, but does not define the physical pathogenesis.

The analysis defines stability and instability, but physical realization comes with consideration of the anatomy and the pathology of the lesions resulting from the instability. This is true of all joints.

At the pastern the obvious joint is that between the proximal and middle phalanges, but the proximal phalanx also articulates with the fibrocartilaginous proximal extension of the palmar proximal edge of the middle phalanx. The combined joints show limit cycle behavior. Excessive dorsiflexion or palmar/plantar flexion leads to instability and pathological changes of the pastern joint.

The distal phalanx and the dorsal surface of the navicular form a double joint with the same considerations as above. The navicular/deep flexor joint is of particular interest as the site of navicular disease. This joint is limit cycling and becomes unstable as the coffin joint rotates too far. Destructive changes of the surfaces of the navicular bone and the deep flexor tendon, simulating those of spontaneous navicular disease, can be produced in vitro (Thompson et al. 1991). The pathogenesis is considered to be toe-first impact of the foot with the ground, with angular movement of the coffin joint in a direction opposite to normal. This causes a momentary abnormal increase in tension of the deep flexor tendon, resulting in an increased normal force (perpendicular to the joint surfaces). The increase of normal force entails increased friction of the surfaces, and that is considered to be the cause of the destruction of the fibrocartilage.

The stability analysis indicates that the navicular-deep flexor joint becomes structurally unstable if the navicular bone is pulled too far distally. This displacement is realized physically by the wrong way angular displacement of the coffin joint with toe-first impact. Toe-first impact is characteristic of horses landing from a jump and for horses walking long hours on hard surfaces, two major predispositions for navicular disease. Repeated toe-first impact, vibration and bouncing, particularly on hard surfaces, would be relevant in the case of carriage and police horses. While the amount of impulse and the frictional damage would be very small for each impact of the foot on the surface, the cumulative effect would be significant. As has been emphasized, stability analysis does not provide all the information necessary to understand the pathogenesis, but does indicate the necessary conditions for damage to occur.

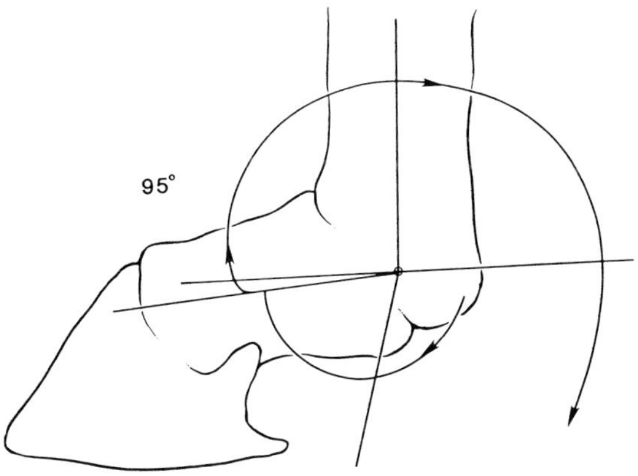

10.14. The fetlock joint is unstable when dorsiflexed beyond its normal anatomical range, 95° here. The behavior of the middle and distal interphalangeal joints is essentially identical to that of the fetlock.

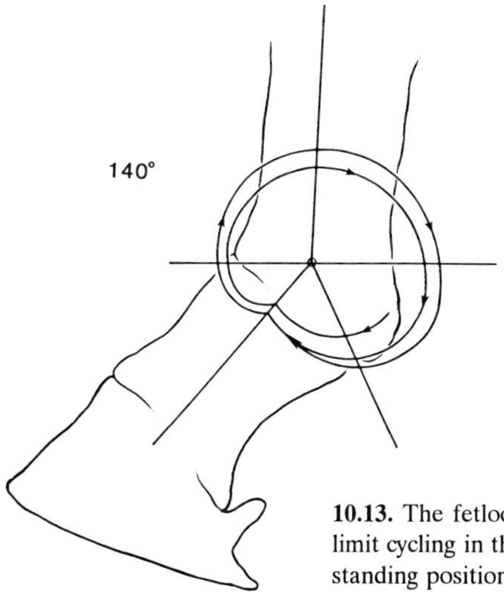

10.13. The fetlock joint is limit cycling in the normal standing position.

Pathogenesis, general

Unstable is undesirable. The potential for instability is either reduced or controlled by trajectories forming or joining limit cycles. This is accomplished by dissipation and/or storage of energy. There can be too slow/inadequate storage of energy as a result of muscular fatigue, for example. There can be too little dissipation (damping) of energy as the "radiator" system of the leg becomes too hot—the rate of energy production exceeding the ability of the system to store or dissipate that energy. There can be too much energy delivered to the system as with a jumping horse or a misstep with overloading of a leg. The control of energy, then, is basic to proper function of the system. In most cases instability of the horse is structural in character. Loss of ordinary stability (initial conditions) characterizes neurological disease.

Earlier studies (Rooney 1969) have suggested that third-order (abnormal) acceleration and entropy are useful concepts in the pathogenesis of lameness. The entropy equation stated that the time behavior of applied and resisting forces described the overall pathogenesis of the lesions of lameness. Abnormal acceleration provided the physical damaging mechanism. Stability theory incorporates both of those theories, as well as a modification of the entropy equation (Rooney 1991b). The trajectories of the system in the phase plane describe the energy relationships. The asymptotic trajectories indicate that energy is being dissipated from or stored in the system. Limit cycles indicate that energy is stored in the musculotendinous system during the first part of support and recovered during the second part: self-excited limit cycling.

Unstable trajectories, specifically those seen with individual joint segments, show that too much energy is present for stable or cycling behavior. As already indicated, there may be too much energy delivered in unit time, or the energy may not be properly stored or dissipated, in unit time.

Gait–lesion–gait principle

This principle was formulated by Rooney (1969): *The gait abnormality caused by a specific lesion is the gait abnormality which caused the lesion.* The gait abnormality may be obvious to the unaided eye, such as the toe-first impact characteristic of navicular disease or more subtle, for example, the slope change, third-order acceleration, of the leg with bowed tendon (Dow et al. 1991). A number of examples have been given in Rooney. Certain lesions, such as arthrosis of the carpus, are not obvious examples of the principle but are expected to fit when examined by more sophisticated analyses such as that for bowed tendon (Dow et al. 1991).

In terms of stability theory, the gait–lesion–gait principle may be restated. The unstable state leads to and is synonymous with the damaged state. Once damaged, and until repair is completed, the system remains unstable. Thus, the gait-lesion-gait principle is the overt, clinical manifestation of the unstable state and the damage inevitable with that state.

CHAPTER 11

Female Reproductive System

Ovary
- Normal
- Cystic
- Hemorrhage

Oviduct
- Collagen masses
- Retention of eggs

Uterus
- Endometritis
- Metritis/pyometra
- Neoplasia
- Rupture of the uterine, ovarian, iliac arteries

Vagina
- Coital exanthema
- Contagious equine metritis
- Neoplasia

Hypocalcemic tetany

Rupture of the prepubic tendon

Embryonic and fetal loss
- Normal placental variations

Hippomanes

Loss up to 4 months

4- to 6-month loss

Bacterial septicemia

Undetermined

6- to 11-month loss

Leptospiral abortion

Bacterial and mycotic placentitis

Chronic placental insufficiency

Twin pregnancy

Chorionic villous hypoplasia

Body pregnancy

Chronic placentitis

Premature aging

Amnion

Viral abortion

Salmonella abortus-equi

Mycobacterium spp.

Fescue toxicity

Extrauterine pregnancy

Ovary

Normal

The ovary of the mare is covered by peritoneum except at the ovulation fossa. The medulla and cortex are not clearly demarcated, the ovary comprising tracts of highly cellular connective tissue with follicles scattered throughout. While the connective tissue of the ovary does not appear organized, careful examination and the ovulation pathways show radial organization from the capsule toward the ovulation fossa (Zietzschmann and Krölling 1955). The radial organization is clearest in the young ovary.

The fetal ovary is small before about 40 days, at which time it grows rapidly because of the proliferation of lipid-rich interstitial cells. True ovarian tissue is present as a thin, subcapsular rim, which is white as compared to the olive green of the interstitial cellular tissue. The fetal ovary is as large as the fetal kidney and often larger than the ovaries of the mare. Both fetal ovary and testis are not infrequently mistaken for kidneys. Aristotle (Peck 1979) made the mistake. During the later stages of pregnancy the interstitial cells regress and are nearly gone at birth. The small neonatal ovary shows the future site of the ovulation fossa. Continued growth and differentiation during the first 2 months converts the ovary to a small adult form with a distinct elliptical ovulation fossa. Growth continues slowly, but without follicular activity until about 1 year. Some yearling fillies, in the spring and early summer, may show one or two small follicles. Rarely, a filly may show multiple, large follicles at this time without overt signs of estrus.

By 2 years of age the ovary is adult size. It is usually small, firm, and inactive during the anestrous period. During the spring and summer variable degrees of follicular activity are seen, depending upon the phase of the estrous cycle at the time of death. The follicles are variable in size and can be very large.

A follicle enlarges, pushing against the capsule and driving its way along the radial pathways of connective tissue toward the ovulation fossa. Depending upon the distance from the capsule at which the follicle begins to develop, there is either a marked, fluctuating bulging of the capsule or only a slight, hardly palpable fluctuant area. When the follicle reaches the ovulation fossa and ruptures, the tense capsule collapses and reexpands as the cavity fills with blood—the corpus hemorrhagicum. There is no evidence that ovulation ever occurs other than through the ovulation fossa.

The path of the follicle to the ovulation fossa is tortuous and can be reconstructed by serial slices of the ovary. Mares ovulate from the left ovary 60% of the time (McEntee 1985). Brendecke (1926) noted that the left ovary, on average, was 1.3 times heavier than the right.

As corpora hemorrhagica form, they bulge, buttonlike, into the ovulation fossa, often with strands of the fimbriated end of the oviduct entrapped in the bulge. These strands are to be differentiated from a fine network of fibrin lying on the surface of the button and adhering to the walls of the ovulation fossa.

The ovary is of variable appearance at any given time during its active months. In the pregnant mare up to 45–50 days, one large corpus luteum will be present. In addition, there may be regressing corpora lutea from a prior estrus, and deeply pigmented, linear traces of corpora lutea from even earlier estrous periods, **corpora atretica**. As well there may be one or more variable, but small, follicles in one or both ovaries. Corpora albicans are described in the equine ovary (Ginther 1992). It is certainly the case that the corpus luteum regresses, becoming narrower and more deeply colored as regression proceeds to disappearance. While an argument in semantics, the regressing corpus luteum does not become white, so that the term *albicans* is inaccurate, *atretica* perhaps being preferable.

As day 50 approaches numerous small follicles develop on one or both ovaries. After about 50 days there is the primary corpus luteum, few follicles, and one or more supplementary corpora lutea. The corpora lutea remain until about 150 days when they regress along with the primary corpus luteum. Work cited by Ginther (1992) clearly shows that the primary corpus luteum does not regress at 50 days, as previously believed. For the remainder of pregnancy the ovary appears inactive, perhaps with a few small follicles.

One often sees small, usually linear, luteinized foci close to the ovulation fossa. Their origin is not known. They may simply be small follicles, which have either ovulated or are undergoing partial luteinization and atresia. They might be the source of the numbers of eggs that can frequently be recovered from the oviducts (Van Niekerk and Gerneke 1966).

Cystic

As mares age the pieces of fimbria entrapped and drawn into the ovulation fossa by the contraction of succeeding generations of corpora hemorrhagica may form **inclusion cysts** in greater or lesser numbers. These cysts bulge into the fossa or, more deeply placed, cause a slitted appearance of the surface of the fossa. The cysts are distinguishable from follicles by their location, small size, and white, opaque lining. Follicles generally have a glistening, pink, velvety lining with the perifollicular blood vessels showing through. Microscopically, the cyst lining is a flattened epithelial layer, often with areas of cuboidal or columnar cells, which may be ciliated. Some, presumably early, cysts are completely lined with ciliated, columnar epithelium (O'Shea 1968; Rooney 1970). The follicle, on the other hand, is lined by columnar epithelium and several layers of spheroid to polyhedral cells.

O'Shea (1968), working with ovaries of unknown age, suggested such cysts derived from ingrowth of the columnar epithelium of the cranial aspect of the ovulation fossa, an epithelium ciliated like that of the fimbriated end of the oviduct, and possibly of Müllerian duct origin. While O'Shea's observations are convincing, it is difficult to understand why these cysts adjacent to the ovulation fossa increase in number with age. That is explained if the cysts originate from the fimbriated end of the oviduct. Further study is required. It is possible that cysts arise by both mechanisms.

It is suggested that the cysts, if present in sufficient numbers, block or delay the passage of the ovum, so that it is nonviable when it reaches the oviduct. McEntee (1990) presented a case where large numbers of such cysts had destroyed much of the normal ovarian parenchyma, and agrees that large numbers of such cysts can block ovulation.

There is no bona fide evidence for pathological **cystic ovary** in the mare. Clinical evidence, however, indicates that follicles may persist for considerable periods of time. New follicles continue to form, the ovary becoming a mass of varying size follicles. This can be called: **follicular detention/retention syndrome**. A sufficiently dense mass of inclusion cysts could be one cause for such retention. Clinical evidence indicates that many of these ovaries eventually return to normal, probably as the follicles undergo atresia.

The pathologist cannot confirm a diagnosis of "cystic ovary," only that there are numerous follicles in the ovary. It is for the clinician to say "follicular detention/retention syndrome."

Hemorrhage

Hemorrhage into follicles, as distinct from corpora hemorrhagica, have been reported (Ginther 1992). They are more frequent in the autumn and are associated with, perhaps causing, anovulatory periods. The cause is not known.

Ovulation sclerosis

As in other species, ovulation sclerosis occurs in the arteries of the equine ovary (Cohrs 1961) (Fig. 11.1). There is fibrous tissue thickening of the intima with elastosis, fragmentation, and reduplication of the internal elastic lamina. In old, multiparous mares the muscle of the media may be largely replaced with fibrous tissue and irregular elastic tissue strands. This occurs in the extraovarian part of the ovarian artery, as well as in the extrauterine course of the uterine arteries and, to a lesser extent, in the arteries within the muscular wall of the uterus. Since there are few muscular arteries within the endometrium, the change is not seen there. The relationship of these changes to prepartum and postpartum rupture of these vessels will be discussed with the uterus, below (Popp 1940).

Paraovarian cysts

Paraovarian cysts, remnants of the Müllerian and Wolffian ducts, are routinely present and of any size from barely perceptible to fist size. The Müllerian (Morgagni) remnants are in the fimbria, while the Wolffian duct remnants are in the mesosalpinx. They are of no functional significance. Small, firm, brownish masses of accessory adrenal cortical tissue may be found in the mesovarium. Ono et al. (1969) found these masses, many very small, in 59% of the mares examined, a high figure in our experience.

Ovarian tumors

Ovarian tumors, specifically **granulosa cell tumors**, are seen with some frequency in mares (Fig. 11.2). They may be encountered incidentally at postmortem or discovered by rectal examination. In some cases there is a history of infertility, and

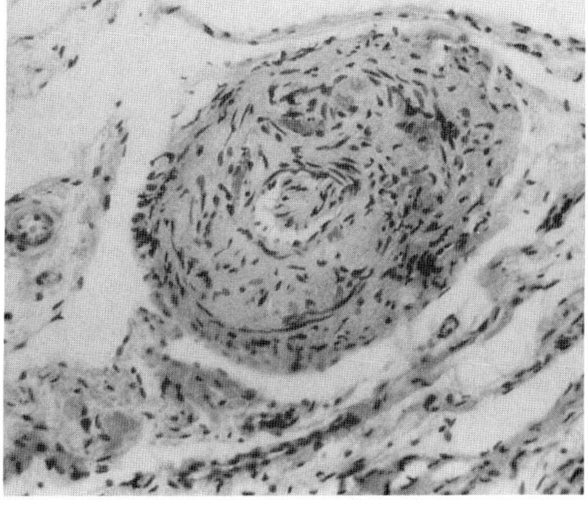

11.1. Middle power, H & E of artery with senile elastotic degeneration. Endometrium.

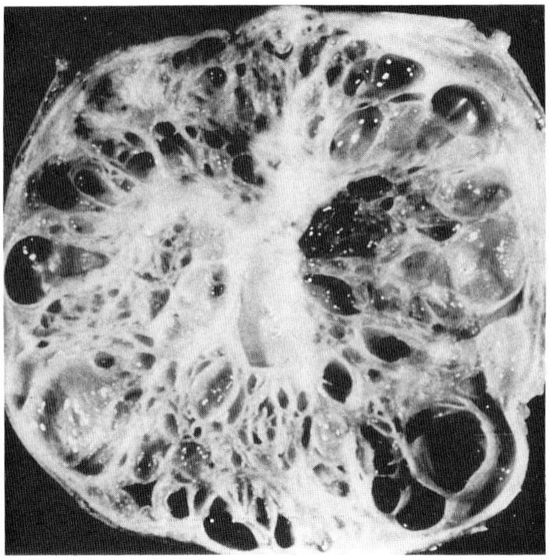

11.2. Granulosa cell tumor.

the tumor is removed. There have been few follow-up studies of the breeding performance of such mares. Meagher et al. (1977) found that 30 of 39 mares from which the tumor had been removed, and that were bred, produced live foals. Metastasis or recurrence have not occurred in our experience, and McEntee (1990) indicates that malignancy is rare. These tumors have long been recognized in mares (Debrade 1892/93). McEntee found 45 granulosa cell tumors, 3 dysgerminomas, 2 teratomas, 1 cystadenoma, and 1 malignant lymphoma, among 52 equine ovarian tumors.

The granulosa cell tumor may be quite small, up to lobulated masses larger than a soccer ball. On section the tumor comprises multiloculated cysts with clear, yellow fluid or blood in a moderate fibrous stroma. Histologically, the cysts are usually lined by flattened epithelium, but areas with characteristic granulosa cells can be found.

Oviduct

The oviduct is remarkably free of pathological changes. A few cases of unilateral hydrosalpinx of undetermined cause have been seen. Henry and Vanderplassche (1981) found no example of hydrosalpinx in 2297 reproductive tracts. They did find a high frequency of adhesions in the infundibulum, more often on the right. In no case was the infundibulum obstructed by the adhesions, which are probably the result of organizing hemorrhage as discussed above. Focal or light and diffuse infiltrations of lymphocytes in the epithelium and lamina propria are not uncommon and may or may not represent inflammation (Henry and Vanderplassche 1981).

Collagen masses

Collagen masses have been reported in the oviduct in 20%–87% of mares (Van Niekerk and Gerneke 1966; Liu et al. 1990). The masses were globular, white, and free in the lumen. There were no changes in the oviduct itself. The source of the masses was not determined. Oguri and Tsutsumi (1972) and Van Niekerk and Gerneke (1966) thought they arose from gelatinous material in the follicles. Onuma and Ohnami (1975) saw similar masses thought to derive from tubular epithelium. Neither explanation is consistent with the presence of collagen fibers in the masses. One may speculate that they arise from the organizing of the fibrin that is regularly deposited on the buttonlike surface of the corpora hemorrhagica. The somewhat greater frequency of these masses in older mares is consistent with that speculation. The significance, if any, of these masses in the migration of ova within the oviduct is unclear.

Retention of eggs

Retention of eggs in the oviduct is apparently a normal, unexplained phenomenon in mares, as reported and discussed by a number of authors (Ginther 1992; McEntee 1990).

Uterus

The young endometrium is grayish red with small, soft, velvety folds. With age the endometrium becomes whiter, even translucent or transparent, the folds atrophy and may disappear, and there can be varying degrees of gross and microscopic cystic change (Fig. 11.2).

From about 45 to 150 days of gestation, numerous, elevated, whitish-gray **endometrial cups** are present at the junction of the uterine horn and body. They disappear about 100 to 150 days as the allantochorial villi form and implantation occurs. After the period of embryonic wandering the initial contact of yolk sac placenta is at the junction of body and horn (Ginther 1992).

Gygax et al. (1979) studied the postpartum involution of the uterus, showing that the microcotyledons within the uterine endometrium disappear in about 7 days. The microcotyledons underwent karyolytic and pyknotic changes (apoptosis) and quickly disappeared, usually without significant inflammatory reaction. Steven et al. (1979) provided ultrastructural details of the involuting uterus.

Endometritis

There are two forms of endometritis in the mare. **Acute endometritis** typically is seen in younger mares. The endometrium is hyperemic, perhaps with scattered petechial hemorrhages. The normally small amount of clear, glistening fluid is increased and gray-white, flaky, or frankly purulent. Histologically, there is marked infiltration of neutrophil leucocytes into the endometrium and lumen. Any one of a variety of infectious agents may be present, for example, *Streptococcus, Klebsiella, Pseudomonas,* or *Rhodococcus.* The infections usually are self-limiting, the uterus returning to normal in a few days to a week.

The second type is usually called **chronic endometritis**, although **recurrent endometritis** may be more appropriate. The endometrium resembles that of acute endometritis, but the hyperemia is patchier: reddish areas interspersed with white or gray areas. The normal small amount of clear, glistening fluid is somewhat increased and contains yellow or white flakes of inspissated purulent material. In keeping with the incidence in older mares, endometrial folds are reduced or absent in areas, and cysts may be present. Unlike acute endometritis, recurrent endometritis persists for long periods of time. Treatment may affect clinical recovery, only to have reinfection at the next estrus.

The argument for recurrent rather than chronic is that chronic infection implies the continued presence of an organism or agent that is not readily removed or destroyed, for example, fungi, *Mycobacteria.* In recurrent endometritis, the infecting agents are the same as in acute endometritis and not necessarily persistent. They may be cleared from the uterus, only to reinfect shortly thereafter. It would appear that either the uterine defense mechanisms cannot rid the endometrium of these agents or cannot prevent reinfection, for example, during estrus.

While the *lesions* produced by these infections may, indeed, be chronic, it may be, in any given case, misleading to say that the *infection* is chronic. Kenney (1978) correlated reproductive effectiveness and biopsies of the endometrium of mares. He grouped the changes into three categories: normal, affected, and severely affected. The changes included inflammatory cell infiltration with neutrophils and with mononuclear/lymphoid cells, particularly in the more severe cases. In the affected and severely affected categories there was increasing fibrosis of the endometrium, particularly periglandular fibrosis, and increasing numbers and size of glandular cysts. Atrophy—loss of glands and thinning of the endometrium—increased in severity in parallel with the other changes. Kenney's criteria and classification facilitate clinical evaluation and prognosis and are compatible with the statements made above (Fig. 11.2).

Perineal conformation as a predisposing factor for endometrial infection has long been recognized. When the anus is farther forward than the vulva, postevacuation drippings from the anus provide a supply of infectious material. While such conformation develops in older, multiparous mares, it also occurs frequently in young Thoroughbred mares as a conformation defect.

Metritis/pyometra

These are uncommon in mares. A particularly dangerous form of metritis is that associated with near-term or term *E. coli* infection. The fetus has lesions of septicemia and startling hemorrhagic enteritis. All layers of the uterus are intensely hemorrhagic, and the lumen contains bloody fluid. *E. coli* are present in large numbers. This can be rapidly fatal. *E. coli* may invade damaged tissues following a difficult parturition with similar results.

Mares rarely develop frank pyometra. A few cases have been seen with thick, yellow-white, tenacious viscid material filling and distending the uterus. Cultures were negative in these few cases and histology offered no insights as to cause.

Neoplasia

Tumors are rare. We have only seen small leiomyomas at autopsy, often previously recognized by rectal examination. Cohrs (1961) mentioned a case of carcinoma with multiple implantation metastases on the peritoneum.

Rupture of the uterine, ovarian, iliac arteries

Prepartum and postpartum rupture of these arteries appears to be unique to the mare (Rooney 1964). The ovarian artery may rupture about the 7th month of pregnancy, while the uterine and internal or external iliac arteries rupture during parturition. Rupture of the uterine artery is by far the most common, followed by the ovarian. Rupture of the external and internal iliac arteries is much less common (Martin 1899/1900). The ruptures are distinctly age related, the probability increasing with each succeeding pregnancy beyond 10 years of age (Meyer 1948). In keeping with the higher frequency of right horn pregnancy, the right uterine and ovarian arteries are more often ruptured.

The clinical picture is acute, hemorrhagic shock immediately after a usually uneventful foaling. Martin's one case of rupture of the internal iliac followed dystocia. The mare may die very quickly or appear to recover for 24 hours, only to lapse once more into profound shock and die. An occasional animal survives rupture of the uterine artery and may repeat the process, fatally, in a subsequent year. We have seen no example of survival after rupture of the ovarian or iliac artery. The mare that survives has a heavily encapsulated hematoma in the broad ligament, which can be found up to 2 years after the event either by rectal examination or at postmortem. Some of these mares fail to conceive again, but, given their years, the cause of the infertility cannot be certainly related to the hematoma.

At postmortem the carcass is anemic and large quantities of unclotted and partially clotted blood escape from the peritoneal cavity. A massive hematoma is present: cranial third of the broad ligament with ovarian artery, middle third with uterine artery, lateral retroperitoneal with external iliac artery, and dorsal retroperitoneal and pelvic with internal iliac artery rupture. Careful examination shows that the hematoma has split open, releasing blood into the peritoneal cavity.

The clinical picture correlates with these findings. The initial shock occurs with the hemorrhage and formation of the hematoma within the confines of the serosal membranes. Apparent recovery occurs as the pressure exerted by the membranes on the hematoma increases, slowing the outflow of blood, followed by fatal relapse as the membrane splits open and massive bleeding resumes.

The site of rupture may be found by tracing the relevant arteries. Relationships are best maintained and the process facilitated if the dissection is done with the urogenital tract in situ. When it appears that the internal iliac artery is affected, the dissection must be done in situ, tediously removing the pubis and ilium as necessary for adequate exposure.

With ovarian and uterine artery rupture the lesion can be found by finger dissection into the largest point of the hematoma, searching for dry, brown, friable strands and lumps of fibrin. These are followed by careful blunt dissection and lead directly to the site of rupture. The latter is usually a simple longitudinal split of the wall, but may be a berry aneurysm that has split open, in both cases with fibrin adherent to the margins (Fig. 11.3).

Histologically, there are multiple focal areas of moderate to marked intimal fibrosis and elastosis (Fig. 11.3). The media is usually thinner than normal. These changes are seen both at the rupture site and elsewhere. In the few cases in the iliac arteries, there is infiltration of neutrophilic inflammatory cells into a normal or moderately thickened intima. The damage in these particular vessels may be caused by partial or complete occlusion of the vessels, with mechanical damage to the intima just before and during parturition.

The lesions in the arteries are clearly senile, aging changes as found in all species with repeated pregnancies (Popp 1940). The predilection of the mare for catastrophic rupture can be related to the advanced ages at which they are bred and the violence of the foaling process. Copper deficiency has been bruited as predisposing, but there is no evidence.

Vagina

The vestibule, vulva, and vagina suffer parturient injuries of startling variety. The **vestibular bulbs**, in the lateral walls of the vagina, are frequently engorged with blood, bulging into the vaginal lumen, in mares dying in shock. Remnants of the hymen may be apparent. Complete, **persistent hymen** is very rare and associated with aseptic

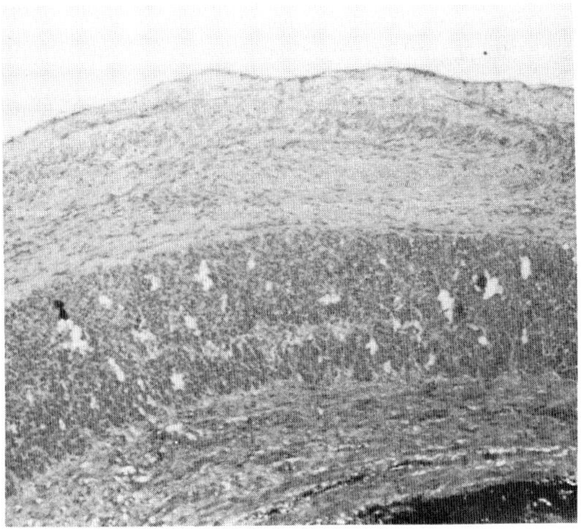

11.3. Low power, H & E of uterine artery with marked endarteritis obliterans, thickening of the intima (*above*) with fibrous tissue.

hydrometra. McEntee (1990) says that, "complete hymen is the most common major congenital defect of the tubular genital system of the mare. . . ." While that may be true, congenital defects of any sort are exceedingly rare in the genital tract of the mare.

Coital exanthema

This disease, caused by equine herpesvirus (EHV)-3, is usually transmitted by breeding. The incubation period is about 3-6 days, but, rarely, can occur within 24–48 hours or as long as 10–11 days (Hutyra and Marek 1920; Krogsrud and Onstad 1971).

There is reddening and, exceptionally, petechial hemorrhages in the vagina, around the clitoris, and on the inside of the vulva. In the horse the lesions appear around the urethral opening and, less commonly, on the inner surface of the prepuce, and the surrounding skin. Lesions may occur on the mouth and nostrils as well.

Within 2-3 days vesicles appear in the reddened, swollen membranes. Small grayish nodules may also appear, which later become vesicles. The vesicles become purulent and burst to form yellowish or brownish erosions or ulcerations. The erosions heal completely, while the ulcers heal with smooth, white scar tissue, which later becomes yellowish red. Histologically, there is hydropic, ballooning degeneration of the epithelium, with infiltration of neutrophils and lymphomononuclear cells, particularly in the vicinity of solitary lymphoid nodules (Cohrs 1961). The regional lymph nodes may be enlarged. Uncomplicated cases heal in 2–4 weeks.

Contagious equine metritis

There is a voluminous literature on this condition; we confine ourselves to pathology. Platt et al. (1978) described the lesions in experimental cases, while Ricketts et al. (1978) studied the lesions by serial biopsy in natural cases. No lesions have been reported in the carrier stallion. The mare develops an acute endometritis, characterized by proliferation, vacuolation, and necrosis of the uterine epithelium with infiltration of neutrophils. The process is most marked toward the tips of the uterine horns. Small foci of neutrophils may be found in the fimbriated end of the oviduct. The epithelial changes are limited to the surface, not extending into the uterine glands. There may be variable amounts of edema in the uterine wall and purulent exudate in the lumen. Focal accumulations of mononuclear cells, lymphocytes, plasma cells, and eosinophils appear as the acute inflammatory response subsides. The mononuclear cell accumulations can persist for some months after experimental infection. The course of the inflammatory process was that expected with any bacterial infection (Acland and Kenney 1983).

Neoplasia

Tumors of the vagina and vulva are very rare, only an occasional squamous cell carcinoma of the vulva has been seen and only in aged mares. Varicose veins in the vagina are discussed with the cardiovascular system (see Chapter 1, "Cardiovascular System").

Hypocalcemic tetany

This has been seen most frequently in the pregnant mare; it is uncommon in the modern era. There is muscle fibrillation, tonic-clonic spasms, neighing, pressing against objects, pawing, and sweating. It appears when the mare is put up in a box before foaling, during the nursing period, or at the time of weaning. Railroad transport was said to precipitate the condition. Hutyra and Marek (1920) suggested sudden decrease of food intake, together with calcium loss in the milk as causative. They reported normal serum calcium of about 13 mg/dl with levels of 4.9%–6% in affected mares. No pathological studies have been reported.

Rupture of the prepubic tendon

This is illustrated in older texts but hardly discussed. Williams (1905/06) indicated that it was more often seen in well-fed, pregnant draft mares. We have seen no case in light horses. Preuss et al. (1972) described the anatomy of the prepubic area and inguinal region of the horse in detail. The **prepubic tendon**, per se, is formed by crossing fibers of the tendons of origin of the pectineus and adductor longus muscles with contributions from the external oblique, gracilis, obturator, and an inconstant portion of the internal oblique. The rectus abdominis does not primarily insert on the prepubic tendon, as stated by Sisson and Grossman (1953). Rather, the tendons of insertion of the rectus abdominis cross to form the **accessory ligaments** of the hip joints, joined by a large component of fibers from the external abdominal oblique, the tunica flava abdominis, and deep pelvic fascia. The rectus tendons also insert indirectly on the pelvis as part of the prepubic tendon (Habel and Budras 1992).

In light of these findings the suggestion of Preuss et al. (1972) that the *Lig. accessorium ossis femoris*—accessory ligament—should be *Tendo femoralis recti* may be apropos. Habel and Budras present evidence for retaining the older name. Rupture of the prepubic tendon, then, is a misnomer, the rupture primarily affecting the components of the *Tendo femoralis recti* cranial to the pubis.

The insertion of the rectus abdominis, much of the external abdominal oblique, and the tunica flava abdominis into the head of the femur via the *Tendo femoralis recti* is unique to the horse among animals examined. The other Perissodactyla would be of interest. Preuss et al. (1972) make several functional suggestions, including that contraction of the rectus and external oblique could assist the ventroflexion of the lumbosacral area during galloping. While that may be true, the iliopsoas would appear to play a larger role.

The attachment to the moveable head of the femur, rather than directly to stationary bone, provides for greater *play* in a muscular system subjected to the heavy, fluctuating load of the abdominal viscera, a view consistent with the well-developed tunica flava abdominis. *Play* means that fluctuating loads on the rectus and external oblique would cause rotation of the head of the femur, a rotation resisted by the muscles around the hip joint. The fluctuating load, then, would be equilibrated not only by the abdominal muscles, but by muscles around the hip joint. Although the amount of energy dealt with may be small, energy peaks during movement could be of sufficient magnitude to compromise tendon directly inserted into bone rather than into the moveable femoral head.

Embryonic and fetal loss

Embryonic and fetal losses occur during three overlapping periods: before 4 months, at 4–6 months, and at 6–11 months. The last period overlaps the neonatal period, which is considered separately. Overall loss is about 10% of all mares bred or about 12.5% of all mares diagnosed pregnant (Ginther 1992). While an anatomical diagnosis can be made in about 50%–60% of abortions, an etiological diagnosis is less often achieved.

Normal placental variations

First are common gross and microscopic features of the placenta, not to be mistaken for abortion-related pathological changes. Whitwell and Jeffcott (1975) provided a detailed description of the term placenta.

That portion of the chorion applied to the internal os of the cervix is devoid of villi and generally white to gray-white. There are often irregular gray thickenings as well as hyperemic patches. Similar, though smaller, bare areas are found at the tips of the horns, the uterine orifices of the oviducts. Oikawa et al. (1990) mistook these for pathological changes. The tips of the horns, particularly the pregnant horn, are often thickened with fluid of no known significance.

Small, 0.1–1.0 cm, bare foci may be scattered at random over the chorial surface. They have raised, irregular brownish centers of homogenous necrotic debris and may be calcified. There can be areas where the allantochorion appears to have folded upon itself, tucking in the chorial surface (Fig. 11.4). The fold can, with care, be pulled out, revealing chorial surfaces devoid of villi. The lack of villi here, as with the cervical star and tips of the horns and with twin placentation, indicates that contact between developing chorion and endometrium is necessary for villous formation (Ginther 1992).

Autolytic changes of the placenta are important. When abortion occurs soon after death of the fetus the chorial villous surface is velvety red with a reasonably uniform texture. With autolysis, whether within the uterus or after expulsion, this surface becomes brown and dry. This will be considered further with the term foal. A small quantity of viscid, reddish material is normally present on the chorial surface of the term placenta.

Hippomanes

The allantoic surface may be smooth and unremarkable or have one or more polyploid

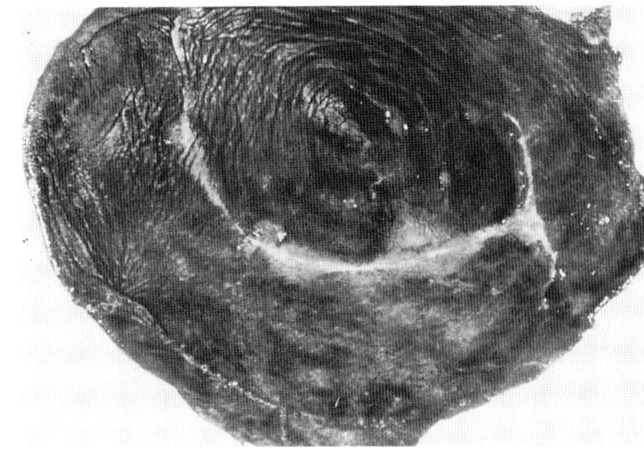

11.4. Allantochorion with folds devoid of villi.

whitish or grayish masses of varying size. Hippomanes are common in the allantoic cavity. According to Zietschmann and Krölling (1955), after Thieke (1911), three forms of hippomane may be distinguished:

1. Single, fingerlike outpouchings of the allantoic epithelium. There is serous content within the mesenchymal-connective tissue wall, which is surrounded by allantoic epithelium. With attenuation of the stalk, the pouch undergoes necrosis and becomes encrusted with salts of the allantoic fluid, becoming the classic hippomane (no. 3, below). Similar outpouchings form in response to regressing endometrial cups. Thieke (1911) provided numerous photographs and drawings of this type of developing hippomane.
2. A warty, verrucose, often stalked outpouching of the allantochorion. The loose, outer allantoic epithelium surrounds a tight connective tissue layer, with chorionic epithelium in turn surrounding a mass of proliferated chorionic epithelium and connective tissue, which undergoes degeneration. This appears as a dent on the chorionic surface and is less frequent than the fingerlike outpouchings (no. 1).
3. Flat, somewhat rounded, more or less olive bodies, which take origin from the outpouchings (see no. 1) of the allantoic surface. These are usually found free in the allantoic fluid but take their origin as described for no. 1. Once the stalk is sufficiently attenuated it tears or disappears, the hippomane floating free in the allantoic cavity. Triple phosphate, oxalic acid, and uric acid accumulate on the surface, increasing the size of the hippomane. This form of the hippomane was known to Aristotle and often described since that time [Ruine (1603) cited by Thieke (1911)].

The sloughing endometrial cups may be enclosed in folds of allantoic epithelium (Zietzschmann and Krölling 1955; Whitwell and Jeffcott 1975; Ginther 1992). These polypoid structures are located near the junction of the body and pregnant horn, the area of the endometrial cups. They contain amorphous necrotic debris, as compared to the serous content of those outpouchings that form elsewhere on the allantoic surface.

Dickerson et al. (1967) and King (1967) have a different version of the formation of the type of hippomane described in no. 3: that it is an allantoic calculus not derived from the pouches as described by Thieke (1911). Our observations support the Thieke mechanism since we have seen type 1 pouches with attenuated stalks, necrosis, and salt encrustation, as shown in Figure 142 of Zietzschmann and Krölling, one of the several illustrations from Thieke, and one of our cases (Fig. 11.5). It is possible that hippomanes may form by both mechanisms.

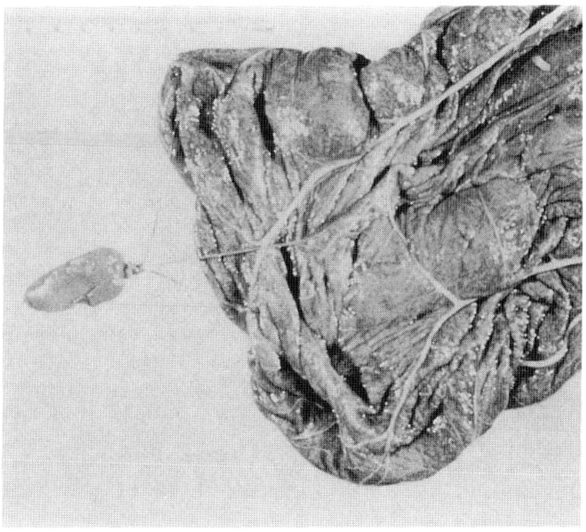

11.5. Hippomane developing from the allantoic surface of the allantochorion.

The surface of the umbilical cord is often studded with calcified plaques, polyps, and, occasionally, a large pedunculated ball composed of plates of calcium and coarse-fiber bone. This is often mistaken for a fetus but apparently is a remnant of the yolk sac. The other changes probably are of the same nature as the type 1 and 2 structures described above. In any event, they have no abortifacient potential.

A frosting of lacy, whitish granular material may be adherent to the surface of the amnion, as well as the skin of the unhaired fetus. This is crystalline material precipitated from the amniotic fluid and is of no known pathological significance.

The umbilical cord is normally twisted, and the postmortem pooling of blood in the loops can be striking. Statements in the literature to the contrary notwithstanding, there is no evidence that twisting of the cord, no matter how startling, is abortifacient. Rarely, the umbilical cord may be wrapped around the neck or a leg with clear evidence of passive vascular stasis both in the cord and the strangulated part. This certainly is a lethal and rare cause of abortion.

Histological changes of the allantochorion are not uncommon and increase with advancing age of the placenta. It is to be remembered that the placenta has an 11-month life span and, so, is expected to show aging changes. Degeneration and fusion of villi, thrombosis and necrosis of small blood vessels in the villi, and hyalinization of vessel walls and the connective tissue stroma are all common. Antemortem, dystrophic calcification is focal, occurring in and often obscuring necrotic vessels and villi. Postmortem or agonal calcification is common and more diffusely scattered, often appearing as plugs in the placental blood vessels. The media of many muscular arteries of the amnion and allantochorion normally contain lakes or islands of basophilic, metachromatic material similar to that in the interstitium of the amnion and allantochorion.

Loss up to 4 months

While the numbers vary from year to year, an average of 5%–10% of mares in foal at 45 days will be barren at 150 days. Recent studies have shown that the loss between conception and 45 days is even higher. Pathology has little to offer since most of the concepta are not found. Of the few examined between 45 and 150 days, most were found in the vagina and all partially decomposed. Bacteria, primarily *Streptococcus zooepidemicus,* were cultured and the tissues saturated with organisms without inflammatory reaction. This does not establish bacterial infection as the cause of death and abortion of the fetus, since bacteria are always present in the environment and invade the fetus after death once the cervix opens.

The strikingly large gonads of the equine fetus have been mentioned. They increase in size from about 30 up to a maximum at about 60 days and regress slowly to term. The enlargement is largely by proliferation of interstitial cells that closely resemble luteal cells. Although there have been studies on the structure, biochemistry, and hormonal content of these cells, their function is unknown (Cole et al. 1933). The decrease in size occurs as the interstitial cells undergo degenerative, apoptotic changes.

4- to 6-month loss

There are three groups: a small number of twins, small numbers of bacterial septicemias and/or placentitis, and, the largest group, cause undetermined. Twin abortion is commoner after 6 months and will be discussed below.

Bacterial septicemia

The fetus usually has so-called fetal diarrhea and is obviously septicemic with yellowish red, dirty discoloration of the tissues. *Fetal diarrhea* is a nonspecific sign of fetal distress, invariably anoxic in origin, and present whenever asphyxia occurred before abortion. It has no specific etiological significance. Petechiae are present on serosal and mucosal surfaces. There may be diffuse, intense hyperemia of the mucosa of the gastrointestinal tract, lungs, spleen, and other organs, including synovial membranes. There is minimal evidence of decomposition, suggesting abortion during the agonal period or immediately after death.

The histological picture is dominated by hemorrhage, variable numbers of largely intravascular bacteria, and scattered ischemic necrosis in such organs as the liver and spleen. There is little or no cellular inflammatory reaction. Pure, sometimes mixed, cultures of abortifacient pathogens are usually obtained, for example, *S. zooepidemicus.*

Streptococcus equi may be a cause. It is more commonly a cause of abortion if an outbreak of strangles is in progress. In younger fetuses it causes septicemia, death, and abortion. In older fetuses abscessation occurs in the liver, lungs, kidneys, small intestine, and mesenteric lymph nodes, but not in the cecum and large intestine (Cadeac 1899b).

The placenta usually has no clear-cut changes, at most hyperemia and a few hemorrhages in the allantochorion. Histologically, hemorrhages and bacterial colonies may be seen in and on the allantochorion.

Undetermined

The cause of the majority of abortions during this period cannot be determined. The fetus is variably decomposed. The least autolyzed are characterized by yellowish-red, muddy discoloration of the tissues, an hazy borderline between genuine septicemia and genuine autolysis. Histological examination usually distinguishes the two, but any given case may not be resolved. Even the isolation of acceptable pathogens cannot be taken as proof of antemortem septicemia/placentitis since postmortem invasion and contamination is common.

Advanced autolysis is characterized by exaggeration of the muddy, dirty appearance of the fetus. The liver is mushy, the abdominal viscera are blurred toward a uniform color, and there is dirty, red-tinged, hemolyzed fluid in the abdominal and thoracic cavities. Similar fluid infiltrates the loose connective tissues of the neck, head, and limbs.

Histological examination is usually fruitless if, indeed, any coherent sections can be obtained. The isolation of a pathogen may or may not be significant, with no way to make the distinction.

The waning of the corpora lutea, maintenance of pregnancy being assumed by placental hormones, occurs during this period, suggesting that these abortions are related to asynchrony of transfer (Hetzel 1936; Kostner 1948). The pathologist can offer no opinion.

6- to 11-month loss

Occasional decomposed fetuses overlap into this period. Most septicemic fetuses, however, are aborted in reasonably fresh condition with the lesions described. Placental lesions may be somewhat more obvious as splashes of hemorrhage on the chorial and allantoic surfaces. Hemorrhages on the allantoic surface alone are, however, agonal and anoxic. Bacteria can be isolated and usually found in considerable numbers in either or both allantochorion and fetal tissues. Ischemic necrosis of fetal tissues occurs, but inflammatory reaction is absent or slight, becoming more apparent during the 8–11-month period.

Leptospiral abortion

Various serovars of leptospira can cause sporadic abortion of mares (Ellis and O'Brien 1988). Infected mares may shed the organism in the urine for variable periods of time in the absence of clinical disease other than abortion. Epizootics in bands of mares have not been reported. Over several years in central Kentucky about 2%–3% of all abortions were attributable to leptospira. There are no specific gross lesions, and the diagnosis is not made unless fetuses are routinely examined for organisms. The organism may be stained in fetal tissues, specifically the kidney, with silver stains and fluorescent antibody, and some fetuses have an antibody titer. Cultural isolation is difficult. The epizootology is unclear, and most cases have been in mares not pastured with cattle or swine. It appears that most infection in adult horses is sporadic and subclinical, abortion occurring if the mare is in foal at the time of the subclinical infection.

With the unexplained disappearance of *Salmonella abortus-equi,* none of the bacterial agents cause epizootics.

Bacterial and mycotic placentitis

Bacterial and mycotic infections largely limited to the allantochorion occur during this period. The classic case is severe necrosis and ulceration of the chorial surface of the allantochorion, largely restricted to the area of the cervical star. The chorial lesion is sharply demarcated from the normal velvety chorial surface by a hemorrhagic border and characterized by yellowish-brown necrosis, denudation, and ulceration. A variable quantity of thick, viscid, tenacious, yellowish-brown or gray exudate adheres to the necrotic area. The exudate varies from barely perceptible with bacterial infection to voluminous with mycotic, *Aspergillus* spp., or mixed fungal and bacterial infections (Fig. 11.6).

The histology is dominated by massive necrosis of allantochorial tissue with variably heavy infiltration of polymorphonuclear leucocytes. Causative organisms are usually seen in routine sections, but special stains are helpful and, often, necessary.

Occasionally, this pattern is modified by apparent metastasis from the primary site at the cervical star to random sites over the chorial surface. In a few cases this random focal pattern may be seen without a marked lesion at the cervical star. This is particularly true of infection by *Histoplasma capsulatum* (Fig. 11.7), indicating hematogenous infection from a focus in the mare. Mycotic lesions of the skin or internal organs of the fetus are not common, with the exception of *H. capsulatum,* but do occur.

A variety of bacteria and fungi have been isolated (Dimock and Edwards 1932; Prickett 1967; Whitwell 1988). Among the fungi, aspergillus is most common (Hensel et al. 1961). It appears that by far the greatest number of such infections enter by the cervix. That, in turn, suggests that the pathogenesis of infectious placentitis (and septicemias) be sought in the route of infection rather than the infecting organism. It may be that the organism(s) involved happens to be the one present at the time the cervix is open. It is well known to veterinarians experienced with broodmares that the cervix does, indeed, open and close unpredictably during the latter months of pregnancy. Virtually nothing is known of this phenomenon, and it may be normal,

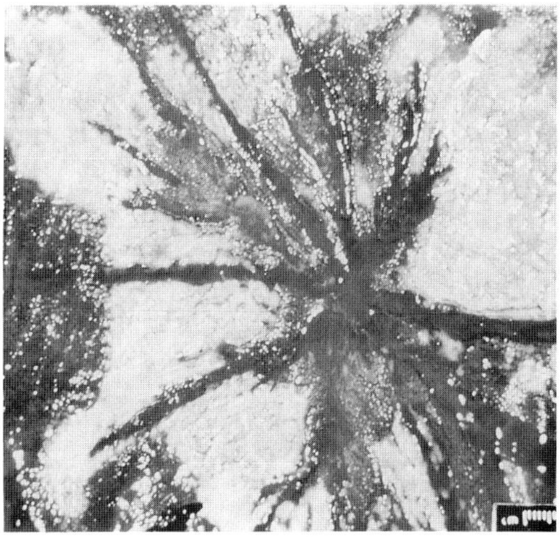

11.6. Mycotic placentitis. Yellow, necrotic masses at the cervical star of the allantochorion.

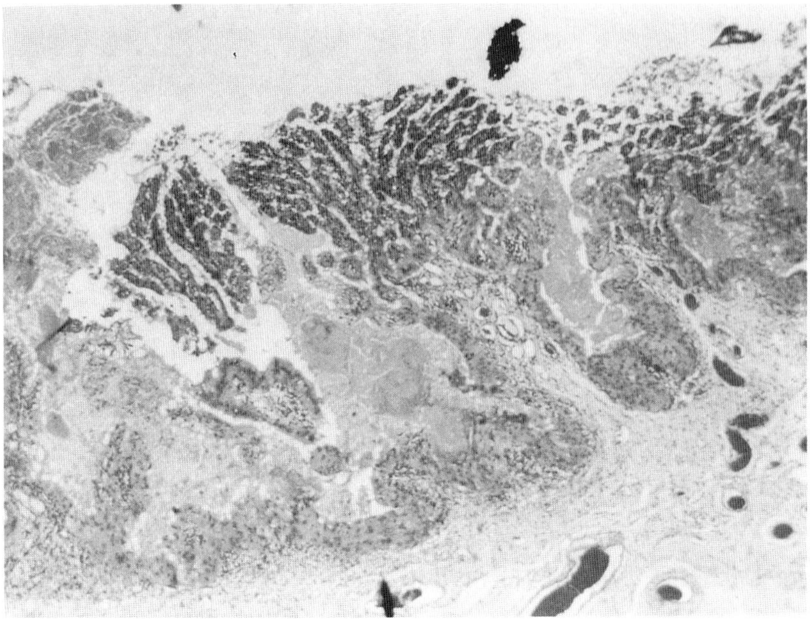

11.7. Low power, H & E of mycotic placentitis. Note the eosinophilic masses, which appear as yellow necrotic areas in the gross. Histoplasmosis.

given that the cervix closes before bacteria or fungi are aspirated into the vagina and onto the chorion. These observations do not eliminate other, possible, sources of infection such as chronic foci of infection in the mare similar to aspergillus abortion in cattle. *Histoplasma capsulatum,* for example, may directly infect through the open cervix or be metastatic to the placenta from a focus(i) in the mare.

Chronic placental insufficiency

This rubric subsumes a number of placental defects, of different or unknown cause, considered to cause abortion. Chronic implies long-term undernutrition of the fetus as a result of inadequate placental function. The appearance of such a fetus is characteristic: it is fresh, smaller than normal for the time of gestation, and emaciated (Fig. 11.8). The tissues are blanched, pale, and pastel rather than of deep, rich, normal color. The liver is characteristically enlarged and discolored. The normal fetal liver is larger relative to body size than in the foal, but is even larger with chronic placental insufficiency. Rather than the normal tan to mahogany color, it is mottled yellowish, gray and, in the extreme, clay-yellow. Pale tan rib impressions are present, but they can be present in the normal fetus as well. Minute, angular white foci are also seen. They are normal **extramedullary hematopoietic foci,** which usually disappear during the 10th to 11th month.

Histologically, these color changes comprise uneven distribution of blood, loss of glycogen, fatty metamorphosis, vacuolar degeneration of hepatocytes, proliferation of sinusoidal lining cells and, infrequently, scattered foci of necrosis of hepatocytes. The changes are, in fact, those of *kwashiorkor*—malnutrition.

Twin pregnancy

The paradigm of chronic placental insufficiency is twin pregnancy. This is pathological in the mare, causing about 20% of abortions in Thoroughbred and Standardbred mares. Hamori (1983) gave an incidence of 0.3%–3% twin pregnancy in mares with considerable variation among breeds. Gylstorff (1985) gave 1%–1.5%. The frequency in Thoroughbreds may be as high as 10%, while draft mares were said to have a much lower frequency, with half breds between the two. Ginther (1992) indicated that draft mares and Thoroughbred mares have similar twinning frequencies, about 1%–3%, while Arabians have about 0.8%, and Quarter horses 0.2%. Pony mares and primitive breeds, so-called, rarely have twin pregnancies (Ginther 1992). Hamori said that twinning is hereditary but provided no data.

As a rule one twin is dead and autolyzed/mummified and the other not autolyzed and smaller than normal, with the lesions of chronic placental insufficiency. Abortion occurs at any time but

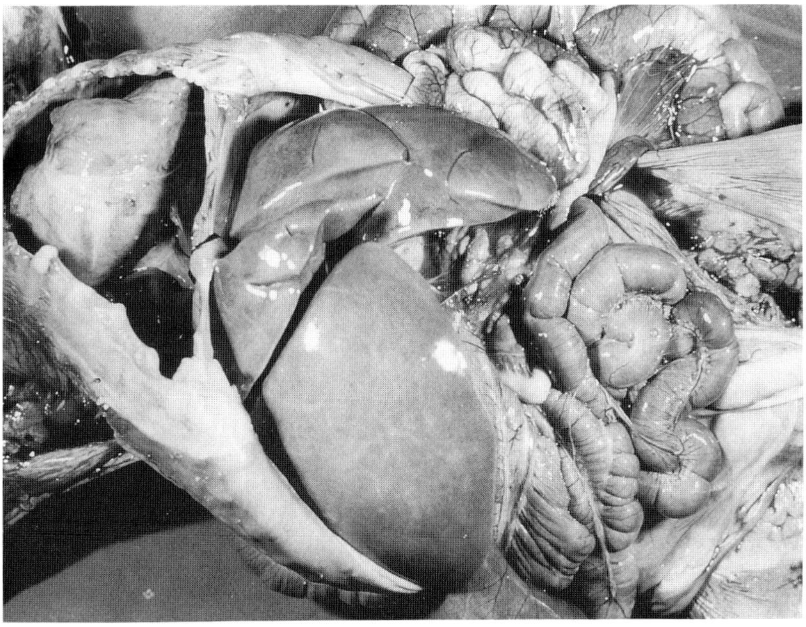

11.8. A "placental disease" fetus, emaciated with enlarged, discolored liver.

usually from about 7 months onward. On occasion both twins reach term and are born alive, though obviously small.

The placenta is characteristic even if only one twin is found or submitted for examination (Fig. 11.9). The two allantochorions are pressed against each other, preventing normal villous formation. They can be separated by careful blunt dissection. This is the classic case of inadequate placental nutrient exchange area, that is, chronic placental insufficiency.

Only one case of identical twinning has been seen. There were two amniotic sacs and a single allantochorion folded upon itself. A second case has been reported (Jeffcott and Whitwell 1973).

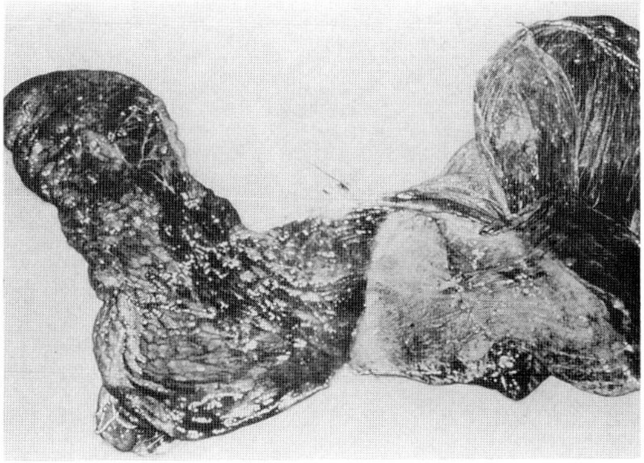

11.9. Twin placenta partially pulled apart with the bare area near the *middle*.

Apparently bona fide cases of **superfetation** have been reported (Gylstorff 1985), but, in most instances, a single mating has resulted in the fertilization of two eggs: true fraternal twinning. In the case of two matings with the same horse no distinction can be made. In the case of matings with different horses blood-typing techniques might make the distinction. There are reports in the 1800s of mares being mated to both horse and jackass and producing twins, one mule and one horse foal.

Chorionic villous hypoplasia

This malformation of the chorion is not common. The fetus has characteristic signs of placental insufficiency. The nonautolyzed chorial surface is paler than normal and less velvety. Variably extensive areas lack villi altogether, while larger areas have less villi than normal. The change may still be apparent after onset of autolysis, but considerably more difficult to appreciate.

While histological examination confirms that there are fewer villi than normal, the determination of villous hypoplasia is best made in the gross. The cause is unknown. While one may speculate about chronic disease of the endometrium—normal endometrium being required for the induction of villi—no correlations have yet been made. It may simply be a congenital defect.

Body pregnancy

This malformation is not uncommon, abortion occurring in the 7th month of gestation. Apparently the fetus develops in the body of the placenta, and the horns do not fully develop (Fig. 11.10). The body appears normal while the horns are thrown into corrugated folds of disorganized villous-covered tissue. The cause is not known. Improper mobility of the conceptus during the early stages of pregnancy (Ginther 1992) might be related.

Virtually every body pregnancy is aborted in the 7th month. The exchange surface represented by the body of the allantochorion appears to be that necessary for the viability of the fetus up until about the 6th–7th month. The exchange surface area of the normal pregnant and nonpregnant horn, then, may be required for about 4–5 months of fetal development.

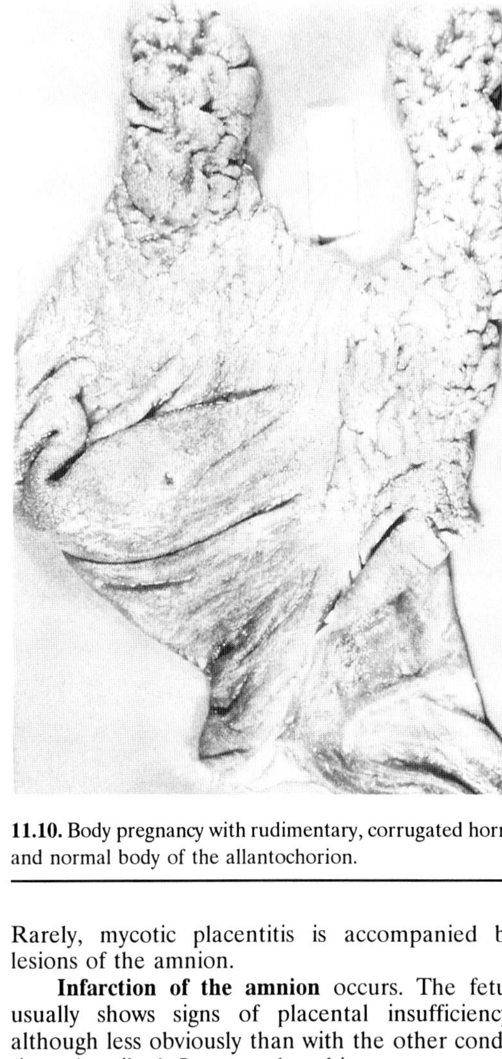

11.10. Body pregnancy with rudimentary, corrugated horns and normal body of the allantochorion.

Chronic placentitis

This uncommon entity is associated with abortion of an emaciated, cachectic fetus. The allantoic surface, in particular, is irregularly thickened, with masses and networks of collagenous scar tissue (Fig. 11.11). Microscopically, this scar tissue contains scattered and focal mononuclear and lymphoid cells, the usual picture of a chronic inflammatory process. No organisms have been seen or cultured. Although speculative, the allantochorion may have become infected earlier in gestation and successfully contained that infection. The scarring, however, compromises nutrient-exchange capability, with eventual abortion as a result of chronic placental insufficiency.

Premature aging

A small number of fetuses are seen with characteristics of placental insufficiency, but without lesions of the placenta. Aging changes are present microscopically, and appear to be earlier and more extensive than expected from the gestational age. This is obviously speculative, and no etiology can be suggested.

Amnion

The amnion is rarely the site of significant lesions. Small calcified plaques of no pathological significance are occasionally present. Either general or localized edema of the amnion is seen both with abortions and at term. The cause is not known. Rarely, mycotic placentitis is accompanied by lesions of the amnion.

Infarction of the amnion occurs. The fetus usually shows signs of placental insufficiency, although less obviously than with the other conditions described. Large, pale, white areas are surrounded by a thin hemorrhagic border. Microscopically, bland thrombi are often, but not invariably, found as the anatomical explanation. The cause of the thrombosis and/or infarction is not known.

Rarely, the only lesion is a thickened, edematous amnion with intense green color, but no other evidence of fetal diarrhea. Microscopically, there is intense inflammation with large numbers of neutrophil leucocytes. No organisms have been seen or cultured, and the cause is not known.

Viral abortion

With the disappearance of *S. abortus-equi,* herpesvirus (EHV)-1 and arteritis virus are the only known causes of epizootic abortion in mares.

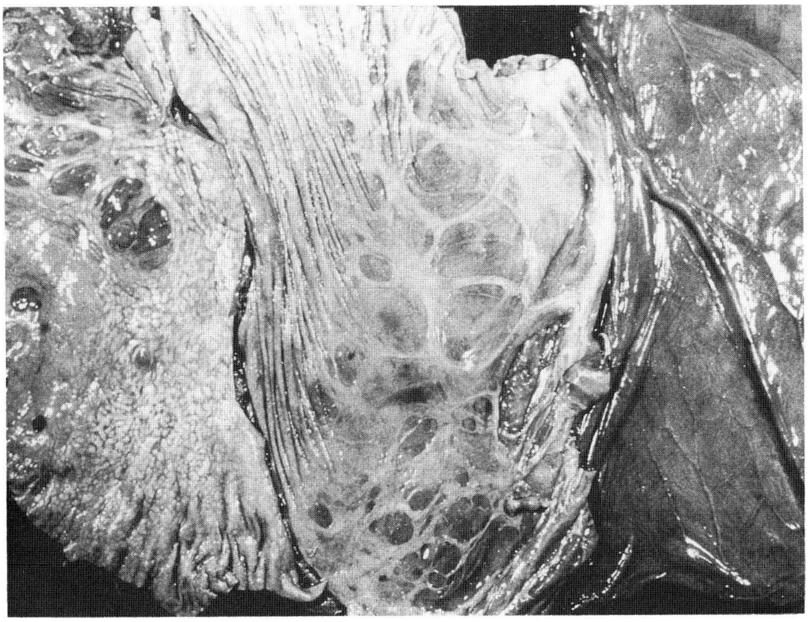

11.11. Chronic placentitis. Normal allantoic surface of allantochorion is at the *right*. The other allantoic surfaces are covered with scar tissue.

Arteritis

Arteritis infection of the pregnant mare frequently causes abortion. The virus can be recovered from the aborted fetus, but there are no lesions of the fetus or placenta. Indeed, the greatest majority of the fetuses are autolyzed.

Herpesvirus (EHV)-1

This is ubiquitous in horse populations and a well-known cause of sporadic and epizootic abortion. As the immune status of a mare population improves, either by natural exposure or vaccination, epizootics are less frequent, though sporadic abortions still occur. As discussed with the nervous and respiratory systems (see Chapters 16 and 2, respectively), herpes is a common cause of respiratory disease in young, susceptible animals and neurological disease in animals of different ages. Reinfection occurs almost routinely in older animals, usually without obvious clinical signs. Vaccination immunity is short-lived as is naturally acquired immunity. While the time from reinfection of the pregnant mare to abortion varies, on average it occurs in 3–4 weeks. Doll (1972) reviewed the disease and its history. It was first recognized in Kentucky in the 1930s (Dimock and Edwards 1933), followed by recognition in Europe, and, eventually, throughout the world. Manninger and Csontos (1941) discerned the relationship between respiratory disease in mares and subsequent abortion.

Abortion may occur at any time during gestation, but is commoner during the 7–11-month period. Abortion is uncommon before 5 months but does occur. Foals may be delivered at term with the infection (see Chapter 12, "Neonate").

The typical case is aborted quickly without premonitory signs and in fresh condition. It appears that the fetus is alive when abortion begins. There is fetal diarrhea, a nonspecific sign of asphyxiation, with greenish, meconium staining of the amnion and fetus. The mucous membranes of the eyes and mouth have multiple, fine petechiae. There may be subcutaneous edema over the nose and forehead, with fine petechiae. Occasionally, this is the only gross lesion. The loose connective tissues of the axillary and femoral spaces are saturated with yellow, gelatinous, edema fluid.

The pleural cavity contains a variable amount of clear, straw-colored fluid. The mediastinal tissues are saturated with yellow, edema fluid. There are multiple, fine epicardial and endocardial petechiae and variable, but usually prominent, bands of interlobular edema of the lungs. Usually, severe hemorrhages are present in the tracheal mucosa, the tissues of the cervical region and thoracic inlet, and, less frequently, in tissues throughout the body. Fluid is normally present in the guttural pouches and is not necessarily part of the disease process.

The liver has multiple, fine white foci of necrosis grossly apparent in about 10% of cases (Fig. 11.12). Yellowish-white angular hematopoietic foci are not to be mistaken for viral lesions. The mesenteric lymph nodes, the root of the mesentery, and the tissues of the portal area of the liver are edematous. The spleen is swollen and dark red. A number of these lesions are simply those of asphyxiation as discussed with neonatal asphyxia (see Chapter 12).

This is classic herpes virus infection of the fetus. Obviously, all of these lesions may not be present with equal severity in any given case. Occasionally, an autolyzed fetus, aborted at 4 or 5 months, may have characteristic histological changes and/or virus isolation. The gross diagnosis of herpes virus abortion, then, is rarely incorrect, but a negative gross diagnosis may be incorrect.

The herpes virus does not cause placental lesions, but the virus can be the immediate cause of abortion in fetuses already suffering from placental disease. The virus is pantropic in the fetus, with distinct predilection for respiratory epithelium and endothelial cells throughout the body. Intranuclear inclusion bodies are readily found in the respiratory epithelium in areas of acute necrotizing bronchiolitis and on the periphery of foci of necrosis in the liver. They may also be found, though with more difficulty, in the spleen in depleted, necrotic germinal centers. Careful search, supplemented with fluorescent antibody, reveals the presence of virus in the endothelium of virtually all tissues.

At the time of abortion the mares show little or no clinical signs. There may be a history of mild upper respiratory infection some weeks earlier, particularly in younger mares, but that infecting exposure usually goes unnoticed. Exposure and abortion is almost inevitable if pregnant mares are shipped any significant distance or gathered in barns for auction sales.

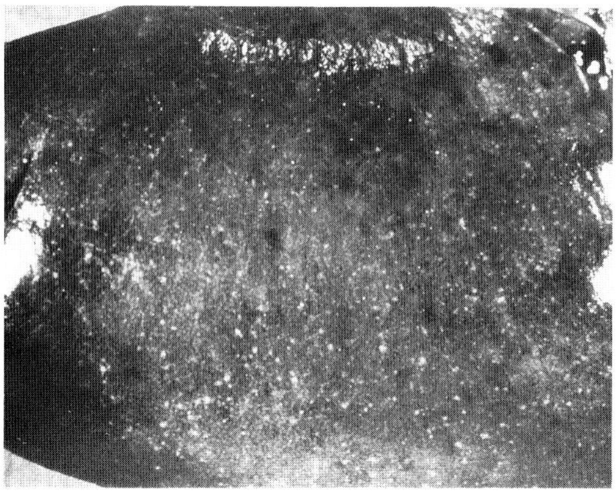

11.12. Foci of necrosis of the liver with herpes viral abortion.

Salmonella abortus-equi

This organism, only known to cause placentitis and abortion of mares, appears to have disappeared, though cases may still occur in southeast Asia. It was, at one time, a significant cause of epizootic abortion in mares.

The allantochorion is the site of an hemorrhagic, purulent, often diphtheritic inflammation. There is marked edema of the allantochorion and, often, multiple foci of necrosis with sharply demarcated hemorrhagic borders. The umbilical cord may also be involved. Histologically, the allantochorion is thickened with edema, multiple hemorrhages, and numerous neutrophil leucocytes. The blood vessels are thrombosed, and the epithelium is necrotic. The chorial surface is bedecked with a necrotic mass of dying neutrophils, red blood cells, and chorionic epithelium. Large numbers of bacteria are present.

The gross and histological picture is that of any bacterial placentitis, but was apparently more severe and more often associated with marked edema than typical of other bacterial infections.

Mycobacterium spp.

There has been one report of abortion caused by *Mycobacterium avium* (Cline et al. 1991). The mare had the disease and the 160-day fetus had multiple granulomatous lesions in a number of organs, as well as in the allantochorion. Stainable bacteria were numerous in the lesions of the fetus. Tasler and Hartley (1981) reported a case of abortion caused by *M. terrae.*

Fescue toxicity

Tall fescue, *Festuca arundinacea,* infected with the endophyte, *Acremonium coenophialum,* is a cause of prolonged gestation, dystocia, poor mammary gland development, agalactia, and foal mortality (Putnam et al. 1991). As many as 90% of mares grazing heavily infected pasturage may be affected. Specific lesions of the placenta and fetus/foal have not been reported. The foal is somewhat larger and the foal and placenta heavier, probably because of the prolonged gestation, about 20 days longer than in mares not grazing such pastures. The foals were large but poorly muscled, with long haircoats, overgrown hooves, and irregular eruption of the incisor teeth (Putnam et al. 1991).

It has been suggested that edema of the placenta is characteristic of fescue toxicity. Edema, specifically of the allantochorion, is seen occasionally with several different types of abortion and is not infrequent in the otherwise normal term placenta with a normal, viable foal. Edema is not characteristic of fescue toxicity, per se. Poor mammary development and agalactia would appear to be the nearly pathognomic findings.

Extrauterine pregnancy

There are a few reports of true extrauterine pregnancy in the mare with the pregnancy terminated at or near term by illness and death of the mare (Powell 1898/99; Perley 1898/99). We have seen no example.

CHAPTER 12

Neonate

Neonatal asphyxia

This specifies a set of lesions caused by asphyxia in the term/neonatal foal, neonatal being the first 24 hours of extrauterine life. Once this set of lesions has been found, one seeks specific lesions and/or clinical information to explain the final common pathological event—asphyxiation. It is hoped that the term *neonatal asphyxia*, with appropriate descriptors, will replace unhelpful jargon such as "neonatal respiratory distress syndrome" and its congeners.

The lesions of asphyxiation in the term and neonatal foal include petechiae of the mucosae of the eyes, mouth, pharynx, larynx, trachea, bronchi, parietal and visceral pleura, endocardium, and epicardium. There may be streaks and splashes of hemorrhage in the loose connective tissues of the ventral cervical region and the thoracic inlet. There is edema of the mesenteric lymph nodes and the root of the great mesentery, as well as the connective tissues of the portal area of the liver. These latter lesions are highly characteristic of asphyxia at this age, but not seen routinely with asphyxia in the older animal. The lungs may be completely atelectatic, partially atelectatic, or fully, even excessively, aerated.

Delayed delivery

This is the most frequent cause of neonatal asphyxia. The foal may either be born dead, failing to breathe after delivery, or born alive, but in weak condition, with or without overt signs of respiratory distress. Delayed delivery is of particular significance with foals as compared to other species. The placenta, on average, is expelled within 15 to 30 minutes after delivery, indicating that separation from the endometrium is early and rapid. The foal, then, is deprived of maternal oxygen early and completely and must reach the ambient air expeditiously.

Dystocia is a clear case of delayed delivery. The variety of such misplacement may be found in obstetrical texts. Overzealous assistance during difficult delivery, or when delivering foals with malformed legs, may cause tearing and/or rupture of the gastrocnemius muscle (Sprinkle et al. 1985). Cox cited by Smith (1976) described such ruptures in 1857.

Specific lesions are associated with delay, whether dystocia was obvious or not. There is almost invariably hemorrhage into the shoulder joints, with reddish staining of the articular cartilage. This indicates that the foal was squeezed during delivery and, so, probably delayed. An apparent cause of such squeezing and hemarthrosis is failure of the forelimbs to extend completely as the foal is being delivered. This increases the effective diameter of the foal and delays delivery. Such a scenario is well known as *shoulder lock* to experienced stud grooms.

Incomplete extension of the fore legs places the elbows in the usual position for fractured ribs, and these are often seen, together with hemarthrosis of the shoulder joints. The fractures occur in or near the middle third of the rib(s) and may be clinically silent or cause lethal contusion of the heart and/or lungs. They are to be distinguished from costochondral fractures, which are very common in light horse foals, heal rapidly, and are of no clinical significance. Costochondral fractures are recognized by localized subpleural hemorrhage and greater mobility and demonstrated by slicing the costochondral junctions.

Placental disease

Cases of bacterial placentitis and chronic placental insufficiency usually do not reach term. It is not uncommon, however, for cases of mycotic placentitis to reach term and delivery. The foal is born weak and in more or less obvious respiratory distress. The placental damage has placed the foal in a precarious oxygen state, and that is exacerbated during delivery.

Allantochorial separation

There are two forms of allantochorial separation, one well known.

Red bag

The first is called *red bag*, accurately describing what the stud groom sees. The body of the allantochorion breaks near the junction with the horns, rather than at the cervical star. Normally, the initial flood of allantoic fluid accompanying rupture of the cervical star is followed by bulging and rupture of the amnion. In this case the body of the allantochorion, with the cervical star intact, is delivered first. Rapid, assisted delivery is necessary if the foal is not to be asphyxiated, since about 60% of the oxygen exchange surface has been lost.

There is usually marked accumulation or infiltration of fluid into the tissues of the cervical star area. This fluid, histologically, is basophilic and metachromatic rather than the usual eosinophilic edema fluid and may, indeed, be an abnormal accumulation of ground substance material rather than true edema. While the cause is not known, the pathogenesis involves failure of the cervical star to rupture, with rupture then occurring at the next possible site.

Premature placental separation

The second form, premature placental separation, is more problematic, or at least less obvious, than red bag. The body and/or part of the pregnant horn of the allantochorion separates some time before delivery. The normally velvet, deep red chorial surface is dry and tan. This determination must only be made on the placenta delivered soon after the foal and quickly examined. If expulsion of the placenta or examination is delayed, the entire chorial surface undergoes this autolytic change. Since, in the case of premature separation, the allantochorion is almost always delivered very quickly, the diagnosis can be made (Fig. 12.1).

The cause(s) of premature placental separation is not known, and light microscopy has been of no assistance. Steven et al. (1979) examined the ultrastructure of placentas of stillborn foals and found degeneration of the chorionic epithelium, characterized by loss of microvilli, fragmentation of the plasma membrane, and chromatolysis of the nuclei. Thickening of the basal lamina, common in normal term placentas, was said to be more frequent than usual, and there was more collagen in the cores of the villi than usual. Capillary endothelium was thickened, with both myelin and lipid inclusions and vacuolation. All these changes were characterized as anoxic. They did not determine causes for the stillbirths, but their observations are consistent with premature placental separation.

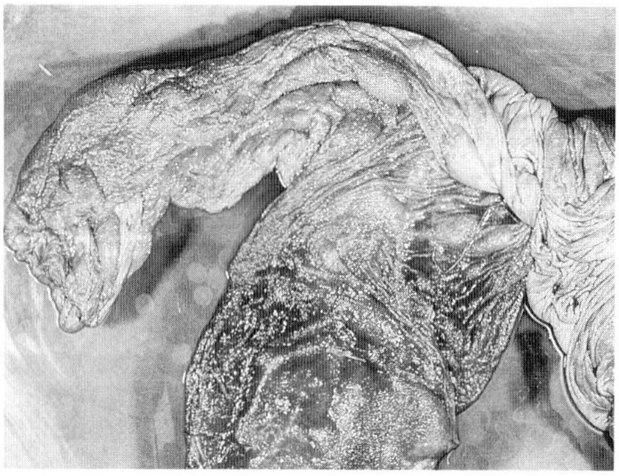

12.1. Premature separation of the horns of the allantochorion, which are brown (*left* and *right*), showing they are dead. The body of the allantochorion is still the normal red color (*center*), indicating it was still alive at the time of expulsion.

Neonatal bacterial infection

There is ample evidence that bacterial infection of the fetus can occur after the cervix opens in preparation for delivery and/or during delivery. Streptococci and *Actinomyces equuli* are the usual organisms. Since the cervix may open some hours before overt signs of parturition, a bacterial septicemia can be present or incubating at the time of birth. The foal so afflicted will present almost immediately with signs of respiratory difficulty. These signs of air hunger can be so striking that the term *barker* has been applied.

The gross findings may suggest septicemia and/or neonatal asphyxia. Culture and histological examination may define bacterial septicemia. In some cases presenting as neonatal asphyxia with pronounced clinical signs of air hunger, an acute bacterial pneumonia is found histologically in the absence of gross lesions of pneumonia. The pneumonic process is characterized by neutrophils, edema, and alveolar emphysema. Organisms can be present in considerable numbers with regular and special stains. Small or moderate amounts of meconium may be found and are quite normal; large amounts indicate asphyxia before rupture of the amnion. It is doubtful that pneumonia is caused by meconium. It should be noted that there is a considerable outpouring of proteinaceous edema fluid with pneumonia and a pseudofibrin membrane may be seen. This is not true hyaline membrane or hyaline membrane disease.

Simpson and Buergelt (1981) described the light and electron microscopic appearance of elongated dense bodies in the alveoli of two aborted foals. These concretions, ranging in size from 10 μm to 40 μm, filled alveoli. They were composed of concentric laminations of fibrillar electron-opaque material. The material was considered to be concretions of amniotic fluid. They are not uncommon.

Foals recovering from acute air hunger, usually with antibiotic therapy, may become so-called *dummys* or *wanderers*. As the terms indicate, the clinical signs are of cerebral cortical damage. Only a few such animals have been seen at postmortem. The asphyxial lesions in the brain are described with the nervous system.

Neonatal herpesvirus (EHV)-1 infection

Herpes virus may infect the fetus late in gestation. The foal is born, at term, with severe respiratory distress and usually dies within 24 hours. Gross lesions are largely restricted to the lungs, which have a characteristic marbled panorama of edema, consolidation, and emphysema. Histologically, there is acute fibrinous pneumonia and necrotizing bronchiolitis with intranuclear inclusion bodies.

Miscellaneous

Not all specific causes of neonatal asphyxia have been enumerated. Few remain. Congenital cardiac defects, such as subaortic septal defect, may be found, though clinical evidence of heart disease is usually not seen until the foal is weeks or months old. The fishnet formaen ovale and the ductus arteriosus are, of course, anatomically patent in the newborn.

Occasionally, the middle lobe of the liver is ruptured in aborted fetuses or newborn foals because of inadequate dilatation of the cervix. In abortion, the rupture is real, though incidental, and usually occurs after the death of the fetus. In the term foal, significant rupture, with hemorrhage into the abdominal cavity, is generally associated with catastrophic dystocia, multiple fractured ribs, and massive hemorrhage into the shoulder joints. Rupture of the middle lobe is seen, uncommonly, as the cause of death in older foals as the result of a kick by an adult horse.

One of the atria, often the right, may be ruptured, with or without evidence of hemorrhage in the torn margins. In the former case, of course, it has occurred after the death of the fetus or foal. The significance is the same as that of rupture of the liver.

Prematurity

The objective determination of prematurity is difficult. Breeding dates may be multiple or wrong, and the foaling dates of maiden mares in particular, are not wholly predictable. On both clinical and pathological grounds, it appears that frank prematurity is associated with marked gaseous distension of the small and large intestine, particularly the former. This bespeaks normally late neuromuscular maturation of the intestine, as does the nearly unique occurrence of intussusception of the small intestine in young foals. Oikawa et al. (1992) found villous hypoplasia in eight neonatal foals. All of their foals were smaller than normal and apparently premature. While immaturity of the respiratory system is the major problem of prematurity in many species, immaturity of the digestive tract seems to be a major defect in the horse.

Infectious diseases of foals

Diseases affecting predominantly a single organ, for example, Tyzzer's and the liver, are considered with that organ. More generalized diseases are included here. Platt (1974) reported that about 98% of Thoroughbred foals born alive in Newmarket, England, survive to 8 weeks of age, a mortality of about 2%. Four percent to 5% of foals die or are destroyed during the first year of life. This is consistent with our experience and that of Oikawa et al. (1991) in Japan. Keiper and Houpt (1984) reported that about 88% of feral horse foals survived to 1 year of age.

Septicemia of foals

Bacterial septicemia has long been, and continues to be, the most important cause of illness and death in foals. Virtually all of the organs and tissues in the body can be involved in a given case. Infection of bones and joints is of particular and lasting importance and discussed below. As pointed out by Platt (1973) many bacterial septicemias of the foal appear to be opportunistic; weak foals and foals that fail to obtain colostrum being at risk. The possibility of immunodeficiency exists in any given case and should be considered, but, with the exception of Arabian foals, has not been adequately studied or defined. Oikawa et al. (1991) found bacterial septicemia to be the commonest cause of death in foals in Japan, with evidence of failure of passive transfer of colostral antibody in about half of the cases. This parallels North American experience.

At postmortem a variable, but characteristic, set of nonspecific gross lesions of septicemia are present. There is often a distinctive sewer-gaslike smell when the abdominal cavity is opened. With experience this can be differentiated from the smell of an autolytic carcass. Once autolysis begins, however, the characteristic odor is masked. The mucosal and serosal membranes, as well as the subcutaneous tissues, are muddy reddish yellow and speckled with petechial and/or ecchymotic hemorrhages. Minimal to moderate dirty yellowish edema may be present in the axillary and femoral spaces. The gastrointestinal tract is muddy yellow or pale with petechial hemorrhages of serosa and/or mucosa. Petechiae are particularly common in the fundic mucosa of the stomach and may be precursors of erosion and ulceration.

The spleen is moderately enlarged, soft, and dark red on section. The liver and kidneys are soft, paler than normal, and have the blurred, somewhat parboiled appearance of cloudy swelling. There are petechial and ecchymotic hemorrhages throughout the respiratory tract, as well as on the parietal and visceral pleura. The lungs are variable, depending upon the presence and degree of pneumonic change. With little or no pneumonia, the lungs are hyperemic, intermixed with alveolar emphysema, particularly along the margins. Histological study is necessary to differentiate early pneumonia, hyperemia, and postmortem change.

The thymus and lymphoid tissue throughout the body are variably affected by hyperemia, petechiae, and edema. Rarely, the thymus and/or other lymphoid tissue is frankly atrophic, suggesting immunodeficiency. Oikawa et al. (1989) reported six Thoroughbred foals with what they considered to be "extremely small thymuses." They could suggest no cause and did no immunological studies.

Significant gross lesions of the central nervous system are uncommon. Variable degrees of hyperemia and blood released during the dissection are not to be interpreted as evidence of "birth trauma." An occasional septicemic foal may develop acute, purulent meningitis, but this is not common.

Histological changes are compatible with the gross findings. Bacteria may be scattered through the tissues or clumped in the tissues and blood vessels. This must be interpreted with care in the autolyzed foal, an inflammatory reaction being required.

Within this general background, specific changes may suggest an etiological diagnosis. Focal accumulations of basophilic bacteria in the renal glomeruli and in the capillaries of the adrenals and, often, other organs, is characteristic of *Actinobacillus equi* septicemia. Frequently, there is significant catarrhal enteritis, as well. The synovitis with this infection is serofibrinous and tinged with blood, rather than frankly purulent as with *S. zooepidemicus* and *Salmonella* spp. *E. coli* septicemia is marked by severe, hemorrhagic inflammation of, particularly, the large intestine. This is uncommon and characteristically seen in the very young foal, often in association with severe hemorrhagic metritis of the mare. *Rhodococcus equi* infection is generally confined to the lungs and/or large intestine, without evidence of septicemia. Salmonellosis is an epizootic disease in foals. Severe catarrhal colitis is seen with erosion and ulceration of the mucosa in prolonged cases.

The age of the affected foal is a guide to probable etiology. *A. equi* and *E. coli* septicemias invariably occur within a week or so of birth. Streptoccocal septicemias can appear this early, but are more common from about 3 weeks to 3 months of age. *R. equi* is not often seen before 2–3 months. Salmonellosis may occur anytime from about a month to 3–4 months. Its epizootic nature is characteristic.

Clostridia

Clostridium perfringens type B has been isolated from cases of severe enteritis in foals in South Africa (Mason and Robinson 1938). The small intestine was markedly hyperemic, with dark, reddish foci. Montgomerie and Rowlands (1937) reported a case in England. Type C has been reported as a cause of hemorrhagic enteritis in one foal (Niilo and Chambers 1982), but the case was not convincing. We have encountered no case of clostridial infection in foals.

Arthritis and osteomyelitis

The term, *arthritis*, is reserved for infectious, inflammatory joint disease. The greatest majority of cases of arthritis and osteomyelitis occur with bacterial septicemia. In the older horse infectious joint disease is usually iatrogenic and osteomyelitis, most often seen in the distal phalanx as the result of puncture wounds of the foot. Firth (1983) reviewed infectious polyarthritis in foals.

Actinobacillus equi characteristically causes acute, fibrinopurulent synovitis, which resolves if the foal survives the septicemic disease (Fig. 12.2). There is no damage to the articular cartilage. *Streptococcus zooepidemicus,* on the other hand, causes erosive and ulcerative damage to the articular cartilage. In the inadequately treated case this damage may become massive and involve, as well, the subchondral bone. Healing can, eventually,

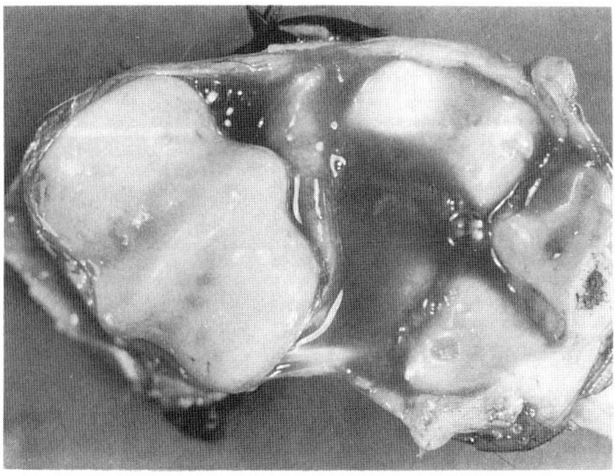

12.2. Acute, infectious synovitis (*A. equi*) of the metacarpophalangeal joint.

occur, but the joint is permanently damaged. During septicemic disease, focal, acute osteomyelitis is not uncommon in the metaphysis of virtually any bone. These foci apparently resolve without sequelae in many cases, but an occasional animal may be lame after recovery from the septicemia as a result of an abscess, so-called solitary bone abscess (Figs. 12.3 and 12.4).

Salmonella spp. can infect both joints and bones as sequelae of an outbreak of septicemic disease. This is not seen in adult salmonellosis. Typically, near or after the end of an outbreak, a few foals develop one, less often several, hot, swollen joints, which respond slowly, if at all, to antibiotic therapy. The stifle seems particularly at risk. The articular cartilage is damaged with the same sequelae as streptococcal joint disease. With or without joint disease, osteomyelitis may occur in virtually any site, but with a predilection for the metaphyses of vertebral bodies. This may not be suspected until pathological fracture and acute spinal cord transection.

Stuart et al. (1973) described a rare case of suppurative meningoencephalitis in an orphan foal caused by *S. typhimurium.*

Although uncommon, massive *Rhodococcus equi* abscesses in the dorsal part of the lung may adhere to the bodies of thoracic vertebrae and cause osteomyelitis. *R. equi* is rarely isolated in cases of purulent synovitis and, then, usually together with *S. zooepidemicus.* An occasional foal with Rhodococcus infection may have increased amounts of synovial fluid, particularly in the stifle joints. This is aseptic and without inflammatory change. The cause is not known. *Klebsiella* spp. is an occasional cause of septicemia in foals and may be isolated from infected joints. *Escherichia coli* may be isolated, with other organisms, but its role as a primary pathogen of joints in the foal is uncertain.

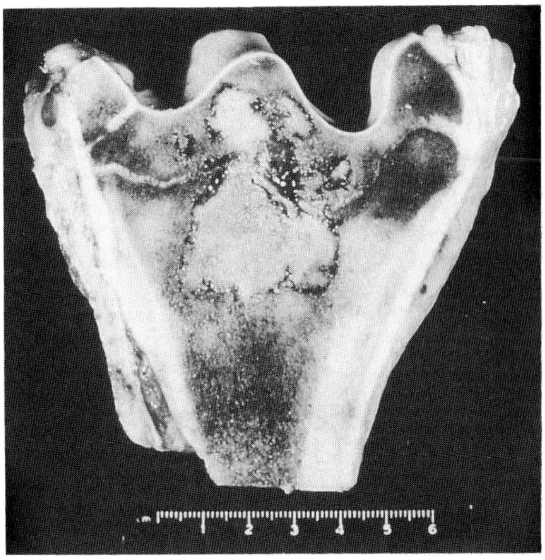

12.4. Bone abscess, localized osteomyelitis, of the distal end of the tibia (scale = centimeters).

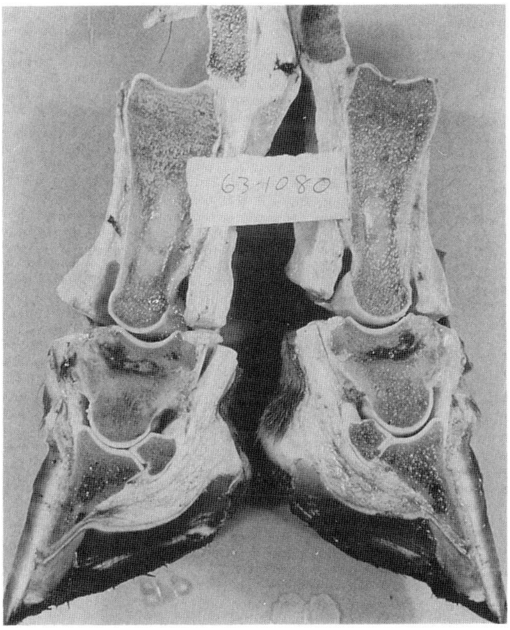

12.3. Purulent osteomyelitis, primarily of the area of the epiphyseal plate of the proximal end of the middle phalanx.

The source of infection is to be sought. Infection of the umbilicus and/or urachus was not uncommon, but has declined in frequency with the widespread use of mild antiseptics. The umbilicus normally weeps fluid for a time after separation of the umbilical cord, a protective function. Strong antiseptics seal the umbilicus and seal in pathogenic bacteria, such as *S. zooepidemicus.* An abscess forms in the urachus and/or the adjacent umbilical arteries and serves as a nidus for recurrent joint infection some months after birth (Fig. 12.5). The stifle is more frequently affected than other joints. Virtually any joint can be infected during septicemia of the young foal, while the stifle joint appears to be predisposed to infection in the older foal.

Most bacterial infections enter by the oral and/or respiratory route, a judgment based on or suggested by the lesions and their distribution.

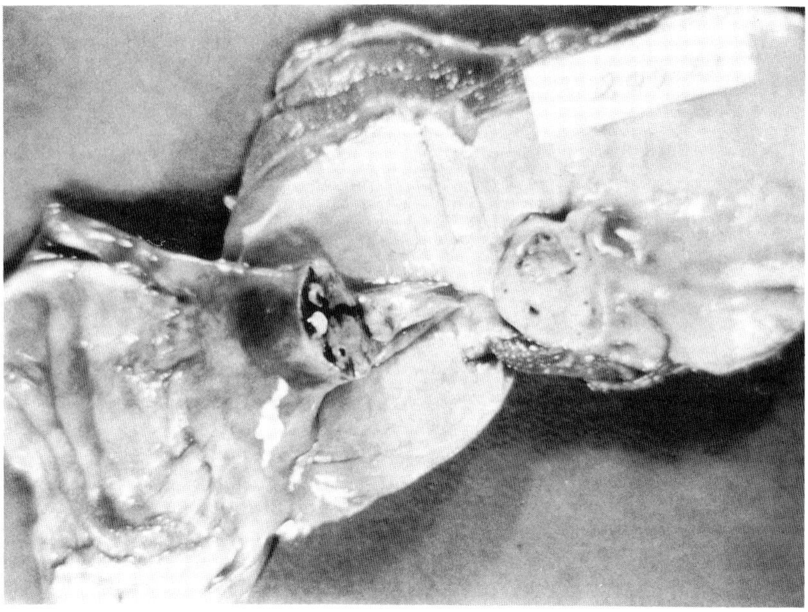

12.5. View of infected urachus from inside the abdomen. The urachus has been transected. Purulent material is oozing from the *left* cut surface and purulent, caseous material is apparent in the *right* cut surface.

Shaker foal

Present evidence indicates that this is botulism, caused by *Clostridium botulinum* type B toxin (Klyza 1983). The clinical signs are characteristic. There is sudden onset of severe muscular weakness and prostration in a 3- to 8-week-old foal, the age range being characteristic. The foal may be found down, unable to rise, after appearing normal a short while before. When aided, it rises, nurses, only to begin trembling, and falls abruptly to the ground. While down the foal appears normal and alert except for dilated, sluggish pupils, and complete cessation of peristalsis. In more severe cases the trembling may not occur, the foal found prostrate and unable to stand even with assistance. Death almost invariably occurs within 72 hours. The disease has been seen in central Kentucky and the Pennsylvania, Maryland, Virginia area for many years (Rooney and Prickett 1967b).

The gross lesions include an empty, contracted large intestine containing small quantities of dry, hard ingesta. There is patchy mucosal hyperemia and hemorrhage. The pericardial sac, in virtually all cases, contains an excessive quantity of clear, yellow fluid with variable numbers of floating fibrin flakes and strands, and is speckled with fine petechial hemorrhages. The histological findings are confined to the hemorrhages noted grossly. No lesions of vessels, muscles, or peripheral nerves, including motor end plates, have been found.

A similar clinical and pathological syndrome was produced in foals by injection of *Cl. botulinum* toxin intravenously. In light of the clinical signs and this observation, a *Cl. botulinum* type B toxoid was developed and is used routinely in broodmares in central Kentucky with virtual disappearance of the disease.

While the pathogenesis is, in part, clarified, questions of the source of toxin and reason for the restricted age range are unanswered. Botulinum toxin given intravenously will produce clinical signs in horses of any age, so it appears that the mode of exposure to toxin is the primary question. Intensive investigations of boxes housing foals that developed the disease have been negative. Culture of smegma and milk from dams of affected foals, after onset of the disease, were noncontributory.

It has been suggested that the toxin comes from an infected focus in the foal or as the result of colonization of the intestinal tract by type B clostridia, so-called *toxicoinfectious botulism* (Klyza 1983). Some affected foals do have urachus abscesses, but most do not, and clostridia have not been isolated from such abscesses. While other foci have been suggested, they have not been found or reported.

Rotavirus infection

Rotavirus infection is common in young of many species, including the foal. It occurs in epizootics, with fever, depression, diarrhea, and leucopenia as leading clinical signs. Morbidity is high and mortality low in the absence of intercurrent disease and with appropriate therapy.

There have only been limited studies on the pathological changes (Conner and Darlington 1980; Wada et al. 1984), and the changes described are essentially identical to those in other species; that is, acute catarrhal enteritis. There is mild edema of the small intestine, with shortening and fusion of villi, necrosis and desquamation of villous epithelial cells, and infiltration of lymphoid and mononuclear cells into the lamina propria and submucosa. There may be mild to moderate necrosis of the lymphoid nodules of the intestine. Wada et al. described epithelial degeneration and infiltration of lymphocytes and plasma cells into the submucosa of the cecum and colon, but the epithelial changes are questionable.

Listeriosis

Listeria infection is rare in horses. Several cases have been reported in the neonate (Krage 1944; Pulst 1964; Mayer et al. 1976). The infections were acquired in utero, with foals born at term and weak. The mares were normal in all cases. The case of Mayer et al. had evidence of neurological disease. There were miliary foci of necrosis in the liver and spleen, and focal areas of vascular and perivascular infiltration of leukocytes in the midbrain. *Listeria monocytogenes* was isolated from the brain.

Listerial septicemia in foals beyond the immediate neonatal period has been reported (Grini 1943; Belin 1946; Svenkerud 1948; Ladds et al. 1974). Clark et al. (1978) reported a case in a 1-month Arabian foal with combined immunodeficiency. There was acute, diffuse, suppurative meningitis, ependymitis, and encephalitis with suppurative and/or granulomatous perivascular cuffing. The organism was isolated from lung, heart, and brain.

Emerson and Jarvis (1968) reported 6 cases in adult ponies, 1 of which died with isolation of *L. monocytogenes* from the brain. The others apparently recovered with penicillin treatment. Belin reported cases in 2-year-old horses with incoordination, cervical spasms, poor mastication, and other clinical signs like that of ruminants. No pathological findings were reported, but the organism was isolated.

Noninfectious conditions

Hernia

While a variety of hernias can occur in foals, the commonest in all breeds is umbilical, followed by inguinal hernia. The variable-sized sac is composed of skin with a peritoneal lining. Incarceration is uncommon, at least in part because of routine surgical repair. Hamori (1983) considers the inheritance of the condition, indicating that it is a monofactorial or bifactorial recessive. Priester et al. (1970) found a 0.5% rate of umbilical hernia, in an assemblage of veterinary clinic populations, probably too low since most cases do not reach academic clinics. They reported 0.1% for inguinal hernia.

Hayes (1974) found umbilical hernias to be about 4 times as common as inguinal hernias. Females were at greater risk for umbilical hernia and at less risk for inguinal hernia than males. Quarter horses were at greatest risk for umbilical hernia.

Rupture of the urinary bladder

Rupture of the bladder is not rare in the young foal. There are three types of rupture resulting in urine accumulation in the peritoneal cavity. In the first, recognized soon after birth and more frequent in the male, there is frank rupture of the dorsal wall of the urinary bladder (Fig. 12.6). This occurs as a result of high pressure within the bladder, presumably because the bladder is full when parturition occurs, and the urine cannot escape through the compressed urethra or the urachus (Rooney 1971). These cases are usually recognized and surgically repaired. The rupture always involves the dorsal surface of the bladder, as the mechanics demand, other statements to the contrary notwithstanding (Maxie 1985).

Less often, there is slow accumulation of urine in the peritoneal cavity over a period of time, with no obvious rupture found at surgery. Careful examination reveals petechiae and pinhole tears in the dorsal wall of the urinary bladder. This type also is seen more often in males.

The third type is abscessation of the urachus, extending into and through the wall of the bladder, with escape of urine into the peritoneal cavity. This occurs with equal frequency in males and females and accompanies other signs of septicemia. This is more often seen in somewhat older foals with streptococcal infection.

Rupture of the urinary bladder of the adult horse is rare and discussed with the urinary system (see Chapter 14).

Contracture

Neonatal

Contracture of the newborn foal is the commonest congenital anomaly of Thoroughbred and Standardbred horses (Crowe and Swerczek 1985). It was well known in heavy horses and, apparently,

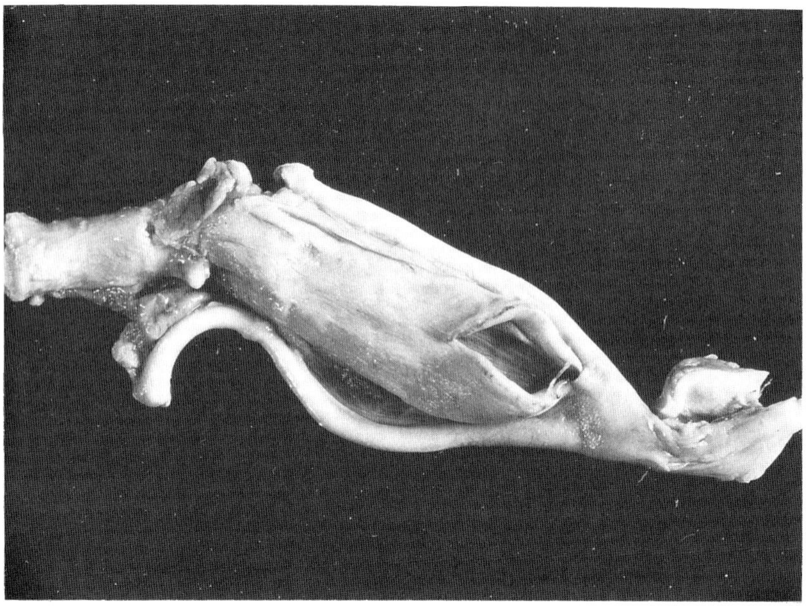

12.6. Rupture of the urinary bladder of the foal in the craniodorsal part.

seen in virtually all breeds. Treatment of contracture by tenotomy was practiced in antiquity (Leclainche 1935), and rediscovered periodically since [Cooper (1850) cited by Smith (1976)]. Hamori (1944) reported a 15% frequency in newborns in Hungary, compatible with our experience.

The syndrome includes contractures of the fore legs, rarely rear legs, scoliosis, less commonly torticollis, and lateral deviation of the nasal bones. Any combination of these lesions may be seen in any given case. It is important to note that many foals are contracted at birth, only to walk out of it in a few days. This is physiological and related to intrauterine crowding. Böhm (1954) suggested that abnormal intrauterine positioning was not a factor in pathological contracture of the newborn, a possibility sometimes bruited, but without evidence.

The pathological changes have been described (Rooney 1969) and are summarized here. Cohrs had already described such changes in one foal in 1929. The scoliosis occurs because of the instability occasioned by unilateral hypoplasia of one or more dorsal intervertebral articular processes of the thoracic vertebrae (Figs. 12.7–12.9). The costovertebral articulations also are hypoplastic. Contracture of the legs is associated with hypoplasias and malformations, specifically of the distal end of the third metacarpal bone (Figs. 12.10 and 12.11). These malformations may sometimes be seen on radiographs (Hertsch 1990). The vertebral and appendicular lesions have been found in fetuses with scoliosis both before and after the appearance of contracture of the legs. There are no histological changes to suggest the reason for these malformations, but it is known that they occur as early as the cartilage model. Although muscular and/or neural lesions are found with contractures in other species, exhaustive studies of the muscles, nerves, and central nervous system have shown no such changes in foals.

The cause of the syndrome is not known. The available evidence does not suggest a genetic cause, mares rarely having more than one such foal despite repeated breeding to the same stallion. Hertsch has suggested that the malformation of Mc3 is the result of lack of pressure from the proximal phalanx, the fetlock being held in palmar flexion in the uterus. As already noted these malformations of Mc3 have been seen in fetuses before uterine crowding could enforce such fetlock flexion.

Hussain (1975) and MacFadden (1992) showed that the sagittal ridge of the distal end of metacarpal 3 was not as well developed in fossil horses, for example, *Mesohippus,* as in later Equidae. As illustrated by MacFadden, the distal end of Mc3 of these early horses would be called hypoplastic in modern Equus. It is suggested, then, that contracture is atavistic, a persistence of distal Mc3 morphology from a pre-Equus evolutionary state. That is, as Equus has evolved from earlier equids, genetic or epigenetic information for a less evolved, less developed Mc3 has persisted, being expressed in about 10%–15% of the modern population.

The pathogenesis of the scoliosis is straightforward. With unilateral instability, muscle/tendon/ligament shortening will inevitably move the verte-

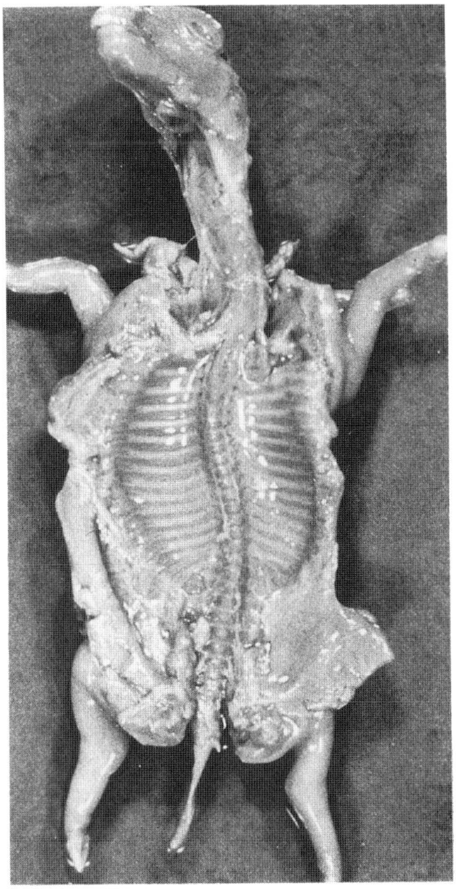

12.7. Scoliosis in an about 3-month fetus. Hypoplasia of the intervertebral articular processes was found.

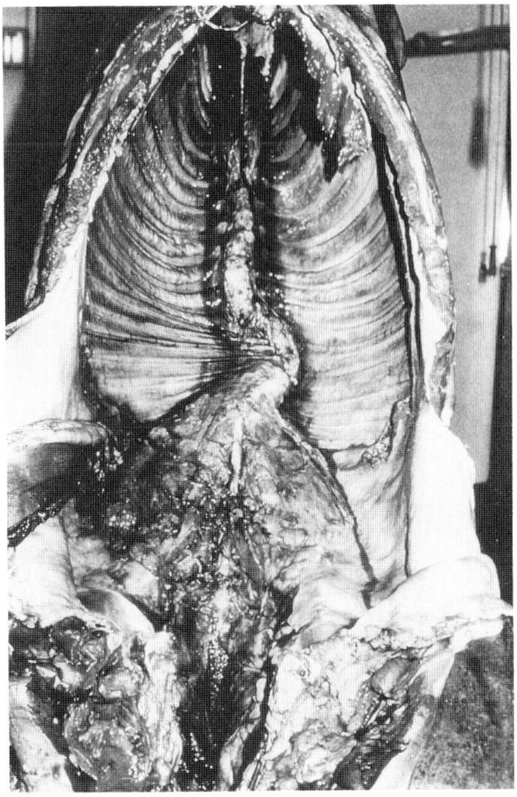

12.8. Congenital scoliosis in an adult horse. The presence of the lesion was not suspected in the live animal.

bral column into scoliosis, with the hypoplastic joints on the convex side of the scoliotic curve. Because of the hypoplasia of the costovertebral articulations, the ribs are inclined more ventrally than normal: drooped. The pathogenesis of the contractures of the legs is not as well understood. It may be suggested that the hypoplasia affects the dorsal aspect of the distal end of Mc3 more than the palmar aspect, and that does seem to be the case. As a result the mechanical moment (turning force) exerted around the fetlock joint by the extensors is less than that exerted by the flexors. In order to regain equilibrium, the flexor tendons shorten, leading over time to flexor contracture.

Prawochenski (1936) reported 8 cases of contracture of the digit of the fore leg among 26 foals sired by one Anglo-Arab stallion. The contracture appeared to affect the distal interphalangeal joint primarily, but no pathological studies were done. The mode of inheritance could not be determined but was not considered a simple recessive.

Nes et al. (1982) described an hereditary lethal arthrogryposis in foals sired by a single Fjörd horse stallion. There was muscular contracture of the rear legs, polydactylia, brachygnathia, and cleft palate.

Extensor

There may be frank flaccidity of the flexor muscles and tendons and the interosseus medius of the rear legs of the newborn foal. The animal stands with difficulty with one, or usually both, rear fetlocks resting on the ground. With or without assistance some of these foals become normal within a few weeks. The digital extensor tendon is normal. No lesions have been found either grossly or microscopically in the few cases examined, and the pathogenesis is unknown. One may propose that the process of collagen cross-linking has been delayed, so that the tendons lack sufficient tensile strength at the time of birth, but the cause of such a putative delay is unknown.

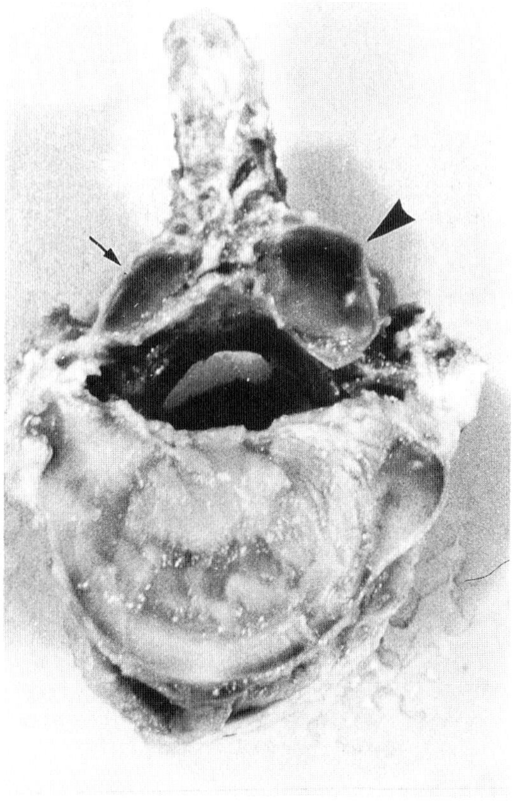

12.9. Hypoplasia of the intervertebral articular process (*small arrow*) compared to the normal (*arrowhead*).

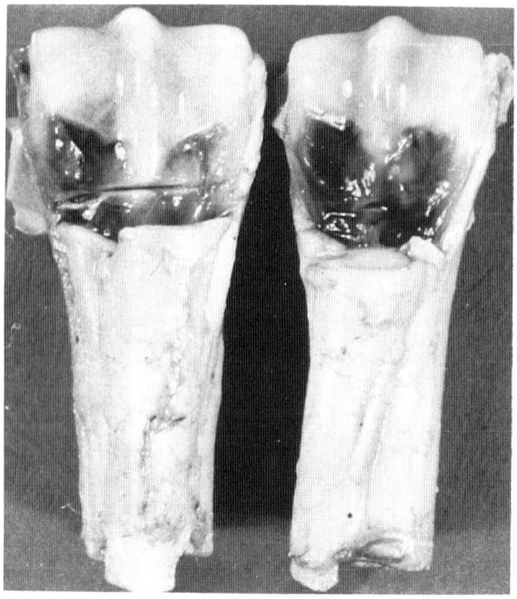

12.10. Hypoplasia of the distal end of third metacarpal (Mc3). The normal is to the *left* and the hypoplasia to the *right*. These were from the same foal; only one leg contracted.

Apparent extensor contracture of the fore legs has been seen in three foals (Conboy et al. 1991), Thoroughbred, Standardbred, and Morgan. The contracture resulted from hypoplasia and malformation of the distal phalanx. In this case the instability leading to shortening of the common extensor would be the result of loss of adequate moment arm for the deep flexor acting around the coffin joint. The articular surface of the distal phalanx was more concave in the dorsopalmar direction, and the distal end of the middle phalanx was modeled with a more obvious than normal distinction between the coffin and navicular portions of the articular surface. The dorsal wall of the hoof was distorted with a coronary to bearing-edge bulge conforming to the smaller distal phalanx.

Postnatal

Contractures, so-called, of the fore legs of young, growing horses have been known for many years. While morphological changes are associated with fetal contracture, there are no such changes, with rare exceptions, in postnatal contracture. Feeding practices have been incriminated (Hintz et al. 1976). Green (1961, 1969) studied the growth rates of horses. It has been suggested that the bones outgrow the tendons, with contracture the result. This ignores the fact that the legs of the foal below the carpus and tarsus grow very little after birth, the metacarpal, metatarsal, and phalangeal bones being nearly of adult length at birth, as was well known, at least to the Greeks [Xenophon in Morgan (1962)].

There are two forms: **deep flexor contracture**, characterized by marked palmar flexion of the coffin joint and acquired "clubfoot"; and **superficial flexor contracture**, characterized by an increasingly upright position of the pastern, that is, greater dorsal angle of the fetlock joint.

A reasonable, if theoretical, case has been made that these contractures are not, in fact, contractures at all, but accommodations of young, immature tendon to pathological modifications of hoof angle (Rooney 1991b). In the case of superficial flexor contracture, it is proposed that the pliant, immature hoof wall is displaced by an excessive rate of loading–weight gain. Such displacement, being greater at the heels and quarters

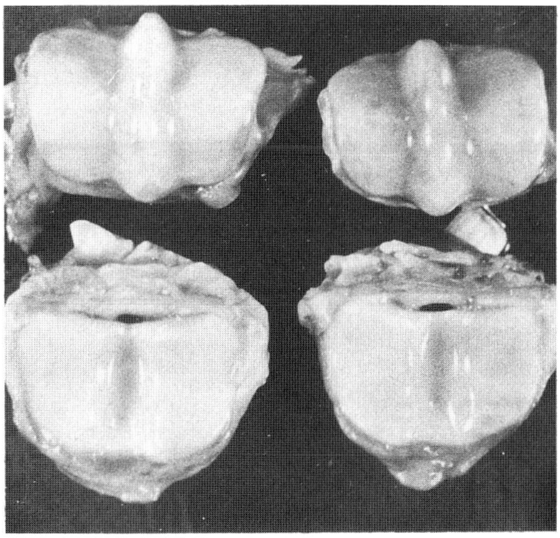

12.11. Normal metacarpal (Mc3) and proximal phalanx to the *left* and hypoplastic to the *right.*

than at the toe, would reduce the hoof angle. Hoof trimming practice would contribute. The hoof angle of the foal is normally greater than that of the adult horse, and there is a tendency to trim the feet of the foal to adult angles rather than the normal and proper larger angles.

A mechanical argument shows that with such decrease of hoof angle the superficial flexor tendon, suspensory ligament, and deep flexor tendon will shorten in order to equilibrate the moments at the coffin and fetlock joints. Genetic factors appear to play a role in this condition. There could be either a propensity for rapid rate of gain and/or slow or delayed maturation of the hoof wall. We have seen examples of full siblings developing postnatal contracture in successive years.

As decreased hoof angle relates to superficial flexor contracture, so increased hoof angle relates to deep flexor contracture. Again, the mechanical argument regarding equilibrium of moments of the coffin and fetlock joints provides an explanation for the process. Preferential wearing of the toe, for example, hard ground, pawing, and pain in the foot, would be the operative factor (Owen 1975).

In the standing animal the flexor tendons and suspensory are in tension because of joint angular changes caused by body weight. When tension decreases, the tendons shorten, eventually to their normal *rest length.* The tendons are maturing, cross-linking collagen during the first year of life. The changes of hoof angle allow shortening, then, and that shortening becomes fixed, or nearly so, as the collagen cross-links at that shortened length. Maturation of the collagen is complete at about 1 year and contractures are rare after that time.

It may be noted that radiographic and pathological evidence of bone atrophy—simple loss of substance from disuse—is often found in animals in which exercise has been limited by contracture persisting for some period of time.

Adult

Rarely, deep flexor contracture of a fore leg occurs in an adult horse. Our few cases have all been associated with severe, perhaps repeated, tearing of the check ligament of the deep flexor tendon (Wintzer 1986). Contracture of the fore leg of the adult horse is said to follow tearing of the superficial flexor as well, though we have seen no example (Ziegler 1969). While contracture of scar tissue is cited (Ziegler; Wintzer) pain causes decreased weight bearing and combines with contraction of scar tissue to cause the contracture.

Angular deformity

Although incidence data is not available, *valgus metacarpus,* outward deviation of the fore leg from the carpus distad, is not uncommon in light horse foals. *Varus metacarpus,* "bow legs," is less common. Some foals show the deformation when first standing, while others develop it during the first week after birth. Comparable deformities of the rear legs are less common.

While there is considerable speculation in the clinical literature [for example, Stashak (1987)], the evidence indicates that hypoplasia and/or delayed development of the carpal bones and/or metacarpal bones 2 and 4 is the basic lesion in most cases (Fretz 1980; McLaughlin et al. 1981). Trauma to the epiphyseal plates, fractures of small bones, or tendo/ligamentous damage can result in angular deformities, though such cases are uncommon. Hypoplasia and delayed development are discussed with osteochondrosis. It is noted here that the angular deformities are the result of too small bones and not the converse. The epiphyseal compression (epiphysitis) usually present in the lateral aspect of the distal epiphyseal plate of the radius is secondary to the deformity, and not a cause of the deformity. Most foals grow out of the less severe deformities without therapeutic intervention. It is virtually impossible to quantitate this observation since almost all animals are subjected to surgery before natural recovery can occur. It is true that before surgical techniques were routinely applied only the most severe cases of angular deformity came to postmortem examination, suggesting that the lesser deformities did, indeed, correct themselves. No controlled studies have been reported in support of the several varieties of surgical intervention.

Other variations of leg structure are usually normal anatomical variations. Occasionally, an extra, rudimentary digit is present, invariably attached to the second metacarpal bone of the fore leg, **polydactylie**. These have been reported by Marsh (1879, 1892) cited by MacFadden (1992), Cartwright (1835) cited by Smith (1976), and Carlens (1927). Gould (1983) has suggested that some of these arise by duplication of Mc3, but we have seen no evidence of that. No rudiments of the first or fifth metacarpal bones are present in the youngest embryos examined, about 4 weeks (Carlens 1927).

Mauderer (1938) reported eight cases of aplasia of both fore legs in highly inbred horses, all by one stallion with all mares related to that stallion. The breed was not mentioned but was probably Cold blood. Mauderer, also, mentioned torticollis as an inherited condition but gave no details.

Hemolytic icterus and neonatal isoerythrolysis

These were first seen in mules and may have first been reported, if not first seen, in Spain in 1744 (Cadeac 1896).

Hemolytic disease of the newborn has been reported in humans, cattle, pigs, and foals. Neonatal isoerythrolysis is apparently commonest in the Thoroughbred. Based on genetic studies of blood group antigens, Scott and Jeffcott (1978) predicted an incidence of about 25%, but found an actual incidence of less than 1% of live births. In their 10-year study only 47 hemolytic foals occurred among approximately 80,000 live births.

Maternal sensitization to fetal alloantigens is believed to be the result of hemorrhage in the allantochorion. Aa, Qa, R/S antigens (Scott and Jeffcott 1978) or A1, R, or C antigens (Becht et al. 1983) are the most immunogenic, depending on the system of nomenclature. Following maternal exposure to fetal red blood cell antigens, agglutinins and hemolysins are present in serum and colostrum. The maternal antibody titers increase from mid-pregnancy to late pregnancy, the amount of antibody apparently related to the amount of exposure to fetal antigen.

The pathogenesis of the disease was worked out by Doll (1941), Bruner (1952), and others in Kentucky, following the observation that neonatal hemolytic anemia was particularly common in foals of mares vaccinated with fetal tissue origin virus abortion vaccine. The vaccine, prepared from the livers of foals aborted with herpesvirus (EHV)-1 infection, virus abortion, was highly effective in producing hemolytic anemia and ineffective in preventing abortion.

The structure of the equine placenta permits small fetal alloantigens to pass from the fetal to maternal circulation but no, or only trace, amounts of maternal antibody pass back to the fetus. Antibody destruction of foal red blood cells does not occur, then, until colostral antibody is ingested. The foal's intestinal mucosa allows the passage of antibody for no longer than 48 hours after birth. These two facts are the basis for prevention of the disease.

Becht et al. (1983) reproduced the disease in eight mares by injection of stallion erythrocytes during the second half of pregnancy. Some of the mares, although sensitized to fetal alloantigens, had foals without isoerythrolysis. Two foals were only mildly affected and recovered spontaneously. Obviously, not all foals exposed to antifetal antibodies develop overt disease, and there is no direct correlation between the amount of colostral allogenic antibody and the occurrence or severity of hemolytic disease.

Anemia usually develops within 24–36 hours after ingesting colostrum containing the antiallogenic antibodies. Severely affected foals are depressed and weak (Scott and Jeffcott 1978). The normal pink mucous membranes become pale or icteric as red blood cells are lysed by antibody. Breathing becomes labored because of decreased blood oxygen-carrying capacity. Some foals have compensatory tachycardia. Severely affected animals may develop hemoglobinuric acute tubular necrosis. There are low erythrocyte counts, markedly decreased packed cell volume, and low blood hemoglobin concentration (Scott and Jeffcott 1978). The clinical course in less severely affected animals may be prolonged and variable.

Gross and microscopic lesions have been described (Coombs et al. 1948; Doll 1952; Jeffcott 1969). The mucous membranes are pale and/or icteric. The spleen is markedly enlarged, depending on the duration of disease, and the liver pale and yellow. The kidneys are red or black-red with hemoglobinuria and the lungs often edematous (Jeffcott 1969). Microscopic lesions include splenic hyperemia and lymphocytolysis. Jeffcott noted that hepatic lesions vary in appearance with the duration and intensity of disease. With severe disease there is centrilobular necrosis, the result of anemic anoxia and exposure to bile pigments. Erythrophagocytosis and Kupffer cell hyperplasia have been seen within 48 hours of onset. With hemoglobinuria there is degeneration of proximal convoluted tubular cells.

Contracture and degeneration of glomerular epithelial cells have been described, possibly the result of hypoxic shunting and exposure to bile pigments and hemoglobin breakdown by-products.

Serum titers of antiallogenic antibodies may be determined in mares, particularly those which have produced an hemolytic foal. Rising titers are an early warning of possible hemolytic disease after birth. Under practical conditions, the colostrum is checked for antibody and, if present, the foal is not allowed maternal colostrum for at least 48 hours.

CHAPTER 13

Male Reproductive System

Anatomical details

Horses may have but three purposes in life—to move appropriately, to breed, and to be a companion. In the modern era, the first two set the economic value of many horses. Diseases of the male reproductive system may alter the breeding value of a stallion and, more importantly, remove valuable genetic material from the population.

Certain anatomical details merit mention. In most Warm bloods, the testis is approximately 10–12-cm long, 6–7.5-cm wide, and 3–6-cm thick. The weight range is 200–300 g (Gebauer et al. 1974; Thomson et al. 1979; Zietzschmann et al. 1943). Woods et al. (1980) measured the testicles of 852 Standardbred stallions during various activities, and found testicular width to be between 4.4 and 6.0 cm, depending on age and type of activity. Heavy training and overmedication reduced testicular width. It is difficult to evaluate such studies unless testicular size and weight are related to body size and weight or, better, to brain weight, since that is reasonably constant.

The tunica albuginea is richly endowed with smooth muscle fibers. The mediastinum testis comprises very delicate connective tissue in the horse. Ninety percent of the weight of the testis is seminiferous tubules. These may be 50–80-cm long, with an outer diameter of 120–240 μm. Variations are expected with differing body size. There are from 12 to 23 efferent ductules leaving the testis.

The vasculature of the testes has many arteriovenous anastomoses, which may have the dual function of controlling pressure within the testes and contributing to the movement of sperm to the epididymis (Krölling and Grau 1960). Sertoli cell tight junctions are a barrier to the movement of cells and macromolecules, such as immunoglobulins, between seminiferous tubules and the circulation. This is a blood–testis barrier and may account for the sequestration of antigens from immunological surveillance in the testis [Dym and Caviacchia (1977) cited by Zhang et al. (1990)].

Inflammatory and infectious diseases

Equine coital exanthema

Equine coital exanthema is a venereal disease of mares and stallions, recognized for over 100 years. It is of worldwide distribution (Craig and Kehoe 1921; Bryans 1968; Pascoe et al. 1969; Bitsch 1972; Gibbs et al. 1972; Uppal et al. 1989). The causative agent is equine herpesvirus (EHV)-3, which is antigenically distinct from equine rhinopneumonitis virus [equine herpesvirus (EHV)-1] and equine cytomegalovirus [equine herpesvirus (EHV)-2].

The clinical signs and lesions in the mare are discussed with the female reproductive tract (see Chapter 11).

Stallions become infected through coitus with infected mares. Early signs of infection include balanitis, with the formation of small vesicles and pustules on the shaft of the penis. Pustules on the urethral orifice were noted within 24 hours of infection in one English stallion (Gibbs et al. 1972). Vesicles and pustules may rupture and scab over in the early stages of the disease. In some animals the ruptured vesicles leave open ulcers on the surface of the penis, which may be secondarily infected (Uppal et al. 1989). Lesions regress within 10–14 days, leaving small foci of scarring and depigmentation. Virus may be isolated during the acute and late stages of the disease, but more commonly from vesicles and pustules in early stages (Gibbs et al. 1972).

Infected stallions are contagious at any stage, and some may be asymptomatic carriers for protracted periods (Uppal et al. 1989). There is no decrease in libido. There have been several reports of abortion or failure to conceive in infected mares (Bitsch 1972). Pustular lesions have been observed in the mouths of infected stallions, and respiratory disease has been associated with infection (Craig and Kehoe 1921; Bryans 1968).

While it is clear that the virus is primarily spread by coitus, the question of transmission by stable flies or contaminated instruments has been raised, though not resolved (Gibbs et al. 1972).

Klebsiella infection

Contagious equine metritis has been recognized as a cause of infertility in horses since the mid-1920s (Dimock and Edwards 1927). It is a venereal disease caused by infection of stallions and mares with strains of *Klebsiella genitalium (pneumoniae)*. More than 80 serotypes have been differentiated by capsular antigens, but types 2 and 5 are considered most virulent (Crouch et al. 1972; Merkt et al. 1974).

The role of stallions in transmission has been debated. While some considered the stallion a temporary transport host, others have shown that the stallion may have a more important role in sustaining and transmitting the disease.

Crouch et al. (1972) studied the infection in a stallion in a Thoroughbred stud. Through several seasons, and despite aggressive antibacterial therapy, the infected stallion continued to infect mares. The organism was isolated from the external genitalia and from the prostate, urinary bladder, and renal pelvis at autopsy.

Merkt et al. (1974) studied the incidence of *Klebsiella* infections in Warm bloods and Thoroughbreds on several stud farms over a 2-year period. Although the stallions were asymptomatic, a high percentage were infected with isolations from nasal secretions, prepuce, and presecretion seminal fluid. Isolations were obtained from the hair and fecal and environmental samples. Although persistently infected, these stallions had a 77% conception rate, suggesting that infection per se does not alter reproductive ability.

Codazza and Sampieri (1973) also found persistent infection of stallions to be a problem in the transmission of disease. They felt that most stallions developed some degree of resistance, self-curing within 3 weeks of infection, and suggested that reinfection by persistently infected mares played a major role. They did not isolate the organism from seminal fluid as did Merkt et al. (1974).

Codazza and Sampieri found that personnel on the farms were asymptomatic carriers of the pathogen, and that there were less equine infections when infected personnel did not come in contact with breeding stock. Contrary to results of German workers, Codazza and Sampieri found that fecundity of mares was dramatically reduced by infection.

Epididymitis

Bacterial epididymitis with infection by *Streptococcus zooepidemicus* has been reported in two stallions (Held et al. 1990). Affected animals were lethargic, anorectic, and had colicky abdominal pain. Ejaculate was blood-tinged and contained numerous neutrophils and organisms. Subsequent examination revealed unilateral enlargement of the epididymis. Abscesses were present in the epididymis and the pathogen was cultured. Granulomatous inflammation of the epididymis and testicular degeneration and fibrosis were seen histologically. Although treated with appropriate antibiotics, the infection persisted.

Seminal vesiculitis

Although inflammation of the **seminal vesicles** and **ampulla** is uncommon, persistent infection with *Pseudomonas aeruginosa* has been reported (Blanchard et al. 1988). The animal infected two mares before being incriminated as the source. The ejaculate was blood-tinged and contained purulent debris. Repeated attempts to eliminate the infection with antibiotics were unsuccessful and the animal was killed. There were no gross pathological changes. Granulomatous vesiculitis and ampullitis were found histologically.

Venereal transmission of *Pseudomonas aeruginosa* from an infected Thoroughbred stallion to a large number of mares was reported by Johnson et al. (1980). Bacteria were cultured from the penis, prepuce, urethra, and urethral fossa. The fertility of the stallion declined. Following extraordinary therapeutic measures, including scrubbing of stallion and mares; antibiotics, antibacterial soaps, and creams applied topically; and inspection with ultraviolet light, the stallion returned to service with a conception/live foal rate of 80%.

Orchitis

Actinobacillus equuli

Actinobacillus equuli is an uncommon pathogen of the male reproductive tract. Only a few cases of genital infection and disease have been recorded, although the organism is ubiquitous in the environment. A case of septic periorchitis was reported by Belknap et al. (1988). A granulating and fibrinosuppurative **orchitis** and **periorchitis** were diagnosed grossly and histologically in a 2-month-old colt with severe, colicky abdominal pain. The colt was castrated and recovered uneventfully.

Mycoplasms and ureoplasms

A number of mycoplasms and ureoplasms have been isolated from genital secretions in mares and stallions, but their role in disease is unknown (Kirchhoff 1982).

Strongyles

The migration of strongyles into male reproductive structures has been reported [Hobday (1917) cited by Cohrs (1961); Bishop et al. (1964); Soulsby (1965); and Smith (1973)]. Larvae of both *S. vulgaris* and *S. edentatus* have been found in the testes as well as in inflamed, hemorrhagic migratory tracts. Smith (1973) noted a higher incidence in abdominal testicles of cryptorchids, but pointed out that cryptorchidism was the primary focus of his study. He correctly discounted the notion of strongyle migration as a cause of equine cryptorchidism. Soulsby (1965) said that thrombosis of the spermatic artery, as a consequence of larval migration, could lead to testicular degeneration, but this has not been reported by others or seen by us.

Genital habronemiasis

A case of genital habronemiasis has been reported, Stick (1981). The prepuce of a 6-year-old Quarter horse was chronically infected, with ulceration, scarring, and induration. The penis was not affected. Histologically, focally extensive granulomatous inflammation was present. *Habronema* infestation is, in fact, not uncommon in geldings (accumulation of smegma), less often stallions, particularly in warm climates. Massive infestations occur, affecting penis, sheath or scrotum.

Viral arteritis

The virus of viral arteritis localizes in several parts of the reproductive tract of carrier stallions. Minimal inflammatory changes accompany the infection.

Other inflammatory diseases

Immune-mediated infertility

There are reports of infertility associated with testicular trauma and antisperm antibodies (Zhang et al. 1990; Papa et al. 1990; Boyle 1990). Sperm components are usually sequestered from immunological surveillance by the blood–testis barrier. Traumatic orchitis disrupts the barrier, allowing an influx of inflammatory cells and sensitization to sperm proteins.

Papa et al. (1990) described steroid-responsive infertility in a stallion. The stallion failed to settle mares following an episode of trauma and orchitis. There was poor sperm motility. Antisperm serum antibodies were found, and they inhibited the motility of spermatozoa from a normal stallion. Following treatment with intravenous prednisolone, sperm motility increased markedly and a 75% conception rate was achieved. When steroid therapy was discontinued, sperm motility dropped.

Zhang et al. (1990) reported antisperm antibodies in the semen of a Thoroughbred stallion after testicular trauma. The stallion had decreased sperm volume, motility, and viability, as well as poor conception. Intravenous dexamethasone reduced the titer of immobilizing antibodies and improved reproductive performance.

In a critical review of these papers, Boyle (1990) identified deficiencies in experimental method and gaps in understanding of the role of immunity in stallion infertility. While correct in concluding that the presence of antibody in either serum or semen is not prima facie evidence for infertility, the therapeutic results clearly suggest a role for immune effects on fertility.

Racetrack infertility

A poorly defined entity is subnormal or absolute infertility of young male horses coming from racing to the breeding stud. Semen examination often reveals many immature spermatozoa or even spermatogonia in the ejaculate. With time the semen usually becomes normal and the stallion fertile. There have been no postmortem or biopsy studies. The cause is not known although the duress of racing and, particularly, drug abuse may be suspected.

Vasculitis in the tunica albuginea

A focal area of reddening and thickening of the tunica albuginea of the testis may be encountered as an incidental finding at postmortem. Infrequent at best, they are more often seen in young horses 1 to 2 years of age. Histologically, the lesion is fibrinoid necrosis of a muscular artery in the tunica, with granulomatous inflammatory reaction. The lesion is identical to that seen with arteritis virus infection, but that has been excluded in these cases.

The lesion is usually solitary in one testis. A single case, a yearling, had severe pain and extraordinary swelling of both testes. At autopsy there were multiple necrotic and thrombosed arteries, with infarction and widespread inflammation of both testes. Arteritis virus infection was excluded. The cause is not known.

Congenital

Cryptorchidism

Retention of one or both testes in the inguinal canal or abdominal cavity is an uncommon defect. Several large surveys of the incidence of the defect have been published [Hobday (1914) cited by Cohrs (1961); Stickle and Fessler (1978); and Cox et al. (1979)].

In their surveys of 350 and 500 cryptorchid cases, respectively, Stickle and Fessler (1978) and Cox et al. (1979) dispelled several fallacies about the defect. They found that left and right testes were equally retained, contrary to the view that the left testis is more often retained: 75.2% of left and 41.8% of right testes were retained in the abdomen; 24.8% of left and 58.2% of right testes were retained in the inguinal canal. Defects in gubernaculum traction, malposition of the vaginal process, and size and time of constriction of the vaginal ring were discussed as causes. In 121 of 350 cases, there were tubular atrophy and aspermatogenesis histologically. We have not seen a cryptorchid testis that did not show these changes.

According to Cox et al. (1979) bilateral cryptorchidism was uncommon (40 of 500 cases) and partial descent of one of the retained testes even more uncommon. In ponies, about equal numbers of right and left testes were in the abdomen, especially in older ponies. In younger ponies there was more retention on the right side. Since the incidence of cryptorchidism decreases with age, some testes may descend as horses mature, but there is no direct evidence. It is important to recognize the large size and the position of the **gubernaculum testis** in the scrotum of the newborn and young foal. It can be mistaken for a descended testis and give rise to the error of thinking a testis had descended and subsequently retracted into the inguinal canal or abdomen. Such a phenomenon is unknown.

In most cases, the retained testis is smaller than normal and is hypoplastic or atrophic as a result of the suppression of spermatogenesis by normal body temperature. There is an increased incidence of seminoma, interstitial cell tumors, and teratomas in retained testes (see below).

The cause of cryptorchidism is not certainly known, though genetic factors must be considered. Stickle and Fessler (1978) found no breed relationship other than a low incidence in the Thoroughbred (see Table 13-1).

Microtubular mass defect in stallion sperm

A defect in the formation of the neck region of sperm in some stallions has been seen in Poland and in the United States [Bielanski and Kaczmarski (1979, 1980) cited by Heath et al. (1985)]. The stallions have low to normal fertility. A mass appears as a protrusion on the neck region of the sperm. The expression is variable: a few percent in some stallions and significant numbers in others. The defect is associated with loose sperm heads. Electron microscopic studies indicate that the mass is composed of **tubulin** and may be involved in the formation or integrity of the nuclear membrane. There is an apparent hereditary predisposition, since some groups of related Standardbred stallions are affected. The defect has been seen in Warm bloods, Anglo-Arabs, Arabians, ponies, as well as a variety of mixed breds. Apart from the microtubular masses and impaired fertility, no other defects have been identified.

Traumatic and mechanical

Torsion of the spermatic cord

Torsion of the testis and epididymis around the spermatic cord has been reported by Pascoe et al. (1981a) and Threlfall et al. (1990). The paucity of reports suggests the lesion is rare, and we have seen no case.

Affected horses suffer mild to severe abdominal discomfort and swelling of the scrotum. Castration is the usual treatment. In one case, unilateral castration for torsion of the left testicle was followed by torsion of the right testicle 4 years later. In order to save this animal for breeding, the testicle was repositioned and tacked in place. Threlfall et al. stated that correction of torsion within 6–10 hours could save the testicle.

Anatomical defects such as laxity of the proper ligament and abnormally long epididymis facilitate testicular torsion and have been found in several cases (Pascoe et al. 1981a; Threlfall et al. 1990).

Inguinal/scrotal hernia

Inguinal hernia is a cause of colic and intestinal obstruction and strangulation (Schneider et al. 1982). Protrusion or prolapse of a loop of bowel

Table 13-1. Incidence of Cryptorchidism

	Population %	Cryptorchid %
Quarter horse	45	49
Appaloosa	6	6
Arabian	10	4
Standardbred	4	3
Thoroughbred	10	1.4
Draft breeds	4	0
Other	26	26

Source: Stickle and Fessler 1978.

into the inguinal ring, with or without torsion, can cause obstruction of blood flow to or from the testis. In 27 cases of acquired inguinal hernia Schneider et al. (1982) found the testis on the affected side swollen and hard. In most cases, the affected testis was edematous and removed during castration and closure of the inguinal ring. Scrotal hernia is simply the exaggerated form of inguinal hernia, the loop of bowel making its way into the scrotum.

Sperm granuloma

Although uncommon in stallions, sperm granulomas can form when rupture of seminiferous or conducting tubules allows sperm to leak into interstitial tissue. There is granulomatous inflammation forming masses of variable size (Held et al. 1989). In one case intermittent, but sudden, pain when ejaculating was noted.

Roberts (1971) suggested that *Strongylus edentatus* larval migration can cause disruption of tubules and granulomatous inflammation. In the few cases we have seen, larvae of *S. edentatus* or *S. vulgaris* had not penetrated the testicular capsule.

Other traumatic and mechanical defects

Paraphimosis

Penile prolapse or paraphimosis has been reported in debilitated horses (Simmons et al. 1985). Usually, penile prolapse has been associated with tranquilizers or anesthetics, as a complication of castration, or following lesions of the spinal cord.

Rupture of the corpus spongiosum

A stallion, presumably kicked by a companion gelding, had a rupture of the corpus spongiosum of the penis, followed by rupture of the urinary bladder (Firth 1976). While traumatic hematoma may occur in breeding stallions, it is uncommon.

Hematocele

Hematocele of one testis was the cause of transient infertility in a Standardbred stallion (Gygax et al. 1973). Testicular trauma was the probable cause. Six months after removing the inflamed, hemorrhagic testis, normal fertility returned. The transient loss of fertility was ascribed to the increased testicular temperature caused by inflammation. The pathology was not described.

Hemospermia

Hemospermia, the result of urethritis in or near the ejaculatory ducts, can cause infertility (Voss and Pickett 1975). Infection with *Pseudomonas aeruginosa,* urethral scars and strictures, trauma, unclassified viral agents, and strongyle infestation have been cited as possible causes of hemospermia.

Ejaculatory and behavioral disorders

Ejaculatory disorders have been reported in stallions (Rasbech 1975). The etiology is complex and appears to involve nervous system deficits, environmental or genetic problems, and psychic states. An overview of ejaculatory dysfunction is given by Rasbech. Abnormalities in mating behavior were reviewed by Pickett and Voss (1975). Since morphological changes are not involved, the reader is referred to their review.

Neoplasia

Neoplasms of the male reproductive tract are uncommon (Trigo et al. 1984; Peterson 1984). Cotchin (1977) found approximately 1% of all equine tumors in the testis in an abattoir survey.

Seminoma

A number of cases of seminoma have been reported, with a higher incidence in retained testes (Becht et al. 1979; Schonbauer and Schonbauer-Langle 1983; Trigo et al. 1984; Hunt et al. 1990b). A case of malignant seminoma was reported in a zebra/mare crossbred (Pandolfi and Roperto 1983). Of 11 cases reviewed, 5 were malignant, with local and distant metastases. Five of 11 cases were cryptorchids, and 4 of the 5 malignant seminomas were in the retained testis. In one case, malignant seminoma was found in the remnant spermatic cord and epididymis of a 22-year-old gelding. All of the horses were 11 years to 22 years old. Clinically, the animals had colicky abdominal pain, scrotal swelling, and loss of weight. Ten of the 11 cases were killed; 1 case was treated by unilateral orchiectomy.

Grossly, the seminomas were large, complex, multilobular masses causing testicular enlargement. In some there was extensive fibrosis surrounding the mass, obliterating the normal architecture. Two horses had torsion of the spermatic cord associated with growth of the mass. Hydroureter and hydronephrosis were reported in 2 of 11 cases. Metastatic masses occurred in nearly half of the cases, with inguinal and distant nodes, abdominal and peritoneal cavities, heart, lungs, and liver infiltrated. The primary and metastatic masses were consistently gray, tan, yellow, or white, with a bulging glistening surface.

Histologically, clusters of polygonal cells with round nuclei, showing some degree of cytologic maturation, are surrounded by bands of connective tissue. Mitotic figures are common and nucleoli prominent. Foci of lymphocytes are often present. Invasion of both lymphatics and veins by tumor cells is a prominent feature of some tumors (Figs. 13.1 and 13.2).

In one case of ours, the affected testis was removed when the tumor was about 5 cm × 5 cm and before clinical signs or evidence of metastasis to the inguinal lymph nodes had occurred. Histological examination showed frank invasion of neoplastic cells into both lymphatics and blood vessels. The animal survived for 2 years, with gradually declining fertility. Metastasis to the inguinal lymph nodes became apparent, and with the appearance of clinical signs of inanition and cachexia, the animal was killed.

Although some reports speak of benign seminomas, our experience, admittedly with a small number of cases, suggests that seminoma is not benign in the horse, only appearing so histologically in the early stages of its development.

Interstitial cell tumor

Gelberg and McEntee (1987) reported 9 interstitial cell tumors from a series of 38 equine testicular neoplasms. Eight of the 9 were in retained testes. The mean age of horses with the tumors was 8.1 years, with a range of 3 to 20 years. Two stallions displayed increased aggression, presumably the result of the synthesis of testosterone or a related androgen by neoplastic cells. In one horse, the behavior abated following removal of the neoplasm.

The masses in the testes ranged from 1 mm to 2 cm in diameter and were firm, gray, and irregularly shaped. Histologically, there was diffuse atrophy of seminiferous tubules. The authors felt that it was somewhat difficult to differentiate

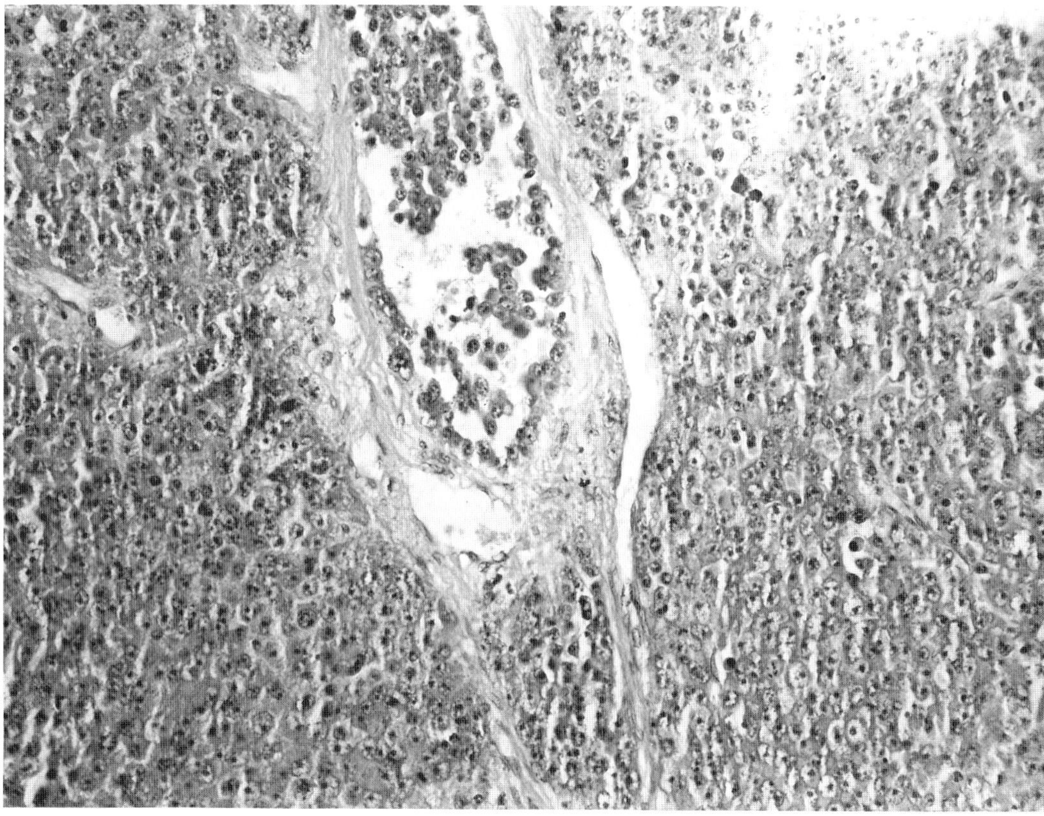

13.1. Seminoma in the testis showing invasion of venule.

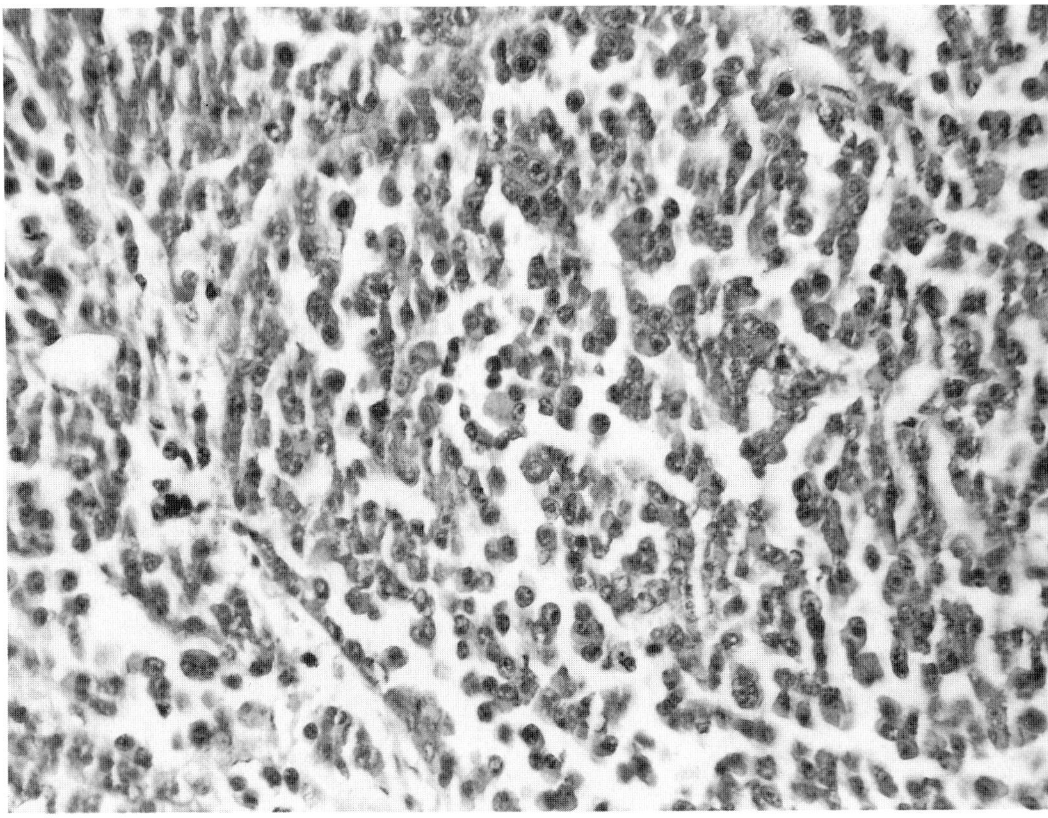

13.2. Moderately well-differentiated seminoma with cells forming cords within neoplastic seminiferous tubules.

hyperplastic and neoplastic lesions, although, in our experience, hyperplasia does not occur in the equine testis.

Two cell populations were seen histologically. In most tumors, large neoplastic interstitial cells with abundant cytoplasm, and somewhat pleomorphic nuclei, were arranged in sheets or nodules separated by connective tissue in an endocrinoid manner. The other cell population was more pleomorphic, with spindle shapes or multinucleate giant cells. Many neoplastic interstitial cells contained brown cytoplasmic pigment, which stained positively for lipid. Inflammatory cells infiltrated many of the lesions. Metastases were not found.

Sertoli cell tumor

A single case of Sertoli cell tumor has been reported (Rahaley et al. 1983). The testes were removed from an 11-year-old Quarter horse stallion with a history of progressive weight loss and poor breeding performance for 2 years. There was diffuse ventral alopecia but no other signs of estrogenism. An encapsulated 2-cm, firm, white mass was found in one testis. There was diffuse degeneration of seminiferous tubules and mild interstitial fibrosis. Some tubules contained clusters of neoplastic or hyperplastic Sertoli cells with well-differentiated characteristic morphology. Individual cells had round vesicular nuclei with prominent nucleoli and lacy eosinophilic cytoplasm. The orientation of cells to the basal lamina was typical of Sertoli cells. There was some cellular anaplasia and a moderate mitotic index, but no evidence of local invasion or metastasis.

Teratomas and teratocarcinomas

Teratomas and teratocarcinomas are neoplasms of the testes, containing cells derived from one or more embryonic germinal layers. Willis and Ruddick (1943) specify that a neoplasm be classified as a teratoma if the tumor tissues are differentiated and unrelated to the tissue of origin. Several authors (Smyth 1979; Stick 1980; Shaw and Roth 1986) described teratomas or teratocarcinomas of the equine testis. All four cases were in retained testes in horses under 2 years old. There were a variety of clinical signs, including weight loss and aggressive behavior. Masses were of variable size and irregular shape. A 122-kg teratocarcinoma was resected from a 330-kg horse. Others were smaller. Some contained multilocular cysts, which required drainage prior to surgical removal. Rebar et al. (1979) reported low levels of estrogen, progesterone, and testosterone in cyst fluid of one teratoma.

All of the neoplasms contained a variety of tissues including bone, adenoid tissue, goblet cells, cartilage, sebaceous glands, and myelin, among others. None of the neoplasms, save the teratocarcinoma, were judged to be highly malignant.

Mixed germ cell tumor

Two unusual testicular neoplasms have been described. Cullen et al. (1987) found a mixed germ cell–sex cord–stromal neoplasm in the testis of a 10-year-old Arabian stallion examined for routine breeding soundness. The unique histological features included proliferation of Sertoli cells and primitive germ cells within a matrix of collagenous fibers.

Embryonal carcinoma

Valentine and Weinstock (1986) found a metastatic testicular embryonal carcinoma in the testis of a 7-year-old Standardbred stallion. Cords of primitive cells formed tubulelike structures. Lack of differentiation of formed elements and positive staining for α-fetoprotein confirmed the diagnosis. Multiple metastases were found at autopsy.

Squamous cell carcinoma

Squamous cell carcinoma of the penis, **prepuce**, and associated structures is not uncommon. Howarth et al. (1991) published a retrospective study of 48 cases. The disease was most common in aged pony geldings with a mean age of 16.5 years. Markel et al. (1988) also noted that the disease was more prevalent in aged animals, the mean age in their 9 cases being 19 years. The external genitalia are common sites for squamous cell carcinoma, 45% of all cases in one study (Strafuss 1973). Hall et al. (1976) cited by Moulton (1985) found that geldings and stallions were equally affected. There was no correlation with coat color.

Lesions generally developed over months or years. Frequently, the predominating clinical sign was foul smelling, blood tinged preputial discharge (Howarth et al. 1991). Gross lesions varied in size and morphology: ulcerated, pendulated, or cauliflowerlike (Howarth et al). In a significant number of their cases squamous papilloma was present. They advised that these lesions be differentiated histologically since this was difficult on gross appearance. The benign papillomas and their transformation to malignant squamous cell carcinoma were discussed by several authors (Howarth et al. 1991). Approximately 10% of cases had histological evidence of metastasis to superficial and regional lymph nodes.

CHAPTER 14

Urinary Tract

Introduction

Disease of the urinary tract, especially primary renal disease, has been considered uncommon in horses and other equids (MacDougall and Ricketts 1987), although Cadeac (1899a) described several forms of renal disease, which we can recognize as nephrosis, glomerulonephritis, and chronic interstitial nephritis.

In the absence of striking gross findings routine histological examination of the kidneys may not be done, and routine hematoxylin and eosin stains may not be informative. Clinicopathological examination—24-hour urine specimens—is cumbersome, and renal biopsy difficult. With improvement in techniques and, particularly, awareness of the rich variety of lesions in other species, it has become apparent that renal lesions are more common in the horse than formerly believed.

Diagnostic techniques

Evaluation of urinary tract disease in horses begins with history and physical examination. In particular, water and food consumption and patterns of urination should be ascertained. Water consumption in healthy adult horses, approximately 450 kg, in a cool environment and fed hay, was 20–25 L/day (Tasker 1967). Mean urine production, catheterized samples, for 13 ponies, mean body weight 152 kg, was 93 mL/h (Rawlings and Bisgard 1975).

Diagnostic techniques for other species can be used in horses: hematology and serum chemistry screening profiles, urinalysis, renal biopsy, radiography, and sonography. Minor modifications may be needed for body size. Recent reviews describe a variety of diagnostic techniques (Bayly et al. 1980; Rantanen 1986; Kohn and Chew 1987).

Routine hematological measurements indicating renal disease may be found in textbooks of clinical pathology. Specifically, anemia indicative of bone marrow hypoplasia may be associated with chronic renal disease in mammals as a result of lack of erythropoietin synthesis by diseased kidneys. This has not been described in horses.

Azotemia

Azotemia is the retention of nitrogenous metabolic waste products, *urea nitrogen* and *creatinine,* in the circulation because of failure of renal excretion. It is an important indicator of urinary tract dysfunction.

Urea nitrogen is a by-product of protein metabolism, while creatinine is produced by the breakdown of creatine phosphate in muscle. Kohn and Chew (1987) discuss factors affecting the production and excretion of these waste products. Prerenal, renal, and postrenal forms of azotemia are recognized.

Prerenal azotemia is usually associated with ineffective renal perfusion caused by hemorrhage and dehydration. Primary glomerular and tubular disease may interfere with effective filtration of nitrogenous wastes, causing **renal azotemia**. Obstruction of the flow of urine and consequent reduction in renal filtration causes **postrenal azotemia**. Prerenal or postrenal causes of azotemia may be suspected from the clinical signs. Timely diagnosis of the predominant form of azotemia is important for appropriate therapy. Values of serum urea nitrogen below 25 mg/dL and serum creatinine below 1.9 mg/dL are within normal physiological limits for horses (Grossman et al. 1982).

The literature suggests that loss of more than 70% of renal function is necessary before detectable elevation of serum urea nitrogen or creatinine. This has not been established for the horse.

Accurate measurements of glomerular filtration rates by inulin and endogenous creatinine clearance are not done routinely in horses because of the difficulty of 24-hour urine collection. As a result, calculated indices or ratios of serum and urine values are used as measures of renal function (Grossman et al. 1982; Kohn and Chew 1987). In 10 horses with renal azotemia, the urea nitrogen index—concentration of urine urea nitrogen divided by concentration of serum urea nitrogen—ranged from 2.1 to 14.3 mg/dL, compared to 34.2–100.8 mg/dL in normal horses. Six horses with prerenal azotemia had urea:nitrogen ratios ranging from 15.2:1 to 43.7:1. Other indices of value in the differentiation of prerenal and renal azotemia include the urine/serum creatinine ratio, urine/plasma osmolality ratio, and fractional excretion of sodium (Grossman et al. 1982). Fractional sodium excretion is calculated:

$$FE[Na] = [Cr]p \times [Na]u \times 100\ [Cr]u\ [Na]p$$

where FE[Na] is the fractional excretion of sodium, [Cr]p is the concentration of creatinine in plasma, [Cr]u is the concentration of creatinine in urine, [Na]u is the concentration of sodium in urine, and [Na]p is the concentration of sodium in plasma. A calculated value of fractional excretion of sodium above 1 indicates renal disease (Grossman et al. 1982).

The concentrations of serum electrolytes—

sodium, potassium, chloride, inorganic phosphorus, and calcium—may reflect altered glomerular filtration, variations in urine production, defects in tubular reabsorption, inadequate ion exchange, and complex interactions of these abnormalities. Although their numbers were small Kohn and Chew (1987) noted that horses with primary renal disease, especially chronic renal failure, were either hypochloridemic, hypercalcemic, or both. Hypercalcemia has been reported in horses with renal failure associated with vitamin K intoxication (Rebhun et al. 1984), and in red maple leaf toxicity (Tennant et al. 1982).

The association of hypercalcemia with renal failure in horses is unique among domesticated mammals. Unlike dogs, for example, horses with renal disease, naturally occurring or experimental, do not develop the profound hyperphosphatemia usually found with acute or chronic renal failure.

Hypoproteinemia and/or hypoalbuminemia and proteinuria may accompany nephrotic syndrome or nephritis in horses (Sabnis et al. 1984), suggesting serum protein and serum and urine electrophoresis as useful diagnostic tools.

γ-Glutamyl transpeptidase is found in equine liver and in the brush border of the proximal convoluted tubule of the kidney. The mean value of urine γ-glutamyl transpeptidase was 3.3 ± 3.0 IU/L in 32 healthy horses of both sexes, 1–16 years old (Brobst et al. 1986). There is apparently no significant sex or age variation in urinary enzyme levels in adult horses.

The size of this enzyme precludes filtration through the normal glomerulus (Brobst et al. 1986). In diseased kidneys, especially with tubular lesions, the enzyme is released into the urine. Brobst et al. (1986) and Barakat and Ford (1988) have shown that the concentration of enzyme in the urine is proportional to the degree of tubular damage (Adams et al. 1985). In some forms of acute tubular necrosis, however, enzyme values did not correlate well with the course of the clinical disease (Roberts et al. 1978a).

While the concentration of enzyme is slightly higher in morning samples, there is little fluctuation during the day. Serum concentrations of γ-glutamyl transpeptidase and urine concentrations of the enzyme are not correlated in disease. In particular, liver parenchymal disease may cause elevation of the serum enzyme without concomitant increases in urinary enzyme. The prognostic value of other enzymes such as urinary 5′-nucleotidase has not been established in horses (Barakat and Ford 1988).

Renal biopsy has not been widely used. Bayly et al. (1980) described percutaneous biopsy of the left kidney and demonstrated its value in several cases of renal disease. Diffuse renal disease may be found in a small, percutaneous biopsy, but focal processes could be missed. Laparoscopic and laparotomy biopsies could be warranted in individual cases.

Radiography is of limited value in the diagnosis of urinary tract disease. Rantanen (1986) described ultrasonography in the diagnosis of equine renal disease.

Inflammatory and infectious diseases

Primary inflammatory renal diseases include glomerulonephritis, glomerulosclerosis, pyelonephritis, hemolytic uremic syndrome, purpura hemorrhagica, and tubulointerstitial nephritis. Acute and chronic forms of some diseases have been recognized in horses.

Glomerular diseases

Mesangioproliferative glomerulonephritis

There are a few case reports of equine mesangioproliferative glomerulonephritis (McCausland and Milestone 1976; Waldvogel et al. 1983; Sabnis et al. 1984; Wilkinson et al. 1985). Horse and pony mares and geldings of several breeds, 1–16 years old, had primary glomerular lesions. In most cases, there was a history of progressive weight loss and peripheral edema of legs, jaw, and face. Clinicopathological abnormalities included nephrotic syndrome with marked proteinuria and hypoproteinemia, azotemia, and multiple electrolyte abnormalities. Several horses had hypercalcemia and hyperkalemia. Most of the animals were killed weeks to months after onset.

The pattern of gross lesions was not consistent. Some horses with nephrotic syndrome had marked edema of the subcutis, gastrointestinal mucosa, and periorbital tissues. The kidneys were either enlarged or smaller than normal (McCausland and Milestone 1976; Sabnis et al. 1984; Wilkinson et al. 1985). Ulceration of the buccal or gastric mucosa was seen in some cases (Sabnis et al. 1984).

Microscopic lesions were consistent. In all cases there was glomerular hypercellularity, mesangial hypercellularity and expansion, fibroepithelial or epithelial crescents, and alterations in the morphology of glomerular basement membranes (Fig. 14.1). Staining for immunoglobulins was equivocal in most cases. The small number of cases precluded evaluation of pathological versus age-related variations in basement-membrane morphology. In sev-

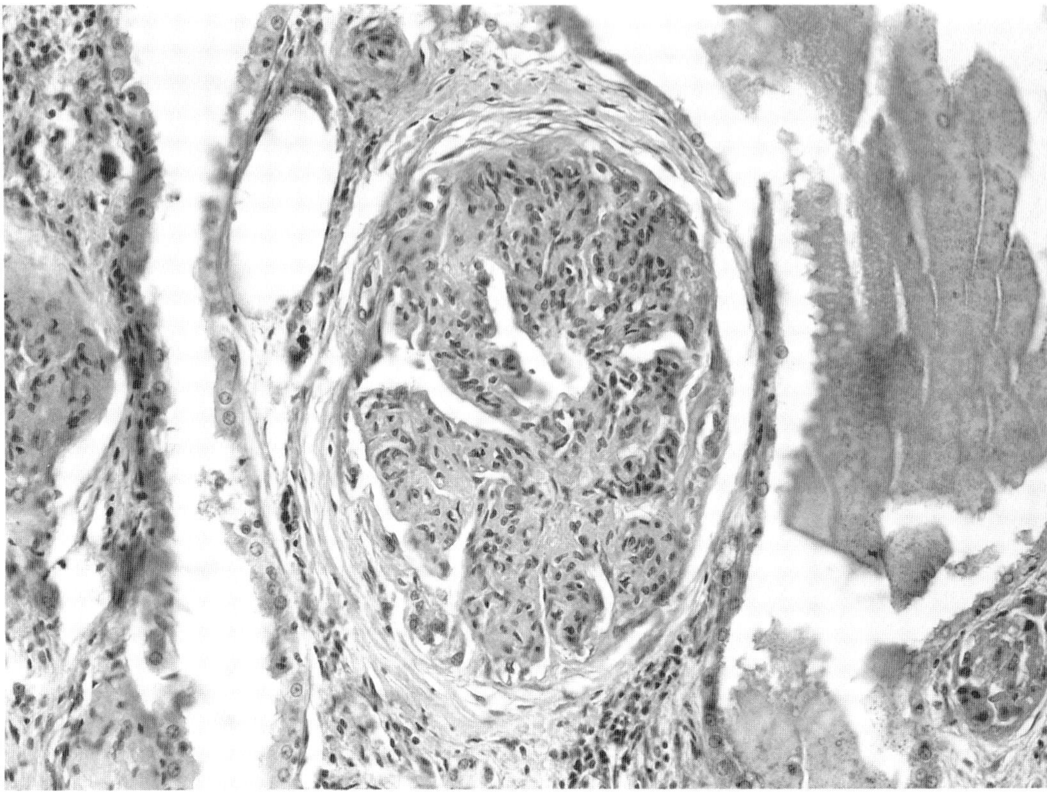

14.1. Mesangiocapillary glomerulonephritis in horses characteristically shows hypercellular tufts with increased synthesis of mesangium.

eral cases, organized fibrillar intramembranous or mesangial deposits were found (Sabnis et al. 1984; Wilkinson et al. 1985). In at least one horse, the deposits in the mesangium and membranes were considered morphologically analogous to those in human cryoglobulinemia (Sabnis et al. 1984).

Glomerulonephritis with purpura hemorrhagica

Mesangioproliferative glomerulonephritis has been diagnosed in one case of purpura hemorrhagica (Roberts and Kelly 1982). There was severe peripheral edema, azotemia, proteinuria, and hypoproteinemia. The kidneys were enlarged and pale. Microscopically, there was marked, diffuse glomerular hypercellularity, the result of mesangial cell proliferation, and a lesser degree of glomerular lymphocytic infiltration. Proteinaceous casts were present in dilated tubules, and there was tubulointerstitial nephritis.

Clearly, renal lesions were associated with the cutaneous and systemic manifestations of purpura hemorrhagica in this one case. Renal lesions have not been seen consistently in other cases, however. Immunologically mediated processes, such as immune complex deposition, have been proposed in the pathogenesis of this condition, but there have been no definitive studies.

Hemolytic uremic syndrome

Two cases of hemolytic uremic syndrome, associated with azotemia, proteinuria and hematuria, and severe glomerular lesions have been reported (Morris et al. 1987). The animals had marked subcutaneous edema and progressive renal failure despite aggressive therapy. At autopsy the kidneys were enlarged, discolored, and there was renal papillary necrosis. Microscopically, glomeruli were enlarged and capillary loops distended with fibrin thrombi (Fig. 14.2). There was marked, diffuse, segmental necrosis of capillary tufts, and prominent lesions were seen in afferent arterioles.

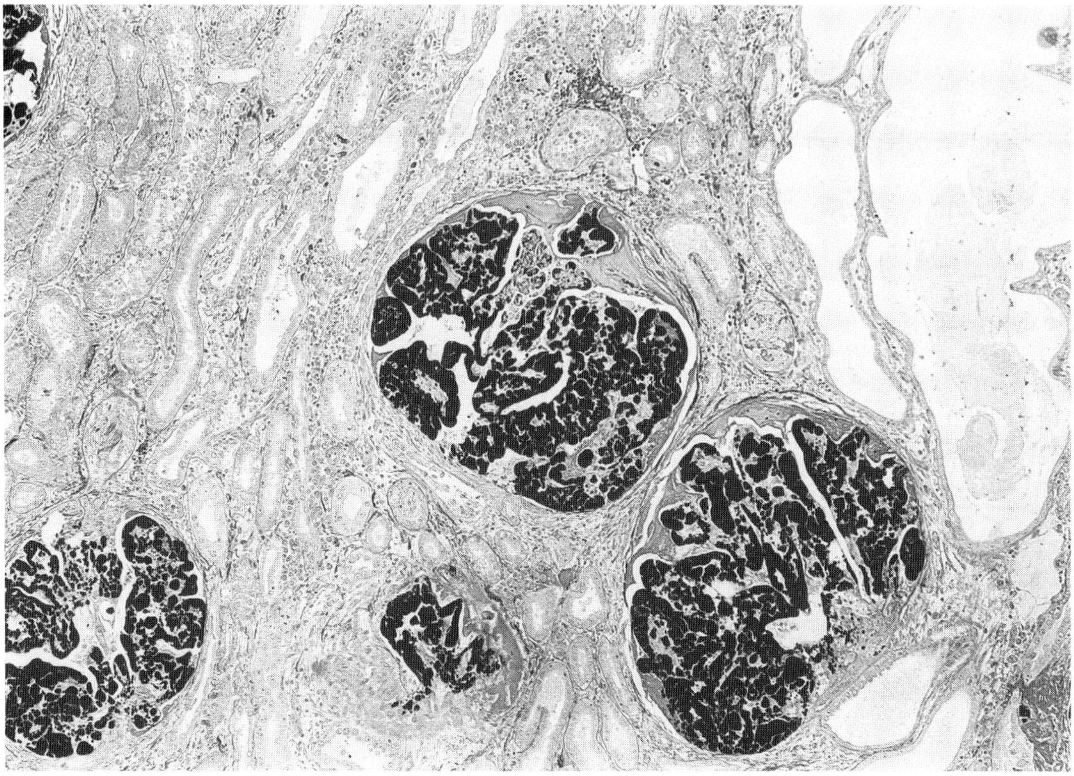

14.2. Fibrin thrombi in capillary loops of a horse with hemolytic uremic syndrome.

There were cortical hemorrhages and interstitial fibrosis and/or nephritis in both cases.

The cause of hemolytic uremic syndrome is unknown, but exposure to coliform toxins and the formation of immune complexes are believed to be significant factors in the development of lesions.

Immune complex glomerulonephritis

Immune complex glomerulonephritis is the commonest immunologically mediated renal disease in humans and a number of domesticated animals. Glomerulonephritis with the deposition of complexes of viral antigen, immunoglobulins, and complement has been seen in experimental equine infectious anemia (Banks et al. 1972a,b).

Baseline renal biopsies were taken from Shetland ponies and Warm bloods. After exposure to infectious anemia virus, sequential renal biopsies and measures of renal function were done from 16 to over 1000 days. Clinical signs and lesions developed within 2 weeks of exposure. Glomerulitis with diffuse tuft hypercellularity and infiltration with inflammatory cells was seen in over 70% of the animals. Granular deposits of immunoglobulin G and complement were present on glomerular basement membranes in all animals, together with glomerular hypercellularity. Irregular thickenings of the membrane were common. Viral elution established that viral antigen, complexed with antibody, comprised the deposits seen by immunofluorescent and electron microscopy. A few horses with immunoglobulin and complement deposits did not have glomerulonephritis.

Despite diffuse and significant glomerular lesions, there was neither azotemia nor proteinuria. The incidence of glomerular lesions in naturally occurring infection with equine infectious anemia virus is not known.

Sixteen percent of the noninfected, clinically normal control ponies and horses in this study also had glomerulonephritis (Banks et al. 1972a,b). Of these normal ponies and horses, 42% had benign deposition of immunoglobulin G and complement, in a granular pattern, along the glomerular basement membrane or in the mesangium. None of the animals were azotemic or proteinuric. As in other species, trapping and removal of circulating immune complexes by the glomeruli are probably normal functions of the equine kidney.

Antiglomerular basement membrane nephritis

Linear deposition of immunoglobulin G and complement along the glomerular basement membrane was reported in 3 of 45 clinically normal horses (Banks et al. 1972b). Antibody eluted from glomeruli bound to normal glomerular basement membrane, but not to other basement membranes in the kidney or other tissues. Thickening and irregular folding of the glomerular basement membrane were also seen.

None of the animals with this unusual change had signs of renal dysfunction, and the relevance of these morphological alterations to clinical disease in the horse is questionable. In humans, the linear deposition of immunoglobulin and complement along glomerular basement membranes is the hallmark of rapidly progressive glomerulonephritis.

Chronic glomerulonephritis

Chronic glomerulonephritis has been reported less in horses than other species (Fincher and Olafson 1934; Frank 1935; Langham and Hallman 1941; Buntain et al. 1979; Tennant et al. 1982). Clinical features included weight loss, dependent edema, and altered food and water consumption. Buntain et al. (1979) reported azotemia, hypoproteinemia, and abnormalities in serum electrolytes, as well as proteinuria and low urine specific gravity. Paradoxical hypercalcemia and hypophosphatemia were seen in five horses with chronic glomerulonephritis (Tennant et al. 1982). Three other horses with advanced renal failure studied at the same time did not have hypercalcemia or hypophosphatemia.

Typical lesions in one case are described (Buntain et al. 1979). The kidneys were symmetrically small, firm, and discolored, and the capsule stripped with difficulty. A variety of glomerular lesions included multifocal, segmental, or global glomerulosclerosis, fibroepithelial crescents and senechia, mesangial hypercellularity, and/or diffuse glomerular hypertrophy (Fig. 14.3). A lymphoplasmacytic interstitial nephritis was accompanied by tubular atrophy, dilation, cast formation, and patchy interstitial fibrosis.

It has been assumed that acute glomerulonephritis progresses in some cases to chronic glomerulonephritis with renal failure, but this has not been unequivocally established in humans or dogs and has not been studied in the horse.

Tennant et al. (1982) discussed the unusual nature of hypercalcemia in horses with chronic renal disease. The horse regulates total body calcium through the combined actions of dietary intake, bone storage, and renal excretion. With kidney disease and loss of renal function there is diminished production of activated vitamin D and decreased absorption of dietary calcium. As well, the kidney loses the capacity to excrete calcium and to cleave and excrete the C-terminal portion of parathyroid hormone (Elfers et al. 1986). These effects may combine to account for the elevation of serum calcium, but hypercalcemia and hypophosphatemia in horses with chronic renal disease is poorly understood.

Glomerulosclerosis

Glomerulosclerosis has rarely been reported in horses (Banks et al. 1972a; Wimberly et al. 1979). Focal glomerulosclerosis was seen in a single young horse with progressive weight loss and multiple signs of renal failure: azotemia, nephrotic syndrome, electrolyte abnormalities, and metabolic acidosis. There was segmental sclerosis of capillary tufts with formation of senechia (Fig. 14.4). Tubular degeneration and interstitial fibrosis were present. No deposits of immunoglobulin or complement were detected.

A horse with diffuse glomerulosclerosis, tubular degeneration, and severe interstitial fibrosis had deposits of calcium oxalate crystals in regenerating tubules and interstitial connective tissue (Andrews 1971). Both the glomerular and tubular lesions were attributed to oxalate deposition, but it is more likely that the scattered crystals formed in the fibrotic kidney well after the parenchyma became fibrotic. Indeed, oxalate crystals are quite regularly present in focal chronic lesions of the equine kidney. The spectrum of glomerular lesions in this case suggests end-stage chronic glomerulonephritis and glomerulosclerosis.

Pyelonephritis

Infection of the renal pelvis and parenchyma is rare in horses and is a consequence of obstruction of the flow of urine and ascending infection. There are reports of pyelonephritis associated with urethral trauma (Roberts 1979), vesiculovaginal reflux (Easley 1988), sorghum cystitis (Adams et al. 1969), postparturient *Corynebacterium renale* infection (Boyd and Bishop 1937), and uroliths (Ehnen et al. 1990). The reason(s) for the low incidence in horses as compared to some other species is not known.

Unilateral or bilateral, acute and chronic forms have been seen in horses, associated with signs of

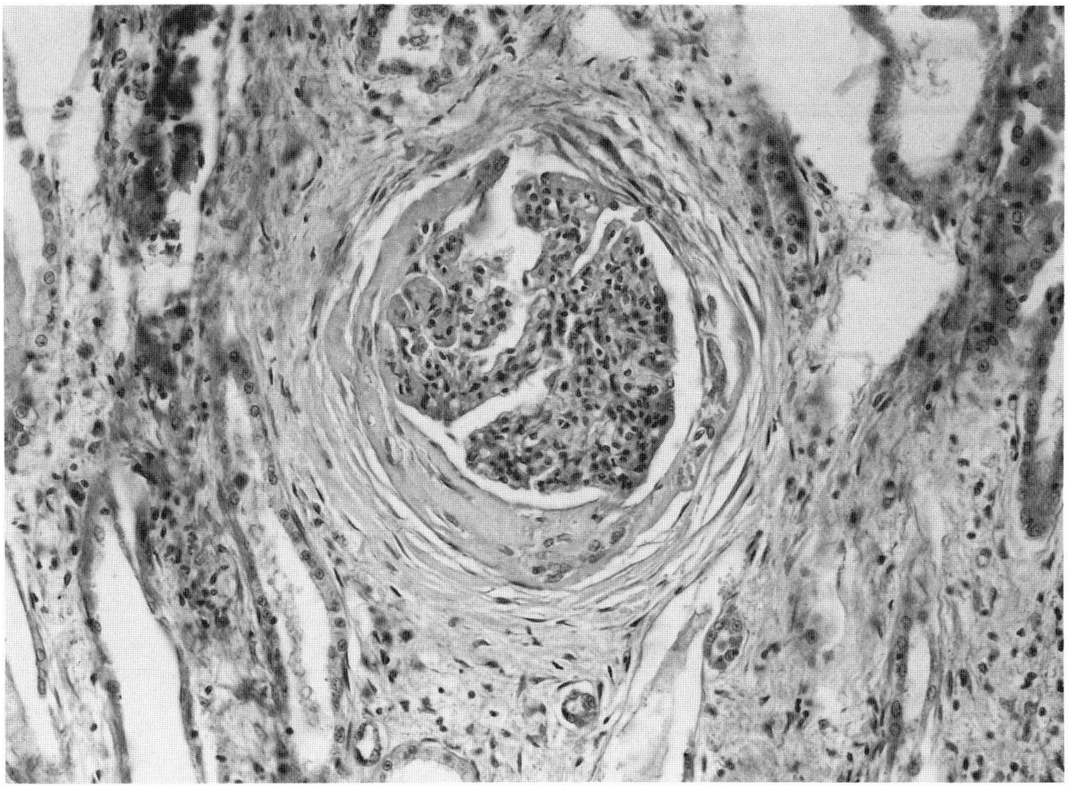

14.3. Fibroepithelial crescent formation in the glomerulus of a horse with chronic glomerulonephritis.

renal failure including azotemia, polydipsia and polyuria, leukocytosis, fever, and abnormal urine (Irwin and Howell 1980; Roberts 1979). In chronic cases scarring and fibrosis may markedly deform the kidneys. Frank abscesses have been reported (Irwin and Howell 1980; Held et al. 1986). *Staphylococcus aureus, C. renale,* and coliforms have been isolated.

Histologically, lesions include intratubular and interstitial inflammatory cells. Tubular degeneration and replacement fibrosis may cause deformation of the pelvis, medulla, and cortex. Focal scarring of the cortex in wedge-shaped rays is common in all species. The inflammatory cells vary with the age of the lesion. There may be glomerular atrophy and periglomerular fibrosis in areas of interstitial fibrosis. In long-standing infections, there is considerable loss of tubules and glomeruli, the result of interstitial fibrosis, bacterial destruction, inflammation, and compromised renal perfusion.

It is not uncommon to find ureteritis, cystitis, and urethritis with pyelonephritis. Horses with chronic pyelonephritis and chronic tubulointerstitial nephritis may form uroliths in tissue, the renal pelvis, ureters, or the urinary bladder. The uroliths can obstruct the flow of urine, further exacerbating the development of chronic lesions (Hope et al. 1989; Ehnen et al. 1990).

Renal coccidiosis

The kidneys of horses and other equids can be infested with the sporozoan parasite *Klossiella equi.* While any equid can be infected, the infestation is almost universal in donkeys and asses. Soulsby (1965) reports infection of equids with *Eimeria leukarti, solipedum,* and *uniungulati.* There is no significant alteration of kidney function, the infestation being found incidentally at postmortem.

Renal coccidiosis is worldwide. Following infection, schizonts are found in epithelial cells in the proximal convoluted tubules and occasionally in glomerular visceral epithelium. Sporogenic and gametogenic forms, in membrane-bound vacuoles, have been seen in collecting duct cells (Lee and

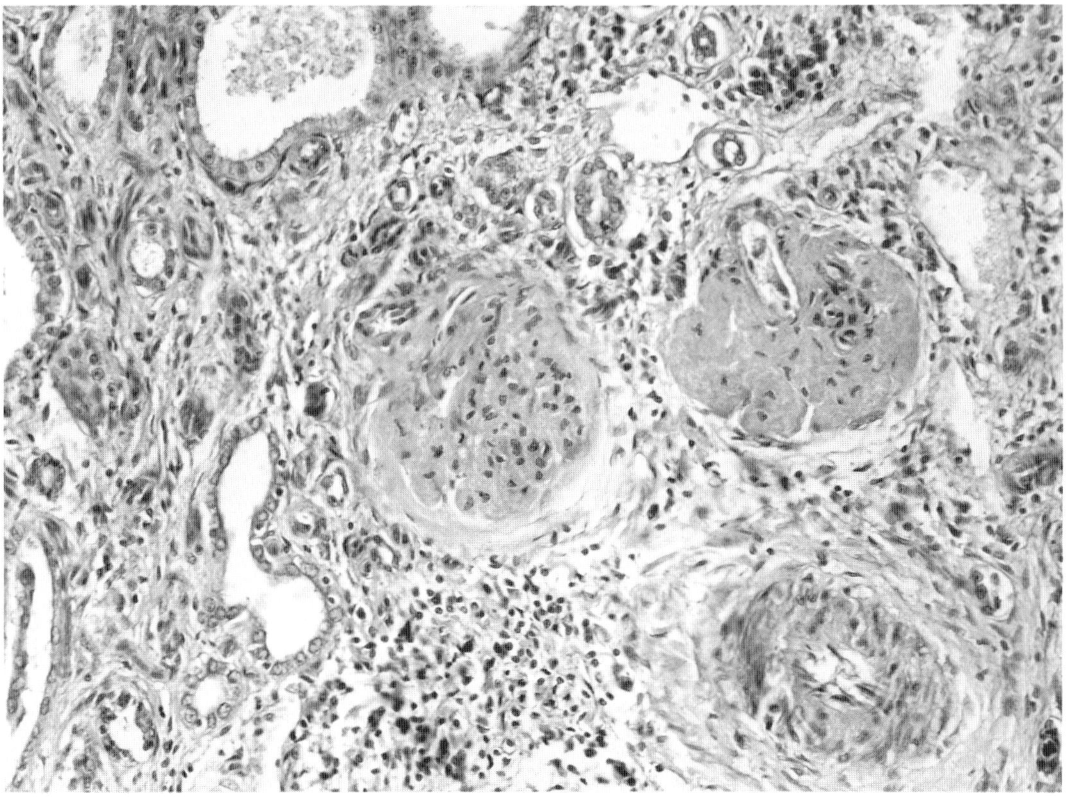

14.4. Sclerotic glomeruli are acellular and have no discernible tuft architecture.

Ross 1977). There is little reaction to the parasites. Some epithelial cells may slough into the lumens of tubules. A multifocal, minimal, lymphoplasmacytic tubulointerstitial nephritis in the kidneys of infected horses has been described. No reaction has been seen in the kidneys of infested donkeys and asses.

Leptospirosis

This disease has long been an enigma in horses. Serological surveys indicate that antibodies for a number of different serovars are present in horses in many, if not all, parts of the world (Ellis and O'Brien 1988). The confirmed clinical disease in horses is uncommon and sporadic (Bryans 1972a). It is perhaps the case that massive exposure and/or partial disabling of the immune system is necessary for clinical disease. Leptospira of several serovars have been associated with sporadic abortion in mares (Ellis and O'Brien) (see Chapter 11, "Female Reproductive System: Leptospiral abortion").

The clinical disease in horses is acute, with fever for several days, anorexia, mild depression, leucocytosis, and, occasionally, icterus. Leptospiremia and clinical signs disappear with the appearance of antibody at about the 7th or 8th day after onset (Bryans 1972). Urinary shedding continues for a variable period after the cessation of clinical signs. There are no reports of pathological findings in postnatal animals.

Strongylus vulgaris thrombosis

Focal or multifocal infarction of the kidneys occurs with parasitic thrombosis of the renal arteries. While there are thrombi in the renal artery, the focal infarcts and histological study show that embolization of the arteries near and at the corticomedullary junction is the immediate cause. We have not seen massive infarction and, in no case, was there clinical disease of the urinary system.

Congenital

Renal hypoplasia

All mammals are born with structurally and functionally immature kidneys. The degree of immaturity varies by species (Zicker et al. 1990). Function tests and morphology indicate that horse kidneys are essentially mature at birth (Zicker et al. 1990; Andrews et al. 1986). There have been reports of diffuse nephron hypoplasia or dysplasia in foals and young horses causing acute or chronic renal failure.

There usually is a short history of wasting, anorexia, failure to thrive, retarded growth, and signs of acute renal dysfunction. Anemia was caused by ineffective erythropoiesis in at least one case. There are abnormalities of serum electrolytes. Urea nitrogen and creatinine are elevated, and there is abnormal renal clearance and fractional electrolyte excretion. The urinalysis is abnormal. Increased fractional sodium excretion, indicative of renal sodium wasting, has been seen. In animals with necrosis of nephrons there are elevated urinary levels of γ-glutamyl transpeptidase (Zicker et al. 1990).

Virtually all animals with severe congenital or early developmental dysplasia develop renal failure and die or are killed soon after azotemia appears. The kidneys, bilaterally affected, may be small or of normal size and pale or brown. There may be hemorrhage and/or necrosis of the medulla and papilla. Both medulla and cortex are thin and attenuated.

Histologically, there is segmental dysplasia and degeneration of portions of the nephron, particularly the medullary tubular segments. The cortical tubular segments are normal with the exception of dilation in most cases. In young animals there is little interstitial fibrosis, and glomeruli are quite normal. An increase in interstitial myxomatous connective tissue has been seen. In several cases of bilateral renal dysplasia in older animals tubular degeneration, interstitial fibrosis, mineralization, and glomerular degeneration were seen.

Polycystic disease

Another form of renal dysplasia is polycystic kidney. In humans, two forms are recognized—polycystic disease of the newborn and adult polycystic disease. Although urinary tubular retention cysts are commonly caused by interstitial fibrosis and interruption of urine flow in diseased nephrons, diffuse cyst formation as the result of genetically programmed dysplasia of tubular segments is rare.

Ramsay et al. (1987) reported the clinical and pathological features of a case of adult polycystic disease in a 9-year-old Warm blood. The mare had a 3-week history of anorexia and weight loss. She had successfully carried two foals, but had aborted the last two pregnancies. She was markedly azotemic with decreased serum sodium, chloride, and calcium. At postmortem, the kidneys were markedly enlarged, with numerous thin-walled cysts filling the cortex and medulla. Microscopic examination showed the cysts were lined by flattened epithelium. Tubular segments that were not cystic had flattened epithelium, and most glomeruli were atrophic or sclerotic.

Adult polycystic kidney disease is an autosomal dominant disease in humans. Unfortunately, the two live foals could not be traced.

Toxic/metabolic

Acute renal failure

There are two types of acute renal failure. One, ischemic acute renal failure, is caused by failure of adequate renal perfusion. The other is caused by tubular intoxication by nephrotoxic chemicals.

Ischemic acute renal failure

Acute blood loss, shock, sepsis, and vascular calamities such as thrombosis can decrease renal perfusion with ischemia and/or hypoperfusion, causing acute tubular necrosis. Conditions causing dehydration may directly cause acute renal lesions or contribute to the pathogenesis of lesions caused by other agents.

In horses, colic is a significant cause of acute renal failure. The combined effects of shock, peripheral blood pooling, dehydration, and fluid shunting to the gut may precipitate ischemic acute tubular necrosis. The absorption of toxins from devitalized areas of the gastrointestinal tract, electrolyte imbalances, nephrotoxic antibiotics, and nonsteroidal antiinflammatory drugs may further compromise the ischemic kidney. Alterations in renal perfusion caused by mechanical obstruction to blood flow and consumptive coagulopathies may be factors in any given case of colic (Seanor et al. 1984).

Ischemic acute renal failure was seen in 6 horses, 2 to 18 years old, with nonspecific signs of diarrhea, myositis, colic, and/or sepsis (Divers et al. 1987). There was azotemia, low urine specific gravity, oliguria, hyponatremia and hypochloremia, and evidence of consumptive coagulopathy in most cases. Renal tissue in 4 of 6 animals had varying degrees of tubular necrosis, swelling, dilation, and inflammation. In several cases thrombi were found in segmental arterioles in the kidneys with infarction of renal parenchyma.

Toxic acute renal failure

The second type of acute renal failure is toxic acute renal failure caused by damage to tubular segments. This has been seen in horses exposed to a variety of toxic materials, including heavy metals (mercury) in blistering agents, myoglobin, red maple leaves, nephrotoxic antibiotics such as gentamicin, some nonsteroidal antiinflammatory drugs, and others.

Although the clinical signs of toxic and ischemic acute renal failure are similar, the morphology of the tubular lesions is different. In ischemic renal failure, there is a distinctive disruption of nephron segments with lysis of tubular basement membranes and epithelium. This is referred to as **hypoperfusion acute tubular necrosis with tubulorrhexis**. Those portions of the proximal and distal tubules with high metabolic activity are most sensitive to ischemia, and it is here that lesions are localized.

Tubular intoxication in toxic acute renal failure causes acute tubular necrosis, with damaged cells in the proximal and distal tubular segments undergoing necrosis and sloughing from basement membranes. The tubular basement membrane is generally preserved and provides a scaffolding for orderly cellular regeneration. The severity and localization of lesions in toxic acute tubular necrosis is dependent on several factors including sites of toxin metabolism in tubules, inherent tubular cell metabolism, renal perfusion, and localization of toxin-binding proteins within tubular cells.

Mercury

Inorganic and organic mercury causes significant renal damage. Horses may eat feedstuffs contaminated with mercury fungicides, drink water contaminated with organic forms of mercury, or ingest material applied to the skin as a blister. In earlier days mercury and other heavy metals were commonly used for treatment of various diseases and, no doubt, were a not infrequent cause of renal disease (Cadeac 1899a).

Acute renal failure occurred in a 4-year-old Standardbred horse to which a mercuric iodide blister had been applied 5 days earlier. Gastrointestinal signs, depression, dementia, and weakness were seen. The animal was markedly azotemic, hyperkalemic and hyperphosphatemic, but hyponatremic and hypochloremic. At postmortem the kidneys were pale and enlarged. Severe, diffuse tubular necrosis was present, with cells and cellular debris filling the tubular lumens.

Horses receiving other forms of inorganic and organic mercury developed similar renal lesions (Roberts et al. 1982; Seawright 1982). Bayly et al. (1986a and b) studied acute renal failure in Shetland ponies induced by the daily intravenous administration of mercuric chloride and potassium dichromate. Elfers et al. (1986) described the pathogenesis of lesions within 2–5 days of exposure to relatively low doses of inorganic mercury. Early signs of acute tubular necrosis and renal dysfunction included transient elevations in urinary γ-glutamyl transpeptidase and marked proteinuria. These serum biochemical changes appeared early and were considered the most sensitive indicators of renal damage. Alterations in serum urea nitrogen and creatinine developed only after profound renal damage. Convoluted tubular epithelium was necrotic and sloughing in some tubules, but regenerating in others after five doses of inorganic mercury. Another horse given low doses of mercuric chloride developed granulomatous interstitial nephritis and tubular necrosis.

Cadmium

Another heavy metal with a propensity for renal localization is cadmium. Several cases of cadmium-related nephropathy in horses had intraparenchymal deposition of calcium salts at the corticomedullary junction (Gunson et al. 1982). Experimental and epidemiological evidence in humans and laboratory animals has shown that cadmium binds preferentially to renal tubular metallothioneins, causes proteinuria, and fosters the deposition of calcium phosphate in the renal parenchyma. Such deposits are, apparently, benign.

Gentamicin

The nephrotoxicity of therapeutic levels of the antibiotic gentamicin is well known in horses. Filtration of the antibiotic and accumulation in tubular epithelial cells causes the death of these cells by direct cellular cytotoxicity. Risk factors for the development of nephrotoxicity in horses and ponies include concomitant administration of other potentially nephrotoxic drugs, frequent or prolonged administration of high doses, impaired renal perfusion, disseminated bacterial infections, endotoxemia, and dietary deficiencies of minerals such as calcium, magnesium, and sodium (Riviere et al. 1982; Sweeney et al. 1988; Schumacher et al. 1991).

Experimental horses on a calcium-poor diet developed biochemical signs of gentamicin nephrotoxicity within 5 days of high intravenous dosing

(Schumacher et al. 1991). Animals on a calcium-enriched diet were resistant to the nephrotoxicity, as indicated by urinary γ-glutamyl transpeptidase values and indices of tubular function. Calcium ions may compete with gentamicin molecules for binding sites on proximal tubule brush borders, and decrease gentamicin reabsorption and concentration in tubular cells.

The kidneys of animals with gentamicin nephrotoxicity may be slightly swollen. Microscopically, proximal tubular cells may be enlarged, contain vacuoles and cytoplasmic bodies, and undergo degeneration. Necrotic cells may slough and fill tubular lumens. There is little inflammation. These lesions appear to be reversible with drug withdrawal.

Vitamin K3

Administration of vitamin K3 (menadione) to horses at doses of 2.2–11 mg/kg produced signs of renal colic, stranguria, azotemia, and hematuria within 24 hours of injection (Rebhun et al. 1984). In spontaneous cases, the drug had been given for treatment of pulmonary epistaxis. In six horses, the drug was given experimentally to study the pathogenesis of lesions. Animals were proteinuric and had low urine specific gravity at the onset of clinical signs. There was no evidence of vitamin-induced hemolysis or hemoglobin nephropathy.

Four animals were autopsied, and the kidneys were enlarged and pale in all. Diffuse or multifocal tubular necrosis, tubular dilation, and proteinaceous casts were seen consistently. Foci of tubular epithelial cell regeneration were seen in 1 horse, while another had minimal, multifocal tubulointerstitial nephritis, fibrosis, and interstitial edema.

One horse died with clinical and biochemical signs of chronic renal failure 20 months after an acute episode of vitamin K3 nephrotoxicity. At autopsy, there was glomerulosclerosis and parenchyma fibrosis.

Renal papillary necrosis

Therapeutic levels of nonsteroidal antiinflammatory drugs such as phenylbutazone, in horses and ponies with hemoconcentration, will cause necrosis of the renal medullary crest and papilla (Read 1983; Gunson 1983; Gunson and Soma 1983). Retrospective analysis was done of 51 horses of both sexes, various breeds, 3 months to 18 years of age (Read 1983; Gunson 1983). The common factor was repetitive administration of nonsteroidal drugs—phenylbutazone, flunixin meglumine, dipyrone, acetyl salicylic acid, or combinations—with increased hematocrit prior to death. Decreased water intake was observed directly or inferred from hospital records. The relationship of drug administration and hemoconcentration to the lesions was confirmed experimentally (Gunson and Soma 1983).

A variety of clinicopathological abnormalities was seen in both spontaneous and experimental cases of papillary necrosis. There was mild to marked azotemia. In some horses, the loss of renal concentrating ability was shown by persistently low urine specific gravity. Hematuria and crystalluria were present to varying degrees.

Gross lesions in both spontaneous and experimental cases included prominent discoloration of the renal medullary crest and papilla, papillary friability or detachment, medullary and peripapillary congestion and hemorrhage, and mineralization. Necrotic sequestra in the renal pelvis were common. Lesions were usually bilateral.

Histologically, there was coagulation necrosis of portions of the medulla and papilla. Blood vessels adjacent to areas of necrosis were congested, or frank hemorrhage was present. Neutrophile leukocytes surrounded and infiltrated necrotic tissue. Interstitial edema, fibrosis, and mineralization were also seen.

The pathogenesis of the lesions has been debated. Experimental work suggests that medullary and papillary ischemia caused by vascular shunting and decreased perfusion is responsible. Other factors may include preferential direct cell cytotoxicity in long loops of Henle, and compromise of peritubular vasa recta (Gunson 1983; Gunson and Soma 1983; Read 1983).

Renal tubular acidosis

Type I

The kidney is one of the two organs responsible for control of systemic pH, the other being the lung. Defects in the ability of distal tubular and collecting duct cells to secrete hydrogen ion adequately cause systemic acidosis. This defect, type I renal tubular acidosis, has been seen in two horses (Ziemer et al. 1987a). Both Quarter horses were profoundly depressed and anorectic. Clinicopathological findings included systemic acidosis, hyperchloremia, dehydration, and alkaline urine pH despite profound systemic acidosis. The defects were corrected by aggressive fluid, electrolyte, and acid–base therapy and by supplementation of the diet with bicarbonate. Neither the cause of type I renal tubular acidosis in these horses nor the pathogenesis is known.

Type II

A single case of type II renal tubular acidosis has been reported in an Appaloosa mare (Trotter et al. 1986). There was anorexia and depression. Arterial blood pH was low, pH 7.04. There was mild hyperchloremia and azotemia. A defect in the ability of the cells of the proximal convoluted tubule to reabsorb filtered bicarbonate was detected by a bicarbonate loading test. In this test, systemic pH remains low in response to a bolus of bicarbonate, but there is abnormal bicarbonaturia. Dietary supplementation with bicarbonate was continued after the mare responded to aggressive therapy. No cause for the defect was found. In humans, this type of reabsorption defect may have a genetic basis or be the result of disease or exposure to nephrotoxins.

Diseases of the urinary bladder

Urolithiasis

Equine urine is a complex mixture of solutes and solvents. Horses regulate body electrolyte composition by excretion of electrolytes in the urine. Normally, equine urine contains abundant amounts of calcium salts, principally calcium carbonate, occasionally calcium oxalate and calcium phosphate. The urine is normally turbid and alkaline, as is generally true of herbivores. The solubility of the solutes in urine is dependent on the total ionic load, concentration of solutes, mixing, rate of urine flow, temperature, pH of the urine, and presence of proteins.

Stones or uroliths form when physicochemical conditions favor the precipitation of solutes from solution in the urine. Cadeac (1899a) noted that calculi were 69%–85% calcium carbonate with calcium oxalate, magnesium carbonate, and organic materials. Common events, such as infection of the urinary tract, alteration in urine pH, increase in relative solute concentration, and urinary stasis, favor mineral precipitation and stone formation. The stones may form anywhere in the urinary tract, including the renal parenchyma and pelvis, ureter, urinary bladder, and urethra. The most common site is the urinary bladder (Holt and Pearson 1984). At best, in our experience, urinary tract calculi are rare at postmortem and usually found incidentally in the renal pelvis of old animals.

Clinical signs in horses with uroliths are somewhat dependent on location. Calculi in the renal parenchyma may cause no signs. At other sites, there may be mechanical irritation of sensitive structures, hematuria, and pain. Incontinence and frequent or painful attempts at urination may be noted (Holt and Pearson 1984; Kaneps et al. 1985; Holt and Mair 1990). Obstruction can lead to hydronephrosis and hydroureter or to total anuria if the calculus occludes the urethra. Rarely, severe, protracted colicky pain and laminitis can be traced to a calculus broken off from a stag horn calculus in the renal pelvis and temporarily or permanently lodged in the ureter. Cadeac described this in 1899, and we have seen several examples.

Several reviews of equine urolithiasis are available (Holt and Pearson 1984; Holt and Mair 1990). Calculi are more common in the bladder of geldings. In cases with a single stone, usually of calcium carbonate, the prognosis was good with surgical removal. With bladder atony or paralysis, sabulous calculi formed, and the prognosis was poor. Causes of bladder atony and paralysis were listed as neuritis of the cauda equina, infection with equine herpesvirus (EHV)-1, spinal trauma or neoplasia, hybrid sudan or sorghum in the diet, and fungal toxins (Holt and Mair 1990). In our experience atony and paralysis of the bladder are almost always the result of damage to nerves of the pelvic plexus whatever the cause. (See Chapter 16, "Nervous System: Peripheral nervous system.")

Cystitis

Cystitis is uncommon in horses except in the presence of damage to the nerves of the pelvic plexus. The cystitis associated with bladder paralysis in hybrid sudan and sorghum poisoning is a function of such neural damage. (See Chapter 16, "Nervous System: Peripheral nervous system.")

Sabulous deposits of epithelial debris and calcium carbonate crystals form a greenish, granular sludge in the bladder. Grossly the mucosa may be thickened, discolored, or covered with fibrinopurulent debris. Mucosal erosions and, rarely, indurated ulcers are present, together with thickening of the bladder wall. Occasionally, benign mucosal polyps project into the lumen of the bladder.

Greenish, granular sludge in the bladder is not uncommon in old horses or horses with long-term chronic disease and is to be differentiated from true cystitis.

Microscopic lesions include acute and chronic inflammatory cell infiltrates, fibrinopurulent exudate adherent to the mucosa, mucosal erosion and ulceration, and intracellular crystal deposition.

Blister beetle poisoning

Schoeb and Panciera (1979) described the clinical signs and pathology of poisoning of horses by cantharidin, the active principle of the blister beetle, *Epicauta*. These beetles infest alfalfa, particularly irrigated alfalfa in the American Southwest. Modern hay-making techniques include cutting and crushing the alfalfa for rapid drying, so that many beetles can be crushed and included in the baled hay.

The horses show pain, fever, depression, frequent urination, synchronous diaphragmatic flutter, and shock. Lesions are somewhat variable in severity from horse to horse. There is sloughing of epithelium of the esophageal portion of the stomach because of necrosis of the basal and prickle cell layers. Neutrophils appear with the loss of the epithelium. There is enterocolitis, varying from catarrhal to fibrinous. The myocardium has multiple isolated and confluent foci of necrosis, which may be apparent grossly.

The urinary bladder is hemorrhagic and may have multiple mucosal ulcerations. The kidneys appear somewhat enlarged and pale in some horses and quite normal in others. Histologically there is segmental tubular epithelial necrosis, particularly in the collecting tubules, together with proteinaceous casts. The neural lesions are discussed with the peripheral nerves (see Chapter 16, "Nervous System.")

Epizootic cystitis in Australian horses

An outbreak of acute and chronic cystitis with hematuria, pyuria, and urine scalding was reported in horses in Australia (Hooper 1968). Over 200 of 1000 horses at risk died. Incontinence was common. Gross lesions consisted of acute catarrhal or chronic ulcerative and fibrosing cystitis. While toxins from *Crotalaria* sp., *Salsola kali,* or a fungal toxin like sporidesmin were considered as etiological agents, and the influence of seasonal rain discussed, the cause was not discovered.

Rupture in foals

Leakage from, or rupture of, the urinary bladder, ureters, or urachus can cause uroperitoneum in foals (Rooney 1971; Behr et al. 1981; Richardson and Kohn 1983; Richardson 1985; Pankowski and Fubini 1987; Adams et al. 1988b). The condition is more common in male foals. Congenital weakness in these structures, or pressure-induced rupture of full bladders during parturition, or combinations of these factors may cause rupture and/or leakage (Rooney 1971). Neonatal septicemia, multiple congenital anomalies of the urinary and gastrointestinal tract, and localized infections of the urinary tract may also predispose to urine leakage (Adams et al. 1988b). Extensive retrospective reviews are available (Richardson and Kohn 1983; Adams et al. 1988b).

Affected foals are in metabolic crisis 3–7 days after birth. Scant urine production, dysuria, abdominal distention with urine, and depression are common clinical findings. Hyponatremia, hypochloremia, and hyperkalemia occur. The electrolyte abnormalities are considered the result of equilibration of urinary electrolytes with serum and plasma electrolytes across the peritoneum. The presence and degree of azotemia are variable; some foals have normal serum creatinine values, while others' are elevated.

Rupture of the bladder of foals is also discussed with neonatal diseases (see Chapter 12, "Neonate").

Rupture of the urinary bladder has been seen in parturient mares. The combined effects of increased intraabdominal pressure, fetal movement, and direct impact on the distended bladder are thought to be involved (Nyrop et al. 1984). Rarely, the bladder may rupture in a male animal with obstruction of the urethra by a calculus.

Renal neoplasia

Primary renal neoplasms have been reported with increasing frequency in the past 15 years, although Struck recognized a renal adenoma in the kidney of a horse in 1934.

Renal carcinoma in horses may present with vague clinical signs. Hematuria has been consistent in a number of cases (Haschek et al. 1981; Brown and Holt 1985; Van Mol and Fransen 1986; West et al. 1987). Other signs include weight loss and anorexia, or horses that collapse unexpectedly when friable neoplasms bleed profusely. In at least two cases, abdominocentesis yielded bloody fluid rich in neutrophils, the result of tumor necrosis and hemorrhage.

The tumor is rare. At the New York State Veterinary College, renal carcinoma represented 0.11% of the autopsy population between 1953 and 1976 (Haschek et al. 1981). A 0.15% incidence among 40,000 postmortem cases was reported by Cesari (1922) cited by Haschek et al. (1981). We have seen one case among over 10,000 postmortems of light horses.

Most renal carcinomas are unilateral, arising from one pole of the kidney and growing by invasion. Several bilateral cases have been reported. The affected kidney may be deformed or obliterated by growth of the neoplasm (Haschek et al. 1981; West et al. 1987). Implantation metastases on peritoneal viscera have been reported, but the tumor usually metastasizes to the liver, lungs, and regional lymph nodes. The tumor is usually friable and pale tan to white. In at least one case, rupture caused hemoperitoneum and sudden death (Brown and Holt 1985).

The microscopic appearance is variable. In well-differentiated areas groups of low cuboidal to cuboidal cells form tubules and pseudotubules surrounded by bands of fibrous connective tissue. Less-differentiated areas or tumors are pleomorphic and anaplastic. Papillary formations are seen. Mitotic activity is variable, as is the tendency to invade vasculature or form connective tissue capsules.

Urinary bladder neoplasia

There have been few reports of neoplasms in the equine urinary bladder. Six cases were reviewed by Fischer et al. (1985). Prominent clinical signs included stranguria, hematuria, weight loss, and depression. In general, affected horses were over 13 years, and more mares than stallions or geldings were affected. Four of the 6 tumors were squamous cell carcinomas, 1 showing evidence of local spread and metastasis. One was a transitional cell carcinoma and 1 a fibromatous polyp. Three of the 6 horses had pyelonephritis, presumably related to obstruction of urine flow.

CHAPTER 15

Integument

Dermatopathies, unknown cause
- Anhidrosis
- Subcutaneous emphysema

Neoplasia
- Equine sarcoid
- Melanoma
- Cutaneous lymphosarcoma
- Papilloma
- Squamous cell carcinoma
- Mastocytosis and mastocytoma
- Keratoma
- Hemangiomatosis
- Apocrine gland adenocarcinoma

Skin disease is common in horses, and immediately visible lesions quickly receive attention by veterinarian or owner. Owner therapeutics may not control, and may even aggravate, the disease process. Topical therapeutic agents often obscure the gross or microscopic appearance of lesions, compounding the already considerable difficulties of pathological diagnosis (Stannard 1972; Devriese et al. 1983; Pascoe et al. 1981b).

McGavin and Fadok (1984) considered factors determining the value of biopsies in equine skin disease. Many dermatoses have similar clinical signs and histology. Breed, sex, age, skin color, biopsy site, clinical history, presumptive clinical diagnosis, and differential diagnoses are necessary background for useful histological evaluation. Biopsies should be representative, include several areas, be carefully handled, and adequately fixed. Full-thickness biopsies are essential since deep-lying lymphoid aggregates occur in 4.5% of equine skin biopsies and are significantly associated with immune-mediated dermatoses (Scott 1989).

There are a number of useful sources on equine dermatology, and the reader is referred to them for clinical and therapeutic information (Pascoe 1973; Thomsett 1984; Scott et al. 1980).

Infectious dermatoses, viral

Coital exanthema

Coital exanthema, equine herpesvirus (EHV)-3 infection of the reproductive tract, is discussed with the male and female reproductive tracts (see Chapters 13 and 11, respectively).

Vesicular stomatitis and horse pox

Vesicular stomatitis and horse pox are diseases of both skin and oral mucosae and are discussed with the mouth (see Chapter 3, "Gastrointestinal Tract and Adnexa"). Although there were reports in the old literature of equine infection with **foot-and-mouth disease**, it is probable that these were vesicular stomatitis [Olitsky et al. (1927) cited by Cohrs (1961)]. **Grease**, a chronic dermatitis of the plantar aspect of the pastern, usually of the rear leg, caused by the horse pox virus, has other causes as well.

Molluscum contagiosum/Uasin Gishu disease

Molluscum cantagiosum is a benign dermatopathy of horse and man. Outbreaks in central Africa have the name Uasin Gishu disease (Kaminjolo and Winqvist 1975). It is caused by a poxvirus antigenically distinct from cowpox virus.

Horses develop lesions weeks to months after presumed exposure. They consist of numerous 2- to 20-mm nonpruritic cutaneous nodules of firm consistency. Common sites are the groin, ventral abdomen, axilla, and pectoral region, but lesions may be diffuse anywhere on the body. The raised nodules lack hair and are covered with scabby or powdery white material (Kominjolo and Winqvist 1975; Rahaley and Mueller 1983; Cooley et al. 1987; Moens and Kombe 1988).

Histologically, there is ballooning degeneration and hyperplasia of the epidermis with rete pegs penetrating into the dermis (Kaminjolo and Winqvist 1975). Characteristic eosinophilic intracytoplasmic inclusions, **molluscum bodies**, containing abundant pox virions, are present in proliferating and desquamating epithelium (Moens and Kombe 1988).

Cooley et al. (1987) reported molluscum contagiosum in a filly debilitated by granulomatous enteritis and protein-losing enteropathy. Immunocompromised animals are more susceptible to the poxvirus. Molluscum contagiosum in horses is poorly contagious and self-limiting, as immunity develops over a period of months.

Infectious dermatoses, bacterial

Bacterial diseases are common. Diseases such as rain scald (dermatophilosis), grease (bacterial dermatitis), ulcerative lymphangitis, folliculitis and furunculosis, and eczematoid dermatitis have been recognized for hundreds of years (Cadeac 1905; Markel et al. 1986). Most of these conditions, recognized and treated appropriately, heal with little or no residua.

Staphylococcus

Infection with various species of *Staphylococcus* causes cellulitis, cutaneous and deep tissue abscesses, pyoderma, folliculitis and furunculosis (Scott and Manning 1980). In 1905 Cadeac recognized bacterial pyoderma as small nodules or pustules, folliculites pilaires, which formed in warm weather under harness and saddles.

Although *Staphylococcus aureus* was thought to be the common pathogen, *S. intermedius* and *S. hyicus* have been defined as important equine pathogens (Devriese et al. 1984/85). Trauma, hot, humid conditions, excessive sweating, and contact with contaminated tack favor the development of staphylococcal skin infections (Scott and Manning 1980). Infections usually appear as folliculitis and furunculosis, with no age, breed, or sex predisposition. They are commonest in areas rubbed by harness and saddle as pustules and discharging, crustose foci of alopecia. Microscopically, there is acute and subacute folliculitis. Reactive keratosis may be present. In more severe lesions, there can be large areas of pyogranulomatous dermatitis with damage to sweat glands and hair follicles, and formation of intradermal abscesses (Scott and Manning 1980).

Spontaneous and experimental *S. hyicus* infections in 21 horses were characterized by exudative and crustose lesions at various sites on the skin (Devriese et al. 1983). Lesions of the hock and pastern were typical of those known as "greasy heel" (Stannard 1972). Grease or greasy heel is simply a chronic, active dermatitis caused by a variety of infectious and noninfectious agents (Scott 1988). (See Chapter 7, "Fore Leg.")

Markel et al. (1986) isolated coagulase-positive *S. aureus* from the skin and subcutaneous exudate of 9 Thoroughbreds with sudden onset of limb swelling and multifocal epidermolysis. Microscopically, there was cleavage and separation of the epidermis, acantholysis, and neutrophilic infiltration of the epidermis and dermis (Devriese et al. 1983). There was minimal multifocal microabscess formation in the stratum spinosum and colonies of Gram-positive cocci throughout the lesions. Five of the 9 horses developed laminitis and were killed.

Devriese et al. (1984/85) biotyped over 100 strains of *Staphylococcus* from dermal lesions in horses. Different biotypes were isolated from healthy skin, suggesting differences in pathogenicity of the several strains.

It is reasonable to observe that staphylococcal skin infections occur in equine veterinarians (and pathologists), particularly in a stud farm area, during the fatiguing duress of the foaling season.

Corynebacterium pseudotuberculosis

Focal, extensive folliculitis and crusting alopecia was seen in a mare with *Corynebacterium pseudotuberculosis* dermatitis. Although this organism is commonly associated with ulcerative lymphangitis, it can cause infections of the skin per se. Histologically, there was multifocal pyogranulomatous dermatitis, which responded rapidly to antibiotics and topical cleansing (Heffner et al. 1988). The condition may run for weeks to months as pustules and papules form, rupture, and become encrusted. The condition appears sporadically in enzootic form in California.

This bacterium also induces large, deep abscesses in the musculature of the chest, pectorals, axilla, and abdomen. Well recognized for years, the condition has been known as Mae West disease, pigeon breast, Colorado strangles, and chest abscess (Reid 1965; Liu et al. 1977; Mayfield and Martin 1979; McMullen 1982). It appears sporadically in enzootic form in California under certain environmental conditions and is especially prevalent in the late summer and autumn. Reid (1965) reported the occurrence of lesions in several horses on a single farm and associated it with migration of *Habronema* larvae. He presumed that the larvae carried the bacterium into the affected tissues. McMullen noted that, in some cases, antibiotics tended to retard the healing process, slowing the drainage of the abscess cavity. (See also Muscle in Chapter 6, "Locomotor System.")

An uncommon cause of cellulitis and abscess formation in young horses is infection with *Rhodococcus equi.* In one case an ulcerated plaque formed on the hock of a 3-month-old filly, followed by multiple abscesses in the inguinal and mammary subcutis. The organism also causes abscesses of the splenic and inguinal lymph nodes in older horses.

Dermatophilus

Dermatophilosis is an acute, subacute, or chronic exudative dermatitis, of horses, humans, and other animals (Hyslop 1980). Often enzootic, it occurs throughout the world in warm, moist climates and is caused by *Dermatophilus congolensis*, a pleomorphic, Gram-positive organism, forming septate filaments and with coccoid and motile forms. The disease has also been called *rain scald* or *streptothricosis*. Small accumulations of sebum are seen on the muzzle, nostrils, and around the ears. Papules and crusting alopecia and ulceration occur on the back, withers, rump, and tail (Hyslop 1980). The lesions are painful, but not notably pruritic (Kelley and Knappenberger 1968). Histologically, there is bacterial growth in superficial layers of the dermis and epidermis, acute dermatitis, serum exudation, hyperkeratosis, and parakeratosis. Purulent exudate accumulates between the dermis and epidermis, causing sloughing of the epidermis (Hyslop 1980).

Factors favoring the spread of the organism include moisture, high ambient temperature, overcrowding, poor nutrition and husbandry, ectoparasitism, and intercurrent disease (Kelley and Knappenberger 1968; Hyslop 1980). Secondary bacterial infection is not uncommon, causing more chronic lesions (Pascoe 1984). Some horses may become chronic or asymptomatic carriers.

Scott and Manning (1980) say that the organism has never been isolated from soil, and proposed that infection is spread by ticks or fomites. Hyslop (1980) stated that infection from soil was less likely than from asymptomatic carriers since the organisms survived poorly in soil. Pascoe (1984) noted that the pathogen had only once been isolated from soil samples.

Ulcerative lymphangitis

Ulcerative lymphangitis of the lower limbs is caused by infection with *Corynebacterium (Rhodococcus) pseudotuberculosis, C. equi,* and, infrequently, by various species of streptococci (see also histoplasmosis in Chapter 2, "Respiratory System"). Sudden, edematous swelling of the lower limb, usually the hind limb, occurs within 12–24 hours of infection. This may persist for 5–7 days or longer depending upon therapeutic success. Areas of cutaneous ulceration discharge green-tinged purulent debris. The infection often becomes chronic with permanent enlargement of the lower leg, as the result of massive fibrosis shot through with pockets of purulent material (milk leg).

A few cases of dermatitis and fistulous withers have been caused by infection with *Actinomyces viscosus* (Kimball and Frank 1945; Specht et al. 1991). Recurrent nodules on the lumbar skin of a horse formed and discharged over a 2-year period. Biopsy and culture yielded the typical granules of the growth of *A. viscosus*. Specht et al. (1991) said that opportunistic infections with this Gram-positive filamentous bacterium were commoner in humans, cattle, and dogs than in horses.

Brucellosis

Serological surveys suggest varying degrees of exposure of horses, at least to *Brucella abortus*. With the exception of poll evil and fistulous withers, there is no hard evidence of a role for brucella in any pathological process in horses. Reports purporting to correlate serological titers with generalized, localized, and shifting lameness have no pathological or bacteriological confirmation. Given the pathogenesis to be described for poll evil and fistulous withers, it might be possible for brucella to localize in synovial structures and cause transient, self-limiting bursitis (Roderick et al. 1948). It is not clear that such localization does in fact occur, or, that if it did, recognizable disease would occur.

Poll evil

Poll evil is a purulent, suppurative process arising in the *bursa subligamentosa nuchalis cranialis/caudalis* between the funicular ligamentum nuchae and the atlas and/or axis. Similarly, **fistulous withers** arises in the *bursa subligamentosa supraspinalis* between the funicular ligamentum nuchae and the highest spines of the thoracic vertebrae (*Nomina Anatomica Veterinaria* 1983).

The pathogenesis of both conditions was worked out in the classic studies of Roderick et al. (1948). It seems certain that both *Brucella abortus/suis* and *Actinomyces bovis* are required to establish the infection, and that horses that reside with brucella-infected cattle are at risk. We hardly see these conditions in light horses, and only then in animals in routine contact with brucella-infected cattle.

Merillat (1917) suggested that the disease could begin as an aseptic bursitis or wound infection. Roderick et al. dissected nine cases before fistulation had occurred, showing that bursitis was primary. The bursa was distended with a viscid, ochre-colored fluid. Fibrin gradually accumulated in the bursa, frank suppuration appearing with fistulation. Histologically, the bursa had chronic proliferative inflammation with fibrosis, lymphocytes, plasma cells, macrophages, fibroblasts, and an occasional giant cell. Neutrophils were uncommon before the lesion opened to the surface. Both *B. abortus* and *A. bovis* were isolated from the lesions, and the latter, at least, was more successfully cultivated from the inner lining of the inflamed bursa than from the fluid.

Fistulous withers, identical to naturally occurring cases, was produced experimentally by injection of *B. abortus* or *suis*, together with smooth strains of *A. bovis*, directly into the supraspinous bursa. The remaining question, probably never to be answered, is whether the two organisms reach the bursa by extension through skin harness wounds, or by the bloodstream, or both.

Fungal dermatopathies

Superficial and deep fungal infections are common causes of skin disease in horses (Cadeac 1899c). Clinical signs are nonspecific in most cases and laboratory examination is needed. Deep dermal mycoses and systemic mycoses with dermal manifestations are more often seen in immunocompromised animals and animals with neoplasms or receiving antibiotic, corticosteroid, or antiinflammatory drugs. Mixed fungal, bacterial, and parasitic infections can occur and complicate diagnosis and therapy. Normal equine hair and skin may be colonized by over 20 species of saprophytic or potentially pathogenic fungi, and culture may be needed to differentiate nonpathogenic from pathogenic organisms (Gravesen et al. 1978; Takatori 1981; Ihrke et al. 1988).

Trichophytosis

Most **superficial dermal mycoses** are caused by *Trichophyton equinum, T. verrucosum, T. mentagrophytes, Microsporum gypseum,* and *M. equinum* (Blackford 1984). There are two subspecies of *Trichophyton equinum*: *T. equinum* var. *equinum* is present in Europe and America, while in Australia, New Zealand, and Asia, *T. equinum var. autotrophicum* predominates. Different requirements for nicotinic acid characterize these variants (Pascoe 1976, 1979; Blackford 1984). Fungal infections previously diagnosed as *M. canis* were probably caused by *M. equinum*, which has recently been definitely classified (Aho 1987).

Transmission is usually by contact, although infection of wounds by soil saprophytes can occur. A role for asymptomatic carriers has been proposed (Ihrke et al. 1988). Moist environments favor fungal growth and increase the risk of infection. Pascoe (1979) found an increased incidence of *Trichophyton equinum* var. *autotrophicum* infections in racehorses during the rainy season in Australia, corroborating earlier observations on the seasonality of the disease by Pepin and Austwick (1968). Contamination of tack and grooming equipment is important in transmission. Lesions of *T. equinum* are commonest in the saddle and girth area (Pascoe 1976, 1979). Recovered horses are resistant to reinfection and heal more quickly if reinfected (Pascoe 1979). Horses older than 4 years appear less susceptible than 2 and 3 year olds (Brocq-Rousseau et al. 1927; Pascoe 1979). Rodents and biting insects apparently do not transmit these fungal pathogens (Kral 1960; Pascoe 1979).

Epizootic spread of *T. equinum* in racing stables and riding academies has been reported (George et al. 1957; Devries and Jitta 1973; Pascoe 1976). Among 568 horses in training for racing, Pascoe (1976) found dermatomycoses in 32%, with *T. equinum* var. *autotrophicum* the pathogen in the majority of cases. Only 1.1% of horses in breeding stables had the disease, suggesting a link of training duress and stabling conditions with susceptibility to the pathogen. Pascoe and Connole (1974) reported similar findings with *M. gypseum.*

Within 7–14 days of contact, *T. equinum* and other dermatophytic fungi colonize the shafts of hairs (Pascoe and Connole 1974; Pascoe 1976). Fungal colonies develop on the outside of the hair (ectothrix growth pattern) or within the hair (endothrix growth pattern) (Pascoe 1976). As fungi grow, the hair shafts are weakened and break and fall away, causing alopecia. Abnormal epidermal desquamation appears as flaking of the skin. By-products of fungal growth cause inflammation by allergic sensitization or direct damage. In some animals, the allergic inflammatory response to soluble fungal toxins may be severe enough to cause edema, dermal necrosis, and pus formation (Stannard 1976). There are often scattered foci of alopecia surrounded by encrusted rims. The inflammation in the center of such lesions destroys the fungi, and spread is circumferential and away from this central zone of inflammation and healing. Pruritis is a common clinical sign. Many lesions will resolve within 30 days. Gross lesions, other than patches of alopecia with peripheral encrustation, are nonspecific.

Batte and Miller (1953) report that *T. equinum* infection causes vesicles that rupture early in the infection. We have not seen this in a limited number of cases. They described the lesions as "girth itch." *Trichophyton verrucosum,* a cause of fungal dermatopathy in cattle, may localize on the back of the pastern, that is, greasy heel (McMullan 1982).

Phycomycosis

Cutaneous and **osseous phycomycosis**, a fungal granulomatous dermatitis, has been reported with increasing frequency since the mid-1960s. Originally described at the turn of the century [Drouin (1896) cited by Haan and Hoogkamer (1903)], it has also been called swamp cancer, leeches, bursattee, and hypomyces destruens equi (Campbell 1990). There are three organisms, *Pythium insidiosum, Basidobolus haptosporus,* and *Conidobolus coronatus* (Miller and Campbell 1984). Although the lesions are similar, the organisms are widely different in morphology, taxonomy, and distribution.

Cases are commoner in wet subtropical and tropical environments such as Australia, New Guinea, Indonesia, northern South America, Central America, the southern United States, New Guinea, and Japan (Haan and Hoogkamer 1903; Connole 1973; Murray et al. 1978a; Miller and Campbell 1984; Owens et al. 1985; Berrocal and van den Ingh 1987; Alfaro and Mendoza 1990).

Pythium insidiosum is a motile, funguslike protist, while both *Basidobolus* and *Conidobolus* are true fungi (Campbell 1990). Both *Pythium insidiosum* and *Basidobolus haptosporus* grow in the skin and subcutis of the legs and abdomen, while *Conidobolus coronatus* prefers the nares, nasal cavity, and pharynx (Miller and Campbell 1982a, 1984). Bone lesions, including lysis and reactive exostoses have been reported in four chronic *Pythium* infections (Alfaro and Mendoza 1990). Secondary bacterial colonization of the fungal lesions is common (Miller and Campbell 1984).

Characteristic gross lesions, to be differentiated from cutaneous habronemiasis, are caused by infection with all three organisms. Large, branching coagula composed of fungal hyphae, necrotic debris, and inflammatory cells form within several weeks of infection (Campbell and Miller 1984; Berrocal and van den Ingh 1987). These masses of coagulated debris have been called "kunkers." In a review of 266 cases in Australia, Miller and Campbell (1982a, 1984) described coagula, inflammatory cell infiltrate, and type of pathogen, as well as sites of lesions as aids in the differential diagnosis. Discrete coagula were present several millimeters below the surface of ulcerated lesions and normal epidermis with *Pythium insidiosum* infection. Coagula in *Basidobolus* infections were surrounded by an indistinct layer of edematous tissue, and those of *Conidobolus* were within edematous and necrotic foci. Vascular invasion with thrombosis and fungal growth in regional lymph nodes was seen in *Pythium* infections, but rarely with either *Basidobolus* or *Conidobolus* (Murray et al. 1978a). Other minor differentiating characteristics included the presence or absence of multinucleate giant cells, less common with *Pythium* infections, and the presence or absence of eosinophil collars around *Basidobolus* and *Conidobolus* hyphae. There is an immunohistochemical staining method for differentiating *Pythium insidiosum* from other phycomycetes (Brown et al. 1988). Miller and Campbell (1982b) developed agar gel immunodiffusion, complement fixation, and intradermal sensitization tests for *Pythium insidiosum.*

The rapid growth of lesions demands rapid treatment since some phycomycotic granulomas may increase in size tenfold in a 4-week period (Owen et al. 1985). Regrowth of incompletely resected lesions occurs (Mendoza and Alfaro 1986).

Maduromycosis

Maduromycosis, caused by *Madurella mycetomatis, Curvularia geniculata,* or *Pseudoallescheria boydii* has been seen in South Africa and North America (Boomker et al. 1977; Van Amstel et al. 1984; McEntee 1987). These saprophytic fungi may cause mycotic abortion and may also cause discrete cutaneous granulomas at sites of trauma (McEntee 1987). Granulomas may be present for long periods of time and grow slowly. It has been speculated that the slow growth is a phase of adaptation to the host (Mariat et al. 1977). The granulomas had fibrous connective tissue capsules and septae separating pockets of proliferating fungal elements. Invariably, darkly pigmented fungal granules were present within the inflamed and necrotic tissue. A variety of inflammatory cells, including neutrophils, lymphocytes, macrophages, giant cells, and plasma cells, infiltrates the lesions. Although morphological criteria are available to differentiate organisms in appropriately stained sections, culture and speciation of the organism affords the definitive diagnosis (Boomker et al. 1977; McEntee 1987).

Other pathogens have been isolated from a few cases of dermatomycosis. Simpson (1966) described draining cutaneous nodules in the ventral neck region of a mature Palomino horse caused by *Hormodendrum* sp. Multifocal dermal ulcerations and raised cutaneous plaques were caused by the saprophytic fungus *Dreschlera spicifera* in a 2-year-old Quarter horse (Kaplan et al. 1975). A mixed infection of *Dermatophilus congolensis* and the saprophytic fungus *Alternaria tenuis* caused nodular dermatitis in a 7-year-old Quarter horse (Coles et al. 1978).

Fungal pathogens may be missed with routine

staining and can be overlooked when they occur in unusual geographical areas.

Parasitic dermatopathies

A variety of flies, biting midges, mites, nematodes, lice, and ticks parasitize equids and cause dermatopathies ranging from mild irritation to severe, deforming ulceration, hemorrhage, and profound illness. Hypersensitization, pruritis, and self-inflicted trauma are common causes of skin lesions induced by parasites. Anaphylactic reactions to the decomposition products of ectoparasites such as *Habronema* have reportedly killed horses (Soulsby 1965; Fadok 1984; Foil and Foil 1986), but this is uncertain.

Excellent reviews of parasitic skin diseases in large animals, especially horses, are available for details of life cycles and treatment (Fadok 1984; Foil and Foil 1986).

Flies

Flies cause lesions by several mechanisms. Some tabanid flies, horse flies, such as *Tabanus, Chlorotabanus, Hybomitra, Leukotabanus,* and *Whitneyomyia,* and *Chrysops* spp., the deer fly, feed on horse blood as part of the life cycle (Soulsby 1965; Foil and Foil 1986). Their bites are annoying and painful. Edematous dermal nodules and wheals may be allergic reactions to fly bites. These flies transmit the virus of equine infectious anemia and *Trypanosoma evansi,* the cause of surra, during feeding.

Horn Flies

Horn flies, *Hematobia irritans,* are primarily ectoparasites of cattle and horses pastured with or near cattle. Their bite may induce hypersensitivity. Horn flies may also be the cause of equine ventral midline dermatitis, preferring to feed on the thin, lightly haired skin of the abdomen.

Stables flies and face flies

Stable flies, *Stomoxys calcitrans,* feed on the abdominal skin and legs of horses. Stable flies, house flies, *Musca domestica,* and face flies, *M. autumnalis,* may transmit habronemiasis, bacterial diseases, and eye worms, *Thelazia* spp. Face flies, in particular, are a significant annoyance to pastured horses.

Black flies

Black flies, *Simulium* sp, feed on all large animals, including horses and cattle. They require blood meals for completion of reproduction. These flies tend to swarm and will attack and even kill large animals. According to Soulsby (1965) swarms of *S. indicum* killed over 20,000 horses, cattle, sheep, goats, and pigs on the river Danube in 1923. The southern buffalo gnat, *S. pecuarum,* has inflicted serious lesions in cattle and mules in the Mississippi River Valley (Soulsby 1965). Fatal black fly attacks have also been seen in subarctic regions.

Foil and Foil (1986) comment that livestock may die of exsanguination or hypersensitivity to toxins in fly saliva, but provide no corroborating evidence. *Simulium* sp. mechanically transmit onchocerca microfilaria, as well as other disease agents (Soulsby 1965).

Hypersensitivity to black fly salivary toxins and the trauma associated with bites are considered the cause of **aural plaques** (Stannard 1972). These are white to gray, flaking, hyperkeratotic plaques in the ears of horses. The pathogenesis includes bites, pruritis, self-trauma, and eventual hyperkeratosis and desquamation (Foil and Foil 1986). Plaques of similar appearance have been seen near the anus and vulva with, apparently, the same pathogenesis. Thomsett (1984) felt there was insufficient evidence to consider black fly bites the cause of aural plaques. Irritation by *Psoroptes* spp. mites caused similar aural lesions in stud farm horses in New Zealand (Shaw 1966).

Mosquitoes

Mosquito bites are a minor annoyance for horses. In hypersensitive individuals, the bites can cause epidermal swelling, erythema, and pruritis. The main importance of the mosquito is as vector for equine encephalomyelitis.

Midges

Biting midges, *Culicoides* and *Leptoconops,* feed on horse blood. Their bite is painful, causing pruritis, self-inflicted trauma, and subsequent alopecia and hyperkeratosis. Hypersensitivity to proteins in midge saliva may lead to hypersensitization in certain families of horses (Greiner and

Fadok 1985). These insects are the primary cause of "sweet itch," a seasonal eczematoid dermatopathy. Culicoid midges are considered primary biological vector of *Onchocerca cervicalis* (Rabalais and Votava 1974).

Myiasis

Several genera of flies can cause myiasis or "fly strike" in equids. Fly larvae infest wounds or may require residence in the skin as part of their life cycle. The cattle screw worm, *Cochliomyia hominivorax,* can infest skin wounds of horses, feeding on devitalized tissue for 3–5 days before falling to the ground (Soulsby 1965; Foil and Foil 1986). *Hypoderma bovis* larvae infest the skin of horses pastured with cattle, but do not complete their life cycle in horses (Foil and Foil 1986). Migrating larvae may be found near the esophagus, rarely in the spinal canal, and in the skin of the back. *Hypoderma* infestation of horses is more common in the British Isles than in North America.

Other species of flies causing nodular or ulcerative dermatopathies include blow flies (*Phormia and Phaenicia*), torsalo larve (*Dermatobia hominis*), and secondary screwworms (*Cochliomyia macellaria*) (Soulsby 1965; Fadok 1984; Foil and Foil 1986). A number of nematodes may infest skin during part or all of their life cycle. Gravid females and eggs of *Oxyuris equi,* the pinworm, infest the perineum and anus, causing irritation and pruritis (Fadok 1984). Rubbing of the tail and anus causes breakage and loss of hair from the tail and rump.

Habronemiasis

Cutaneous habronemiasis is an infestation of the skin of equids with the larvae of *Habronema majus* (*microstoma*), *H. muscae,* and *Draschia megastoma.* The disease is worldwide and most common in warm months, and so the name, *summer sores.* Eggs shed in the feces develop as larvae in several species of flies, *Stomoxys calcitrans, Musca domestica,* and are transmitted to horses in feed or by direct deposition of the infective spiurid larvae on moist membranes or in wounds.

Lesions are commonest in untreated wounds on the lower part of the legs, the medial canthus of the eye, and the urethral process and prepuce (Foil and Foil 1986; Mohamed et al. 1989). The lesion is a granulomatous dermatitis with masses of necrotic debris, foci of calcification, and caseated pus. The foci may be walled off by connective tissue (Mohamed et al. 1989). Foil and Foil (1986) note that the lesions can grow rapidly, masses and whorls of fibroplasia suggesting equine sarcoid or phycomycosis. The lesions may be pruritic and secondarily traumatized (Mohamed et al. 1989). Multiple, massive, and life-threatening infestations have been seen, particularly in Arabian horses in the southern United States, although the breed involvement may be fortuitous.

The lesions may be hypersensitivity reactions to *Habronema* larvae or their waste products, regression being a manifestation of an immune response (Foil and Foil 1986). In endemic areas, the Sudan for example, lesions do not heal and there is no seasonal pattern (Mohamed et al. 1989), suggesting that the life cycle of the fly vectors determines infection of skin wounds, not an immune response.

The gastric lesions of *Habronema* and *Draschia* sp. are discussed with the gastrointestinal tract (see Chapter 3).

Onchocerciasis

Onchocerciasis is a parasitic skin disease of horses, cattle, and other mammals worldwide. The primary pathogen of horses is *Onchocerca cervicalis,* a filarid nematode living as an adult in the ligamentum nuchae (Soulsby 1965). Microfilaria of *O. cervicalis* circulate in the bloodstream and localize on the ventral midline, flank, and chest where they are ingested by biting *Culicoides* midges. *Aedes aegypti* and some species of anopheline mosquitoes may also serve as intermediate hosts (Yoeli et al. 1948; Schmidt et al. 1985). After maturation and transformation for about 30 days, infectious microfilaria are introduced into susceptible horses by midge blood-feeding. Rabalais and Votava (1974) examined biopsies from live and dead horses and found the highest concentrations of preinfectious microfilaria in those skin sites where the vector was most likely to feed, confirming earlier work in Australia (Riek 1953) and Britain (Mellor 1973).

There was no seasonal variation in the distribution of the parasite in the dermis (Schmidt et al. 1985), as already shown by Mellor (1973) and McMullan (1972), and more recently in Louisiana by Foil and Foil (1986). There is no relationship between numbers of dermal microfilaria and the presence of dermatitis (Foil and Foil 1986).

Pruritic dermatitis with alopecia, depigmentation, and ventral midline crusting and excoriation is common (Foil and Foil 1986). Firm subcutaneous nodules may be present in various sites. The lesions may be an allergic reaction to antigens released by dead or dying microfilaria (Foil and Foil 1986).

Schmidt et al. (1985) studied the relationship between dermal histopathology and microfilaremia. Microfilaria localized around the base of hair follicles and sweat glands and were surrounded by lymphocytes and macrophages. Perivascular mononuclear dermatitis was seen in 90% of horses with dermal microfilaria, but in only 5% of those without dermal microfilaria. Eosinophils were frequently present in biopsies of horses with dermatitis, but were also seen in roughly a third of horses without dermatitis.

Ivermectin rapidly eliminates microfilaremia, but not the adult worms in the ligamentum nuchae (Foil and Foil 1986). Recurrence is common 2–8 months after treatment.

Lice

The infestation of equids with lice is an age-old problem. Two species, *Hematopinus asini* and *Bovicola equi,* can infest the coat of debilitated animals and/or those housed in substandard conditions. These parasites feed differently; *H. asini* ingests blood, while *B. equi* lives on cutaneous debris. Infection is by direct contact, contaminated blankets, tack, and grooming brushes spreading lice from horse to horse. The hair of the head, neck, mane, and tail may be heavily infested before the rest of the coat is colonized (Foil and Foil 1986). Pruritis and secondary trauma cause alopecia and excoriation. Heavily infested horses may become anemic and cachectic. The heaviest infestations are seen during the winter in overcrowded stabling.

Mites

Mites parasitize the skin and cause dermatitis. The straw itch mite, *Pyemotes tritici,* caused nonpruritic papular dermatitis in 12 horses and human contacts in Florida (Kunkle and Greiner 1982). Lesions occurred on the neck, head, and thorax following exposure to parasite infested alfalfa hay. Histologically, there was epidermal ulceration, infiltration of the dermis and epidermis with a mixed population of inflammatory cells, and perivascular eosinophilic cuffing. The lesions were not pruritic and resolved spontaneously. A similar dermatopathy has been reported following contact with another grain mite, *Acarus farinae* (Norval and McPherson 1983).

Ticks

Equids may be infested with ticks of the genera *Dermacentor, Amblyomma, Ixodes, Boophilus,* and *Anocentor* (Fadok 1984; Foil and Foil 1986). While tick bites in themselves are only a minor nuisance, they may transmit several serious infectious diseases, including equine babesiosis (Knowles et al. 1980), equine ehrlichiosis (Foil and Foil 1986), and Lyme disease.

Tick bites may become infested with other ectoparasites, *Habronema,* or bacteria, causing focal pyoderma. Hypersensitivity to toxins and components of tick salivary secretions could cause allergic pruritis, but this has not been demonstrated. Tick paralysis in horses has been suggested anecdotally, but no references have been found. The spinose ear tick, *Otobius megnini,* parasitizes the ear canal, causing irritation, head-rubbing, and secondary infections (Fadok 1984). Foil and Foil (1986) described papular dermatoses in horses exposed to chiggers.

Mange

Demodex

Demodectic mange is caused by *Demodex equi* or *Demodex folliculorum* var. *equi* (Soulsby 1965; Scott and Manning 1980; Fadok 1984; Foil and Foil 1986). Two forms are recognized clinically: scaling alopecia and pustules with discharge of debris and pus from infected hair follicles (Soulsby 1965; Fadok 1984). Mange mites colonize hair follicles, deriving nutrition from secretions and digestion of keratin debris (Ihrke and Schwartman 1975). The condition is uncommon in healthy horses, being seen in those debilitated by disease, poor nutrition, or treated with corticosteroids (Besch and Griffiths 1956; Scott and White 1983). As in other species, demodex mites may be found incidentally in the hair follicles of otherwise normal horses.

Sarcoptes

Sarcoptic mange in equids is uncommon (Fadok 1984). Soulsby (1965) considered it a disease of animals in poor condition. The mange mite, *Sarcoptes scabei,* is transmitted by direct contact (Fadok 1984), although fomites and environmental contamination have been mentioned (Soulsby 1965). Female mites burrow in tunnels in the dermal connective tissue, laying eggs and causing significant pruritis. Pruritic lesions and alopecia with secondary hyperkeratosis develop primarily on the head and neck. There is an intense eosinophilic and mixed inflammatory cell dermatitis.

Psoroptes

Psoroptic mange may present with focal alopecia and formation of papules at the base of the mane and tail, on the forehead, and within the ear canal (Shaw 1966; Fadok 1984). Secondary trauma leads to hyperkeratosis, hyperpigmentation, and epidermal erosion. Several species of psoroptic mange mites, including *Psoroptes equi, P. ovis,* and *P. cuniculi,* can cause dermatitis in horses and other equids (Soulsby 1965). Unlike sarcoptic mange mites, these ectoparasites do not burrow within the dermis, preferring to live on the epidermis. They may persist on the animal for up to 3 weeks, providing ample opportunity for environmental contamination and transmission.

Chorioptes

Chorioptic mange is caused by *Chorioptes bovis* (*equi*). It has been called "foot mange" or "itchy leg" (Soulsby 1965). Pruritic and encrusted lesions occur on the fetlock and pastern. Pustules and scabs are characteristic. Secondary trauma caused by mite-induced pruritis is significant.

Noninfectious inflammatory dermatopathies

Pemphigus foliaceus and bullous pemphigoid

A dozen or so cases of immune-mediated vesiculobullous skin disease have been identified in horses. Most have been pemphigus foliaceus, in which binding of antibodies to intracellular cement substance causes acantholysis and intraepidermal vesicle formation (Scott 1983; Scott et al. 1983; George and White 1984; Day and Penhale 1986; Pfeiffer et al. 1988). Anderson and Findlay described pemphigus foliaceus in a horse in 1902, but this may not be the condition described more recently (Pfeiffer et al. 1988).

Lesions in typical cases may be present for months and include alopecia, swelling, and dermal ulceration of the coronary band and pastern (George and White 1984). Lesions continue to enlarge with exudation of serum from ruptured vesicles, cracks, and fissures. Secondary bacterial infection occurs. Direct immunofluorescent examination of skin biopsies shows binding of immunoglobulin G within and around cells of the acanthocyte layer. Some horses have circulating levels of antinuclear antibody (Scott and White 1983). Pfeiffer et al. (1988) found electron-dense deposits in the acanthocyte layer and suggested they were antigen–antibody complexes. With antibody binding, there is lysis of acanthocytes, vesiculation, and infiltration of acute inflammatory cells. Subcellular alterations precede vesicle formation and include enlargement of intracellular spaces in the acanthocyte layer, dyskeratosis, dilatation of rough endoplasmic reticulum, cytoplasmic vacuolation, and mitochondrial damage (Pfeiffer et al. 1988).

There are a few reports of bullous pemphigoid (George and White 1984). In one, a 5-year-old Quarter horse, bullous vesicles formed at mucocutaneous junctions and on the oral mucosa over a 1-month period. Separation of epidermis from underlying dermis was noted both clinically and on biopsy. Rupture of the fluid-filled bullae caused ulceration, secondary bacterial infection, and acute inflammation. Direct immunofluorescent staining showed deposition of immunoglobulin G on the epidermal basement membrane, typical of bullous pemphigoid in other species. Treatment with antibiotics and topical and systemic corticosteroids was ineffective, and the horse was killed. At autopsy multiple bullae were found at mucocutaneous junctions throughout the body, together with pleuritis and laminitis.

Systemic lupus erythematosus

Several cases of systemic lupus erythematosus with dermatopathy have been reported (Vrins and Feldman 1983; Geor et al. 1990), but this disease is rare in equids.

Geor et al. described lupus dermatopathy and multisystemic dysfunction in a 2-year-old Standardbred filly. The clinical signs included weight loss, anemia, bilaterally symmetrical alopecia, and generalized seborrhea, developing in 3 weeks. There were multiple cutaneous ulcers, punctate ulcerations at mucocutaneous junctions, and generalized lymphadenopathy. Biopsies revealed superficial and deep dermatitis with necrosis and inflammation at the epidermal basement membrane and around adnexa. There was orthokeratotic hyperkeratosis and parakeratosis. Immunoglobulin G was deposited at the epidermal basement membrane.

The filly had Coombs-positive hemolytic anemia and elevations of serum alkaline phosphatase and aspartate aminotransferase. A urine specimen had protein and blood, indicative of glomerulopathy. An immunoperoxidase antinuclear antibody test on a section of mouse liver (indirect test) was positive. The skin lesions were refractory to high-dose corticosteroid therapy, and the animal was killed. There was extensive ulceration at mucocutaneous junctions throughout the body, as well as membranous glomerulopathy with immunoglobulin deposition on renal basement membranes, thrombosis and fibrinoid necrosis of vessels in lymph nodes, fibrinous synovitis, and hepatitis.

Vitiligo

Vitiligo is a dermatopathy with progressive depigmentation of skin caused by selective destruction of melanin-containing cells. Because of the depigmentation the animals are prone to solar skin damage. The disease has been seen in Lippizaner and Arabian horses (Lerner and Cage 1973). Experimental evidence suggests an immune-mediated process modulating the melanocyte destruction (Naughton et al. 1986). For example, immunization with melanoma cells, as immunostimulant therapy for cutaneous melanoma, will induce antibodies against melanocytes and cause vitiligo in several species. Sera from normal humans and several animal species, including horses, had high levels of circulating antibodies to a specific antigen in melanoma cells, as assessed by immunoprecipitation and cell-labeling techniques.

Leukotrichia and leukoderma

Leukotrichia and leukoderma are related disorders of skin and hair depigmentation. Several forms, such as **reticulated leukotrichia** of Quarter horses, Thoroughbreds, and Standardbreds, and **spotted leukotrichia** of Arabian horses, probably have an hereditary component. In some forms of leukotrichia there is only patchy focal depigmentation of the coat, while in others there may be papules and pustules. Secondary trauma and inflammation are seen (Scott and Manning 1980).

Nodular panniculitis

Six cases of sterile nodular panniculitis have been reported in horses in the recent literature (Scott 1985; Karcher et al. 1990). There are a number of reports in the old literature, usually with the name **xanthoma**, which appear to be the same entity.

There are firm subcutaneous nodules ranging from 1 to 6 cm in diameter. In more severely affected horses, the nodules ruptured and discharged through ulcerations and fistulous tracts in the skin. No breed or sex predisposition was seen, although 2 of 6 cases occurred in Morgan horses. Lesions occurred in horses with normal serum selenium and tocopherol levels and are not part of the generalized steatitis seen with vitamin E–selenium deficiency in horses (Kroneman and Wensvoort 1968; Dodd et al. 1960; Foreman et al. 1986). Subcutaneous nodules increase and decrease in size periodically with variable response to corticosteroid therapy (Karcher et al. 1990).

Histologically, the nodules are confined to the subcutis and are a focally extensive to diffuse pyogranulomatous panniculitis. There is fat necrosis and lymphocytic inflammatory cell infiltration with variable fibrosis. Dystrophic mineralization and ceroid deposition, common in vitamin E–selenium deficiency dermatopathy, are less common in sterile nodular panniculitis. Pathogenic organisms have not been recovered and an immune-mediated etiology is suspected (Karcher et al. 1990).

Skin and vitamin E–selenium deficiency

Generalized necrosis and inflammation of fat deposits in the subcutis, internal fat as well as myodegeneration were noted by Hartley and Dodd (1957) in Thoroughbred foals in New Zealand. The condition was more fully described in Thoroughbreds by Dodd et al. (1960) and Shetland ponies by Kroneman and Wensvoort (1968), and in ponies, a Przewalski horse, and two donkeys by Platt and Whitwell (1971).

The clinical course is highly variable, ranging from gradual onset of vague signs of anorexia, weight loss, depression, and pyrexia, to diarrhea, proteinuria and azotemia, localized and generalized pain, edema, and death. Platt and Whitwell (1971) commented that signs may persist from 4 to 30 days. At autopsy there is diffuse yellow discoloration of fat because of the deposition of ceroid, an autofluorescent pigment. There is focal fat degeneration of subcutaneous and internal fat deposits, often with calcification. Subcutaneous fat of the back and hindquarters is commonly affected. There may be calcification and fibrosis of the ligamentum nuchae, although this may have been onchocerciasis. Histological and other features are considered with the muscular system.

Idiopathic granulomatous dermatitis

Generalized granulomatous disease in horses is a multisystemic disease associated with lymphadenopathy, weight loss, exercise intolerance, low-grade fever, and exfoliative dermatitis. Heath et al. (1990) described a variant in which a horse developed primary cutaneous signs. This 14-year-old Thoroughbred had a year-long period of progressive lymph node enlargement and recent signs of depression, stiffness, and pitting ventral edema. The haircoat was poor and easily shed, and there was bilaterally symmetrical alopecia. Focal cutaneous depigmentation was prominent along the lips and eyelid margins. Multiple punch biopsies showed diffuse granulomatous dermatitis, with mixed perivascular infiltrates of inflammatory cells.

Tests of immune function, including Coombs' test for autoimmune hemolytic anemia, antinuclear antibody, lupus erythematosus cell preparations, and intradermal mycobacterial tests for delayed hypersensitivity were normal. Several courses of corticosteroid therapy caused some decrease in size of the lymph nodes. Similarities to human sarcoidosis (unrelated to equine sarcoid) were discussed by Heath et al. (1990).

Eosinophilic dermatitis

Eosinophilic dermatitis is morphologically similar to idiopathic granulomatous dermatitis. Cases have been seen with chronic eosinophilic enteritis (Gibson and Alders 1987), or with multisystem eosinophilic granulomatous disease (Nimmo-Wilkie et al. 1985).

Two horses were in poor condition with recent history of weight loss and diarrhea (Gibson and Alders 1987). In 1, there was generalized alopecia, lichenification, and crusting of the skin. Histologically, this animal had multifocal dermal eosinophilic granulomata, perivascular eosinophilic infiltrates, and crustose hyperkeratosis. The other horse had small, patchy and pruritic skin lesions and pitting edema. A biopsy of the skin of the leg showed diffuse eosinophilic dermatitis, hyperkeratosis, and acanthosis. Lesions resolved after prolonged corticosteroid therapy.

In five horses without eosinophilic enteritis and diarrhea, there was a crustose dermatitis of the coronary band, diffuse scaling and flaking dermatitis, and epilation and alopecia (Nimmo-Wilkie et al. 1985). Histological lesions of variable severity ranged from multifocal to diffuse eosinophilic granulomatous dermatitis, acanthosis, hyperkeratosis, and parakeratosis, formation of eosinophil-containing subcorneal pustules, and dermal cracks and fissures. Ulceration, excoriation, exudation, and secondary purulent inflammation were seen in severely affected animals. All horses had significant chronic pancreatic disease with enlargement and fibrosis. In 3 of the 5 horses, there was hyperkeratosis of the esophageal and gastric squamous mucosa. Eosinophilic granulomas or eosinophilic infiltrates were found in pancreas, liver, gut, uterus, lungs, lymph nodes, and salivary glands. See also Pancreas in Chapter 3, "Gastrointestinal System" and eosinophilic myositis in Chapter 6, "Locomotor System"; nonspecific dermatitis does occur with primary parasitic pancreatic disease.

Necrotizing vasculitis

Two cases of necrotizing vasculitis with dermal manifestations have been reported (Morris et al. 1983; Werner et al. 1984). Both horses had crustose, ulcerative, and granulomatous dermatitis of the legs with edema. In 1 animal, lesions developed slowly over an 18-month period, while they were present for only 5 days in the other. There were areas of alopecia and hypopigmentation at the sites of healed ulcerated lesions. The histology of skin biopsies from both horses was similar, including acute necrotizing dermatitis, cellulitis, and varying degrees of acanthosis, hyperkeratosis, and epidermal hyperplasia. A prominent deep dermal vasculitis was present in both cases. In 1 animal there was fibrinoid necrosis of vessels associated with eosinophilic and granulomatous vasculitis. In 1 horse, immunoglobulin deposits were localized along the basement membrane while, in the other, granular immunoglobulin deposits were present within the vascular endothelium. Antinuclear antibody test values were equivocal in the chronic case, but elevated in the horse with acute necrotizing vasculitis.

Cutaneous allergy

Allergic contact dermatitis

Allergic contact dermatitis is common in areas such as the face, neck, and saddle. Virtually any area of the horse's body contacting sensitizing materials can react. Chemicals, such as insecticidal sprays, preservatives, saddle soaps, grooming products and shampoos, can combine with haptenic proteins in the skin to cause both acute and chronic dermatitis (Byars 1984). Home remedies such as pine tar hoof conditioners and topical antibacterial dressings may cause exuberant contact dermatitis (Salsbury 1970). Affected horses have circumscribed lesions in the contact areas: alopecia, pruritis, hyperkeratosis, papules, erythema, and exudation of serum and cells, often with self-mutilation. Biopsies are usually a mixture of inflammatory cells, congestion, and edema.

Allergic contact dermatitis is to be differentiated, when possible from the history, from **simple contact dermatitis** caused by exposure to caustic agents such as urine, feces, serum, and cellular debris (Byars 1984).

Immunoglobulin E

Clinical observations suggest that horses may develop cutaneous lesions as the result of inhalation or ingestion of allergens. Immunoglobulin-E-mediated acute hypersensitivity may be the result of ingestion of drugs such as penicillins, phenylbutazone, acetylsalicylic acid, and tetracycline (Byars 1984). The animals can develop typical wheal-and-erythema with edematous cutaneous nodules.

Nodular collagenolytic granuloma

Griffin (1982) described nodular collagenolytic granulomata in the skin of horses. Firm, nonulcerating dermal nodules were found on the neck, back, and girth and were more common in warm weather. Cutaneous hypersensitivity to insect bites or dietary components ("sweet feed bumps") were suspected, but this was disputed and not resolved (Thomsett 1984).

Allergic dermatitis

A well-known form of cutaneous hypersensitivity is allergic dermatitis: summer eczema, Queensland itch in Australia, summer mange or kasen in Japan, Sommerekzem in Germany and Scandinavia, and sweet itch. Allergic dermatitis occurs throughout the world. It is an intensely pruritic, common, chronic, seasonal dermatopathy primarily of the mane, tail, and withers. It is an insect bite hypersensitivity, especially biting midges of the genus *Culicoides.* Ponies and light and heavy horses of all ages and breeds are affected, although the disease tends to be more severe in older horses (Brostrom et al. 1987; Halldordsottir and Larsen 1991). There is significant individual variation in severity and clinical signs.

Riek (1953) reported this dermatitis in over 60% of horses in Queensland, Australia. Nakamura et al. (1956) reported 4.43% in a survey of over 43,000 Japanese horses. McCaig (1973) reported 2.79%, based on a postcard survey of British pony owners and club secretaries. Brostrom et al. (1987) found a lower incidence in native-born Swedish horses than in horses imported to Sweden from Iceland.

Halldordsottir and Larsen found an incidence of 17.6% in 391 Icelandic horses in Norway. The incidence of allergic dermatitis was higher in imported Icelandic horses (26.9%) than in Icelandic horses born in Norway (8.2%).

Baker and Quinn (1978) described the clinical and histological features of the disease in Irish horses: seasonal dermatopathy characterized by intense pruritis, self-mutilation, alopecia, focally extensive hyperkeratosis, and secondary dermal excoriation. The lesions were most common on the back, the preferred feeding site of certain species of *Culicoides* in Ireland. Others have reported distributions of lesions consonant with preferential feeding sites of other species of biting insects (Riek 1953; Braverman 1988). Baker and Quinn (1978) produced lesions characteristic of allergic dermatitis by intradermal injection of *Culicoides* extracts. Skin biopsies of both spontaneous and induced cases had subepidermal edema, perivascular inflammatory cell infiltration, hyperkeratosis and acanthosis, eosinophilia, and focal mast cell degranulation. Morrow et al. (1987) failed to associate the cutaneous distribution of mast cells with lesions of allergic dermatitis.

Fadok and Greiner (1990) studied the incidence of insect bite hypersensitivity in horses in Florida, confirming and extending earlier work in Ireland of Baker and Quinn (1978). Large numbers of horses in subtropical Florida have dermatopathies of insect bite origin since such insects are present virtually year-round. They reported over 50 species of *Culicoides,* 65 species of mosquitoes, 18 species of black flies, and 44 species of tabanid flies in Florida (Wirth and Blanton 1970; Pinkovsky and Butler 1978).

Intradermal skin tests for hypersensitivity to insect, mold, and grass antigens were done on 44 horses with allergic dermatitis and 21 controls (Fadok and Greiner 1990). Over 80% of both groups reacted to the insect antigens, either with immediate or delayed hypersensitivity reactions. A number of horses reacted to multiple antigens (*Culicoides,* black flies, and yellow jackets, for example). While of interest, the difficulties of interpretation of multiple reactive intradermal sensitivity tests must be kept in mind.

Skin biopsies had superficial and deep perivascular dermatitis with infiltration of eosinophils, lymphocytes, and macrophages (Fadok and Greiner 1990).

Certain families have shown predisposition for allergic dermatitis (Ishihara and Ueno 1957a,b, 1958; Ueno and Ishihara 1957; Frost 1974; McCaig 1973). As noted, Brostrom et al. (1987) found that Icelandic horses living in Sweden were more susceptible to the disease than native-born Swedish horses. They speculated that Icelandic horses are not exposed to *Culicoides* antigens in Iceland and, so, are sensitive when transported to areas where these insects feed on horses.

Potatoes and potato trimmings have caused dermatitis that might be allergic, although the condition has not been defined pathologically (Hutyra and Marek 1920). A mild, erythematous and vesicular eczema develops on the distal parts of the legs 2–3 weeks after starting to feed potato material. The lesions weep serum, become crusted, and begin to heal in 2–4 weeks. The animal may have ill-defined systemic signs.

Congenital and developmental dermatopathies

Mechanobullous dermatopathy

Congenital abnormalities of the skin are uncommon in horses. Kohn et al. (1989) described mechanobullous dermatopathy in 2 Belgian foals. Between 2 and 6 days of age they developed pronounced fluid-filled bullae on the coronary band, stifle, fetlock, carpi, and hocks. Even minor trauma produced such bullae. In 1 foal the lesions progressed until over 30% of the body was covered either by bullae or by inflamed and granulating ulcers created by ruptured bullae. The hooves delaminated and sloughed from all four feet. Biopsies showed fluid-filled bullae beneath the basement membrane of the dermis, although a portion of the basement membrane remained adherent to the underlying collagenous tissue. In intact bullae, there were few, if any, inflammatory cells in the fluid. Electron microscopy showed defects at the basement membrane and underdevelopment of hemidesmosomes (Johnson et al. 1988). Oral bulla formation and ulceration were observed at autopsy, as well as widely distributed cutaneous lesions. Scott et al. (1980) and others have suggested that the production of collagenase and destruction of the basement membrane is important in the pathogenesis of this condition. Only 2 of these animals have been studied and the pathogenesis remains uncertain although the condition closely resembles human junctional epidermolysis bullosa.

Hyperextensible and fragile skin

Hyperextensible and fragile skin has been reported by several investigators (Lerner and McCracken 1978; Solomons 1984; Gunson et al. 1984). A typical and well-investigated case was a 2-year-old Arabian-cross filly (Gunson et al. 1984). The horse bruised or lacerated easily with minor trauma. Not all of the skin was thin, lacerations and rugose scarring being most prominent on the shoulders. Biopsies showed a paucity of dermal collagen, the result of degradation of collagen and associated fibroblasts by phagocytosis. Epidermal architecture was unaffected. The dermal collagen defect had been seen since birth, but no information on related horses could be obtained. Gunson et al. concluded that this unique disease was unlike Ehlers-Danlos syndrome of humans or dermatosparaxis of cattle, sheep, cats, and mink.

Hyperelastosis cutis

A similar condition was diagnosed as hyperelastosis cutis by Lerner and McCracken (1978) in two foals and by Solomons (1978) in one foal, these authors considering their cases comparable to Ehlers-Danlos syndrome of humans.

Lethal dominant white

Sturtevant (1912) and Wriedt (1924), both cited by Pulos and Hutt (1969), described a condition now known as lethal dominant white. While this is not a dermatopathy per se, the association with coat color merits discussion here. Pulos and Hutt (1970) found, through breeding studies and genetic analysis, that white horses with pink skin, white mane, coat, tail, and hooves were invariably heterozygous for the dominant gene W for white coat color. Homozygous fetuses (WW) were either resorbed or failed to survive after birth.

Dominant white heterozygotes may produce white progeny, but they also produce progeny with colored coats, skin, and hooves. Some horses, like the Lippizan, carry a skin and coat color gene G, which causes progressive silvering with aging, and these animals are not homozygous for the W gene (Pulos and Hutt 1970). A recessive form of the condition has been reported in the progeny of two overo parents (Schneider and Leipold 1978; Jones 1979).

Congenital porphyria

Rare cases of congenital porphyria have been reported in cattle, horses, and cats. Accumulation of photodynamic porphyrin pigments in dermal cells, and subsequent irradiation and chemical activation of these pigments destroys dermal cells and vessels, leading to dermal necrosis and inflammation.

Toxic dermatopathies

Primary photodermatitis

Two types of photodermatitis occur in equids. Primary photodermatitis follows ingestion of photodynamic plant materials such as hypericin from St. John's wort, or pigments from lucerne and trifolium, and drugs (Thomsett 1984). When such photodynamic materials absorb radiant energy, they become chemically reactive (by free radical formation, for example) and destroy dermal cells. Primary direct photodermatitis is most prominent in white areas of the coat and on those parts of the horse most exposed to sunlight (Thomsett 1984). White or gray horses are more susceptible. There may be focal or extensive areas of epidermal and dermal necrosis, cutaneous erythema and edema, cutaneous ulceration, and serum and cellular exudation. Secondary bacterial, fungal, and parasitic infection of open wounds occurs. Horses with substantial cutaneous pigmentation are protected from this type of photodermatitis since normal skin pigments such as melanin absorb radiant energy without chemical transformation.

Secondary photodermatitis

Secondary (indirect) photodermatitis can occur in equids suffering significant liver damage, which prevents the normal conjugation and excretion of the chlorophyll metabolite, phylloerthyrin (Thomsett 1984). This photodynamic pigment becomes chemically reactive when exposed to radiant energy, producing lesions as described above. Horses with secondary photodermatitis may have jaundice if there is severe liver damage. It is to be remembered, however, that icterus of mucous membranes is often nonspecific in horses, reflecting only minor illness or inappetence.

Plant and diet dermatopathies

Ingestion of the legume *Leucaena glauca* leads to alopecia of the mane, tail, and distal limbs. Abnormal hoof growth, laminitis, and signs of hyperthyroidism have been reported (Owen 1958; Thomsett 1984). This is a tropical legume consumed by horses when more desirable feedstuffs are unavailable.

Chronic consumption of seleniferous plants or selenium can cause dermal signs of **selenium toxicity**. The horses have poor quality haircoat, abnormal hoof growth, and loss of mane and tail. In Ireland, with high levels of selenium in the soil in some areas, horses may suffer delamination and shedding of the hoof wall (Crinion and O'Connor 1978). This was seen in seleniferous areas in the western United States as "alkali poisoning." Exposure to arsenical medications also causes poor quality coat. In neither case are there specific pathological findings.

Granulomatous dermatitis

Granulomatous dermatitis, together with systemic granulomatous disease, has been seen in a horse grazing hairy vetch, *Vicia villosa* (Anderson and Divers 1983). Cattle grazing this plant will develop papular dermatitis within 2 weeks of consumption.

Endocrine dermatopathies

Endocrine dysfunction is a common cause of dermal disease in dogs and cats, but less so in horses and other equids.

Hypothyroidism

Stanley and Hillidge (1982) reported bilaterally symmetrical alopecia and hypoplastic skin associated with hypothyroidism in a 2-year-old Paint horse. The animal was lethargic, cold intolerant, with poor quality haircoat. A defect in the conversion of thyroxine to triiodothyronine was shown by stimulation tests. Other endocrinopathies, such as adrenocortical suppression, were eliminated. The colt had underdeveloped testes and low plasma testosterone values. Skin biopsies showed epidermal hypoplasia and dermal edema and collagenization, considered strongly suggestive of suppressed thyroid function. Supplementation with thyroid hormones caused a rapid, 3-week, resolution of coat abnormalities and an increase in testicular size and function. The testicular abnormalities in this colt were at variance with the normal function in a group of thyroidectomized horses studied by Lowe et al. (1975). Grossly abnormal haircoat and epidermal hypoplasia were seen in most, but not all, foals with hypothyroidism as a result of kelp feeding of their dams (see Chapter 4, "Endocrine System").

Hyperadrenocorticism

Hyperadrenocorticism has not been defined in the horse.

Dermatopathies, unknown cause

Anhidrosis

With expansion of Thoroughbred racing after the First World War, Britain exported horses to tropical and subtropical climates. It was in these warm, moist areas that anhidrosis was first seen. The syndrome is characterized by inability to sweat and dissipate heat. As the primary mechanism for heat dissipation in horses is sweating, anhidrosis can result in life-threatening hyperthermia. The pathophysiology of this syndrome was reviewed by Warner and Mayhew (1983).

Classically, animals not adapted to warm environments have episodic profuse sweating, followed by progressive diminution of sweat production. This is usually seen in horses in training, but can occur in nonexercising horses. There is no correlation with sex, coat color, or breed (Warner and Mayhew 1983; Mayhew and Ferguson 1987). In a survey in central Florida, the incidence was slightly over 6% (Mayhew and Ferguson 1987). Some horses may have a dry or unthrifty coat, while others have focal or generalized alopecia, depressed appetite, and poor performance. Hyperthermic horses may become tachypneic in an effort to dissipate core heat. Barnes (1938) reported that horses that were moved to cooler climates eventually regained the ability to sweat, but this is not always true.

A multifactorial etiology was proposed by Warner and Mayhew (1983). Potential causes included hypothyroidism (Correa and Calderin 1966), hypochloremia from loss in sweat (Gilyard 1944), elevation of blood epinephrine levels coupled with sweat gland epinephrine receptor exhaustion [Evans (1957) and Evans et al. (1957a,b)], high protein diets, or atrophy and obstruction of sweat glands (Jenkinson et al. 1985). Jenkinson et al. found that sweat gland cells of anhidrotic horses were depleted of vesicles, flattened, and surrounded by or attached to a thickened basal lamina. These ultrastructural changes are probably cell atrophy rather than primary disease. Mayhew and Ferguson (1987) showed a relative chloride conservation in anhidrotic horses. The cause or causes of this condition are, in fact, not known.

Subcutaneous emphysema

Leblanc (1902) reported cases of subcutaneous emphysema following cutaneous trauma. Cadeac (1905) saw several cases of spontaneous subcutaneous emphysema with no evidence of trauma or respiratory lesions. We have seen several cases in which no skin wound could be found either in the live horse or at postmortem. The lesion usually resolves spontaneously, with no long-term ill effects, effectively eliminating gas-forming infection.

Neoplasia

Cutaneous neoplasms are not uncommon in horses and other equids. Strafuss et al. (1973) reported that 55.6% of all equine neoplasms were sarcoids. A variety of skin tumors have been seen, but the commonest are sarcoid, fibroma, papilloma, squamous cell carcinoma, and melanoma. The incidence is somewhat variable, depending on geographical location, type of equids surveyed, interests of the pathologists, diagnostic criteria for classification of tumor types, and other, ill-defined factors.

A number of surveys have been published (Table 15-1; Messow 1952-53; Misdorp 1967; Baker and Leyland 1975; Murray et al. 1978a; Pascoe and Summers 1981; Miller and Campbell 1982c; Bastianello 1982). Few or no epidemiological studies have been done.

Equine sarcoid

The classic description of this transmissible neoplasm was given by Jackson (1936), following its earlier recognition by Cadeac (1901) and Montpelier et al. (1939), among others. Equine sarcoid, by most estimates (Table 15-1), is the commonest neoplasm of the skin of horses, mules, and donkeys, worldwide. The incidence ranges from 15% to over 60% of all skin tumors, depending on the diagnostic criteria used (Strafuss et al. 1973; Baker and Leyland 1975; Murray et al. 1978a; Pascoe and Summers 1981). Although sarcoids occur anywhere, the largest number are on the extremities, head, and ventral abdomen. Thirty-five percent of all sarcoids in one study of 153 tumors occurred on the head, neck, eye/adnexa, and shoulder; 28.1% on the hind leg; 24.2% on the fore leg; and 12.4% on the trunk

Table 15-1. Incidence of cutaneous neoplasms in equids, expressed as a percentage of cases studied

	Reference:	Baker et al. 1975	Murray et al. 1978	Pascoe et al. 1981	Miller et al. 1982
	Location:	UK	Australia	Australia	Australia
Tumor type	No. of cases	96	97	409	205
			(%)		
Fibroma		46	21	1	77
Sarcoid		17	60	35	*
Squamous cell carcinoma		20	10	14	12
Papilloma		11	1	34	4
Melanoma		6	3	8	3
Cutaneous lymphosarcoma		-	-	<1	-
Hemangioma/sarcoma		-	4	1	2
Adenoma/carcinoma		-	1	<1	<1
Mast cell tumor		-	-	-	<1
Lipoma		-	-	<1	-
Neurofibroma		-	-	4	1
Basal cell tumor		-	-	<1	-

*The diagnosis of fibroma and sarcoid have been lumped into a single category by Miller and Campbell, 1982c.

(Strafuss et al. 1973). It is generally recognized that sarcoids occur at sites of earlier trauma in some horses, and this may explain the distribution of lesions. Recurrence following surgical resection is common and estimated at 30%–50%.

Sarcoid is commonest under 7 years of age, with Strafuss et al. (1973) reporting that over 70% occur in horses 4 years or less. They occur in foals as young as 6 months (Ragland et al. 1966). Multiple lesions are common but metastasis rare. There is no sex or coat color predisposition. Sarcoids occurred as an epizootic in five young, closely related horses and ponies in a herd in eastern Washington, perhaps suggesting heritable predisposing factors (Ragland et al. 1966).

In an analysis of 120 cases, Angelos et al. (1988) found Quarter horses at twice the risk of Thoroughbreds and Standardbreds at half the risk of Thoroughbreds. This is in general agreement with the data of Miller and Campbell (1982c). A relationship among sarcoids and certain equine leukocyte antigens, W3,B1 (also known as W13), W5, and W11, was suggested by Lazary et al. (1985) and Meredith et al. (1986). Irish, Swiss, and French Warm bloods with sarcoid are more likely to have the W3,B1 antigen than unaffected horses. An increase in the W11 haplotype in Irish Warm bloods and W5 in French and Swiss horses was also associated with an increased incidence of sarcoids. The W3,B1 antigen is uncommon in Standardbred horses, perhaps accounting for their low incidence of sarcoids (Angelos et al. 1988). Brostrom et al. (1988) found an increase in certain equine leukocyte antigen haplotypes in 69 Swedish half-breeds with sarcoid. From their genetic studies, and earlier work by Brostrom et al. (1979), they proposed an hereditary predisposition, related to an autosomal, dominant equine leukocyte antigen-linked gene with incomplete penetrance. Current thinking is that these equine leukocyte antigens do not control expression of the major histocompatibility complex, but are associated markers.

Despite the recognition of sarcoid for over 90 years, the etiology is not surely known. A virus, distinct from the bovine papilloma virus, is presumed to be the cause. Jackson (1936) suggested that the growth pattern and incidence were characteristic of neoplasms of viral etiology. Cadeac (1905) recognized that fibromas (sarcoids) were related to papillomas and could be transmitted by inoculation.

Voss (1969) transmitted the tumor in horses with explants, minced tumor suspensions, and centrifuged, cell-free supernatants of sarcoid suspensions. Growth latency of 14–170 days was thought consistent with a viral agent adapting to its host. Transplant success was greatest with whole tumor explants; 90% of the homologous explants grew in recipient horses. Approximately 6% of sites injected with cell-free sarcoid supernatant developed tumors. Most transplanted sarcoids regressed within 6 months. Spontaneous regression is also seen in the natural disease.

Early investigators speculated that equine sarcoid was induced by bovine papilloma virus. In a series of experiments Ragland and Spencer (1969) injected the virus into the skin of 21 horses and eight young Shetland ponies. Fibroblastic tumors formed at over 90% of the sites, but the tumor in horses was histologically and behaviorally distinct from equine sarcoid. Major differences included the lack of the epithelial component, infiltration of the fibroblastic tumors with mixed inflammatory cells, collagen deposition and maturation, and lack of regrowth of any of the fibroblastic lesions following surgical excision. Some tumors induced in ponies resembled equine sarcoid at some point in their growth, but only 3 of 24 tumors were judged indistinguishable from sarcoid after 6 months. By 12 months they were biologically and histologically quiescent. Although the authors felt that the bovine papilloma virus could be considered a candidate for equine sarcoid, their data did not support that view.

Work by three groups, Amtmann et al. (1980), Lancaster and Olsen (1982), and Trenfield et al. (1985), has identified papilloma DNA viral sequences in sarcoids, but it is not known if this represents a facultative viral regulatory genome or is actually involved in cell transformation. Peculiar tubuloreticular inclusion bodies, not found in normal skin cells, are found in the dilated endoplasmic reticulum of some sarcoids (Madewell and Munn 1989). Attempts to isolate a causative virus intensified when England et al. (1973) identified viruslike particles in electron micrographs of Mc-1 cells derived from an equine sarcoid. Injection of these cells into an immunodeficient Arabian foal caused tumors, but the morphology and location of the tumors were not adequately described. A malignant cell line, T-77-4, was derived from the foal, and these cells produced viral particles characteristic of C-type retroviruses, with similar viral morphology, RNA genome, and manganese-dependent reverse transcriptase activity (Cheevers et al. 1982). Injection of Mc-1 cells into athymic nude mice produced undifferentiated sarcomas and viral particles (Fatemi-Nainie et al. 1984). However, Fatemi-Nainie et al. showed that Mc-1 did not transform equine dermal fibroblasts, as previously reported, but did induce release of an endogenous retrovirus from normal equine cells. The role of this endogenous virus in the pathogenesis of equine sarcoid is undefined.

Sarcoids are of variable appearance: flat, raised, sessile, pedunculated, or verrucous, and varying from 1 to over 20 cm (Ragland et al. 1970; Angelos et al. 1988). They are firm, adherent to surrounding skin and underlying connective tissue, and may be ulcerated. The rate of growth is highly variable from slow to very rapid. Lesions that ulcerate may form granulation tissue at the margins, increasing the size of the lesion and making it more likely to bleed when traumatized. Baker and Leyland (1975) proposed histological criteria to differentiate sarcoids from dermal fibromas and fibrosarcomas based on their evaluation of 124 cutaneous neoplasms. Fibromas were classified as collagen-producing neoplasms, while sarcoids had both fibroblastic and epithelial components. The formation of long rete pegs penetrating deeply into the substance of sarcoids was thought an important differentiating feature from fibromas. A third of the fibromas "shelled out" easily from surrounding tissue, while sarcoids had no sharp boundary with surrounding tissue. Baker and Leyland noted that the whorling fibroblastic cellular component of sarcoids was oriented at right angles to the epithelial component, unlike fibromas, which had no distinct organization. Sarcoids were considered more vascular than fibromas. There is no universal agreement on these features or the system of differentiation and classification. The connective tissue composition of sarcoids and normal skin were considered similar by Williams et al. (1982), except that more type III collagen was organized into fibers in sarcoids than in normal skin.

Of some interest is that experienced medical pathologists almost invariably consider equine sarcoids to be fibromatous tumors with strong suggestions of neural organization.

Melanoma

Melanoma has been recognized in horses for hundreds of years. Leblanc et al. (1902) cites reports by Brugnone (1781) and Gohier (1813). In 1832 William Dick, cited by Levene (1971), discussed melanosis in horses and questioned whether they were more common in aged humans with dark complexions when their hair turned gray! Levene recounted a case of Gollety-Latournelle in France in 1809 associating coat color and melanoma. The possible heritable nature of the tumor was discussed and attempts made to transmit it. An important treatise on melanosis in horses was published by Cornil and Trasbot (1867) cited by Leblanc et al. (1902).

Equine melanoma is not well understood by some. Jubb and Kennedy (1985), for example, report that melanomas in horses occur in two forms, both biologically benign. In fact, they consider most melanomas to be manifestations of a dermal melanocytosis that is questionably neoplastic. Stannard and Pulley in Moulton (1978) emphasized the prevalence of melanomas in old gray horses, citing earlier work by McFadyean (1933), Runnells and Benbrook (1941a), and Mangrulkar (1944). They say that melanomas are rare in horses under 6 years of age. Most believe that these tumors are an inevitable consequence of aging in gray and dilute coat color horses, especially Arabian and Percheron horses (Levene 1971; Lerner and Cage 1974). Recent work by Dye et al. (1993), Stiers et al. (1993, personal communication), and Valentine and Cooper (1993, personal communication) has improved our understanding of equine melanoma. It is certainly true that melanin pigment and melanocytes preferentially accumulate in the perineal subcutis and in the parotid lymph nodes of gray horses. This can be called melanosis with no implication of future biological behavior. The perineal melanin "locus" is the site of origin for the greatest majority of malignant melanomas, and the parotid lymph node a rare site.

The incidence of melanoma is 3%–15% (Cotchin 1960; Baker and Leyland 1975; Murray et al. 1978a; Pascoe and Summers 1981; Miller and Campbell 1984; Table 15-1). Such figures under-represent since many melanomas are not recorded. The association with dilute coat color is unquestionable. In a study of 67 melanomas, we found that over 30% occurred in non-white/gray horses (Dye et al. 1993), and this has been confirmed by Stiers et al. (1993, personal communication) and Valentine and Cooper (1993, personal communication).

The frequency of melanoma increases after 6 years of age, approximately 80% of gray horses over 15 years old having dermal melanomas [Van Dorssen (1903) cited by Levene (1971)]. In 67 horses, the mean age was slightly over 6 years (Dye et al. 1993). Runnells and Benbrook (1941a) found a range of 4–18 years in their 16 cases. Levene (1971) reported that mounted police horses in Australia frequently succumb to malignant melanoma at less than 10 years of age. There are numerous reports of melanoma in horses less than 6 years old, and several congenital cases have been reported (Hamilton and Byerly 1974; Cox et al. 1989).

The common sites for primary melanomas include the undersurface of the tail, the perineum, and the external genitalia. Other sites include the parotid lymph nodes, mammary gland, paralumbar and neck musculature, feet and legs, eye, mouth, and vertebral column, although some of these may, in fact, be metastatic. While Levene (1971), Stannard and Pulley (1978), and Jubb et al. (1985) consider melanomas to largely be benign, others have found that approximately 30% of melanomas are malignant, metastasizing lesions (Dye et al. 1993; Stiers et al. 1993, personal communication; Valentine and Cooper 1993, personal communication). Metastatic lesions may be found throughout the body, including lymph nodes, body cavities, liver, kidney, heart, and gastrointestinal tract. Melanosis of the parotid lymph nodes is a routine finding in older gray/white horses, and may be the nidus for very rare primary melanoma in this area.

Clinical signs depend on the location of the tumor, rate of growth, and amount and type of tissue compromised. For example, Head et al. (1985) reported that melanoma nodules in the vertebral canal, pelvic canal, and surrounding the ischiatic nerve, among other sites, caused lameness of the rear leg in a 21-year-old gray Arabian gelding. We have seen unilateral stringhalt associated with melanoma compression of the obturator nerve in a number of old horses. Paralysis of the rear legs follows melanoma metastatic to the lumbar vertebral bodies, lumbar dorsal spines, or directly to the meninges of the lumbar spinal cord (see Chapter 9, "Vertebral Column"). Most perineal melanomas extend locally and aggressively and metastasize to regional lymph nodes, the sublumbar chain of lymph nodes, and to the lumbar vertebral column. More distant metastasis is less common.

Primary tumors may range from less than 1 cm to over 20 cm and be flat, raised, verrucous, pedunculated, and ulcerated. Runnells and Benbrook (1941) described a variable amount of pigmentation in tumor cells. In many primary lesions, populations of pleomorphic, melanin-laden cells infiltrate dermal connective tissue and adjacent musculature. The so-called junctional formation, aggregates of neoplastic melanocytes adjacent to and appearing to arise from the stratum germinativum, is infrequent. Some tumors mainly comprise large, polygonal, pigment-laden cells, while others have abundant spindle-shaped and giant cells. Some are amelanotic or contain a substantial number of amelanotic cells. The number and type of inflammatory cells are variable with a preponderance of lymphocytes. Mitotic figures vary, roughly in proportion to the aggressiveness of the tumor. Bleaching of melanin is helpful in discerning nuclear morphology, presence or absence of mitotic figures, and nuclear pleomorphism. Nuclei are generally large, ovoid or round, with marginated chromatin and prominent nucleoli.

There are several theories for the pathogenesis of melanoma in horses (Levene 1971), but there is no viable etiological explanation.

Cutaneous lymphosarcoma

Lymphosarcoma is not rare in horses. Runnells and Benbrook (1944) reported 6 cases in 600 tumor cases. Multicentric, digestive, thymic, cutaneous, and mixed forms are recognized (van den Hoven and Franklin 1983). In 88 cases Jaeschke and

Rudolph (1985) found only 2 cutaneous cases, and van den Hoven and Franklin (1983) saw 1 cutaneous among 16 cases. The low incidence of the purely cutaneous form is consistent with our experience.

Cutaneous involvement is not, however, uncommon with systemic lymphosarcoma (Gupta et al. 1972). A 7-year-old Quarter horse mare had pyrexia and generalized lymphadenopathy, as well as multiple foci of alopecia, cutaneous and subcutaneous nodules, and ulceration of the skin. The skin of the abdomen and neck was thickened and firm. At postmortem all peripheral and internal lymph nodes were markedly enlarged, and tumor nodules were present in the thoracic esophagus, stomach, small intestine, peritoneal cavity and retroperitoneal space, and stifle. Neoplastic infiltration of the skin obliterated the epidermal and dermal architecture and occluded some blood vessels. There was focal ulceration and dermal necrosis, and pleomorphic lymphocytes and multinucleated giant cells were present. Similar patterns have been seen in other cases. As discussed with the gastrointestinal tract, lymphosarcoma of the ileum can cause obstruction, particularly in young horses (see Chapter 3).

Specialized techniques, such as electron microscopy, immunocytochemistry. and lectin cytochemistry, have allowed differentiation of the cell populations of dermal lymphosarcomas. Detilleux et al. (1989) labeled lymphocytes and histiocytic cells. With the use of lectin cytochemistry in a 15-year-old Standardbred mare, they found that the histiocytic cell population was primarily reactive and nontransformed, while the lymphoid component clearly was neoplastic, contrasting with the general view by light microscopy that most lymphoid tumors of horses are histiocytic.

Papilloma

Cutaneous papilloma of equids is a neoplastic disease induced by infection with equine papilloma virus, a DNA-containing papovavirus (Fulton et al. 1970). The tumors are most common on the muzzle and lips of 1- to 3-year-old horses (Baker and Leyland 1975). Cases of congenital papillomatosis have been reported by Garma-Avina et al. (1981). Single papillomas on the head or neck are occasionally seen in aborted fetuses and newborn foals. There is no breed or sex predisposition. Lesions may persist for 1–9 months and then spontaneously regress (Sundberg et al. 1985). Cadeac (1910) reported transmission of papilloma from one horse to another. Papillomas are irregularly shaped, multiple, discrete nodules, ranging from 2 mm to over 1 cm, and gray, white, or multicolored, and mottled. The verrucous character of this tumor develops as the tumor matures. Hamada et al. (1990) studied the growth of 78 spontaneous papillomas on 50 horses, and of 54 tumors induced experimentally in 3 Thoroughbred horses. Spontaneous lesions had been present for weeks to months when biopsied. Papillomas developed in experimental horses within 19 days of viral inoculation. There were three proliferative phases based on histology: growth, development, and regression. In the initial phase, basal cells are swollen and hypochromic. There is minimal to moderate acanthosis, hyperkeratosis, and parakeratosis. Intranuclear inclusion bodies and minimal cytolytic changes are seen in the stratum spinosum and stratum corneum. Mild lymphocytic infiltration of the margins of lesions may occur. In the developing phase, all layers of the epidermis become hyperplastic. The basal cell layer becomes multilayered, folded, and hypomelanotic (Hamada and Itakura 1990). Ballooning degeneration of the stratum spinosum has been reported, and numerous intranuclear inclusion bodies are present in nuclei of the stratum spinosum and granulosum. There are long rete pegs of hyperplastic epidermis. Congestion, edema, minimal lymphocytic infiltration, and fibroblastic proliferation are all seen in the developing lesion. Finally, lesions enter the regression phase with the epidermis returning to normal with only a few viral inclusions in cells. Fibroblast proliferation and collagen deposition occur during this phase.

Squamous cell carcinoma

This tumor is common (Table 15-1). Usual sites include the face, external genitalia, and mucocutaneous junctions [Stannard and Pulley in Moulton (1978)]. Squamous cell carcinoma occurs commonly in skin lacking pigmentation and, so, susceptible to solar radiation. Baird and Frelier (1990) reported a squamous cell carcinoma at the site of a healed wound in the gluteal skin.

Squamous cell carcinomas are ulcerated, raised, or verrucous, nodular growths of variable size from 3 mm to over 20 cm. The tumor is locally invasive and spreads readily to adjacent lymph nodes. Distant metastases occur but are uncommon.

Histologically, variably well-organized anastomosing cords of neoplastic epidermis penetrate into the dermis. The tumor may be well differentiated or anaplastic from tumor to tumor and within a given tumor. The margins are typically indistinct. Keratin production and mitotic activity are highly variable and roughly proportional to the degree of differentiation. In our experience, squamous cell carcinoma in the horse has less keratinization than in dogs or cats, keratin pearls being infrequent. Secondary inflammation is common in ulcerated tumors, which can be the site of myiasis and/or habronemiasis.

Mastocytosis and mastocytoma

McEntee (1991) precisely defined equine cutaneous mastocytoma based on 30 cases with good demographic profiles. It is a benign, usually solitary, lesion of the skin and subcutis characterized histologically by sheets of mast cells. The lesion had been reported sporadically in the literature since 1908 (Sabrazes and Lafon). There has been confusion about the neoplastic nature of the lesion and the related cutaneous mastocytosis (Altera and Clark 1970; Prasse et al. 1975).

Mastocytoma is a benign neoplasm of horses 1–18 years old, McEntee (1991). A case of congenital mastocytosis has been seen (Prasse et al. 1975). The mean age in McEntee's group was 9.5 years. Ten of 30 horses were Arabians; no other breed was prevalent, and there was no sex predisposition. Tumors were commonest on the trunk and head, less so on the neck and extremities.

Gross lesions ranged from 5 mm to 8 cm in diameter, average of 3.5 cm. The majority were firm, tan, raised cutaneous nodules. Surface ulceration and foci of caseous debris were seen (Doran and Collins 1986; McEntee 1991). Microscopically, 70% of the lesions were either partially or fully encapsulated. There was compression of adjacent soft tissues. Sheets and nests of well-differentiated mast cells were found, together with variable numbers of eosinophils and bundles of necrotic collagen. McEntee recognized three phases: initiation and early growth, inflammation, and regression. In the initial phase, there was proliferation of mast cells in mitotically active nests and nodules. In the inflammatory phase, lesions were infiltrated with eosinophils with necrosis of collagen and mineralization. In regression, fibroplasia and granulomatous inflammation predominated. There were no recurrences after surgical removal in over 90% of cases followed for 6 years or more (McEntee 1991). Metastasis was not seen.

Keratoma

Keratoma has been seen in the hooves of horses for many years. Lloyd et al. (1988) reported 7 cases causing lameness in horses ranging from 2–20 years old. Six lesions were in the hoof wall, 1 in the sole. Grossly, they were firm, solitary lesions, 1–5 cm in size. Microscopically, they consisted of cores of mature keratin and debris surrounded by a rim of neoplastic squamous epithelium. Inflammation, secondary infection, and necrosis, was common. Surgical excision was curative on 1 year follow-up. Keratoma is also discussed with the foot (see Chapter 7, "Fore Leg").

Hemangiomatosis

There are a number of case reports of **cutaneous hemangioma** and **hemangiosarcoma** (Trasbot 1876; Montane 1890; Hargis and McElwain 1984; Johnstone 1987). In a large series, Hargis and McElwain described 21 such tumors. Eight were hemangiomas and 3 hemangiosarcomas. Twelve of 18 horses with hemangioma were 1 year old or less, and 6 horses had definitely congenital lesions. Johnstone (1987) saw an hemangioma and an hemangiosarcoma in 2 horses less that 1 year old. Hargis and McElwain reported that 3 horses with cutaneous hemangiosarcoma were from 8.5 to 13 years old. Lesions were most common on the head, neck, and extremities. Six of 18 horses were Arabians, with lesser numbers of Thoroughbreds, Quarter horses, and Appaloosas, among others. Grossly, lesions ranged from 1.5 cm to 31 cm, and most were ulcerated and bled easily.

Histologically, the lesions were classified as capillary hemangiomas, cavernous hemangiomas, and hemangiosarcomas. Tumors excised from eight horses did not regrow.

Vascular tumors of the skin and other tissues, meninges, muscles, nasal mucosa (ethmoid hematoma) are not uncommon and usually occur in young horses. In any given case the diagnosis may be hemangioma, cavernous hemangioma, hemangiosarcoma, capillary hemangioma, and so forth. Some tumors are virtually unclassifiable other than as mixed masses of abnormal vascular tissue. It appears that the several forms are variations of a basic, congenital hemangiomatosis peculiar to the horse. The biological behavior is variable with complete recovery after extirpation to locally aggressive recurrence. While the picture is not unclouded, it is our opinion that all of these vascular tumors belong to a single congenital category, which we prefer to call **hemangiomatosis**.

Apocrine gland adenocarcinoma

Single occurrences of apocrine gland adenocarcinoma and carcinosarcoma have been reported in aged animals (Anderson et al. 1990b). The animals had advanced disease with weight loss and anorexia.

CHAPTER 16

Nervous System

Central nervous system—brain

Viral encephalitides

Viral encephalitides are common and significant causes of morbidity and mortality in horses, donkeys, mules, and other equids. The *Alphaviruses* (formerly group A arboviruses—Eastern, Western, and Venezuelan encephalomyelitis viruses) are the most important in the Western Hemisphere, causing encephalomyelitis and high mortality in horses. These viruses also cause encephalitis in humans.

Some viral agents—Japanese B encephalitis, Powassan, Murray Valley, Ross River, Main Drain, Borna/Near Eastern, and louping ill viruses—cause encephalitis in discrete geographical areas.

Alphavirus encephalomyelitis (Venezuelan, Eastern, and Western equine encephalomyelitis)

Venezuelan equine encephalomyelitis

Venezuelan equine encephalomyelitis has been recognized since the late 1930s, when periodic epizootics occurred in northern South America and Central America. In 1969 an epizootic in the southern United States killed over 50,000 horses in 2 years (Gibbs 1976). There have been periodic epizootics in Colombia (Roberts et al. 1970), typically occurring in low lying, swampy areas with marked seasonal variation in rainfall.

Infection and disease follow exposure of susceptible equids to mosquito-borne virus. Four subtypes, with eight serological variants of this RNA togavirus, have been identified. The A, B, and C variants of subtype I are most virulent and produce serious clinical disease. Infection of humans, ruminants, pigs, dogs, and rabbits has been reported. Only partial cross-protection is provided by immunity to Eastern equine encephalomyelitis virus, despite some degree of cross-reaction (hemagglutination inhibition) with Eastern and Western equine encephalomyelitis.

Variants D and E of subtype I, and subtypes II, III, and IV cause enzootic infection of horses in Florida and Central and South America. Infected horses do not become viremic and have few clinical signs. Human infection with enzootic viral strains has been reported. Enzootic forms of the virus have been found in wild rodents, but the role of such reservoirs in epizootics of more virulent strains is unclear (Gibbs 1976). Walton and Johnson (1972) and Byrne (1972) stated that horses were dead-end hosts for enzootic viral strains, but amplifier hosts for epizootic strains. It is unclear if epizootic strains exist in reservoirs such as dogs or domestic pigs, or if they arise by mutation of enzootic strains.

Horses infected with virulent strains may have viremia within 24 hours, which persists an average of 4 days. Virus may be isolated from oral, nasal, and conjunctival secretions, and milk, but has not been found in feces or urine. The virus probably proliferates in hematopoietic and lymphoid tissue since both are destroyed in experimental infections in guinea pigs (Gleiser et al. 1962). Viral neutralizing antibody can be detected approximately 24 hours after viremia disappears and is usually present before neurological signs.

Walton (1972) and others described three clinical forms of Venezuelan equine encephalomyelitis. In the mildest, horses develop inapparent infection with low fever. In one more severe form there are pyrexic and viremia with profound depression, anorexia, weight loss, diarrhea or constipation, sawhorse stance, falling, paddling, and grinding of teeth. The other encephalitic form is characterized by hyperexcitability, convulsions, aggressiveness, circling, and salivation.

Mortality of 40%–80% in natural cases has been reported (Gibbs 1976), and similar rates occur with experimental infection (Kissling and Chamberlain 1967).

Clinicopathological diagnosis involves detection of specific antibody by hemagglutination inhibition. Neutropenia has been reported in more severe cases. In about 50% of fatal cases virus can be isolated from the brain and assayed in mice by complement fixation.

There are no gross lesions. Microscopically, a spectrum of lesions may be present, depending on duration and severity of disease. Roberts (1970) felt that necrotizing vasculitis predominated, unlike the more diffuse inflammatory disease of Eastern equine encephalomyelitis. Kissling and Rubin (1951), however, found that vascular lesions were prominent in peracute cases of Eastern equine encephalomyelitis.

Roberts (1970) described neutrophilic or mixed inflammatory cell, perivascular infiltrates in the brain and spinal cord. Severely damaged vessels were necrotic, contained thrombi, and adjacent neural tissue was malacic. Perivascular and perineuronal neutrophilic or mixed inflammatory cell infiltrates were present in the cerebral cortex, corpus striatum, basal ganglia, thalamus, and caudate nucleus. Glial nodules may form in the cortex and cerebellum with perineuronal astrocytic satellitosis.

Monlux and Luedke (1973) studied the pathogenesis of lesions in the brain and spinal cord caused by the American and Trinidadian epidemic strains of the Venezuelan virus in 18 experimental horses. As in naturally occurring cases, the experimental horses developed fever, anorexia, leukopenia, and central nervous system depression within 10 days. Severely affected animals had ataxia, circling, altered behavior and excitability, rage, salivation, convulsions, paddling, and recumbency. Focal hemorrhagic and liquefactive cortical necrosis were seen grossly in the brains of some severely affected horses. In less severe cases no gross lesions or only minimal focal discolorations were apparent. Few gross lesions were seen in spinal cords. The authors specifically noted liquefactive necrosis of the lobus orbitalis portion of the external olfactory tract and portions of the claustrum and external capsule.

A variety of microscopic lesions were described (Monlux et al. 1973). Foci of mixed inflammatory cells and liquefactive necrosis were found in various parts of the brain. Demyelinating lesions occurred in concert with foci of necrosis and inflammation. There were scattered foci of myelitis and minimal, diffuse meningitis of the spinal cord, less severe in more caudal portions of the cord. Unlike natural cases, significant or consistent vascular lesions or neuronal necrosis was not seen in experimental animals. There were no substantial differences in pathogenicity between American and Trinidad epidemic strains.

As with other forms of equine encephalitis, horses recovering from Venezuelan encephalomyelitis may have permanent neurological deficits. Moderately severe, diffuse, patchy alopecia of unknown cause has also been reported in recovered animals.

Eastern equine encephalomyelitis

An epizootic of equine encephalitis was reported in Massachusetts in 1831. One hundred horses were affected and 75 died. Other outbreaks were reported on Long Island in 1845 and in Kansas in 1912 (Hanson 1972b). Periodic epizootics occurred in nonvaccinated horses until the early 1960s (Byrne et al. 1961). In 1933 Giltner and Shahan isolated the virus from brain and cord of horses in Virginia, Maryland, and Delaware and demonstrated antigenic differences from the Western equine encephalomyelitis virus isolated in the California epizootic of 1930. Later work showed that there was considerable overlap in the distribution of these viruses, both being present in North and South America and in the Caribbean. Eastern equine encephalomyelitis, like Western equine encephalomyelitis, is morphologically and antigenically similar to Venezuelan equine encephalomyelitis, but does not have enzootic and epizootic strains. There is some antigenic variation among strains of Eastern equine encephalomyelitis in North and South America.

Eastern encephalomyelitis is a seasonal disease with peak incidence in late summer, coinciding with large populations of mosquito vectors (Gibbs 1976). A number of birds and mammals are susceptible to infection. Humans and horses are not considered definitive hosts although vector-mediated, horse-to-horse transmission can occur during viremia. Pheasants and other birds are highly susceptible to infection; mortality in pheasants may reach 75%. Numerous studies have suggested that in most epizootics, infection of wild birds (ringneck pheasants, English sparrows) precedes equine cases by 2–4 weeks (Byrne et al. 1961). Human cases are generally seen about 2 weeks after horse infections peak.

Viral proliferation occurs first in the regional lymph nodes after the bite of an infected mosquito. A secondary cycle of proliferation occurs in viscera before infection of the central nervous system and clinical signs (Hanson 1972; Kissling et al. 1954).

The clinical course is usually 2–3 days, with a morbidity of 25%–30% and a mortality of 75%–90% in nonvaccinated horses and mules (Giltner and Shahan 1933). Byrne (1972) described three clinical forms. Some horses had clinically inapparent infection with slight fever and minimal viremia, while others had high fever and viremia without neurological signs. The most severely affected had high fever, viremia, and typical clinical signs: depression, ataxia, circling, head-pressing, and hyperexcitability.

There are no gross lesions. Kissling and Rubin (1951) described microscopic lesions in the brains and spinal cords of 21 horses. They recognized two basic patterns. Horses dying peracutely (within 1 day of the onset of neurological signs) had diffuse infiltration of gray matter with neutrophils. Vascular damage, including swelling and necrosis of endothelium, thrombosis, and perivascular edema and hemorrhage, were seen. Mixed inflammatory cell infiltrates were present in the vascular adventitia and Virchow-Robin spaces. Neuronal necrosis and neuronophagia were minimal.

Animals dying 2 or more days after onset of neurological signs had less neutrophilic infiltration and lower incidence and severity of vascular lesions. Nodules of microglia and mononuclear cells were scattered through the gray matter, and there was diffuse microgliosis and perivascular lymphocytic infiltration.

Lesions were distributed throughout the gray matter of the brain and cord, but were more prominent and severe in frontal and occipital cortices, hippocampus, hypothalamus, and dorsal medullary nuclei. The pattern of lesions suggested hematogenous, rather than neurotropic, spread of virus.

The routine use of polyvalent vaccines has dramatically reduced the frequency of this disease since the 1940s.

Western equine encephalomyelitis

An epizootic of encephalomyelitis killed an estimated 25,000 horses in Nebraska, Kansas, Oklahoma, Missouri, and Colorado in 1912 [Udall (1913) cited by Doby et al. (1966)]. The Western equine encephalomyelitis virus was first isolated from horses during the California epizootic of 1930 [Meyer et al. (1931) cited by Doby et al. (1966)]. Periodic epizootics in nonvaccinated or poorly protected horses continued to occur into the mid-1960s (Doby et al. 1966).

An epizootic in 263 horses and ponies in Illinois, with 25% mortality, was described by Doby et al. in 1966. Clinical signs included fever, incoordination, staggering, drowsiness, anorexia, lip droop, and recumbency. Some horses were depressed, ataxic, falling, or circling. Seventy-eight percent with these clinical signs died within 4 days of onset; 42% of the survivors improved within 4 days of onset; and less than 2% had residual neurological signs. Fewer young animals less than 2 years old died—12%—compared to horses and ponies over 2 years—24%. Approximately 10% of the horses and ponies had a history of, probably inadequate, vaccination. A small number, less than 2%, had antibody titers for St. Louis and Murray Valley viruses.

Hurst (1934), cited by Sponseller et al. (1966), described the gross and histological lesions of naturally occurring cases, and Sponseller et al. (1966) described experimental infection. The latter inoculated groups of ponies with 1 of 4 strains of Western virus by intracerebral or subcutaneous routes. There was variation in severity of disease, depending on the strain/isolate of virus used.

A low degree of viremia occurred within 1–5 days of infection, regardless of the route. All ponies inoculated intracerebrally developed encephalitic signs, including sawhorse stance, hyperesthesia, depression, teeth-grinding, and muscular twitching.

Gross and microscopic lesions, comparable to those reported by Hurst (1934) in spontaneous cases, were found in 2 of 13 ponies. Both animals were killed in moribund condition following intracerebral injection of BFS 1703 strain virus. In both there was gross meningeal congestion. There was patchy vascular congestion and perivascular cuffing with lymphocytes and neutrophils, as well as perivascular hemorrhage. Glial nodules and foci of neutrophilic infiltration were present in both gray and white matter. Focal gliosis was present in the spinal cord. In one pony satellitosis and neuronophagia occurred in areas of neutrophilic infiltration. Lesions were more severe in frontal and occipital cortices.

As with Eastern and Venezuelan encephalomyelitis, prophylactic vaccination has dramatically reduced morbidity and mortality.

Murray Valley and Ross River encephalitis

Epizootics of viral encephalitis caused by Murray Valley and Ross River viruses occurred in Queensland and New South Wales, Australia, in 1971 and 1974 (Gard et al. 1977). Clinical encephalitis had not been seen previously, although neutralizing antibody to Murray Valley virus had been detected in horses since 1952 (Anderson 1952). Of six or so enzootic arthropod-borne viruses in Australia, only Murray Valley and Ross River are known to cause encephalitis in horses. Limited data suggest that the rate of infection is high (many serologically positive horses) but the mortality rate slow to moderate: 25%–50% (Gard et al. 1977). Both viruses cause encephalitis and polyarthritis in humans. Brief descriptions indicated muscle stiffness, reluctance to move, and joint pain and swelling as primary clinical signs.

There are no characteristic gross lesions. Microscopically, there is a spectrum of lesions including nonsuppurative meningomyelitis and encephalomyelitis and encephalomalacia of the internal capsule, pons, cerebral peduncle, and midbrain. Ross River virus may produce more severe lesions than Murray Valley virus (Gard et al. 1977).

Attempts to reproduce these two diseases experimentally have had limited success; horses developed serological evidence of infection, but rarely developed clinical signs.

Japanese B encephalomyelitis

Sporadic cases and epizootics of encephalomyelitis in Japan and Southeast Asia have been described since the late 1800s. Japanese B encephalomyelitis virus was shown to be the cause of epizootics in 1935–1937. Epizootics occurred in Japan in 1947 and in Singapore in 1951. In affected areas approximately 85% of horses had been exposed to the virus and developed neutralizing antibodies (Burns et al. 1949). Neutralizing antibodies were found in approximately 33% of horses in Malaya (Hale and Witherington 1953). Young horses, less than 3 years old, are apparently more susceptible to infection, perhaps reflecting exposure of naive animals (Kii et al. 1942). Pigs, goats, cattle, rabbits, and some dogs, had antibodies against the virus.

The virus is transmitted by culicine (*Culex* sp., *Aedes* sp.) mosquitoes with a predilection for feeding on large domestic animals (Burns and Matumoto 1949a,b; Rosen 1986). In enzootic and semienzootic areas, the disease is seasonal in early autumn when vector populations are largest. The disease is common in low-lying swampy areas where the vector is common (Burns and Matumoto

1949a,b). Heavy rainfall increases the incidence of disease in enzootic areas (Wang et al. 1982).

The Japanese B virus is a flavivirus and an important human pathogen. It was first described in 1933 as a cause of epidemic seasonal encephalitis in humans in Japan (Rosen 1986). It causes abortion and neonatal death in pigs in enzootic areas. Swine are an important source of virus for human infection, but horses are not. While birds are considered to be definitive hosts for viral propagation, their role in transmission is unclear (Rosen 1986).

Burns et al. (1949) and Burns and Matumoto (1949a,b) reviewed the literature and described the clinical signs in 2 severely affected, fatal cases. The initial signs in 1 animal were fever, anorexia, and listlessness. The horse subsequently developed submandibular swelling and periorbital scleral congestion. Rear leg weakness and staggering gait, as well as excitation and disorientation, were seen. The animal died on the 3rd day. The other horse was febrile, anorectic, and became recumbent, disoriented, and blind, and died in 3 days.

Three forms of Japanese B encephalomyelitis were recognized clinically by Hale and Witherington (1953): transient, lethargic, and hyperexcitable. The transient form was characterized by 2–3 days of fever and congestion of mucous membranes. The lethargic form was more severe, with fever, difficult eating and swallowing, lethargy, ataxia, abnormal stance and hypermetria, muscle rigidity, and collapse. Some animals had jaundice and congestion of mucous membranes. The most severe form, the hyperexcitable, was characterized by high fever (105°–107°F), mania, loss of vision, tooth grinding, ataxia, and collapse. Death within a day of onset was not uncommon.

The hyperexcitable form is similar to the fatal case of Japanese B encephalomyelitis reported by Kheng et al. (1968) in a Malaysian racehorse. Fever and anorexia were followed by hypersensitivity of head and neck, photophobia, tremor, ataxia, unconsciousness, and death in respiratory failure.

Fever and anorexia were seen by Gould et al. (1964) in an experimental case of Japanese B encephalomyelitis, but the animal recovered after a period of ataxia and incoordination.

Hale and Witherington (1953), Kheng et al. (1968), and Burns et al. (1949) gave the gross and microscopic findings. They all found marked meningeal vascular congestion grossly. Hale and Witherington and Kheng described petechial and ecchymotic hemorrhages on the pericardium and myocardium and congestion of the lungs. Cerebral cortical vessels were congested in all four cases. There was perivascular lymphocytic cuffing and foci of microgliosis. Burns described marked perivascular edema and focal neuronal degeneration, necrosis, neuronophagia. Malacia and neuronal degeneration was not found in Kheng's case. Kii et al. (1935), cited by Burns and Matumoto (1949a,b), studied the pathogenesis of the disease in a variety of experimental animals and horses with similar morphological findings. There have been reports of intranuclear or intracytoplasmic inclusions in hippocampal neurons (Burns and Matumoto 1949a,b).

Serological evidence suggests that Japanese B encephalomyelitis is enzootic in domesticated species in areas of Japan and Southeast Asia. Kheng found that horses newly imported to Malaysia were at greatest risk of developing the disease within a few months of arrival. Hale and Witherington (1953) concluded that horses became infected within 6–12 months of arrival in enzootic areas, and that nearly 100% of horses had either complement-fixing or neutralizing antibodies to Japanese B encephalomyelitis virus after 12 months in Malaysia.

The virus seems poorly pathogenic since Hale and Witherington found that only 4 of 60 horses infected in their series had to be destroyed. Kheng et al. examined records of racehorses with episodes of high fever. They found that approximately 50% became infected during transport or stabling at tracks, and that few, if any, died. Gould et al. (1964) reported low levels of viremia during infection, and this may be a factor in the low pathogenicity.

Burns and Matumoto (1949a) reported that the equine mortality rate in the 1947 Japanese epizootic of Japanese B encephalomyelitis was over 50%. Some strains of the virus may be more pathogenic than others, or enzootic infections protect against epizootic forms of the disease.

Burns et al. (1949) showed that Japanese B encephalomyelitis virus is antigenically related to the St. Louis encephalitis virus. Convalescent serum from Japanese B encephalomyelitis horses may cross-react with Murray Valley virus in complement fixation tests (Hale and Witherington 1954). No relationship was found between equine enzootics of Japanese B encephalomyelitis and human epidemics, unlike Eastern and other encephalitic viruses. Wang et al. (1982) also found no correlation.

Louping ill encephalitis

Louping ill is a tick-borne viral disease of ruminants in the British Isles. Timoney et al. (1974) found neutralizing antibodies to this flavivirus in approximately 11% of Irish horses. In 1976 Timoney et al. described 3 cases of louping ill encephalitis in pastured horses in Ireland. The horses were reluctant to move, ataxic, or recumbent. Muscle tremors were seen in 2 of 3 animals, and one was hyperexcitable, incoordinated, and had opisthotonos. One animal lost body condition and had only transient clinical signs. Similar signs in a young draft horse were reported earlier by Fletcher (1937).

Two of the 3 horses died. There was congestion of meningeal blood vessels in 1, and both had microscopic evidence of viral encephalitis, including neuronal degeneration, perivascular lymphoid infiltration, and focal gliosis in the midbrain nuclei and cerebellum. Louping ill virus was recovered from the brain of 1 horse. The lack of polymorphonuclear leukocytic infiltration was considered an important differentiating characteristic from Eastern equine encephalomyelitis. Louping ill encephalitis causes focal disease of the midbrain red nuclei rather than of the oculomotor nuclei as in Borna disease [Innes (1965) cited by Jubb and Kennedy (1985)].

Experimental horses had serological evidence of infection but did not show neurological signs (Alexander et al. 1935).

Powassan viral encephalitis

Nonfatal viral encephalitis, perhaps caused by tick-borne Powassan flavivirus, is seen sporadically in horses in southern Canada. The first human case of this encephalitis was identified near Powassan, Ontario, and has been diagnosed in southern Ontario, Quebec, British Colombia, and the eastern seaboard of the United States. Little et al. (1985) found serological evidence of infection in 13 of 101 horses and a high incidence of antibody in dogs, skunk, groundhog, fox, raccoon, rabbit, hare, and opossum.

The pathogenicity of Powassan virus was studied by Little et al. (1985) in horses and ponies infected by intracerebral and intravenous routes. Within 8 days 3 horses showed variably severe neurological signs. One horse had abdominal tenderness, repetitive chewing movements, ataxia, staggering, and recumbency. The signs progressed over a 5-hour period, and the horse was killed. Another horse, infected by intracerebral injection, had chewing movements, head and neck tremors, ataxia, and marked proprioceptive deficits within 8 days of infection. The animal was killed 24 hours after onset. A third horse, infected intravenously, was depressed, ataxic, and hyperesthetic for 10 days, but the signs resolved. The animal was killed after 39 days.

Two horses infected intracerebrally developed the most severe gross and microscopic lesions. Both had gross meningeal congestion and hemorrhage around spinal nerve roots. Microscopic lesions included severe nonsuppurative necrotizing encephalomalacia at the site of injection, lymphocytic perivascular cuffing and meningitis, focal gliosis, neuronal necrosis, and neuronophagia. There were axonal spheroids in the medulla and mesencephalon and lymphocytic perivascular cuffing in the fifth cranial nerve. Minimal meningitis and scattered lymphocytic perivascular cuffs were seen in the brain (basal ganglia, corpus callosum, thalamus, hippocampus, and medulla) and cord of one horse infected by intravenous injection.

While clinical signs in these experimental animals were similar to those in other viral encephalitides, the distribution, character, and severity of the microscopic lesions were different. Powassan viral encephalitis produced a nonsuppurative meningoencephalomyelitis with most severe lesions in the medulla and mesencephalon. Gasserian ganglioneuritis, seen characteristically in rabies encephalitis, is not a feature of Powassan viral encephalitis. Inflammatory lesions in equine encephalomyelitis are more prominent in cortical gray matter unlike the medullary/mesencephalic lesions in Powassan viral encephalitis. The necrotizing vascular lesions of herpesvirus (EHV)-1 myeloencephalitis are not seen in Powassan encephalitis.

Main Drain viral encephalitis

A single case of equine encephalitis caused by Main Drain virus was reported by Emmons et al. (1983). This is an arbovirus carried by biting midges in California. Main Drain virus occurs naturally in rabbits and several species of wild rodents and infects sheep, cattle, pigs, and horses, as indicated by the presence of antibodies.

In the one case, a 1-year-old Quarter horse suddenly developed progressive neurological signs including ataxia, reluctance to move, chewing movements, inability to swallow, and head-pressing, over a 2-day period. There were pyrexia and increased heart rate as well as increased values for serum creatinine, creatine kinase, and blood glucose. The animal was killed. Gross and microscopic lesions were not described, but Main Drain virus was isolated from brain tissue and caused neurological disease and deaths in a mouse bioassay. Tests for the presence of rabies, Saint Louis encephalitis, Venezuelan equine encephalomyelitis, Eastern equine encephalomyelitis, and Western equine encephalomyelitis were negative.

Borna disease/Near Eastern encephalitis

Borna disease is a tick-borne arbovirus encephalitis of equids and other animals: sheep, cattle, and rabbits. The disease is named for the town in central Germany where it was first seen by Joest and Degen in 1911 [Joest and Degen (1911) cited by Cohrs (1961)]. A nearly identical disease occurs in sheep, cattle, goats, horses, mules, and donkeys, in eastern Europe, the Mideast, northeastern

Africa, southern Russia, and Kazakstan and is known as Near Eastern encephalitis. The virus has been isolated from a number of species of wild birds in the Near East and Egypt, and these birds are, presumably, the reservoir for the enzootic form of the disease in equids and other animals. Periodic epizootics of Borna disease/Near Eastern encephalitis have been described since the early 1940s. The disease has seasonal peaks in early and late summer, coinciding with peak activity of the tick vector. Transovarian viral transmission in ticks has been described. The presence of the virus in central Germany is thought related to migration of birds from the Near East and Mideast (Daubney 1967).

In horses, donkeys, and mules three clinical types have been described in both spontaneous and experimental cases: hyperacute and fulminating, acute, and chronic and/or relapsing. Young horses are most susceptible. Mortality may approach 90% in animals with neurological signs (Daubney and Mahlau 1967; Daubney 1967).

Following a variable incubation of greater than 20 days, horses and mules become febrile and colicky. In the hyperacute form animals are excitable and vicious and rapidly—within 12–18 hours—become ataxic, paralyzed, and die. Animals with the acute form of the disease have muscle tremor, unsteadiness, weakness, paraesthesia, and facial paralysis for a few days before death. More chronic cases have the same signs but are ataxic or paralyzed for longer periods of 20–40 days. Relapse and death have been seen in experimental animals as late as 170 days after resolution of neurological signs.

Meningeal congestion has been seen consistently, and meningeal petechiae have also been described. The myocardial hemorrhage and pericardial transudate described in some North African cases were probably related to African horse sickness rather than Borna disease/Near Eastern encephalitis (Dabney and Mahlau 1967).

Microscopically, there is encephalitis with lymphocytic perivascular cuffing. Jubb and Kennedy (1987) say that lesions are found in the meninges and from olfactory bulbs to medulla, with more prominent lesions in gray matter and nuclei of the cerebral axis. The cerebellar cortex is usually spared. Intranuclear inclusions, *Joest-Degen bodies,* are seen in neurons (especially Ammon's horn), and are unusual for viral encephalitides. Some authors have described intracytoplasmic inclusions (Daubney and Mahlau 1967). Glial nodules are present in the cerebral cortex, together with neuronal satellitosis and neuronophagia.

Although the lesions, clinical signs, and morphological characteristics of Borna disease and Near Eastern encephalitis are similar, these diseases may not be identical. Antigenic cross-reactivity of the two viruses by immunodiffusion in gel and by complement-fixation has not been established (Daubney and Mahlau 1967).

Rabies encephalitis

Despite the worldwide occurrence of rabies and the nearly uniform fatal course of the disease in mammals, there is surprisingly little literature on rabies in horses and other equids. There are approximately 60–90 cases of confirmed rabies in horses each year in the United States (Communicable Disease Center 1983). The routine use of vaccines in enzootic areas has, in part, limited the threat to horses. There are, however, a large number of nonvaccinated horses, and recent carnivore enzootics in the northeastern United States and southern Canada have increased the likelihood of equine exposure. The virus has been successfully eliminated from Great Britain and Scandinavia and was never introduced to Australia or New Zealand (Jubb and Kennedy 1985).

Rabies, a rhabdovirus, is most commonly transmitted by the bite of infected animals—primarily canids, skunks, raccoons, and bats. Rare instances of human and bat-to-bat infection by aerosols have been reported in bat caves or laboratory accidents. The virus is neurotropic and the sequential propagation of virus in nerve trunks, paravertebral ganglia, peripheral nerves, spinal cord, and brain are well documented in naturally occurring and experimental infections in many species. Various strains of the virus have been identified, differing in biological properties and ability to proliferate in salivary glands.

The clinical course in horses and other equids is variable, depending on the site of infection and the strain of rabies virus. Both the furious and the dumb or paralytic forms can occur. Schroeder (1969) briefly described a case in which a horse, bitten on the coronary band by a rabid skunk, developed rapidly progressive neurological signs 51 days after exposure. Over a 2-day period, the animal became anorectic, incoordinated, and died. The animal received two postexposure doses of vaccine, but not until 24 days after the skunk bite. There was microscopic evidence of rabies, but this was not described.

Ferris et al. (1968) infected 2 donkeys with virulent rabies virus, 1 by a single intramuscular injection in the neck and the second by injection in the left foreleg. Within 11 days the first donkey developed signs of rabies, including depressed attitude, leaning against a wall, torticollis, and sternal recumbency. The animal died on the 13th day.

Postmortem examination revealed no gross lesions. Microscopically, there was nonspecific, nonsuppurative encephalitis. Perivascular cuffing, foci of neuronal degeneration, and neuronophagia were present in all parts of the brain examined. Negri bodies were not found. Neuronal degeneration of the Gasserian ganglia, considered to be common in rabies, was found.

The second donkey developed neurological signs 11 days after infection. For 11 days this donkey had colicky pain, stiff-legged movements, leaning against the walls of the stall, and intermittent recumbency. It then gradually recovered without residual neurological deficits. Paired sera, prior to infection, and after recovery 39 days after infection, showed that animal had been infected by rabies virus and recovered.

An unusual rear leg hyperesthesia was reported in 2 rabid horses (Meyer et al. 1986). Both animals had fascicular muscular twitching, progressive unilateral and bilateral rear leg weakness, hyperesthesia, and progressive loss of reflexes. The clinical course was 2–3 days, before the animals were killed or died. There were no gross lesions. Tissues of 1 horse were examined microscopically. A nonsuppurative meningomyelitis and ganglionitis was present, with inflammation most severe in the lumbar spinal cord. Marked perivascular lymphocytic cuffing, gray matter gliosis, and vascular congestion were seen in lumbar cord sections. There was swelling and lysis of neurons, minimal spongiform degeneration of white matter, and leptomeningitis. Characteristic of infection with rabies virus, there was marked ganglioneuritis with dense lymphocytic infiltration around nerve cell bodies. There were no cord lesions cranial to the sixth cervical vertebrae. Negri bodies were not found, although sections of brain and sciatic nerve were positive for virus by fluorescent antibody.

Fluorescent antibody tests on a variety of tissues collected at autopsy from the second horse also were positive for rabies virus. Of particular interest was that both sciatic nerves were positive. Meyer and colleagues believed that initial infection in one sciatic nerve spread to the other, and to the cord, simultaneously. In both cases the authors believed that clinical signs were produced by localized infection of cord gray matter before the virus traveled to the brain.

Herpesvirus (EHV)-1 myeloencephalitis

Sporadic outbreaks of ataxia and paralysis in horses have been definitively associated with infection by EHV-1 since the early 1970s. The literature strongly suggests that EHV-1 neurological disease has been seen since the mid-1800s in Europe and North America. Stockfleth (1855) and Comeny (1888), both cited by Platt (1980), described ataxia and paraplegia in horses with clinical descriptions indicative of EHV-1 infection. Little and Thorsen (1976) saw epizootics of ataxia and paralysis in both young and mature horses in Ontario between 1958 and 1976. Outbreaks of neurological disease in mares, geldings, and stallions on stud farms have been described (Crowhurst 1981; Platt et al. 1980b; Greenwood 1980; Thomson et al. 1979; Bitsch and Dam 1971; Charlton et al. 1976).

In companion papers, Greenwood and Simson (1980) and Platt et al. (1980b) described the clinical and pathological features of a typical outbreak of EHV-1 in horses on a British Thoroughbred stud farm. Eighty-two horses (39 mares, 39 foals, and 4 stallions) were exposed to infection after abortion of a 10-month fetus. Of this number, 35 of 39 mares, 5 of 39 foals, and 2 of 4 stallions developed neurological signs, primarily ataxia. The signs appeared within 14 days of initial exposure in some horses, but the investigators felt that an incubation period of approximately 7 days was more typical. Initial clinical signs in mares and stallions included pyrexia, ataxia, urinary incontinence, atony of the bladder, and nasoocular discharge. Infected foals, on the other hand, showed respiratory signs including nasal discharge, pyrexia, and respiratory rales. Ataxia, limb dragging, and paresis with recumbency occurred in most horses within 1–6 days after onset of pyrexia. Similar clinical signs and patterns of onset were seen by Crowhurst et al. (1981) during an outbreak of EHV-1 on another stud farm and by Thein (1981) in Germany. We have seen a number of outbreaks in different parts of North America with virtually identical clinical signs and courses.

Platt et al. (1980) described the gross and microscopic findings in 8 mares that died spontaneously or were killed shortly after onset of neurological signs. There were petechial and ecchymotic hemorrhages in the subcutis and nasal mucosa. Four of 8 had hemorrhagic cystitis and enlarged, hemorrhagic lymph nodes. There was leptomeningeal congestion in 4 of 8 animals, and foci of malacia and hemorrhage in the brain and spinal cords.

Microscopically, disseminated necrotizing vasculitis of small arteries, arterioles, and venules was seen in the brain and spinal cord. Acute inflammation, endothelial swelling and necrosis, fibrinoid mural necrosis, and thrombosis were observed in the vessels of the cerebral cortex and the brainstem, surrounding spinal nerve roots, trigeminal nerve, ileocecal mesenteric ganglia, and cauda equina. Vascular lesions were focal or segmental, and thromboses formed in only the more severely inflamed and damaged vessels. Perivascular hemorrhages were present. Damage to nervous tissue was most prominent in proximity to vascular lesions with malacia of both gray and white matter.

The degree of inflammatory cell reaction

varied according to the amount of affected tissue and the duration of the lesion. Horses dying acutely or killed shortly after the onset of neurological signs had a few neutrophils in malacic lesions. Macrophages, plasma cells, lymphocytes, and gitter cells were seen in resolving malacic foci in horses surviving for longer periods. Axonal swelling was seen near foci of cord degeneration and was a consistent lesion in many horses. These authors saw no evidence of neuronophagia and only minimal demyelination.

Lesions in other tissues included a single case of degeneration in the outer nuclear layer of the retina, and minimal focal hepatic necrosis.

Little et al. (1976) described similar clinical and pathological findings in a 3-year-old Standardbred filly. There were foci of necrosis in the corpus callosum, mesencephalon, septal nuclei, and occipital cortex, with giant cells in Virchow–Robin spaces and malacic foci adjacent to degenerate, inflamed arterioles in the leptomeninges. Little et al. noted that most cases of EHV-1 infection occurred in the autumn, and most horses recovered.

Thein (1981) found spinal cord lesions of demyelination and mononuclear cell infiltration. There was spongiform encephalopathy in the rhombencephalon. Herpesvirus (EHV)-1 was isolated from neural tissue. In most reports of spontaneous disease the virus was not isolated, perhaps because of the presence of neutralizing antibody.

Edington et al. (1986) infected eight mares with EHV-1 and described progressive vascular and neurological lesions over 28 days. Within 4 days of infection, there was viral infection of and thrombosis in nasal and spinal cord arterioles. The platelet counts decreased as early as 2 days after infection, and circulating immune complexes were seen from 2 days postinfection onward, peaking at 28 days. Infected, circulating mononuclear cells were found within 2 days of infection near vascular lesions and also in regional lymph nodes, suggesting a role in viral dissemination. Clinical neurological dysfunction was seen within 8 days.

Edington et al. proposed that an endotheliotropic strain of EHV-1 was more likely to produce neurological disease than was type 2 herpes. They felt that vascular damage was the primary cause of lesions, and that immune/inflammatory events following production and deposition of immune complexes were less important. They acknowledged that antecedent infection and/or vaccination with EHV-1 and EHV-2 might play a significant role in priming horses for neurological disease.

Jackson and Kendrick (1971) had similar findings in a study of seven mares inoculated with EHV-1. Pregnant mares were more likely to develop neurological disease than nonpregnant mares, and affected animals had increased protein levels in cerebrospinal fluid.

Thomson et al. (1979) noted that the vascular tropism and pathogenesis of lesions in equine EHV-1 infection is like malignant catarrhal fever in cattle and unlike the neurotropism of herpes infections in other species, an observation made earlier by Charlton et al. Their study of paresis in vaccinated horses emphasized the limitation of current vaccines in preventing respiratory infection, abortion, or neurological lesions. This confirmed earlier observations by Bitsch and Dam (1971) who believed that EHV-1 neurological disease was the result of reinfection of partially immune horses rather than a primary infection.

Equine infectious anemia

Ataxia has been the primary clinical sign of neurological disease in horses infected with equine infectious anemia virus. Such signs, and associated lesions of granulomatous meningoencephalomyelitis, have been described for over 40 years. There seems to be no data on the frequency of neurological involvement in equine infectious anemia.

McClure et al. (1982) described equine infectious anemia neurological disease in 4 horses. All had a history of lameness or ataxia. Several had a history of progressive weight loss and pyrexia unresponsive to therapy. Neurological signs included symmetrical proprioceptive defects, especially of the rear legs. The animals tended to circumduct the legs when circled, and several had difficulty pacing, or knuckled or stumbled when walked over obstacles. Some had atrophy of gluteal musculature, and/or loss of anal sphincter or tail tone. Three of the 4 horses had positive agar gel immunodiffusion tests for equine infectious anemia.

Gross lesions in the central nervous system included scattered foci of malacia in the gray and white matter of the cord (1/4 horses), meningeal opacity and thickening (1/4), and petechial hemorrhages on the cord and brainstem (1/4).

Microscopically, there was a spectrum of lesions in the central nervous system, with variations in the degree, location, and type of inflammatory reaction and tissue destruction. Two horses had severe, nonsuppurative, granulomatous ependymitis; meningitis; and encephalomyelitis. Lymphocytes, plasma cells, and macrophages infiltrated portions of the cerebellum and spinal cord. There was almost total obliteration of the central canal of the spinal cord and severe granulomatous meningitis. Lesions were less severe and more focal in two other horses.

Tajima (1953) found similar histological lesions in the central nervous system of experimental ponies. Neurological signs and lesions were described by Held et al. (1983) in a 16-year-old

Thoroughbred gelding. There was nonsuppurative leptomeningitis of the spinal cord and aggregation of mixed inflammatory cells around nerve roots. This animal had no other signs of equine infectious anemia. The protein content of cerebrospinal fluid was elevated—greater than 250 mg/dL—as was the white blood cell count—greater than 95 cells/mm^3.

Most cases have positive cerebrospinal fluid agar gel immunodiffusion tests. Other hematological and biochemical abnormalities are consistent with the clinical phase, acute or chronic, of the infection. McClure et al. (1982) suggested that infectious anemia antibody in cerebrospinal fluid was very helpful in confirming the etiological relationship of equine infectious anemia to neurological disease, since infectious anemia horses without neurological signs did not have this antibody.

Bacterial diseases

Botulism

Botulism in the horse, as other species, is not accompanied by specific gross or microscopic lesions. The condition appears in horses of any age as single cases or in epizootics (see shaker foal, grass sickness, below). *Clostridium botulinum* B, C, and D toxins have been isolated (Mayhew and MacKay 1982).

The clinical signs include sudden onset, generalized muscular weakness, loss of ability to swallow, dilatation of the pupils, ileus, and rapid heart rate. There may be frank paralysis of the tongue and dripping of saliva. Prostration and death are usually rapid but may be delayed some days, apparently depending upon the amount of toxin. In less fulminant cases slow intravenous infusion of parasympathomimetic and sympathomimetic drugs may provide at least temporary remission of signs.

There are no pathognomonic lesions, although the fibrinous hydropericardium of the shaker foal is strongly suggestive. While lesions were suggested in the central nervous system in the earlier literature, it is clear that the toxin only acts at motor endplates without morphological changes. Examination of the motor endplates of the muscle of shaker foals with cholinesterase stains revealed no changes. The clinical signs and the postmortem evidence of ileus suggest a search for toxin and its source. It is difficult to recover toxin from the animal, greater success attending the search for the environmental source. Silage safe for cattle has long been known to be dangerous for horses because of the presence of botulinum toxin, which, in moderate amounts, can apparently be destroyed in the forestomach of ruminants. A number of epizootics have been associated with feed contaminated by dead animal carcasses (Mayhew and MacKay 1982), and one major epizootic was traced to toxin in silage produced by an anaerobic storage system.

So-called toxicoinfectious botulism has been bruited as a cause of shaker foal and botulism in older horses. This implies a focus of infection in the animal in which the organism can proliferate, and from which toxin is liberated. This has not been confirmed, and we have seen no example.

Tetanus

Tetanus is a major neuromuscular disease of equids throughout the world, recognized as a cause of morbidity and mortality since ancient times. Fortunately, the disease is no longer common with the widespread use of tetanus toxoid.

Infection of wounds with infectious spores of one of the 10 strains of *Clostridium tetani* and subsequent vegetative growth leads to toxin production. Penetrating, deep wounds in the hoof are a major site of infection since the infectious spores are ubiquitous in soil. Neonatal wounds are also readily infected. The organism is a moderately fastidious anaerobe. Anaerobic conditions, devitalized tissue, disruption of tissue blood supply, and growth of facultative aerobes favor vegetative proliferation. The toxin, *tetanospasm,* is produced during bacterial growth and gains entry to the circulation by diffusion. Some studies have shown that vegetative forms of the bacteria may enter the circulation and colonize internal organs. The toxin probably cannot penetrate intact mucosa or mucous membranes, but intercurrent disease might facilitate absorption by disrupting these barriers.

Tetanospasm is readily bound to neurons at myoneural junctions. Binding of toxin to these junctions disables inhibitory control of synaptic transmission, so that synapses are continuously activated with consequent tetanic muscular contraction.

Clinical signs may occur from a few days to months after infection. Prolapse of the membrane nictatans is the first clinical sign. Progressive muscle stiffness and tremor soon follow, and spasms of maxillary and mandibular musculature interfere with eating. Tetanic spasm of oppositional muscles causes rigidity and the characteristic sawhorse stance. Affected animals may fall and be unable to urinate or defecate.

Barton and Knight (1972) reported that mortality is approximately 80% in nonvaccinated animals.

There are no gross or microscopic lesions in the nervous system. Prolonged muscle spasm causes generalized muscle congestion and bruising. A characteristic and not infrequent terminal lesion is fracture of one or more thoracic vertebrae. (See Chapter 9, "Vertebral Column.")

Borreliosis (Lyme disease)

A case of encephalitis in a 6-year-old Morgan gelding, suspected to be infection with *Borrelia burgdorferi,* was reported by Burgess and Mattison (1987). The animal had a week-long history of progressive neurological impairment, including circling and constant pacing, profuse sweating, dysphagia, flaccid paralysis of the tail, and head tilt. Serological and fluorescent antibody tests for Eastern and Western encephalomyelitis and rabies were negative, but there was a moderately high serum titer for *B. burgdorferi.* The organism was isolated from the brain. No gross or histological examinations were done, the isolation of *Borrelia* considered sufficient for the diagnosis.

Melioidosis

In Australia, France, and Malaysia serological data suggest that melioidosis is a common disease of horses and other livestock. Infection of horses with *Pseudomonas pseudomallei* has caused minor epizootics of gastrointestinal disease in France (Desbrosse et al. 1978). Some chronically infected horses had ataxia and pyrexia.

Ladds et al. (1981) described suppurative meningoencephalomyelitis in a 15-month-old colt with *P. pseudomallei* infection. The animal was recumbent with facial paralysis and opisthotonos. Neurological signs progressed concurrently with pyrexia and clinical deterioration. The animal was killed 9 hours after onset of clinical signs.

Grossly, there were focal thickenings of the meninges and suppurative foci between cerebral hemispheres. Malacic and hemorrhagic foci were seen in the brainstem and cervical spinal cord. Microscopically, a mixed inflammatory cell infiltration was present in malacic and hemorrhagic foci. There was mononuclear cell cuffing of vessels, focal vasculitis, perivascular hemorrhage and edema, swollen axons, scattered foci of gliosis, and neuronal degeneration. *P. pseudomallei* was isolated from the brain and cord.

Streptococcal brain abscess

Streptococcus equi can produce abscesses in a variety of tissues. Raphael (1982) described three cases of abscess of the brain caused by either *S. equi, S. zooepidemicus,* or other, unidentified Gram-positive organisms.

The horses had various clinical signs including head tilt, ataxia, circling, head-pressing, and/or loss of vision or sensation. Elevated protein and inflammatory cell content was seen in cerebrospinal fluid in 2 of 3 horses. At autopsy there were discrete, large abscesses in the cerebral cortex and adjacent structures, compressing and displacing adjacent brain parenchyma. Inflammatory cells and macrophages were present in and surrounding abscessed areas.

S. zooepidemicus infrequently causes diffuse cerebrospinal meningitis in foals with septicemia. Opisthotonos and hyperesthesia are common clinical signs. The purulent process is obvious on gross examination of the brain and spinal cord.

Actinobacillosis and Actinomycosis

Rare cases of meningitis and abscessation caused by *Actinobacillus lignieresi* and *Actinomyces sp.* have been reported. Both infections caused progressive neurological deficits and death.

Chladek and Ruth (1976) described progressive paralysis caused by an epidural abscess in a 3-year-old Appaloosa filly. The filly had difficulty moving, then standing, and finally was recumbent. At autopsy, an 8-cm-long epidural abscess extended caudad from the fifth cervical vertebra. A mixed inflammatory cell infiltrate was present in a large focus of malacic cord. A mixed culture of *A. lignieresi* and *S. zooepidemicus* was isolated.

Disseminated septic meningitis was the cause of neurological signs in a 3-year-old Morgan mare described by Rumbaugh (1977). The animal had pyrexia, depression, and nasal discharge, and soon developed rear leg ataxia, difficult neck flexion, and hypermetria. Some improvement was noted with sulfonamide treatment, but the mare suddenly became quadriplegic and recumbent and was killed. A large abscess was present in the meninges adjacent to the pituitary gland. The meninges were acutely inflamed from the olfactory bulbs to the sacral spinal cord. A species of *Actinomyces* was isolated.

Klebsiella meningitis

Klebsiella pneumoniae is a primary respiratory and genital pathogen in horses. Prior to the report by Timoney et al. (1983), it had not been reported as a cause of meningitis in horses.

An 8-year-old Thoroughbred mare had retained placenta after aborting twins. Within 24 hours, despite therapy, she was febrile and recumbent. By 72 hours she was ataxic with hyperexcitability, nystagmus, and opisthotonos, and died in convulsions.

There was marked meningeal vascular congestion, and focal areas of meningeal discoloration over the cerebellum and cerebrum. A severe, suppurative meningitis was found microscopically. While there was hemorrhage in the cerebellum, there was no microscopic evidence of encephalitis or encephalomyelitis. *Klebsiella pneumoniae,* capsular type I, was cultured from multiple sites, including the meninges.

Fungal diseases

There are scattered reports of fungal meningitis and encephalitis. In particular, cases of cryptococcal meningitis have been described in the United States and Australia.

Horses with cryptococcal meningitis have a variety of nonspecific neurological signs including depression, anorexia, ataxia, recumbency, hyperesthesia, hyperexcitability, and blindness (Irwin and Rac 1957; Barton and Knight 1972; Steckel et al. 1982).

Steckel et al. (1982) described a typical case. A 7-year-old Quarter horse had a 3-week history of progressive signs including weight loss, ataxia, incoordination, and unilateral blindness. There were proprioceptive defects of all legs, and the horse circled, stumbled over obstacles, and was reluctant to back. A cerebrospinal tap had a high protein and cell content, and *Cryptococcus neoformans* budding bodies were present. Therapy was attempted with corticosteroids and amphotericin B, but the horse succumbed. Terminal signs included recumbency, convulsions, ataxia, hyperexcitability, and severe depression.

There was severe, suppurative leptomeningitis extending from the midbrain to the third cervical vertebra. An acute, fibrinopurulent exudate was seen microscopically. This was attributed, in large part, to intrathecal administration of an excessive amount of amphotericin B. However, there were lesions clearly attributable to *Cryptococcus.* These included foci of chronic inflammation in the right cerebral hemisphere, choroid plexus, and fourth ventricle, as well as deep within the brain along vessels. The chronically inflamed areas were infiltrated with lymphocytes and macrophages, and a few giant cells and cryptococcal budding bodies were present.

Similar clinical signs, neurological deficits and gross and microscopic findings, were reported in a case of cryptococcal meningitis in a 3-year-old Standardbred gelding (Barclay and de Lahunta 1979).

As in most cases of fungal infection in the central nervous system, the prognosis for cryptococcal meningitis is grim (Barclay and de Lahunta 1979; Steckel et al. 1982). The route of infection is probably respiratory with subsequent hematogenous spread, although there is the potential of direct spread from infected sinuses and nasal granulomata (Scott et al. 1974).

Protozoal diseases

Diseases with established or presumed protozoal etiology have been found in horses and donkeys. Of these, equine protozoal myeloencephalitis is the most common and well recognized.

Equine protozoal myeloencephalitis

In 1970 Rooney et al. described focal myeloencephalitis in 52 horses with gait abnormalities, stumbling, recumbency, ataxia, and paresis. The horses fell, dog-sat when backed, and had asymmetrical and progressive motion deficits. Subsequently, other investigators described a variety of other, less common, neurological signs including tremor, asymmetric lameness, weakness, and asymmetrical paralysis of the face (Dorr et al. 1984; Fayer et al. 1990). Elevations in protein and cell content of cerebrospinal fluid has been reported in some cases (Dorr et al. 1984). Peracute, acute, and chronic forms of the disease were described. The disease does not kill, but the neurological deficits are usually permanent.

Several lines of evidence suggest the etiological agent(s) is coccidian protozoa either of the genus *Sarcocystis* or closely related. Various protozoal feeding and motile forms (sporozoites, merozoites, tachyzoites, and bradyzoites) with light and electron microscopic appearances consistent with *Sarcocystis* sp. are found in tissue sections of lesions in approximately one-third to one-half of cases (Simpson and Mayhew 1980; Boy et al. 1990). Recent work has shown that polyclonal antisarcocystis antibody will stain organisms in tissue sections (Granstrom et al. 1991). Fayer and Dubey (1982) found indirect hemagglutination inhibiting antibody against *Sarcocystis* sp. in 9 of 10 horses with confirmed equine protozoal myeloencephalitis, but not in 3 control horses. Therapeutic agents (pyrimethamine, sulfonamides) active against protozoa apparently are helpful in the treatment of suspected cases and decrease the frequency of visible protozoa in tissue sections (Fayer et al. 1990; Boy et al. 1990). Repeated attempts to isolate the etiological protozoa have failed, as have experimental transmission attempts (Fayer and Dubey 1982). An evaluation of various risk factors suggests the disease is more common in young—less than 4 years old—Standardbred, Thoroughbred, and Quarter horses. In a survey of 364 histologically confirmed cases, no sex predisposition, seasonal peaks, or geographical association were seen in the United States (Fayer et al. 1990).

Gross and microscopic lesions are confined to the central nervous system, especially the thoracic and lumbar spinal cord. Grossly, there is focal, segmental hemorrhage and necrosis of gray and white matter (Fig. 16.1). Typically, gross lesions only occur in one, two or more segments of the cord, although multiple sites may be found histologically (Rooney et al. 1970).

Microscopically there is focal nonsuppurative

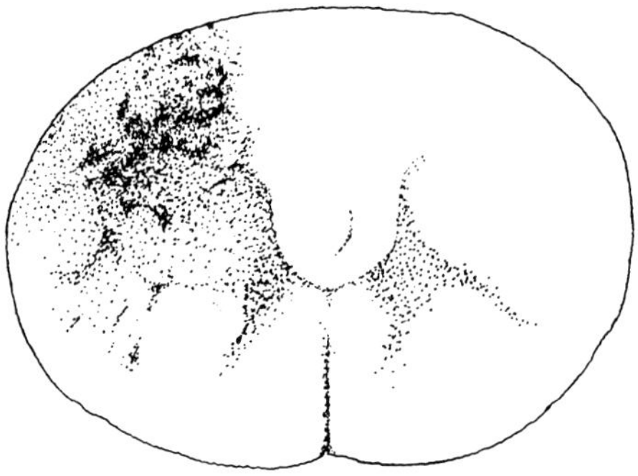

16.1. Diagram showing typical focal distribution of hemorrhagic lesions in protozoal myelitis.

myeloencephalitis, with infiltration by lymphocytes and eosinophils and occasional giant cells. In acute cases there may be small hemorrhages around vessels or larger areas of frank hemorrhage in the gray and white matter (Figs. 16.2–16.5). With longer duration, hemosiderin may be present at the site of old hemorrhage. Rooney (1970) saw marked lymphocytic perivascular cuffing, focal gliosis, and neuronal necrosis. When the organism is found in tissue sections, it is intracytoplasmic in neurons, infiltrating inflammatory cells, and vascular endothelium.

The disease has only been reported in North America, though cases may have occurred in Central and South America. While the etiology remains problematic without successful transmission, an aberrant or unadapted species of *Sarcocystis* is suspected.

Toxoplasmosis

Beech and Dodd (1974) described segmental myeloencephalitis in 8 horses, which they felt was caused by infection with a *Toxoplasma*like organism. McDonald and Cleary (1970) and Cusick et al. (1974) described similar cases. A serological survey of horses in California by Riemann et al. (1975) showed that 20% of the horses had *Toxoplasma* antibodies. No correlation with clinical disease was given.

Beech and Dodd attempted to isolate and transmit the etiological agent to susceptible mice unsuccessfully, and no antibody to *Toxoplasma* was found in cerebrospinal fluid 14–21 days after the onset of neurological signs in horses.

It seems certain that the disease described by Beech and Dodd and others as possible toxoplasmosis is, in fact, protozoal myeloencephalitis.

Trypanosomiasis

Infection of horses with trypanosomes causes systemic and neurological disease. The important equine pathogens are *Trypanosoma evansi*: surra (Hindu—"rotten"), *T. brucei*: nagana in Asia, Africa, and South America, *T. equinum*: mal de caderas in

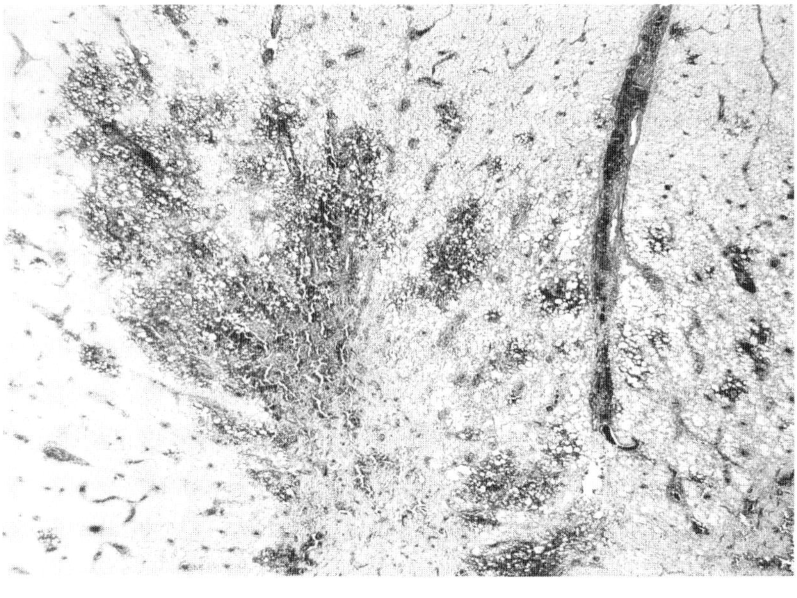

16.2. Photomicrograph demonstrating areas of hemorrhage and malacia in spinal cord of horse with protozoal myelitis.

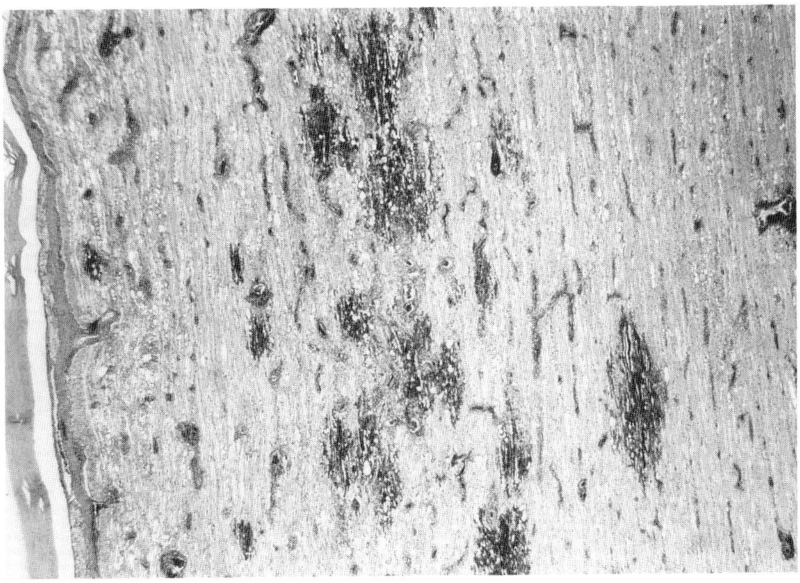

16.3. Focal lesions in protozoal myelitis.

Central and South America, *T. hippicum*: murrina, perhaps identical to mal de caderas, and *T. equiperdum*: dourine (Arabic—"unclean") in Asia, Africa, Europe, and the Americas. Although these diseases have been recognized for hundreds of years, the pathology has not been well described. The clinical signs and venereal transmission of dourine were well known in antiquity. The material here is largely from Hutyra and Marek (1926).

For trypanosomiasis, in general, at the time trypanosomes appear in the blood the horse develops fever, depression, decreased appetite, and rapid/weak pulse. The mucous membranes are injected; there is profuse lacrimation, and edema

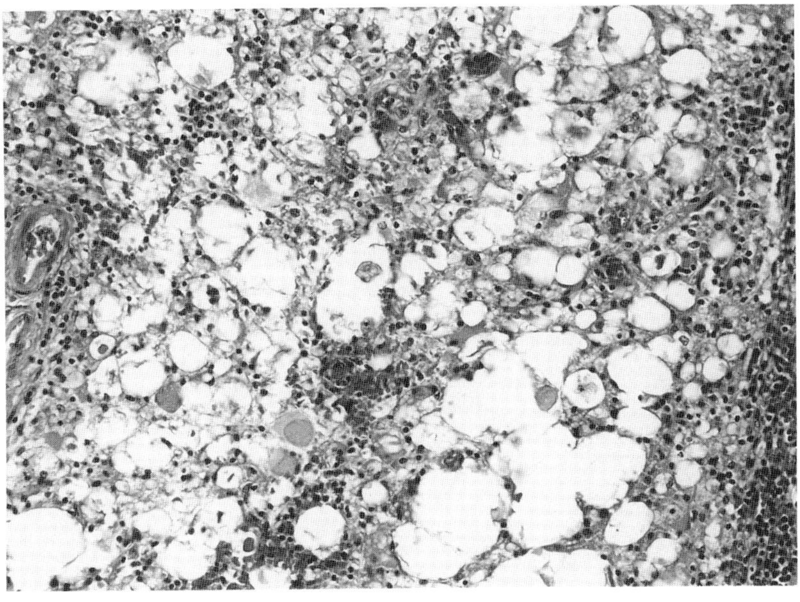

16.4. Swollen axons in area of malacia in cord of horse with protozoal myelitis.

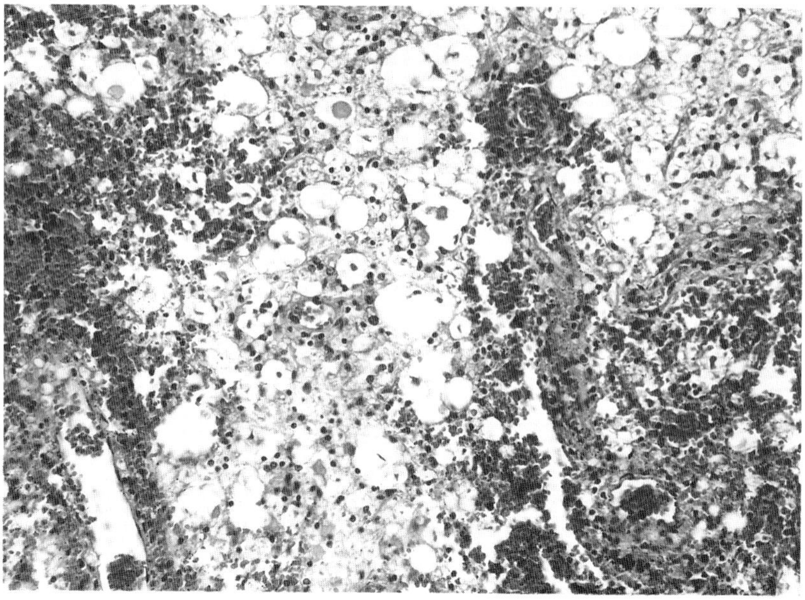

16.5. Cellular debris, inflammatory cells, and necrosis of nerve tissue is typical of focal lesions in protozoal myelitis.

appears on the legs, ventral abdomen, and around the genital organs. After 2 to 3 days the fever abates, other signs improve, and the animal appears to be recovering. Clinical signs recur, however, after a variable period, with the reappearance of trypanosomes in the blood. The subsequent clinical course varies with the individual case and is characterized by progressive emaciation, weakness, and recurring episodes of illness and partial recovery. Most animals die in about 1-2 months, though some may last longer.

Surra (T. evansi infection)

Meningoencephalitis was described in five naturally occurring infections of Malaysian horses with *T. evansi* (Seiler et al. 1981). The authors discussed the worldwide distribution and importance of the disease and the lack of description of neurological lesions prior to their report.

Cadeac (1899a) indicated that age resistance or selection for resistance with increasing age had been shown for surra (see Table 16-1).

The clinical course of disease was over 2 months from initial signs to death. Pyrexia was followed by progressive lethargy, ataxia, emaciation, anemia, and subcutaneous, edematous plaques.

At postmortem, there was emaciation with ventral subcutaneous edema, enlarged lymph nodes, and scattered hemorrhages on serosal surfaces. The meninges were congested. Microscopically, infected horses had diffuse, nonsuppurative meningoencephalitis of gray and white matter, with perivascular lymphocytic and histiocytic cuffing, patchy gliosis, and minimal axonal degeneration in severely inflamed areas.

In enzootic areas of Asia and Africa, cattle, water buffalo, and chronically infected camels are the main reservoir species for equine infection. In South America the capybara is the main reservoir species for horses. The parasite is mechanically transmitted by biting flies (Soulsby 1968).

Nagana (T. brucei infection)

Nagana (debilitated) is a disease of African horses transmitted biologically or mechanically by the Tsetse fly. A detailed description was presented in companion papers by McCully and Neitz (1971). Trypanosomiasis was induced in 6 adult horses and 3 were treated with subtherapeutic doses of two

Table 16-1. Age resistance for surra (*Typanosoma evansi* infection)

Attack rate (%)	Age (years)
39–45	5-9
31–36	10–14
13–15	15–19
2–3	20–24

Source: Cadeac 1899a.

antitrypanosomal drugs, Berenil and Antrypol. This suboptimal regimen was designed to induce chronic disease.

The animals became anemic, depressed, and ataxic. There was unilateral or bilateral blindness. By the end of 9 months, during which chronic disease developed, the affected horses had *T. brucei* in the cerebrospinal fluid and macroscopic lesions in the brain and spinal cord.

Gross and microscopic lesions were present in a number of tissues. There was moderately severe myocarditis and epicarditis, pulmonary endarteritis and thrombosis, interstitial nephritis, diffuse reactive hyperplastic lymphadenopathy, and skeletal myositis. The liver had focally extensive to diffuse centrilobular atrophy, fatty change, degeneration, and necrosis of hepatocytes. These lesions were presumed to be anoxia secondary to anemia. There was mixed inflammatory cell infiltration, bile stasis, and hemosiderosis of the liver. Variable amounts of hemosiderin were found in the lungs, spleen, lymph nodes, and myocardium.

A detailed description of gross and microscopic pathology in the central nervous system was presented by McCully and Neitz (1971). Horses with chronic nagana had severe, diffuse, nonsuppurative meningitis (meningeal pleocytosis), extensive subpial gliosis adjacent to inflamed areas of the leptomeninges, segmental demyelination of optic tract fibers and other areas of white matter, vasculitis, and extensive lymphoplasmacytic perivascular cuffing in white and gray matter. Neuronal necrosis and degeneration were not important features. It was felt that the neurological lesions could be attributed to anoxia, vasculitis, and nonsuppurative inflammation of the meninges.

Mal de caderas (T. equinum infection)

Infection with *T. equinum* causes systemic and neurological disease in horses, mules, and donkeys in Central and South America. The disease is enzootic in Argentina, Bolivia, and Paraguay and is a significant cause of morbidity and mortality in wet, swampy areas. The protozoan parasite is transmitted mechanically by biting flies. The capybara is thought to be the primary wildlife reservoir for equine infection (Soulsby 1968).

The common form of the disease is chronic wasting, emaciation, and weakness of the rear legs. More acute cases die in a few weeks. Progressive weakness leads eventually to recumbency. Keratoconjunctivitis and periorbital edema have been seen in terminal animals. Death from chronic disease occurs in 2–6 months.

Gross lesions of splenomegaly, lymphadenomegaly, and edema are similar to those with *T. evansi* infection. Edematous swelling of soft tissues may be present around the spinal cord.

Dourine (T. equiperdum infection)

Primarily a venereal disease of horses and asses, dourine often causes paralysis in the terminal stages. It occurs in Asia, North and South Africa, and southern Europe. It was successfully eradicated from the United States by the mid-1960s. Although the protozoan parasite is generally transmitted during coitus, it may also be spread mechanically by biting flies and fomites. The mortality rate can approach 70%. Jackasses may be asymptomatic carriers.

Dourine is a three-phase disease. In the first, following coital exposure, lesions are restricted to the genitalia. The stallion develops nonpainful edema of the sheath, scrotum, and contiguous abdominal wall. After some days yellowish-red nodules appear in and adjacent to the urethra, on the glans, and on the body of the penis. These nodules ulcerate and heal as prominent, white scars. There are signs of inflammatory irritation of the penis: frequent urination and erections.

The mare develops edematous swelling of the vulva, white then yellow, slimy, purulent vaginal discharge, and reddening and swelling of the vaginal mucous membrane. Nodules develop in the mucosa as in the stallion with progression to ulceration and healing. There may be spotty loss of pigmentation of the skin of the labia (toad spots). There are estral signs and frequent urination. In both the stallion and the mare the severity of clinical signs varies widely from barely perceptible to severe.

The second stage usually follows in several weeks either with or without transitory improvement. The characteristic *dollar spots* appear on the sides of the chest, croup, less often neck, withers, and other areas. The dollar spot is round or irregular in outline and up to 15 cm in diameter. The periphery is a ring of edematous tissue 1–3-cm wide, with the hair standing on end or disarranged. Within the peripheral edematous ring, the hair is smooth, and there is no edema. There are several variants, including irregular zig-zags of edema and disarranged hair, bean-sized nodules, and plaques of edema resembling urticaria. These lesions are not hot, painful, or itching. They persist for some days, disappear, and are replaced by a new crop.

The third, neurological, stage is characterized by generalized and localized hyperesthesia of the skin and variable paresis, paralysis, and localized muscular atrophy. Stringhalt or shiveringlike signs may occur, progress inexorably, or disappear. Affected animals died anywhere from 3 weeks to 1–2 years after onset.

The rich set of clinical signs would suggest equally rich pathological findings. The descriptions, however, are slender and usually of nonspecific cachectic changes. No description of the histology of the skin lesions has been found. Edema of nerve roots with mononuclear cell infiltration, fibrosis, and loss of peripheral nerve fibers is mentioned. Marek (1904), cited by Fankhauser (1968), found inflammation and infiltration of cells in the nerve roots, spinal ganglia, and peripheral nerves, particularly of the rear quarters. The changes in the peripheral nerves decreased with distance from the spinal cord. Degenerative changes were also seen in the spinal cord, presumably secondary to the peripheral nerve damage. Similar changes have apparently been seen in horses with mal de caderas [Torres et al. (1944) cited by Fankhauser and Luginbühl (1968)].

Toxic and metabolic neurological diseases

Mycotoxic encephalomalacia

Mycotoxic encephalomalacia is a neurotoxic disease of equids caused by *Fusarium moniliforme* toxins. It has been recognized since 1902 when Butler [Butler (1902) cited by McCallum and Buckley (1904)] described the clinical signs and characteristic brain lesions. An epizootic of mycotoxic encephalomalacia was reported in Maryland in 1904–1905 (MacCallum and Buckley 1904). Buck et al. (1979) described a small epizootic in horses in Illinois, Nebraska, Iowa, Kentucky, and Tennessee during a 15-month period in 1978–1979. Mycotoxic encephalomalacia has been the presumptive or established cause of outbreaks of equine neurological disease throughout the world being described in Argentina, China, Egypt, New Caledonia, South Africa, Greece and other parts of Europe, and the United States (Marasas et al. 1988; Jubb and Kennedy 1985). The disease has been known as equine leukoencephalomalacia, moldy corn poisoning, cornstalk disease, and blind staggers.

Mycotoxic encephalomalacia is caused by exposure to and metabolism of toxins liberated by the growth of *Fusarium moniliforme* on damaged corn kernels and cobs (Wilson et al. 1973 and 1990; Marasas et al. 1976; Buck et al. 1979; Masri et al. 1987; Uhlinger 1991b). Corn, corn products mixed in feed, and contaminated commercial feed have been incriminated. Although a number of *Fusarium* toxins and metabolites have been suspected, it has been established that fumonisin B_1 produces the neurological lesions (Marasas et al. 1988; Wilson et al. 1990). Oral doses of crude *Fusarium* extract, 1.25- 2.5 g/kg of body weight for 7 days, produced early mycotoxic encephalomalacia lesions in two horses. The intravenous administration of purified fumonisin B_1 toxin at 0.125 mg/kg body weight daily for 8 days caused bilaterally symmetrical malacic lesions, consistent with early mycotoxic encephalomalacia, in the medulla of one experimental horse. Wilson et al. (1990) correlated levels of fumonisin B_1 in contaminated feed with lesions in 18 Arabian horses and verified the relationship of disease to toxin levels.

The roles of closely related toxins, fumonisin B_2, and moniliformin is not known. Buck et al. (1979) injected repeated small quantities, 1 mg/kg, of moniliformin intravenously into a donkey. The animal died suddenly after 26 daily injections, but lesions were equivocal. It has been suggested that different *Fusarium* toxins or metabolites cause the brain and liver lesions (Haliburton et al. 1979; Gelderblom et al. 1986; Brownie and Cullen 1987; Marasas et al. 1976). Some have suggested that the same toxin produces both brain and liver lesions with the duration of exposure and concentration of toxin determining the prevalence and severity of lesions (Brownie and Cullen 1987; Marasas et al. 1988). In the absence of dose-response studies, the question is moot.

Horses appear to be one of the most sensitive species for *Fusarium* toxins (Wilson et al. 1973; Hintz 1990). Rats exposed to crude *Fusarium* extracts develop hepatocellular carcinomas (Marasas et al. 1984). Some rodents and ruminants develop no disease when exposed experimentally to *Fusarium*-contaminated feed at levels causing profound lesions in horses. Older horses may be at higher risk, but there is considerable individual variation. Epidemiological and experimental studies have shown an attack rate of 14%–25% and fatality in excess of 60% (Brownie and Cullen 1987; Wilson et al. 1990; Uhlinger 1991).

Mycotoxic encephalomalacia occurs most commonly in the United States from September to May. Certain growing and harvest conditions (dry summers and/or drought, followed by rainy autumns) increase the amount of *Fusarium moniliforme* on feed corn. Epizootics have occurred in years in which corn was harvested during periods of high humidity (Schwarte et al. 1937; Badiali et al. 1968; Masri et al. 1987).

There are a variety of clinical signs including colic, ataxia and weakness, unilateral or bilateral blindness, mania and hyperexcitability, anorexia, recumbency, convulsions, icterus, and sudden death (Masri et al. 1987). Marasas et al. (1976, 1988) reported trembling, profuse sweating, sawhorse stance, reluctance to move, and circling. They reported that several affected horses became violent and attempted to run through fencing or stall walls. Signs may develop within weeks or months after exposure to contaminated feed (Uhlinger 1991). Neurological dysfunction is usually progressive, although there have been reports of partial recovery with permanent neurological deficits. It is apparent that the time of onset and severity of lesions is largely determined by the amount of toxin in the feed, rate of ingestion, and cumulative dose.

Biochemical analysis revealed that aspartate aminotransferase, alkaline phosphatase, and γ-glutamyltransferase levels were elevated (Brownie and Cullen 1987; Masri et al. 1987; Wilson et al. 1990; Uhlinger 1991). Masri et al. (1987) reported elevations in blood ammonia. Elevations of protein and cells in cerebrospinal fluid have also been seen (Masri et al. 1987; Brownie and Cullen 1987; McCue 1989). Brownie and Cullen (1987) reported increased levels of myelin basic protein in cerebrospinal fluid, a consequence of myelin destruction. Uhlinger (1991) saw slightly elevated serum creatinine values as well as anemia. Elevations in serum creatinine values were thought to be prerenal azotemia, a consequence of dehydration and anorexia. Some investigators have failed to detect abnormalities in these parameters in naturally occurring or experimental cases (Buck et al. 1979).

Gross lesions are in the brain, spinal cord, liver, and kidneys. Meningeal and cortical edema with flattening of gyri have been consistently reported (MacCallum and Buckley 1904; Marasas et al. 1976; Brownie and Cullen 1987; Marasas et al. 1988). Foci of vascular congestion, hemorrhage, and yellow-gray discoloration of the cortex, brainstem, and spinal cord are common. Large areas of the cerebral cortex are soft, with a gelatinous texture. The degree and distribution of edema and hemorrhage, as well as the size and distribution of malacic foci in the brain and spinal cord, are highly variable with the most severe and extensive lesions in subcortical white matter (Fig. 16.6). Malacic foci are seen in the subcortical white matter of the frontal cortex, hippocampus, midbrain, and medial geniculate areas (Marasas et al. 1976). Foci of liquefactive necrosis have also been found in the rostral, temporal, and occipital lobes, the thalamus, cerebellum, brainstem, and spinal cord (MacCallum and Buckley 1904; Wilson et al. 1973; Masri et al. 1987). In some cases, the gray matter overlying the malacic foci is compressed and "tented" over the lesion. Many have commented on the symmetrical nature of lesions in the white matter. Some horses with marked clinical signs may show few lesions other than edema, while others with similar dysfunction may have malacia of major portions of the cerebral white matter.

Liver lesions include mottled, brown discoloration and swelling. Perirenal edema and congestion may be present (Marasas et al. 1976). Hemorrhagic and erosive lesions may be seen in the gastrointestinal tract, as well as hemorrhages in the urinary bladder, lungs, thyroid glands, and myocardium

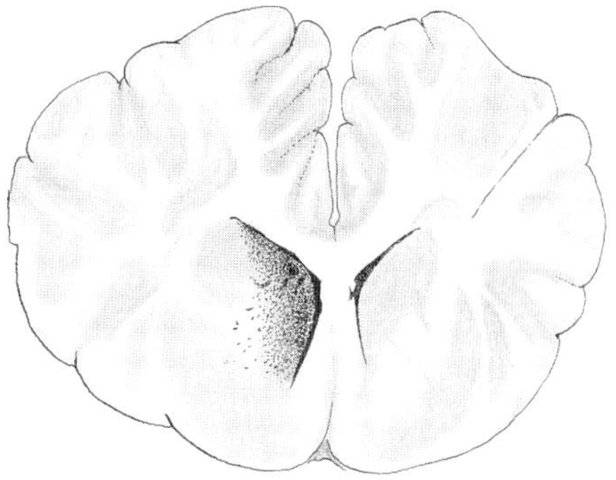

16.6. Diagram of hemorrhagic focus in thalamus in a case of *Fusarium* toxicity.

(Buckley and MacCallum 1901/02; Graham 1936; Badiali et al. 1968).

Microscopic lesions in the brain were described by Marasas et al. (1976) in three horses fed corn contaminated by *Fusarium moniliforme.* All had profound clinical signs. There was liquefactive necrosis of white matter, with complete loss in some areas. There was a gradual transition between liquefied, necrotic areas and more normal areas of the white matter. There was perivascular edema, hemorrhage, and perivascular cuffing in the white matter adjacent to malacic foci. Eosinophils and plasma cells predominated in perivascular cuffs. Foci of myelin degeneration and both glial cell proliferation and degeneration were seen in nonnecrotic areas of white matter. Numerous lipofuscin-laden macrophages probably explain the gross yellow discoloration. Lesions in gray matter included satellitosis and neuronophagia. Leptomeningeal edema was present in some cases.

Liver lesions consisted of vacuolation of hepatocytes, centrilobular necrosis and replacement fibrosis, lipofuscin deposition in macrophages and Kupffer cells, and infiltration with a mixture of inflammatory cells. Focal minimal bile ductule proliferation was seen by Marasas et al. (1976).

The pathogenesis of these lesions is unknown. Several authors suggested that vascular damage was an important factor (Wilson et al. 1973; Marasas et al. 1976, 1988; Brownie and Cullen 1987).

Nigropallidal encephalomalacia

Horses eating Russian knapweed, *Centaurea repens,* or yellow star thistle, *Centaurea solstitialis,* two weeds found in pasture and hay in the western United States, develop a disease characterized by inability to chew or swallow effectively. The disease was first described in California in the mid-1950s (Cordy 1954), and later in other western and northwestern states (Young et al. 1970a and b; Farrell et al. 1971). The plants are members of the genus *Centaurea* (Cordy 1954). Young et al. (1970a and b) described the clinical signs and lesions. Fowler (1965) reproduced the disease in feeding trials. Risk factors have been examined (Fowler 1965; Farrell et al. 1971; Young et al. 1970a and b).

Yellow star thistle and Russian knapweed are common weeds in poor or unimproved pastures. They are durable weeds tolerant of poor growing conditions, such as saline or alkaline soil and require little moisture. Farrell et al. (1971) noted that nigropallidal encephalomalacia was most prevalent in the late summer and early fall during moderately dry conditions. These weeds may be the only green plants in otherwise brown pastures; they do not thrive in competition with healthy pasture grasses.

Clinical signs appear within 1–3 months of eating yellow star thistle and within 1 month with Russian knapweed. Feeding studies by Young et al. (1970a and b) indicate that Russian knapweed is more toxic than yellow star thistle if one considers the cumulative dose. Horses consuming between 1.8 and 2.6 kg/100 kg body weight developed characteristic clinical signs.

The toxic principle has not been identified and is not destroyed by drying. Specific neurotoxins and antimetabolites have both been proposed as classes of potential candidates for the toxic principle. A review of feeding studies and natural cases indicates that younger horses (less than 4 years) may be more susceptible. Horses between 4 months and 10 years have been affected. Suckling foals have been reported, anecdotally, to develop the disease when mares have been unaffected and vice versa. There is considerable variation in individual sensitivity to intoxication.

The clinical picture is stereotypical. Animals are unable to swallow food or to drink water, often within 1–2 days of ingestion. Other signs include partial opening of the mouth, contracture of lip muscles, repetitive chewing movements, rhythmic movement of the tongue, muzzle hypertonia and "grinning," lowered head, depraved appetite (coprophagy), somnolence, widened stance, and mental dissociation. The animals are unable to eat and drink and may attempt to develop strategies to do so without success. They usually die of starvation or are killed in weak, emaciated condition (Fowler 1965; Young et al. 1970a and b; Farrell et al. 1971). Recovery is rare and with permanent neurological deficits (Young 1970b).

There are no consistent clinicopathological alterations. Gross lesions are common in horses with well-developed disease and are characteristic. Symmetrical areas of yellow-tan discoloration are present in the substantia nigra and globus pallidus, sometimes with gelatinous material filling malacic and necrotic cavities. Young et al. (1970b) reported that more frequent and severe lesions are seen with Russian knapweed than yellow star thistle. Horses ingesting knapweed may have gross lesions in the inferior colliculus, mesencephalic nucleus of the trigeminal nerve, and the dentate nucleus. Microscopically, there is neuronal degeneration and necrosis and minimal to moderate gliosis. Axons adjacent to liquefactive lesions may be swollen. Areas of liquefactive necrosis in the substantia nigra and globus pallidus may contain a delicate meshwork of connective tissue, vascular strands, and gitter cells.

Ryegrass staggers

Sheep, cattle, and horses fed heavily on ryegrass as a major component of the diet develop a syndrome known as ryegrass staggers. The disease is worldwide, but uncommon. Both naturally occurring and experimental cases have similar, but individually variable, clinical signs including hyperexcitability, ataxia, hypermetria and dysmetria, and tetany in extreme cases (Hunt et al. 1983; Munday et al. 1985). Ryegrass staggers can begin suddenly, within 3 weeks of exposure to a high percentage of ryegrass, *Lolium perenne,* in the diet.

Hunt et al. (1983) described a spectrum of clinical signs ranging from minimal to severe neurological dysfunction and tetany. The severity was roughly proportional to the percentage of ryegrass, as pellets, in the diet, ranging from 45% to 60% of the total. The signs did not appear to be progressive. No animals fed the diet for 3–8 weeks died. Biochemical and hematological values were normal. There was increased protein in the cerebrospinal fluid. The tremorigenic neurotoxin, *lolitrem B,* has been proposed as a cause of ryegrass staggers. At levels in excess of 2 ppm, this material causes neurological signs in sheep, and levels in excess of 5 ppm cause signs in ponies (Munday et al. 1985). Other tremorigenic toxins are produced during the growth of soil fungi like *Penicillium cyclopium,* for example, penitrem A, verrucologen, and fumitremorigen B. Their role, if any, in the syndrome is not known.

With removal of ryegrass from the diet, signs resolve without residual deficits, and no gross or microscopic lesions have been found (Hunt et al. 1983).

Neurolipofuscinosis

Two discrete types of lipofuscin-associated disease are seen in the equine nervous system. The first, **Gomen disease**, was described by LeGonidec et al. in 1981 as a degenerative disease of the cerebellum in horses on the northwest coast of the island of New Caledonia in the South Pacific. Islanders have recognized the disease since the 1930s in wild (bush)-pastured animals, but not in penned horses.

There are progressive cerebellar signs including incoordination and ataxia, especially of the rear legs, which persist for years. The disease is never seen in horses younger than 1 year, and the variable clinical course may be 1–5 years or longer. Death is usually by slow starvation of animals unable to walk and feed.

At postmortem, there were varying degrees of cerebellar atrophy, most obvious in the dorsal folia of the vermis (LeGonidec et al. 1981; Hartley et al. 1982). Light microscopic lesions in severe cases were complete or nearly complete loss of Purkinje cells and diminution of the granule cell layer. In remaining Purkinje cells, there was marked accumulation of variably stained red/brown/orange pigment. Pigmented macrophages were in the granule cell and molecular layers adjacent to the Purkinje cell layer. The staining characteristics of the pigment were those of lipofuscin. Hartley et al. (1982) saw vacuoles in the white matter of the lateral and ventral funiculi of the spinal cord and suggested these lesions were Wallerian degeneration of peripheral axon segments. Small amounts of pigment were found in kidney, spleen, and liver. By electron microscopy, granules or whorls of membrane-bound and free pigment were found in Purkinje cells and in scattered neurons.

Hartley et al. (1982) compared the deposition of pigment in these nerve cells to lesions in dogs with lipid storage diseases. They also compared the cerebellar lesions with those seen in Arab and Arab-cross horses and Gotland ponies. In those examples, there are genetic links to the deposition of pigments. Purkinje cell and neuronal pigmentation was uncommon in horses under 10–15 years old, a complicating factor since such pigmentation normally becomes more and more frequent with age. The cause is unknown, with the strong suspicion that a plant or mineral toxin may cause the disease in horses grazing in the bush and on unimproved pastures. LeGonidec et al. (1981) found a high concentration of heavy metals in the soil of New Caledonia and poor growing conditions on the northwest coast, which would favor the growth of some types of hardy weeds. Plants, such as *Swainsona, Astragalus, Oxytropis, Trachyandra,* and *Solanum kwebense,* produce neurovisceral lesions and storage disorders in other geographical locations and species, raising the likelihood that Gomen may have a similar etiology and pathogenesis. The relationship of stored pigment to cellular degeneration is not clear. Excessive pigment may cause cellular atrophy or be quite incidental to other processes compromising the Purkinje cells and neurons.

Horses and sheep foraging in areas of abundant *Trachyandra divaricata,* branched onion weed, develop a severe paretic syndrome with storage of lipofuscin in neurons of the brain, spinal and peripheral ganglia, and other tissues such as the kidney, liver, splenic macrophages, lung macrophages, and intestinal mucosa. Huxtable et al. (1987) described the clinical signs and lesions in horses and sheep in Western Australia. A similar syndrome in grazing livestock in South Africa was described by Newsholme et al. (1985) and Grant et al. (1985).

In the Huxtable et al. report, 12 horses showed progressive rear leg ataxia and paresis, hunched stance, muscle tremors, and recumbency. Brain, spinal cord, and liver of 7 animals had diffuse deposition of lipofuscin in neurons and Kupffer cells. Axonal swelling and axonal dystrophy were present in segments of the spinal cord. In 5 cases, in which brain and cord samples were not procured, there was lipofuscin in autonomic ganglia of the gut (Huxtable et al. 1987).

Although a neurotoxin from *Trachyandra* was not specifically identified, Huxtable et al. (1987) felt that dietary exposure to the plant for 4–6 weeks was sufficient to cause lipofuscin storage and neuroaxonal degeneration. In feeding experiments with karakul sheep and one horse Grant et al. (1985) were able to produce the disease within 6 weeks to 4 months.

As already noted lipofuscin pigmentation of neural and other tissues is a common aging phenomenon; its pathological significance in any given animal or disease must be carefully weighed. When seen in large amounts in young, diseased animals, the process may well represent or be described as accelerated aging.

Swainsona neuropathy

A few cases of neuropathy caused by ingestion of *Swainsona galegifolia* (Darling pea), have been reported in horses in New South Wales, Australia. The disease is a significant problem in weanling cattle that develop a preference for the plant (Hartley and Gibson 1971).

On a farm with numerous calves affected by *Swainsona* toxicity ("peastruck"), an 8-month-old foal was ataxic with hypermetric, stiff gait, circling, and hyperesthesia. After several days, the foal was killed.

No gross lesions were described, and microscopically the corpus callosum was said to be atrophic and the hippocampus hypoplastic. Numerous vacuolated neurons were seen at various levels of the brain including the cerebral cortex, rostral brain stem, midbrain, pons, cerebellum, and spinal cord. Eosinophilic spheroids were present in gray matter throughout the central nervous system. Parenchymal cells in the choroid, pancreas, liver, and kidney were vacuolated. There were vacuolated and lipofuscin-containing macrophages in several lymph nodes. Similar morphological changes were found in calves with similar clinical signs.

Contrast medium neuropathy

Hubbell et al. (1988) described metrizimide-associated complications of cervical spine myelography. A retrospective study of 131 equine neurological cases that received metrizimide while under general anesthesia was reported. Sixty-seven percent of the horses had significant neurological deficits (ataxia, gait deficits, and paresis) prior to myelography. After myelography, the neurological condition of 8.3% worsened. Complications included depression, progressive ataxia, recumbency, fever, and/or seizures. One horse developed meningitis, a known complication of metrizimide myelography (Nyland et al. 1980). Unfortunately, gross and histopathological examinations were not done.

Congenital and developmental defects

Cerebellar abiotrophy

Abiotrophy is the state of a congenital error being expressed during postnatal life. Cerebellar abiotrophy is loss of organization and substance of the cerebellum. This is to be differentiated from congenital cerebellar hypoplasia and atrophy as might be caused by in utero viral infection, for example. The distinction is not always clear.

Cerebellar hypoplasia and abiotrophy have been recognized for nearly 40 years. The cause is unknown, but the frequency in highly inbred horses and ponies (Arabian and part-Arabian horses, Oldenburg horses, and Gotland ponies) has suggested a combination of heritable and environmental factors [Hippen (1949), cited by Björck et al. (1973); Sponseller (1967); Björck et al. (1973); Palmer et al. (1973); and Baird and MacKenzie (1974)].

Hippen (1949), Koch and Fischer (1950, 1952a,b), and Weyers (1954) described rapid onset of ataxia in Oldenburg foals 4- to 8-weeks old. They died within 1–2 weeks of onset. There were few macroscopic lesions. Hippen described degeneration of ganglion cells in the hippocampus. Weyers reported cerebellar lesions. No conclusions were reached about the etiology. The condition is obviously hereditary, but the possible role of viral infections, dietary and environmental factors, or specific toxins was not excluded.

A high incidence of cerebellar hypoplasia and ataxia in Gotland (Sweden) ponies was described by Björck et al. (1973). Foals with cerebellar hypoplasia had movement deficits shortly after birth. In about 30% neurological dysfunction did not appear until 4–8 weeks of age, as with the Oldenburg foals. There was fore leg hypermetria, unstable and base-wide stance, and stiff movements. Ataxia was seen as the disease progressed, and some ponies were unable to rise. Affected foals would fall backward when the neck was dorsiflexed. There were no alterations in hematology, serum analyses, or cerebrospinal fluid composition.

Meticulous autopsy examinations were done. By measuring and weighing various structures in the brain, they found that the ratio of cerebellar to cerebral weights was decreased in ponies with ataxia. The surface of the cerebellum was more convoluted than in normal ponies. Cerebellar width and height were less in ataxic ponies than in normals.

Histologically, the cerebellum had a narrow molecular layer, irregular architecture of the granular cell layer, and loss of Purkinje cells with gliosis.

Pedigrees strongly suggested inheritance by an autosomal recessive factor with incomplete penetrance, but possible complicating effects of extragenetic factors could not be excluded. Cerebellar hypoplasia/abiotrophy has been extensively described in Arab and part-Arab horses (Dungworth and Fowler 1966; Sponseller 1967; Palmer et al. 1973; Baird and MacKenzie 1974). Sponseller found the incidence in some groups of Arabs with high consanguinity to be approximately 80%. Foals show clinical signs typically by 4 months of age. Palmer et al. described 6 foals, of which 4 had clinical signs at birth. They saw fine head tremor, ataxia and hypermetria, and defective blink reflex. There were no gross lesions. Microscopically there was thinning and disorganization of the granular cell layer, attenuation of cerebellar folia, and decreased numbers of Purkinje cells. The severity of lesions was not related to age of onset or to the duration of disease. As with the Gotland ponies and Oldenburg horses, the defect in Arabs and part-Arabs is thought to be hereditary. Indeed, virtually all North American cases, at least, could be traced to a single Arabian stallion of great popularity.

Vascular malformations

A small number of vascular malformations have been reported as causes of neurological dysfunction. Ataxia of the rear legs caused by venous malformations or benign vascular neoplasms (angioma) in or on the spinal cord have been reported in a Thoroughbred (Palmer and Hickman

1960) and a Welsh Cob pony (Gilmour and Fraser 1977). Progressive rear leg ataxia was seen in both cases. Hemorrhage, compression, and malacia at the site of the malformation were seen in both cases.

Miller et al. (1985) reported ataxia, dysmetria, and weakness in two 4-year-old Thoroughbreds with vascular anomalies and hematomas in the fourth ventricle. Hemorrhage and compression-induced malacia and herniation of the cerebellum were seen in both animals. The cause of the hematomas was felt to be small vessel degeneration, a microvascular parallel of basilar aneurysm as described by Mayhew et al. (1978). In our opinion these vascular lesions probably are part of the general spectrum of **angiomatosis**, congenital vascular malformation/ tumors of many tissues in horses (see Chapter 15, "Integument.")

A single case of hepatic encephalopathy related to a portal vein anomaly was reported by Beech et al. (1977). The 11-month-old filly had episodes of ataxia, stupor, and dissociation for months. Elevated blood ammonia levels were consistently related to the neurological dysfunction. A vascular anomaly in the portal vein was found at autopsy. Histologically, there was minimal hepatic fatty change and fibrosis. Diffuse astrocytosis was seen in sections of the brain, and the predominating cell type was Alzheimer type II cells, *leberglia.*

Neonatal asphyxia

Millar (1959) reported Thoroughbred foals developing "characteristic" neurological deficits within hours of birth. Palmer et al. (1973, 1984) and Palmer and Rossdale (1975, 1976) gave the syndrome the unfortunate name *neonatal maladjustment syndrome*. According to Rossdale (1972a,b) it occurs in about 0.75% of full-term births. The birth may have been normal, or there may be history and evidence of dystocia and fetal distress (such as fractured ribs or contusion of the heart).

Within 1–24 hours after birth, the foals become incoordinated, with jerking head movements, inability to stand, convulsions, stupor, and opisthotonos (Palmer and Rossdale 1975, 1976). Hyperexcitability, inspiratory stridor, peculiar vocalization (barking), apparent blindness, and inability to nurse have been reported.

Palmer and Rossdale (1975, 1976) examined the brains of some of these foals. There was diffuse or localized frank hemorrhage or edema in approximately 50% of the cases with lesions. Microscopically there was hemorrhage and/or laminar, ischemic necrosis of neurons of the cerebral cortex, diencephalon, cerebellum, midbrain, or combinations thereof. Animals surviving for several days had reactive gliosis. In less severely affected foals, hemorrhage and cortical edema predominated, with patchy perivascular hemorrhage in the subcortical white matter, subcortical gray matter, cerebellar molecular layer and mesencephalon/brainstem.

While many choose to see this as a self-standing syndrome, the clinical signs and lesions are those of neonatal asphyxia. The histology of the lungs of many of the first reported cases was reviewed years after the initial reports. In most cases there was clear-cut bacterial pneumonia, which had evidently been overlooked on the earlier examinations. It is our firm conviction that "neonatal maladjustment syndrome" is jargon and better called neonatal asphyxia, often but not necessarily caused by neonatal bacterial pneumonia. Neonatal septicemia, for example, of whatever cause, often shows these clinical signs, and the asphyxial lesions described by Palmer and Rossdale are routinely present in the brain.

The Palmer and Rossdale (1976, 1977) reports are of value in confirming that ischemic lesions in the brain of the asphyxiated foal are comparable to such lesions in the brain of any other animal or human that has been asphyxiated by whatever means.

Optic nerve hypoplasia

Gelatt et al. (1969) described a case of congenital blindness associated with bilateral optic nerve hypoplasia and retinal defects. The retina was attenuated with a paucity of ganglion cells, pseudorosette formation, and abnormal vasculature. Glastonbury and Day (1985) described optic nerve degeneration and demyelination in an adult pony.

Dummkoller

This condition is peculiar to the European, specifically German, literature (Hutyra and Marek 1926; Nieberle and Cohrs 1961). Despite many years of thought and writing, it remains an enigma and may remain so since no more cases seem to occur. Hutyra and Marek (1927) suggested the disease was one of heavy horses only, which might explain its virtual disappearance.

The acute signs are those of stupefaction alternating with excitement, together with ataxia. The acute phase often goes over into an inexorable, fatal chronic course characterized by profound dullness, sleepiness, reluctance to move, and apparent blindness. There may be periods of apparent improvement. The signs are not unfamiliar, suggesting the profound damage of fatal encephalitides and mycotoxic encephalomalacia.

The characteristic gross change is protrusion of the medial parts of the occipital lobes backward toward the cerebellum—the *druckwulst* of Dexler.

The corpora quadrigemina are flattened and shifted caudally. The cerebellum is pushed backward to the foramen magnum, its rostral face flattened, and its caudal part formed into cone shape. The cerebral gyri are flattened and the cerebral cortex appears pale. Changes in the aqueductal system are mentioned but are unconvincing. The third and lateral ventricles may be slightly enlarged, with very slight increase of cerebrospinal fluid pressure. The septum pellucidum is stretched, thinned, and often perforated.

These changes were ascribed to chronic edema of the brain: hydrocephalus interna acquisita. The histological changes were widening of pericapillary lymph spaces, small, slitlike fluid-filled spaces in white and gray matter, and hydropic swelling of the ganglion cells and nerve fibers. Neuronophagia, microglia proliferation, subpial and subependymal gliosis, and noninflammatory pial fibrosis were also described. There can be an apparent increase of capillary density because of shrinkage of tissue.

Modern neuropathology casts doubt on these histological changes as indicative of edema and, so, internal hydrocephalus. The gross lesions and their depiction in the old literature are, however, convincing for, at least, pathological change. The cause was not and is not known and with the absence of present-day cases, may never be known. It is considered here in case those still concerned with large horses may have the opportunity for further study.

Central nervous system—spinal cord

Equine degenerative myeloencephalopathy and neuroaxonal dystrophy

Equine degenerative myeloencephalopathy is a common cause of spinal cord disease. Dill et al. (1989a,b) reported that 45% of horses with spinal cord disease at the New York State Veterinary College had equine degenerative myeloencephalopathy. Thirty-one percent of the cases were equine protozoal myelitis, and 24% were cervical stenotic myelopathy. These figures may represent the bias of a clinic with an interest in neurological cases. In Kentucky equine degenerative myeloencephalopathy is much less frequent than cervical stenotic myelopathy and equine protozoal myelitis.

Montali et al. (1974b) published the first description of progressive degenerative myeloencephalopathy in equids (zebra) characterized by rear and fore leg incoordination and ataxia in young animals. Montali called the condition in Grant's zebra (*Equus burchelli*) **spinal ataxia** and differentiated it from cervical stenotic myelopathy. In a herd of closely related animals by a single stallion and two unrelated mares, approximately 50% of the progeny developed progressive ataxia before 2 years of age. Neither the stallion nor mares had neurological dysfunction. There was no sex predisposition in the affected foals.

Subtle deficits in rear leg coordination were detected in the young zebras at 4–6 months of age. More severe ataxia and rear leg weakness developed by 1–2 years of age. Ataxia was less common and severe in the fore legs. Severely affected animals stumbled and fell repeatedly.

Neurological, clinical, radiographic, and gross and microscopic examinations of 3 of 8 affected zebras were done. None of the zebras had cervical vertebral stenosis. There were no gross lesions in the spinal cord. Microscopically, there was bilaterally symmetrical demyelination of dorsolateral and ventromedial funiculi, degeneration of axons, and minimal to moderate astrocytic gliosis in the demyelinated areas. When the entire cord was sectioned, lesions were present in all segments. Degenerated tracts ended in nuclei in the medulla. The etiology was not found, but there was an obvious genetic component.

Within 3 years Mayhew et al. (1977) described an identical condition in 5 mixed breed horses and 1 zebra unrelated to Montali's zebras. The animals had ataxic gait and histories of progressive fore and rear leg incoordination and weakness. The gait abnormalities were usually seen by 12 months of age. Neurological signs included rear leg ataxia (5/5 horses), hypertonic foot placement (4/5), abnormally wide stance (4/5), and toe scuffing (2/5). Radiographs were normal. There were no gross lesions in the brains or spinal cords. As in Montali's cases, there were diffuse demyelinating lesions of the dorsolateral and ventromedial funiculi, astrocytic gliosis, dystrophic axonopathy, and axonal spheroids. Lesions were present in all levels of the cord, severity varying among cord segments. Axonal degeneration was present in the gracilis and medial cuneate nuclei, lateral cerebellum, medulla, and red nucleus. Mayhew et al. speculated on the potential role of diet (vitamin E deficiency, copper deficiency), plant poisons, inherited metabolic disorders, and cervical vertebral stenosis in the development of the lesions. No cause was found.

Liu et al. (1983) described progressive degenerative myeloencephalopathy in 6 related Mongolian wild horses. Clinical signs of incoordination and ataxia were seen by 3 months of age in 3 of 6 horses. Clinical signs and neurological deficits were as described by Montali et al. (1974) and Mayhew et al. (1977). There were no gross lesions. Microscopic lesions of degenerative myelopathy, as described above, were found in the spinal cord and brain. Lipofuscin was present in some neurons, perhaps age related. Liu found that plasma α-tocopherol levels in 5 horses were significantly lower than in 7 normal, unaffected wild horses on the same premises and husbandry. The feed contained sufficient levels of vitamin E and selenium for normal horse maintenance.

Genetic studies of related Appaloosa horses with degenerative myelopathy showed familial clustering in some lines (Blythe et al. 1991a,b).

The roles of heritable versus environmental factors in the pathogenesis of this disease are not understood. Low serum vitamin E and selenium levels have sometimes been found, without consistent correlations with incidence, severity, or progression of lesions.

Mayhew et al. (1987) found low serum vitamin E levels in Standardbred and Paso Fino crossbred horses with and without equine degenerative myelopathy on two farms. Many of the affected foals were by the same stallion. A vitamin E supplementation plan seemed to reduce the incidence of equine degenerative myelopathy from 40% to 10%.

Dill et al. (1989a) measured serum vitamin E levels. They used serum glutathione peroxidase levels as an indirect measure of selenium availability. No statistically significant differences were found, effectively challenging a role for vitamin E and selenium in the pathogenesis of equine degenerative myelopathy. In an epidemiological survey Dill et al. found that exposure to topical pyrethroid insecticides or wood preservatives and stabling in dirt lots appeared to increase the risk. A foal from a mare with a previously affected foal also was at greater risk. Access to fresh pasture appeared to decrease the risk (Dill et al. 1990). In another study Dill et al. (1989b) discounted copper deficiency as a factor.

Blythe et al. (1991) measured plasma α-tocopherol during the first year of life in 9 foals sired by an affected stallion and 5 foals by a normal stallion. Eight of 9 foals sired by the affected stallion had gait abnormalities by 1 year, while the 5 normal foals remained normal. Plasma α-tocopherol levels were significantly low in equine degenerative myelopathy foals between 6 weeks and 10 months of age. No significant differences were found in oral vitamin E absorption tests between affected and nonaffected horses and foals. The investigators felt that vitamin E deficiency at some period in the first year of life was a factor in the development of equine degenerative myelopathy in genetically predisposed foals. Vitamin E deficiency, and possibly selenium deficiency, during critical metabolic periods in growing foals, may relate to defective myelinogenesis.

Neuroaxonal dystrophy of the accessory cuneate nucleus

Beech (1984) and Beech and Haskins (1987) described neuroaxonal dystrophy of the accessory cuneate nucleus in Morgan horses. The animals developed rear leg incoordination by 2 years of age, many showing gait deficits by 1 year of age. Demyelinating cord lesions were not prominent. Degeneration of neurons with spheroids and vacuoles were the most striking lesions. There was poor correlation between microscopic lesions and clinical signs. Genetic analysis was not productive.

Cervical stenotic myelopathy

Long known, and still known, as **wobbler**, this primarily affects tall, long-necked horses such as the Thoroughbred and large draft breeds. Smaller individuals and small breeds such as ponies and Arabians are not affected. There is a 3:1 preponderance, in Thoroughbreds, of males to females. The clinical signs have been described and are primarily those of damage to the white matter of the cervical spinal cord with ascending and descending degeneration in proprioceptive tracts (Rooney 1971). All the evidence available suggests that this is an hereditary condition expressed in the tall horse, long-neck conformation.

The focal malacic lesion of the ventral and lateral white matter is caused by functional stenosis with compression of the cervical portion of the spinal cord (Fig. 16.7). The functional stenosis is the result of osteochondrosis of the vertebral articular facets. The development of osteochondrosis, the spinal cord lesions, and an hypothesis relating the two, have been given in detail elsewhere (see Chapter 9, "Vertebral Column") and summarized here (Rooney 1969).

The osteochondrosis of the vertebral articular facets is bilateral, most often at C3-4, or unilateral, more often at C4 through C7. Examination of the cervical vertebrae of over 500 fetuses and foals, mainly Thoroughbred, has conclusively shown that the osteochondrosis develops 2–4 months after birth. Routine examination of foals at postmortem within this period will reveal the stages in the development of marginal osteochondrosis of the articular facets. The case has been made for long neck and asynchronous musculoskeletal development as factors leading to the final common pathological pathway—overloading of the growing articular cartilage, necrosis, and repair with overgrowth of the articular cartilage (Rooney 1969).

Osteochondrosis is present in 10%–20% of Thoroughbreds at postmortem with or without clinical signs of ataxia. Since about 0.5% of the autopsy population is wobbler, it is apparent that

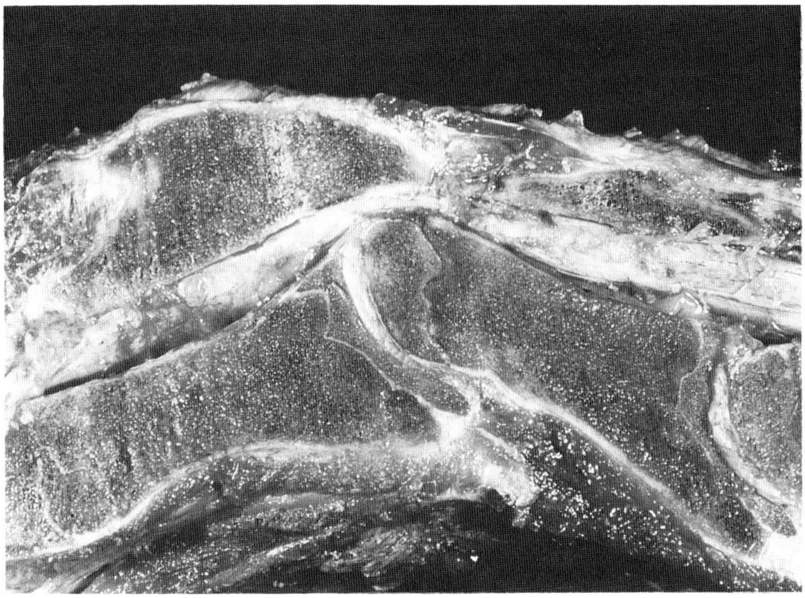

16.7. A focal malacic lesion is present in the ventral and lateral white matter of the spinal cord in a horse with functional stenosis.

many Thoroughbreds have lesions, but do not experience damage to the spinal cord. Unlike osteochondrosis of the appendicular joints where secondary arthrosis is not common, arthrosis does occur in the cervical articulations. It is important, if difficult, to differentiate osteochondrosis and secondary arthrosis. Arthrosis in the absence of osteochondrosis is seen, particularly in older horses, as the intervertebral disks undergo aging degeneration, and this is rarely, if ever, associated with neurological disease.

The primary site of malacic damage will be at the level of most severe osteochondrotic overgrowth of articular facets. If the cervical spinal cord is removed *en toto,* the lesion can be found on gross examination and related to the changes in the facets. It is to be emphasized that the examination should include disarticulation of the cervical vertebrae with preservation of the cord as described in the chapter on postmortem method (see Chapter 19). The dura is removed and the cord laid out carefully, ventral surface up. The moistened finger is lightly drawn along the ventral surface. At the site of the lesion a distinct loss of substance will be appreciated, emphasized if the eyes are closed. A normal depression is felt at each intervertebral space where the ventral nerve roots leave the spinal cord. The depression at the malacic site is greater and easily detected. The malacic lesion extends over about 0.5–2.5 cm, fading off indistinctly at each end.

Histologically, at the primary site, the lateral and ventral white matter, with the exception of a thin rim around the gray matter, has extensive Wallerian degeneration with loss of myelin sheaths and swelling and disappearance of axons. There is an astroglial response. Gitter cells are common in the young lesion. There is a characteristic hyalinizing, perivascular fibrosis only in the malacic area. Ascending degeneration in the dorsal white matter often can be traced for only a few segments. Descending degeneration, in the lateral and ventral white matter, can be traced to the lumbar enlargement.

The pathogenesis entails pressure on the spinal cord because of excessive ventroflexion allowed by the overgrown articular facets. The pressure compromises the venous drainage from the spinal cord, leading to anoxia and the malacic changes. The hypothesis accounts for the damage caused by compression, the surviving rim of white matter next to the gray matter, the absence of damage to the gray matter, and the perivascular fibrosis (venous stasis) (Rooney 1969).

Cerebrospinal nematodiasis

The extensive literature has been reviewed by Innes et al. (1952) and Innes and Saunders (1962). The commonest cause is the microfilaria of *Setaria digitata* with wandering larvae of *Strongylus vulgaris* a distant second. The clinical signs are variable and, often, seem to change from day to day, apparently depending upon sequential lesions caused by the wandering helminth larvae.

Setariosis

Setariosis has been reported most frequently from the Far East in the summer months. The microfilaria produced by the adult worm in the peritoneal cavity of cattle and water buffalo, the major hosts, invade the bloodstream and are transmitted by mosquitoes to the next host. The horse is an abnormal, dead-end host for *S. digitata.* The migration pathway for the microfilaria to the central nervous system is not known, but is probably by the vascular system, although peripheral nerves have been suggested.

Setariosis is an uncommon cause of ataxia in horses in North America and Europe. This despite the fact that adult setaria are not uncommon in the peritoneal cavity of both cattle and horses. About 5% of adult horses coming to postmortem have at least one, and rarely more than one, adult *Setaria equina* in the peritoneal cavity. Somewhat higher frequencies are apparently seen in the southern part of the United States. This species is adapted to the horse and does not seem to be associated with neurological disease. In the few cases of setariosis reported in the United States, only sections of the larvae were found microscopically, and the species could not be determined (Frauenfelder et al. 1980). One can but speculate that the species was not the natural *S. equina* of the horse and may have been *S. digitata.*

Strongylus

S. vulgaris infestation of the central nervous system is uncommon and apparently the result of the far wandering of a single larva in a given case. It has been seen in Europe and North America [Albrecht (1872) and Heill (1874), both cited by Cadeac (1899c); Pohlenz et al. (1965); Stavrou (1967); Swanstrom et al. (1969); and Little (1972)]. The lesions are essentially identical with both setaria and strongyles. There may be no gross lesions in the central nervous system. Occasionally, malacic or hemorrhagic foci are seen. Characteristically, but by no means commonly, these foci are found scattered along the spinal cord as if produced by the wandering of a single larva.

Histologically, the characteristic lesion(s) is a malacic focus in the gray and/or white matter. The softened necrotic center is surrounded by diffuse astrogliosis, variable numbers of gitter cells, and axonal swelling and degeneration. There may be hemorrhage. There is perivascular cuffing with mononuclear cells and eosinophils. Similar infiltrations occur in the meninges adjacent to or continuous with the malacic foci. It seems that the larva(ae) wanders along the surface of the spinal cord, moving in and out of the spinal cord at random.

The malacic foci may appear, after fixation and sectioning, as microcavities. These microcavities are probably created when soft, necrotic tissue drops out of sections during histological processing, and may, therefore, be artifactual. Worm larvae are not readily found on routine examination. Indeed, even multiple sections may not reveal larvae, particularly if the case is of some duration. In some instances (Innes and Saunders 1962) larvae have been recovered by filtering the fixation fluid.

While lesions may be found in any part of the central nervous system, the spinal cord and thalamus seem to be preferred (Innes and Saunders). We have seen several cases with a fulminating clinical history with involvement only of the thalamus by a massive hemorrhagic lesion with large numbers of eosinophils. Worm larvae in those cases were tentatively identified in sections as *S. vulgaris.*

Micronema

Micronema, *Halicephalobus deletrix,* is a saprophytic nematode found in North America, Europe, and Africa. Typically it causes nasal and maxillary sinus granulomas, with kidneys and nervous system sometimes affected (Rubin and Woodard 1974; Jordan et al. 1975; Alstad and Berg 1979; Pohlenz et al. 1981; Darien et al. 1988).

The clinical signs, as in the other parasitic diseases of the nervous system, are variable, depending upon the localization and migration of the agents. Examination of the cerebrospinal fluid sometimes shows xanthochromia, increased cellularity, and increased protein.

Gross patchy discoloration may be seen. Histologically, there is malacia, perivascular cuffing, and granulomatous inflammation. Larvae, ova, and adults have been seen in sections in some cases. Larvae can be present without an attendant inflammatory reaction.

Other parasites

Olander (1967) reported *Hypoderma lineatum* infestation of the brain of a 2-year-old Quarter horse. Ataxia and eventual paralysis were related to malacic and hemorrhagic tracks in the cerebral peduncles and pons. The larva was found in the left cerebral peduncle.

Mayhew et al. (1982) reported a case in a Paint horse caused by migration of *Draschia (Habronema) megastoma* through the corona radiata, temporal cortex, globus pallidus, hippocampus, midbrain, and so forth. A gravid female *Draschia* was found in a malacic area in the pons. A variety of clinical signs had been seen as the larva migrated through the brain. In both of these cases the microscopic findings were essentially identical to those seen with *S. vulgaris* and other parasites.

Motor neuron disease

Cummings et al. (1991) reported a motor neuron disease with clinical and pathological similarities to the progressive muscular atrophy form of amyotrophic lateral sclerosis of humans. The cause is not known and no viruses or genetic linkages have been found. The disease has been seen in a number of states and Canada, with new geographical recognition still occurring. Virtually all ages appear to be affected, though no cases have as yet been seen in foals. There are some clinical similarities with the syndrome of shivering in horses (Mitchell 1930b), but the pathology of that condition has never been described. Sonnenberg (1912) described eight cases in horses that he considered to be amyotrophic lateral sclerosis.

There were progressive signs of generalized weakness, muscle fasciculation, muscle atrophy, and weight loss in young and old horses of several breeds in the eastern part of the United States. Ataxia was not a feature. While some cases were progressive, the disease apparently arrested in some individuals with at least partial remission of clinical signs. Sonnenberg's description of the clinical signs in his eight cases was similar, though he sometimes found rigidity and stiffness, particularly of the rear legs.

There were no gross lesions of the nervous system. There was degeneration and loss of motor neurons in the spinal cord and brain stem, with subsequent axonal degeneration of the ventral roots of cranial and spinal nerves (Fig. 16.8). Denervation atrophy of muscle followed. The affected neurons were swollen and chromatolytic with neurofilamentous accumulations. Later stages of degeneration were characterized by shrinkage of the cells, neuronophagia, dropping out, and gliosis. Eosinophilic inclusions may be found in the cytoplasm of affected neurons. No inflammatory changes were present. As well as gross muscular atrophy, there was histological evidence of denervation atrophy, partial reinnervation, and muscle regenerative hypertrophy, particularly in the deeper muscles of the thigh.

Sonnenberg did not report pathological findings, but his clinical findings at least suggest the disease described by Cummings et al. Bergmann et al. (1990) reported a neurological disease in 24 of 240 mares between 1984 and 1988. While they concluded the cause was EHV-1, the etiological evidence was not conclusive. The clinical signs essentially duplicated those of Sonnenberg, while both clinical and pathological findings were suggestive of those described by Cummings et al. All three

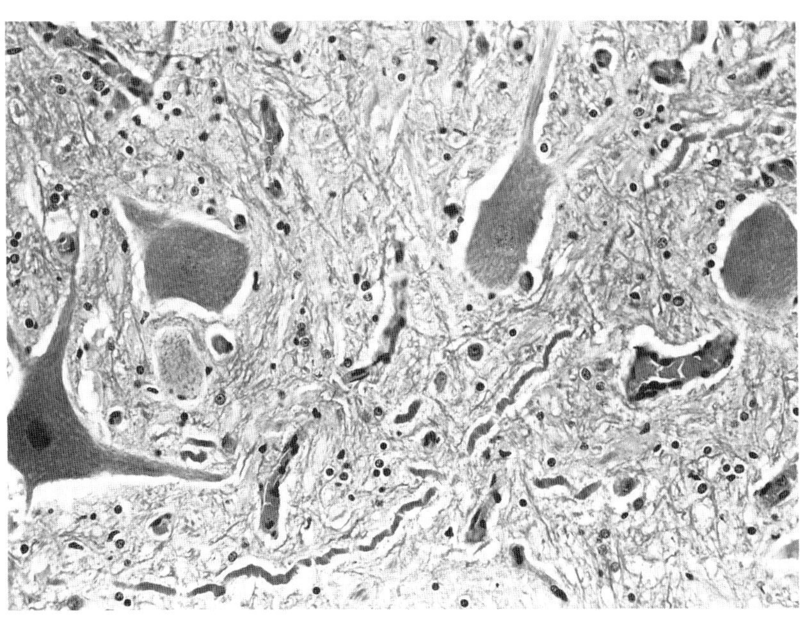

16.8. Degeneration and loss of motor neurons in the spinal cord and brainstem from a horse with motor neuron disease.

reports may be of the same condition, with the etiology unknown and a role for the herpes virus possible, but not established.

Bulbar paralysis

A chronic bulbar paralysis syndrome was described in Belgium, France, and Germany. The clinical signs indicated damage to nerves involved in eating with atrophy of the tongue, paralysis of the tongue and pharynx, and difficulty in drinking. The syndrome may persist for months, 5–6 or more, and was said to be associated with the feeding of turnips, or perhaps rape (weiss ruben) (Hutyra and Marek 1920, 1926). Cohrs (1961) mentions a bulbar paralysis that may be the same entity, noting that Thomassen (no reference) found degeneration and decreased numbers of ganglion cells in nuclei of the medulla oblongata of affected horses. The cause was not identified. The clinical signs are suggestive of botulism, but the chronic course is inconsistent. Cadeac (1899a) provided a clinical description of the same syndrome, noting that it was restricted to one area of Belgium and first described by Laridon and Demeester (1851). He mentioned, but did not describe, alterations of the nuclei of the relevant cranial nerves, and offered no etiology.

Ataxia, other

Infection of the middle and/or inner ear causes marked ataxia of all four legs. As discussed with the vertebral column (see Chapter 9), painful lesions of the cervical region, of whatever origin, are accompanied by ataxia of all four legs, which disappears when the pain disappears.

Peripheral nervous system

Renaut (1881) described pale staining, foamy cell masses of varying sizes in the nerve roots and peripheral nerves of donkeys and horses, stating that they occurred in most large nerves of solipeds and were found in rudimentary form in humans and dog (Fig. 16.9). The function of these **Renaut bodies** is not known, but Renaut suggested that they served a shock-absorbing, protective function in the peripheral nerves of large animals. He described the bodies as gelatinous, incompressible, and elastic in nature. Study with modern techniques would be interesting.

Renaut bodies are often mistaken for evidence of neural degeneration or other more esoteric neural disease [Innes and Saunders (1962); and numerous Japanese authors]. It is not at all clear, though possible, that Renaut bodies increase in size when degeneration of nerves occurs (Duncan et al. 1987).

Cranial nerves

Specific injury or damage to individual cranial nerves is uncommon. Loss of function of a number of these nerves may be seen with several encephalitides. Fractures and abscesses can, in a given case, involve virtually any of the cranial nerves.

Facial paralysis

One discreet entity is paralysis of the facial nerve. This is usually traumatic, the result of pres-

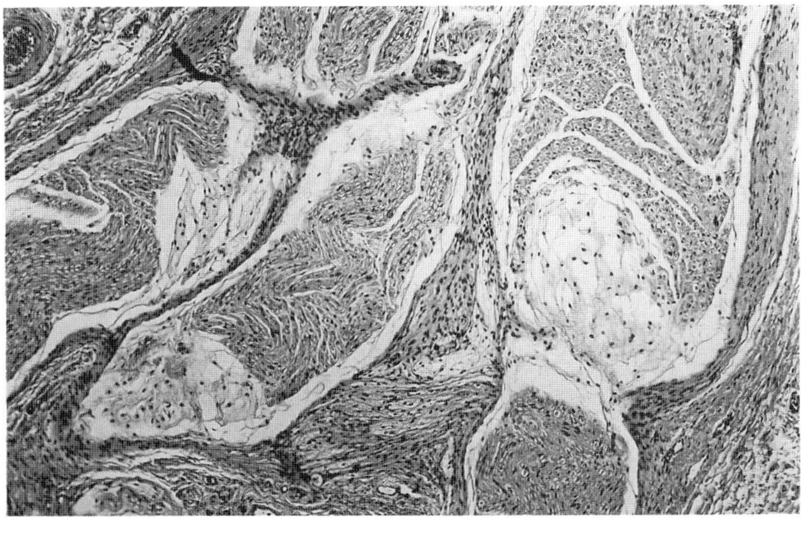

16.9. Renaut bodies appear as pale staining, foamy cell masses in the nerve roots and peripheral nerves of donkeys and horses.

sure on the nerve in its subcutaneous course. Strangles abscesses of the parotid lymph nodes may involve the facial nerve. The glossopharyngeal and vagus nerves may be damaged by extension of guttural pouch mycosis.

Facial and vestibular nerve disease

There are occasional reports of trauma to the skull and otitis media/interna as causes of neurological signs. In 7 cases of cranial trauma, horses had incoordination, head tilt, and nystagmus (Firth 1977). Three of the 7 also had facial nerve paralysis on one or both sides, with exposure keratitis secondary to lid paralysis, lip droop, and altered feeding behavior. Power et al. (1983) reported that 6 horses with earlier respiratory infections had similar signs. In most of these cases tympanosclerosis and osseous proliferative changes were seen in the petrous or temporal bones or in the ear proper.

Since the facial and vestibulocochlear nerves follow similar paths through the temporal bone, pathological processes—trauma, neoplasia, polyneuritis, meningitis, other inflammatory/infectious conditions, and, uncommonly, guttural pouch infection—affecting one nerve, usually affect both (Power et al. 1983).

Laryngeal hemiplegia

This disease was described at least as early as 1754 by Solleysel, but is probably of even greater antiquity [review by Fleming (1882)]. Field (1837) and later Dadd (1854), both cited by Smith (1976), produced the condition by transecting the right recurrent nerve and noted the unilateral muscular atrophy. The clinical, surgical, and pathological features of this condition are well known. Cahill and Goulden (1986, 1987, 1989) have provided recent research and review. In brief, afflicted horses make roaring or whistling sounds at work as a result of paralysis of, in the greatest majority of cases, the muscles supplied by the left recurrent nerve. While all the muscles undergo atrophy, it is the loss of function of the cricoarytenoideus dorsalis that allows the focal fold into the airway and, so, abnormal respiratory, particularly inspiratory, sounds (Fig. 16.10).

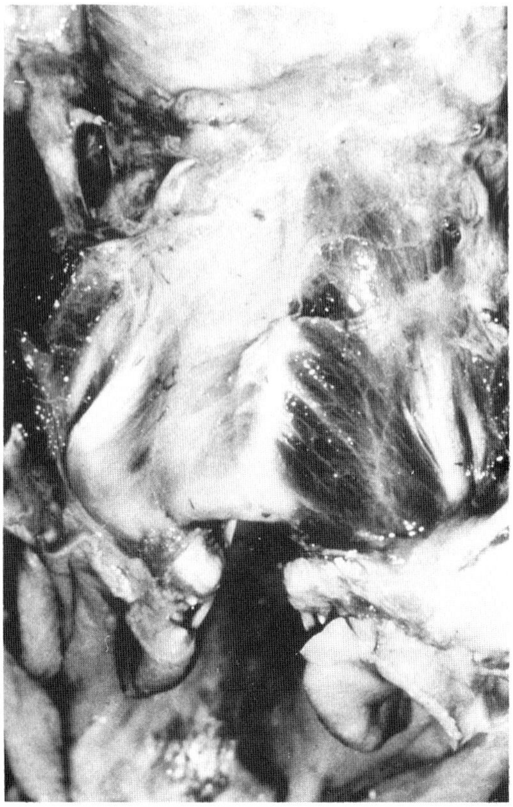

16.10. Atrophy and pale discoloration of the cricoarytenoideus dorsalis in laryngeal hemiplegia.

The histological picture in the left recurrent nerve has been described by several authors (Cole 1946; Duncan et al. 1974; Cahill and Goulden (1987, 1989). There is loss, particularly of larger myelinated fibers, and evidence of ongoing degeneration and regeneration of nerve fibers. This has been characterized as dying-back or distal axonopathy. While that provides a name for the pathological process, it does not provide etiology or pathogenesis. One suggestion is that the pathogenesis is related to direct local axonal damage, a view not incompatible with an ischemic process such as that proposed for suprascapular and radial nerve damage (Rooney 1969) and for the recurrent nerve by Rooney (1970).

The basic facts are that large horses—large in the sense of draft breeds or tall in the sense of Thoroughbreds—are predisposed and that the major damage is of the left recurrent nerve. Navez cited by Hutyra and Marek (1920) reported the incidence of laryngeal atrophy in horses in Belgium: heavy horses 50.8%, full and half bloods 12.5%, and horses of small races 6.5%.

Whether the size—the conformation—is directly related to the neural damage, as suggested by Rooney and Delaney, or is simply a phenotypical indicator of a more occult genetic defect, is moot (Robertson 1910). While there is evidence suggesting a genetic basis, an hereditary mechanism has not been established. That suggests, but does not establish, that the nerve damage may not be primarily genetic but mediated by some aspect of body size. Schaper (1939) was convinced of the hereditary nature of the condition. He reported one Cold blood stallion that produced 32 roarers among 41 offspring, 26 males and 15 females.

It has been suggested that there is a polyneuropathy in roarers, rather than damage only to recurrent nerves, based on changes in the peroneal nerve of the rear leg of two roarers (Cahill and Goulden). The illustrations given, the small number of animals, and the lack of controls are less than convincing evidence for such a polyneuropathy. The same authors have also reported axonal spheroids in the lateral cuneate nucleus of roarers and nonroarers. In sufficient numbers such axonal changes might be significant, but they do occur as aging changes in otherwise normal horses.

As an historical note it may be pointed out that W L Williams, Cornell University, developed the first successful surgery for roarer and taught the technique to English and Continental veterinarians. Subsequently, Sir Frederick Hobday allowed the method to take his name. The tale is clearly written in the *Veterinary Record* and the *American Veterinary Review* of the time.

Neurogenic atrophy, m. gluteus medius

Unilateral atrophy of the gluteus medius is uncommon although long known [Hell in *Bayer-Fröhner* (1900)]. We have seen only a few cases in Thoroughbred horses. There is no significant gait defect, at least at the walk and trot (Fig. 16.11). Pathological study of three cases showed degenerative lesions of the cranial gluteal nerve without apparent etiology. The nerve is grossly normal. Histologically, there was "torpedolike" degeneration of many axons and an apparent loss of axons in the peripheral portions of the nerve.

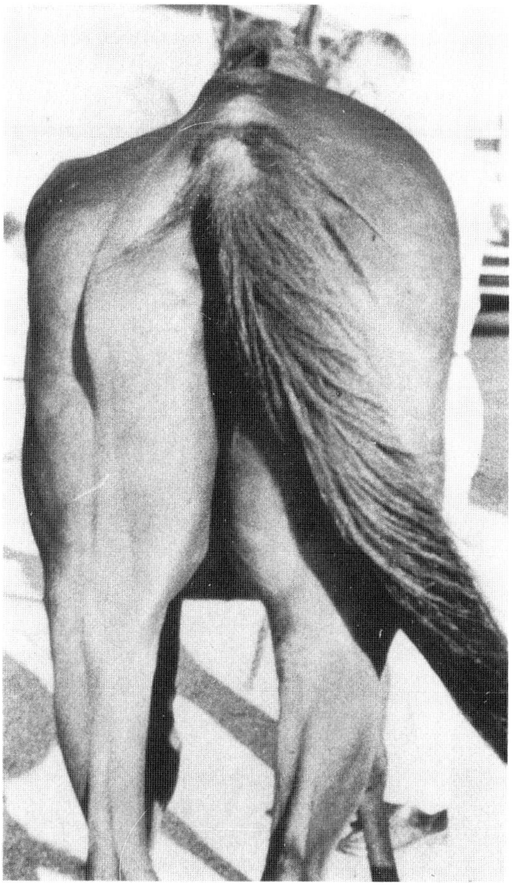

16.11. Unilateral atrophy of the gluteal musculature following degeneration of the cranial gluteal nerve.

Stringhalt

This has been known for many years (Banham 1882). It was referred to as *springhalt* in Shakespeare's Henry VIII. It still awaits complete etiological and pathogenetic definition. Characteristically, it is a disease of the older horse, usually unilateral, though it may be or become bilateral. Recovery is rare if it ever occurs.

It was suggested, based on a single case (Rooney 1969), that a fracture callus compressing the obturator nerve could produce stringhalt. Additional cases of stringhalt with compression of the obturator nerve by callus and melanomas have been seen. Hutyra and Marek (1920) summarized the clinical findings in several cases of obturator nerve damage in horses, describing, in effect, stringhalt. In three cases fracture and callus formation compromised the obturator nerve. Inglis, commenting on a paper by Mitchell (1930a), mentioned that a William Williams had recorded two cases of stringhalt associated with exostosis of the ileum. It is appropriate to repeat the observation of Vaughn cited in Palmer (1965) that pinching the intact obturator nerve of cattle caused the leg to be held quivering in midair. He also saw this in postparturient cattle. The evidence, then, supports the conclusion that some cases of stringhalt involving one rear leg are the result of compression of the obturator nerve.

Some cases, specifically bilateral stringhalt, have not had lesions involving the obturator nerve. Two of these cases have been instructive. The first was a young horse with sudden onset of bilateral stringhalt, which lasted for approximately 24 hours before additional, profound neurological disturbances led to destruction. The animal had a massive area of hemorrhagic destruction in the hypothalamus and thalamus associated with *S. vulgaris* larval migration.

The second case was an old mare with a history of unilateral, then bilateral, stringhalt for an unknown time. At postmortem the only gross lesion was marked, bilateral, yellowish-brown discoloration of the thalamus (Fig. 16.12). Histologically, there was severe siderofibrosis of the arterial vessels. Siderofibrosis is not uncommon in the brain of aging horses (Kikuchi 1928; Saunders 1953). This was the only case of **siderofibrosis** we have seen that was obvious grossly and, histologically, the most severe case seen.

While one cannot establish pathogenesis on two cases, the involvement of the thalamus, a sensory relay and coordination center, is suggestive taken together with the sensory mechanism proposed for stringhalt with compression of the obturator nerve (Rooney 1969). As an historical curiosity there was an Italian report in 1901 of "curing" stringhalt with acupuncture.

Australian stringhalt

This affects horses of any age and recovery is usual. There is an incompletely defined relationship to specific pasturage (Pemberton and Caple 1980). The condition has been seen in Australia, New Zealand, and California and tentatively associated with *Hypochaeris radicata* (catsear, flatweed, dandelion). Experimental induction of the condition has been unsuccessful (Cahill et al. 1985). Pemberton and Caple suggested that a mycotoxin might be involved since cases tended to appear when climatic conditions favored such diseases in other species. The pathological findings have been equivocal as might be expected, with recovery the rule. The results of the report by Slocombe et al. (1992) must be considered in the same light as the discussion of putative polyneuropathy with recurrent laryngeal nerve damage.

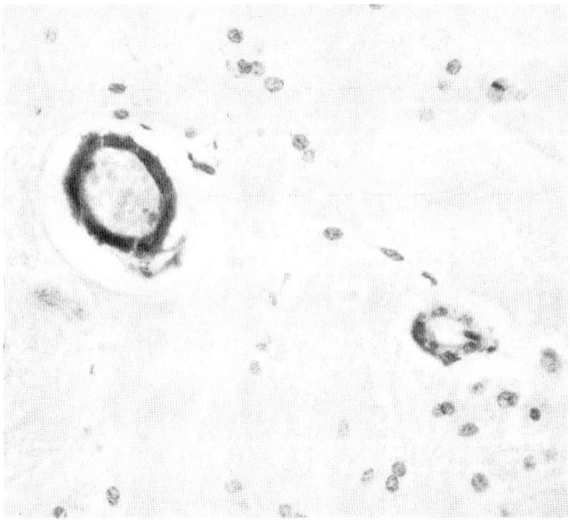

16.12. Siderofibrosis of arterial wall in the thalamus of a horse with stringhalt.

Shivering

This condition may be related to stringhalt, but there are no adequate pathological reports. There are spasmodic contractions and fasciculations of muscles, particularly those of the rear legs in the early stages (thus, the resemblance to stringhalt), which may progress to involve the trunk, foreleg, and facial muscles. The spasms are not usually apparent at rest, appearing when the animal moves (Mitchell 1930b; Innes and Saunders 1962).

This was reported from England in the early 1900s but has not, apparently, been recognized elsewhere. It was said to be more common in draft breeds. In an extensive clinical experience with neurological disease in Thoroughbreds and Standardbreds in North America, no unequivocal cases have been seen. There are at least some similarities between the clinical signs of shivering and the recently described motor neuron disease of the horse (Cummings et al. 1991).

Neuritis of the cauda equina

This condition was well known in Europe for many years before being reported in North America (Innes and Saunders 1962). An early report is that of Raymond (1899/90). It was long thought to affect only the nerves of the cauda equina, but Sjolte (1944) showed that cranial nerves were also affected with or without clinical signs. Wright et al. (1987) have shown that the autonomic nervous system can be affected as well. It would be as well to rename the disease *polyneuritis equi*.

The predominant clinical signs are of damage to the nerves of the cauda equina: paresis and paralysis of the perineum, bladder, rectum, anus, and tail. Cranial nerve signs of muscular twitching and hyperesthesia have been largely restricted to acute cases and the trigeminal nerve, but severe ataxia has been seen with involvement of the vestibular nerves. Incomplete or partial paralysis may be seen in an occasional case, with only part of the cauda equina affected.

Few acute cases have been seen at postmortem. There is marked hemorrhagic inflammation of the nerves of the cauda equina *outside* the dura mater, with deposition of fibrin and matting together of the nerves (Fig. 16.13). Microscopically, there is hemorrhagic inflammation, with striking medial necrosis of the small muscular arteries and slight to moderate infiltration of mononuclear cells.

Chronic cases are more often seen at postmortem (Fig. 16.14). The cauda equina is the site of nodular, granulomatous inflammation with mononuclear cells, eosinophils, giant cells, and fibrosis (Stunzi and Pohlenz 1974). In long-standing cases fibrosis predominates, with numerous mononuclear and lymphoid cells interspersed throughout the fibrous tissue.

Gross lesions have not been seen in the cranial nerves. The histological picture for acute and chronic cases is as described for the cauda equina. The cause of this polyneuritis is not known. An association with outbreaks of respiratory disease and strangles has been noted (Cohrs 1961). Only sporadic cases have been seen in North America, with no such associations reported.

Damaged tail ataxia

Several horses have been seen that had suffered severe damage to the tail by having it caught and virtually torn away from the body. These animals had marked, persistent ataxia of the rear legs. Anecdote also indicates that too-short, deliberate docking of the tail causes ataxia of the rear legs. There are no pathological reports, and the personally observed cases were still ataxic when lost to follow-up. The pathogenesis is unknown. Rarely, there may be a fracture of the caudal part of the sacrum and/or coccygeal vertebrae with either ataxia, as described, or, more often, clinical signs similar to those of neuritis of the cauda equina.

Sorghum neuritis

This has been reported, primarily from the southwestern part of the United States and northwestern Australia, in horses grazing hybrid sorghum or Sudangrass pasture (Adams et al. 1969). Crossbred combinations of sorghum (*Sorghum vulgare*) and Sudangrass (*S. vulgare* var. *sudanese*) were usually involved. Johnsongrass and an Australian hybrid, Sudax, have also been incriminated. Drying the materials as hay apparently destroyed the toxic principle(s). The clinical picture is dominated by complete or partial paralysis of the bladder and ataxia of the rear legs. Lesions of the bladder and kidneys, secondary to neurological damage, are described with those organs.

Equivocal lesions have been reported in the white matter of the lumbar spinal cord (Adams et al. 1969). Morgan et al. (1990) described vacuoles around swollen axons in the brain, as well as gliosis in relation to degenerate axons in the cauda equina. In a personally observed case, there was neuritis of a number of nerves of the lumbosacral plexus, characterized by degeneration of nerve fibers and infiltration of mononuclear and lymphoid cells. No lesions were present in the spinal cord. These lesions, though only one case, are more consistent with paralysis of the urinary bladder than putative lesions of the brain or spinal cord. No further studies have been reported on the pathology or etiology since the condition has virtually disappeared with changes in forage practice.

Suprascapular nerve paralysis

Damage to this nerve causes atrophy of the supraspinatus and, usually, infraspinatus muscles: so-called **sweeny**. The nerve usually does not show gross changes. Histologically, there is a spectrum of degenerative changes of fibers in the peripheral part of the nerve. As seems to be true of most peripheral nerve damage in the horse, the larger myelinated fibers are the earliest and most profoundly damaged. Finer, unmyelinated fibers are less susceptible. These changes gradually disappear as one progresses proximally. In general, the nerve is normal before the turn around the cranial border of the scapula, abnormal after the turn, with an indistinct borderline between the two (Rooney 1969).

Dollar (1920) provided the pathogenesis: "unloaded limb thrusts it back. The cause of paralysis of the suprascapular nerve is violent backward

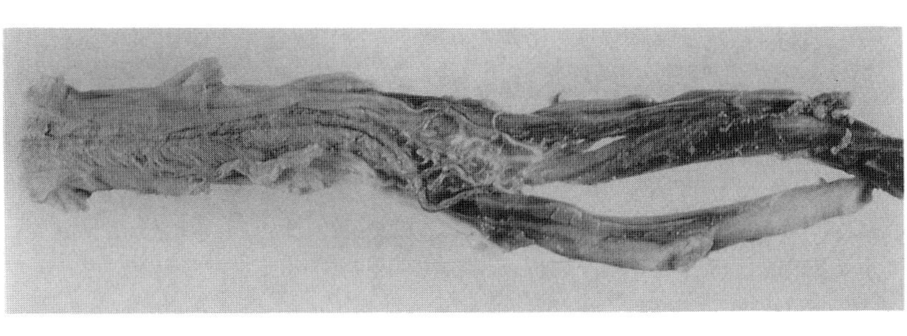

16.13. Hemorrhagic inflammation of the nerves of the cauda equina may be seen outside of the dura mater.

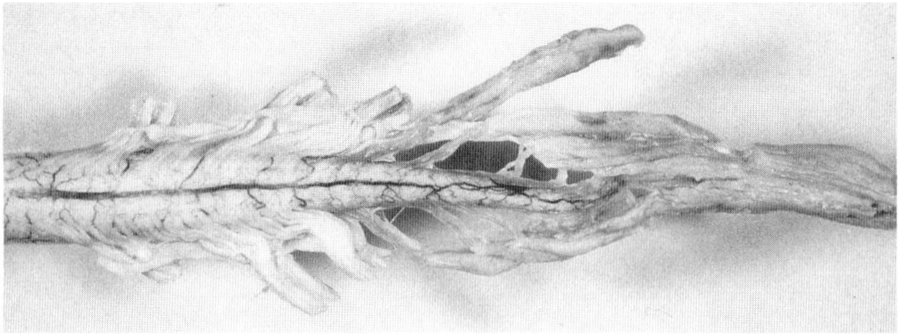

16.14. Chronic granulomatous inflammation may be seen in long-standing cases of cauda equina neuritis.

movement of the shoulder or leg whereby the nerve is overstretched." The limb does not have to be unloaded. Backward slipping of the hoof on insecure footing, for example during spring plowing or on ice, provides the necessary tension in the nerve. Whether the damage to the nerve is the result of direct tensile damage to nerve fibers per se, or, indirectly, through damage to the vascular supply, is not known.

The difference between the backward slipping of the leg causing suprascapular nerve damage and the slipping that causes damage to the biceps brachii tendon has been described (Rooney 1969). In effect, the whole leg slips backward to cause sweeny, while the slipping that damages the biceps is from the elbow distad.

Duncan et al. (1987) reported so-called entrapment of the suprascapular nerve. They indicated that subclinical damage to the suprascapular nerve was found in 7 of 9 normal horses. The damage consisted of remyelinating fibers, onion bulb formation, scattered demyelination, and Renaut body formation. Since Renaut bodies (Renaut 1881) are normal in equine peripheral nerves, their presence may be discounted. The significance of the other changes, in the absence of changes in the muscles and clinical evidence of disease, requires clarification. It appears that whenever equine peripheral nerves are intensely scrutinized, such changes are seen (see also laryngeal hemiplegia and Australian stringhalt, above). Whether they represent true pathological change or are unrecognized normal phenomena requires investigation.

Radial paralysis

This is an occasional cause of severe lameness in horses. In accordance with the motor innervation of the radial nerve, radial paralysis may take one of three clinical forms: loss of function of the extensor muscles of the elbow, the extensor muscles of the carpus and digit, or both. Preuss and Eggers (1951) sectioned the radial nerve at different levels and described the resulting paralyses. Section of the nerve to the ulnaris lateralis alone caused no detectable clinical signs, while more proximal sections did cause clinical signs.

Dollar (1920), cited by Rooney (1969) summarized the clinical findings:

> The foot is advanced forward to a normal position but due to loss of function of the triceps brachii, the horse is unable to extend the elbow joint and straighten the leg to a normal position for supporting weight. As well, the triceps brachii will be flaccid and, eventually, atrophy. If the animal moves slowly and on a smooth surface, nothing in particular may be noticed. In case an obstacle is encountered the foot is not sufficiently extended so it strikes against an obstacle. This lameness is characterized by stumbling, particularly on an uneven surface and later by a sliding motion of the foot when the limb is extended. In complete paralysis of the radial nerve the animal stands with the shoulder and elbow extended and the knee and phalanges flexed. The toe of the foot is the only portion which rests on the ground.

The onset of radial paralysis is almost always sudden. While the prognosis is favorable in many cases, it is not possible to predict the outcome. There are usually no gross lesions of the nerve or structures in its vicinity. Rarely there may be fractured ribs or purulent inflammation of the axillary lymph nodes (strangles) with obvious involvement of the nerve.

Histologically, there are marked degenerative changes: swelling and bulbous formations of axons, degeneration of myelin sheaths, loss of axons, and eventual fibrosis. The Renaut bodies may appear larger than normal. Changes are most marked in that portion of the nerve distal to the shoulder joint, gradually being replaced by normal-appearing neural tissue proximally. These changes appear to be the result of overstretching the radial nerve. Whether such tension directly and physically damages the nerve fibers or acts by damaging the vasa nervorum is moot. While the latter may be a more attractive hypothesis, it is an hypothesis here, as well as with suprascapular and recurrent nerve neuropathy.

While many causes have been suggested, most cases appear to follow overstretching of the nerve as the fore leg slides forward on the surface. Falling on the outstretched leg can contribute by compressing the nerve between the shoulder joint and the ribs. The mechanism has been described by Rooney (1963).

Mixed nerve paralysis

The clinical signs are more profound and widespread than with radial paralysis, suggesting involvement of the median and ulnar as well as the radial nerve. This is seen after prolonged recumbency and is usually transient. The condition was mimicked by compressing the brachial artery experimentally, causing transient mixed paralysis (Marolt et al. 1962).

Other nerves

Paralyses related to the femoral, peroneal, and tibial nerves are described in clinical texts. We have seen no cases at postmortem and have found no pathological descriptions in the literature.

Autonomic nervous system

Periodically, the autonomic nervous system comes to the attention of pathologists. Köhler (1968) has discussed the histology of this system. Despite the efforts of Mollman (1932), Obel (1955), Mahaffey (1959), and others to assign putative lesions of the autonomic nervous system to various diseases, there is no real evidence that recognizable morphological changes of significance occur in any disease of the horse. One need only examine autonomic ganglia, histologically, at random in normal and abnormal horses to realize that the changes that have been reported are within a widely variable range of normal. That any of these changes, at any given time, may be pathological is possible, but there is no way to ascertain that in view of the normal variation of the nerve cells of this system.

The autonomic nervous system is not unimportant in the pathogenesis of disease. At present, however, there is singular ignorance about all but the more obvious aspects of autonomic function and virtually no pathological information. An avenue of assistance may be the elegant concept of the distal terminal network or **neurosyncytium** of the autonomic system of European anatomists (Meyling 1955; Walter 1958; Krölling and Grau 1960). This neurosyncytium seems to be recognized but briefly in American texts as the **sympathetic ground plexus**. Some elegant considerations of the physiological role of the autonomic nervous system are those of Goldstein (1939).

Grass sickness

This still enigmatic disease of the horse was apparently first seen in about 1907 in Scotland (Pool 1928), and subsequently reported in northern England, northern Europe, and Switzerland. Reports from North America, Australia, and so forth, are doubtful. A detailed summary of the clinical and pathological findings has been given by Holman et al. (1944). A recent review is that of Pinsent (1989). While it is far from certain where this disease should be classified, we place it here, arbitrarily, for now.

The onset is almost always in the spring months, with subacute and chronic cases persisting into later months of the year. Pool noted that 60% of the cases appeared in June. It appears that only horses on grass are at risk, though there have been sporadic cases not known to be associated with fresh grass. In one outbreak among coal mine pit ponies hay appeared to be the causative agent (Forsyth 1941). The disease has acute, subacute, and chronic forms. The acute form is characterized by depression, difficulty in swallowing, ileus, rapid heart rate, sweating, tremor of limb muscles, and regurgitation of ingesta. There may be intermittent salivation. Death may occur in 12–72 hours. Animals surviving the acute form are depressed, lose condition, and are dehydrated, apparently being designated subacute or chronic depending upon survival time.

In the acute disease there may be erosions of the esophageal mucosa (regurgitation) and edema of the wall. The stomach is grossly distended with a watery, mucoid, or pea soup consistency, and tan, alkaline content. The small intestine has copious watery content. The cecum and colon, by contrast, are impacted with dry, hard ingesta, these findings characteristic of ileus.

In prolonged cases there is little fluid in the stomach. The small intestine contains foul-smelling greenish or amber colored tenacious fluid. The large intestine and cecum may be empty or contain a thick soupy fluid. The changes are nonspecific, related to lack of food intake.

No specific histopathological changes have been reported. There have been claims of lesions in autonomic ganglia (Obel 1955; Gilmour 1973), but the changes reported are normal features of the cytologically labile autonomic nerve cells. Bishop et al. (1984) examined a variety of regulatory peptides in the gut of subacute and chronic cases and reported decreases, particularly in the ileum. Since secondary damage and depressed function of peripheral nerves is not uncommon in a variety of disease processes in many tissues, the significance of these findings is obscure. No further studies were found.

Despite many years of investigation, the cause and pathogenesis are unknown. The disease was characterized by Grieg (1928) as a sympathicotonia. While that astute hypothesis remains unrefuted, it may be suggested that an autonomic, specifically parasympathetic, blocking agent of some type might be involved. Many of the clinical signs and the pathological evidence of ileus are, at least, reminiscent of botulism. The suggestion, however, that *Clostridium perfringens,* type A, was involved has not been confirmed in the endemic areas.

Neoplasia

Central

Neoplastic lesions in the nervous systems of equids are uncommon. The **cholesteatoma** in the choroid plexus of aged horses is not a neoplasm, but an aggregation of cholesterol and macrophages. There are only sporadic case reports of neoplasms of the nervous system. Surveys have found few central nervous system neoplasms (Runnells et al. 1942; Luginbuhl 1963; Cotchin 1977; Pascoe and Summers 1981).

Cholesteatoma

Cholesteatoma is a nonneoplastic aggregation of cholesterol-laden macrophages in the choroid plexus of the lateral ventricles of aged horses (Moulton 1978). Lesions may be solitary or bilaterally symmetrical. Most are small, clinically benign, and discovered incidentally at autopsy. Some may reach sufficient size to cause space-occupying clinical signs. Early lesions are soft and waxy gray/yellow nodules, composed of foamy macrophages infiltrating the stroma of the choroid. Larger masses may be brown, firm, discrete, and granular. They are primarily composed of cholesterol aggregates in a matrix of connective tissue and granulomatous inflammation. Nothing is known of the pathogenesis.

Meningeal carcinomatosis

Wright and Giles (1986) reported a case of meningeal carcinomatosis in a 12-year-old Hackney pony gelding with progressive ataxia beginning with the rear legs and progressing to quadriplegia over a 6-week period. There was atrophy of the croup muscles. Gross and microscopic lesions were confined to the central nervous system. The meninges of the medulla and cervical spinal cord were thickened and corrugated. The same changes were present in the thoracic cord, together with hemorrhage. A poorly differentiated and infiltrative carcinoma in the meninges was characterized by neoplastic cells infiltrating the perivascular spaces of the dorsal and dorsolateral white matter and causing axonal degeneration. The neoplasm was thought to be metastatic, but no primary lesion was found.

Meningocerebral hemangiomatosis

McEntee et al. (1987) reported a case of meningocerebral hemangiomatosis, considered to be a form of vascular dysplasia and abnormal Schwann cell proliferation in humans: Sturge-Weber-Dimitri disease.

A 3-year-old Quarter horse had recurrent generalized seizures for 2 months. No abnormalities were seen on physical and neurological examination, or on hematological or biochemical tests. Seizures were poorly controlled with barbiturates over a 2- to 3-week period before the animal was killed. Gross and microscopic lesions were found in the brain, spinal cord, and trigeminal nerve and ganglion. The left cerebral cortex leptomeninges were thickened and discolored and the left cortical hemisphere minimally enlarged, with the left pyriform lobe soft and easily deformed. Histologically, there was proliferation of meningoepithelial cells and redundant vasculature in the leptomeninges and choroid. Various layers of the cortex were disorganized with reactive gliosis and loss of neurons. Abnormally large and abundant Schwann cell proliferations around left trigeminal nerve fascicles were seen with light and electron microscopy.

Pineoblastoma

Before the report of Holshuh and Howard (1982) tumors of the pineal body in horses had not been identified. This neoplasm is rare in all species (Fankhauser et al. 1974).

An adult Quarter horse stallion had progressive weakness and incoordination for a 4- to 5-month period. The animal was killed. Grossly, a 4 × 4 × 6-cm, friable, gray-yellow, gelatinous mass enveloped the brainstem from the cerebellum to the pituitary fossa. Portions of the mass invaded the third ventricle and the periventricular parenchyma. Histologically, there were sheets of round-oval, pseudopalisading cells, with areas of hemorrhage and focal necrosis. The histological diagnosis was a neoplasm of neuroectodermal origin. The location of the mass suggested pineoblastoma.

Melanoma

Uveal tract melanomas have been reported in horses (Moulton 1978), but are uncommon. Melanomas in other sites, such as the lumbar spine, do cause neurological dysfunction.

Milne (1986) reported a malignant melanoma of the thoracic inlet that produced Horner's syndrome in an 8-year-old gray pony. The pony had enophthalmos, prolapse of the membrana nictatans, ptosis, and miosis, as well as Horner's syndrome. Grossly, there was a 10 × 6-cm melanoma in the thoracic inlet compressing the cervical sympathetic ganglion and surrounding soft tissues.

Schott et al. (1990) reported two cases of melanoma causing spinal cord compression. A 13-year-old gray Arabian gelding had a history of collapse of the rear legs when exercising. There were numerous cutaneous melanomas in the perineal region with metastasis to regional lymph nodes. A tumor mass at C7-T1 compressed the spinal cord. There was focal demyelination, vacuolation, and reactive gliosis in the spinal cord adjacent to the tumor, which had not penetrated the dura mater. A 22-year-old Arabian mare was found down with weakness and pulse deficit in the left rear leg. Masses were palpated in the pelvic canal, and an area of cord compression at C7-T1 was seen on a myelogram. Melanotic cells were found in cerebrospinal fluid. At postmortem there were multiple melanomas throughout the body, one at C7-T1.

We have seen a number of cases of metastasis of perineal melanoma to the lumbar vertebral body and/or spine, with either compression of the spinal cord or pathological fracture. Less often the perinal melanoma metastasizes to the lumbar meninges, producing cord compression signs.

We have seen one typical **craniopharyngioma** in a young horse that compressed and invaded the hypothalamus.

Peripheral

Melanomas

Apart from nonneoplastic amputation neuromas, tumors in the peripheral nervous system of horses are rare. Melanomas may involve peripheral nerves as already noted. Two cases of presumed **neurofibromatosis** have been seen, with nodular involvement of the thoracic and cervical autonomic nerve trunks and clinical signs of Horner's syndrome. Histologically, in both cases, the tumors were composed of featureless round cells, and the diagnosis was based on topography of the gross lesions.

Neurofibromas of the skin are occasionally diagnosed, but it is difficult, with routine examination, to separate such putative cases from the more common sarcoid.

CHAPTER 17

Shock

Primary shock

There are many causes of primary or acute shock in the horse: electrical (for example, lightning), massive hemorrhage in the postparturient mare, anesthesia, and so on. Characteristic lesions include a greatly enlarged, congested, dark red spleen, variable alveolar emphysema of the lungs, and petechiae and splash hemorrhages throughout the respiratory tract and in the mucosa of the large intestine. This complex, in the timely postmortem examination, indicates shock and search for its cause. Unfortunately, these lesions are quickly obscured by autolytic changes.

The pathogenesis of shock is no more understood in horses than in other species. It is the rapid and complete breakdown or failure of the cardiovascular system. Pathology, accustomed to the study of specific lesions, seems unable to cope intellectually with the sudden and complete change of state from life to death. The "cause of death" always begs the question: drawing a sharp line between life and death is not possible, and the actual transition from the one state to the other cannot be defined. The question is perhaps metaphysical rather than physical, with one approach, perhaps, the sophisticated realm of nonlinear dynamics (Thompson and Stewart 1986).

Exhaustion shock

Exhaustion shock is a sporadic, acute, highly fatal disease. The morbidity is low, mortality high, and there is no evidence of infection or contagion.

The condition is characterized from the onset by signs of shock and either severe diarrhea or severe gaseous distension of the gastrointestinal tract. The diarrhea typically is brief, but massive and watery. There is hemoconcentration and leucopenia with marked dehydration. The animal is depressed, with muddy, discolored mucous membranes; thready, rapid pulse; patchy sweating; dyspnea; and cramping abdominal pain. Death is usually between 3 and 24 hours. Horses of all ages, with the exception of young foals, are affected.

The carcass is dehydrated, the subcutaneous vessels distended, and there are petechiae and ecchymoses in the subcutaneous tissues of the head and neck. The serosal surfaces of the cecum and ascending colon are a dull, reddish-blue, cyanotic color. There is a large quantity of fluid, often foamy, odoriferous ingesta. The mucosa of the cecum and colon varies from hyperemic with fine petechiation in a dull, plum-red background to greenish-black and intensely hemorrhagic (Fig. 17.1). The submucosa is characteristically and markedly edematous and often tinged with blood. Free blood is rare in the gut contents.

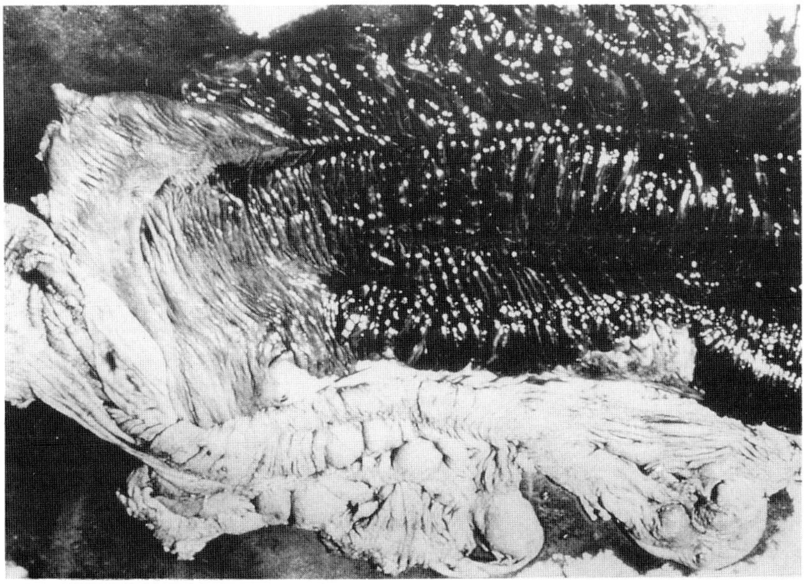

17.1. Intense congestion and edema of the mucosa and submucosa of the ventral colon. Exhaustion shock.

Usually, lesions are most severe in the cecum and ventral segments of the colon, fading to the normal gray-white between the pelvic flexure and the transverse colon (Fig. 17.1). The cecum, only, or the ascending colon, only, may be involved. The descending colon and ileum may show variable, patchy hyperemia. The cecocolic lymph nodes are hyperemic and edematous.

The liver is normal or somewhat enlarged and bluish with dark, fluid blood running out on section. The spleen is normal or slightly enlarged, with a dark red color and loss of follicular markings. There is patchy or massive hemorrhage in the adrenal cortices.

The lungs are hyperemic and emphysematous, with petechiae on the parietal and visceral pleura. The heart may be normal or somewhat dilated with epicardial and endocardial petechiae and ecchymoses. The cut surface may be grayish and cooked in appearance. Varying degrees of petechiation, hyperemia, and ecchymoses are present throughout the respiratory passages.

Histological examination reveals no specific lesions, simply confirming the gross observations, with the exceptions below. While first described under this name in 1965, this condition had been known long before. It was not uncommon in horses off-loaded after long shipment by rail, and was seen in draft animals worked heavily for long periods. Salmonella infection was often suspected but never incriminated. Based on observation and limited experiments, it appears that this condition is, in fact, **exhaustion or secondary shock**, in the sense of Selye (1950). Either a single factor, such as exhausting work or transport, or multiple factors can combine to overwhelm the system and cause shock.

Numerous cases were seen during the A equi-2 influenza outbreak in North America in the 1960s. It became apparent that those animals treated primarily by stall rest recovered uneventfully, while there were numerous cases of exhaustion shock among animals treated aggressively with oxytetracycline. There have been a number of subsequent reports of death in animals under duress and treated with oxytetracycline (Cook 1973; Baker and Leyland 1973; Owen 1975). Oxytetracycline per se can elicit untoward reactions in apparently normal horses, but, in this instance, it combined with an already existing process to cause exhaustion shock. We have seen a number of cases in which evidence for two or more stressing factors was present. These have included multifocal interstitial myocarditis, histological evidence of viral rhinitis, and purulent cholangiohepatitis.

While repeated intravenous infusion of *E. coli* endotoxin caused mild signs of shock, there is no evidence that endotoxin, per se, is the specific cause of any specific disease entity in horses, including exhaustion shock. In summary, the clinical and pathological entity described is, in fact, nonspecific failure of the cardiovascular system—shock—as the result of an overwhelming assault by a single agent or combination of agents. It is not a specific disease entity.

Intestinal clostridiosis

Weirup (1977, 1983) described a disease in horses 2–6 years of age associated with large numbers of *Clostridium perfringens* type A in the intestinal tract. The clinical and pathological features were similar to those of exhaustion shock. A major differential feature, perhaps, was the presence of catarrhal typhlitis and colitis, rather than the hemorrhage and edema characteristic of exhaustion shock.

While Weirup's studies were exacting, the variable presence of *Cl. perfringens* in the equine intestinal tract and the rapid proliferation of the organisms when ileus is present make the existence of intestinal clostridiosis as a specific disease entity uncertain. That clostridia, and other organisms, may proliferate in the distressed intestinal tract and contribute to pathological and clinical disease is certainly possible. The role of *Cl. perfringens* as a primary etiological agent, however, remains uncertain, particularly in view of the absence of experimental production of disease and the fulfilling of Koch's postulates.

Sudden death with equivocal or uncertain postmortem findings is not uncommon in young, working horses (see Chapter 20, "Forensics"). Weirup's observations need to be taken into account in such cases, but the mere presence of clostridial organisms is not sufficient for a diagnosis. This point may be reiterated for the all too common diagnosis of "enterotoxemia" in cases of sudden death of young horses. There is no sound evidence for such an entity in horses, the putative lesions and "characteristic" odor being entirely autolytic.

Anaphylactic shock

This has not been adequately defined in the horse. Two horses were experimentally sensitized with chicken egg albumin and challenged. They died with marked submucosal edema, mucosal congestion, and hemorrhage throughout the gastrointestinal tract. The changes were present from stomach to anus and not limited to the large intestine, as with exhaustion shock. Changes in the lungs were not prominent and were limited to alveolar emphysema. Such a lesion complex has not been seen in spontaneous deaths.

Horses do die shortly after injection with various materials, such as vitamin preparations or antibiotics, either after a single or repeated injections. At postmortem the only lesions are those of acute shock. It is moot if, in any given case, these are allergic or untoward drug reactions (see Chapter 20, "Forensics"). The lesions seen with experimental egg albumin sensitivity have not been seen in spontaneous deaths.

Eyre and Lewis (1973) induced anaphylactic shock in ponies with bovine serum albumin. Apparently none of their animals died but were killed. The lesions were hyperemia and edema of the lungs and patchy edema and congestion in the cecum and colon. The published description, at least, was quite different from our cases of chicken albumin anaphylaxis. Their animals were under anesthesia when the shocking injection was given, which may be relevant. Code and Hester (1939) induced anaphylaxis in 2 horses, 1 with canine serum and the other with egg white. The latter horse died, but no postmortem findings were reported. Ritzenthaler (1924) induced anaphylactic shock with several proteins, including egg white, but no deaths or postmortem findings were recorded. There was acceleration of heart and respiratory rates and increased peristalsis. There was petechiation of the mucous membranes and edema of the legs and prepuce. He demonstrated that the anaphylactic reaction was antigen specific, and that passive anaphylaxis could be produced.

There is no specific shock organ in the horse or any species; rather, shock is generalized failure of the cardiovascular system and manifest in all organs and tissues. In specifying a shock organ, one is simply pointing out an organ or system with a large vascular supply and, so, more obvious failure of the vascular system. In the horse the cecum and ascending colon are of great size and well vascularized. Hyperemia and alveolar emphysema are often taken to indicate that the lung is the shock organ (Cheville 1983). In fact, there is generalized failure of the vascular system, with acute anoxia being the immediate cause of the nonspecific pulmonary changes.

Sudden death after intended intravenous injection may be the result of **injection into the carotid artery**. This may be immediately suspected at postmortem by the presence of severe hemorrhage in the area of injection. Careful dissection will reveal the puncture wound in the artery and may, rarely, reveal the injected material in, particularly, the middle cerebral artery of the injected side (see Chapter 20, "Forensics").

Fire

An unfortunately common cause of death is barn fires. Being constructed of wood and containing inflammable forages and grains, fires spread quickly with little chance for rescue of panic-stricken animals.

At postmortem there will, of course, be varying degrees of burning and charring of the external surfaces. There are few specific lesions. Severe asphyxial hemorrhages are found throughout the respiratory system, pleura, epicardium, and endocardium. Burn ash may be found in the upper respiratory passages and even in the trachea and larger bronchi in some animals. The lesions bespeak the cause of death as asphyxiation, probably because of glottal spasm. The burn ash in the tracheobronchial tree probably enters with the last agonal gasps as the glottal spasm relaxes.

An important forensic point is that barns may be fired to cover malicious killing of one or more horses. The postmortem examination is important in determining the precise cause of death, which may appear superficially as fire.

Drowning

Certainly uncommon, drowning of foals, debilitated animals, and others does occur. Foals may fall or be knocked upside down into water troughs; animals may become trapped in mud and drown after exhausting themselves.

The lesions are nonspecific and those of asphyxiation, presumably because of glottal spasm as with fire asphyxiation. Water and materials in the water, algae, detritus, and so forth, may be found in the upper respiratory passages, but not in the trachea, bronchi, and lungs. Presumably water could enter the bronchial tree after death, but we have seen no example.

CHAPTER 18

Hemolymphatic System

In many diseases of horses, there are changes in the composition and properties of blood and lymph, and many of these changes are included in the discussion of specific diseases. This chapter focuses on disease entities primarily affecting the hemolymphatic system: lymph nodes, thymus, spleen, bone marrow, hematopoietic centers, blood, and lymph.

Normal and abnormal hematopoiesis

Kinetics

The kinetics of hematopoiesis have been thoroughly studied. In Standardbred horses Carter et al. (1974) found the mean life span of normal erythrocytes to be 155 days using radiolabeled selenomethionine. Marcilese et al. (1964) estimated the total blood volume as 10.31 L/100 kg of body weight, red cell mass of 3.98 L/100 kg of body weight, and mean packed cell volume of 42.7% in 31 Thoroughbreds. Unlike humans, horses do not have a distinct fetal hemoglobin. Red cell numbers, hematocrit, and hemoglobin concentration increase from birth to 12 months, when adult values are attained. Mean corpuscular volume and mean corpuscular hemoglobin are lower in Thoroughbred foals less than 12 months old compared to mature horses (Medeiros et al. 1971).

The erythropoietic response to **hemorrhage** and **anemia** was studied by Carter et al. (1974). In response to 63% blood depletion, horses restored approximately 40% of red cell mass within 4 days, and 100% in approximately 100 days. The initial, partial recovery of red cells was attributed to release from the spleen, while complete recovery entailed production and release of up to 7×10^9 red cells per kg per day. Complete restoration of red cell mass following hemorrhage is a function of iron mobilization from body stores. Carter et al. (1974) found that unlike other species, horses do not release immature red cells into the circulation in response to blood loss and anemia, as verified experimentally by Easley (1985) and Radin et al. (1986). There is, however, a macrocytic response, and these new cells have a mean life span of 139 days compared to 155 days for cells released under normal homeostatic demand. Total leukocyte, neutrophil, and platelet counts did not decrease following experimental hemorrhage (Carter et al. 1975). Osbaldiston and Griffith (1972) determined that horses have stable serum iron levels with the bone marrow pools of iron acting to maintain serum levels and total iron binding capacity.

Easley (1985) studied erythrogenesis and the kinetics of the erythroid response in horses and ponies with experimental acute and chronic blood loss and with acute hemolytic anemia induced with acetyl phenylhydrazine. A nearly identical study was done by Radin et al. (1986) with similar results. Both groups found that horses responded most rapidly to the acute anemia caused by drug-induced hemolysis. Heinz bodies were present within 2 days of drug administration. The mean hematocrit declined for 4–14 days, although there was progressive loss of erythrocytes until about day 30. Radin et al. noted that mean hematocrit values correlated poorly with estimated mean erythrocyte production. Significant increases in mean red cell volume were noted with acute and chronic blood loss by 17 and 20 days, respectively. The increase in red cell volume occurred somewhat earlier (14 days) with induced hemolytic anemia. Red cell distribution width, an electronically calculated measurement of erythrocyte distribution, indicated that horses respond to severe, acute blood loss and hemolysis with production of long-lived macrocytic erythrocytes. However, not all horses show this response, and Easley (1985) indicated that ponies and horses respond differently, with the response dependent upon adequate marrow stores of iron. Both studies indicated that some horses may restore lost erythrocyte mass without developing macrocytosis.

Erythrocyte enzymes

Erythrocyte enzymes or biochemical constituents have been used by some investigators to identify immature erythrocytes. Shull (1981) measured creatine and glucose-6-phosphate dehydrogenase, and Smith and Agar (1976) studied adenosine-5′ triphosphatase. These enzymes are present in higher quantities in immature erythrocytes and, so, indicative of anemia or resolving anemia. Only glucose-6-phosphate dehydrogenase has been used as a clinical test, and then infrequently, because of time and expense (Easley 1985).

Serum biochemical tests

Serum biochemical tests such as lactate dehydrogenase and cholinesterase have been unconvincing in the differentiation of anemias (Osbaldiston et al. 1970).

Equine haptoglobin

Equine haptoglobin, a serum protein with multiple functions, is present in utero and after birth. Levels remain high for the first 12 months of life and gradually decrease thereafter (Taira et al. 1992a). Mean serum levels are slightly higher in females than males, regardless of age. The haptoglobulin, classified electrophoretically as an α_2-globulin, binds free hemoglobin for phagocytosis and excretion (Allen and Archer 1971; Taira et al. 1992). By sequestering the iron from hemoglobin and making it unavailable for bacterial growth, haptoglobulin has a bacteriostatic effect. Equine haptoglobin is particularly effective in binding free hemoglobin in intravascular hemolysis. Taira et al. suggested that haptoglobin helped to prevent development of hemoglobin-induced acute renal failure and protected foals from free hemoglobin in neonatal isoerythrolysis. Haptoglobin also functions as an acute phase reactive protein, increasing in numerous inflammatory conditions (Taira et al. 1992).

Serum transferrin

Ek (1981) studied the relationship among various diseases and serum transferrin, another iron sequestering agent. Horses and foals with acute infectious diseases or laminitis had significantly decreased levels of serum transferrin and albumin. Differences in transferrin response among different phenotypes were also reported.

Serum c-reactive protein

Serum c-reactive protein is an acute reactive phase protein thought to act as a chemotactin and opsonizer. Yamashita et al. (1991) found c-reactive protein increased 3–4 times a few days after onset of acute inflammatory lesions, with bacterial infections being the most effective stimulus. Serum c-reactive protein is not present prior to ingestion of colostrum and reached peak, nonstimulated levels by 12 months of age. Other acute reactive phase proteins, such as **α_1-acid glycoprotein** (orosomucoid) and **ceruloplasmin**, show similar activity and age-related distribution (Smith and Cipriano 1987; Okumura et al. 1991; Taira et al. 1992).

Pregnancy and postpartum

Reviews of hemostasis in horses are available (Darien and Feldman 1992; Meyers et al. 1987). Specific defects of hemostatic function are discussed below.

There are significant alterations in blood values in pregnancy and in postpartum foals. Gentry et al. (1992) studied hemostasis in preparturient and postparturient mares and in normal, nonpregnant mares (Gentry et al. 1992). Pregnant mares had increasing levels of plasma fibrinogen, factor VIII: C, and von Willebrand factor from midpregnancy to parturition. Plasma fibronectin increased and fibrin degradation products appeared. There was a rise in antithrombin III concentration. There were no significant changes in factors VII and IX, or in one-stage prothrombin time, or in activated partial thromboplastin time.

Chavatte et al. (1991) studied bone marrow and peripheral leukocyte counts in a group of pre and postpartum foals. They found that neutrophil counts and neutrophil:leukocyte ratios increased with advancing gestational age and immediately postpartum, presumably the result of neutrophil mobilization by corticoids. Premature foals had lower total leukocyte counts than term foals. Failure of effective leukopoiesis and leukocyte mobilization by 36 hours after birth correlated with increased foal mortality. In utero infection with equine herpesvirus (EHV)-1 and severe perinatal bacterial septicemia causes neutropenia.

Lymph

The production and circulation of lymph has been studied for over 200 years. Colin (1886/88) cites work in 1790 in which investigators ligated the thoracic ducts of four horses to study lymph production and circulation. Approximately 40–100 mL of lymph per kg per day were produced. The circulation of lymph through the skin varied with anatomical site. Ferrocyanate injected near the foot reached midthigh in 20 minutes, while a similar injection near the nares of an eating horse reached a cannulated lymphatic in the neck within 7 minutes.

Spleen

The spleen, of great physiological importance, is as often a source of confusion as enlightenment at postmortem. It varies markedly in size because of its function as a blood cell reservoir. Primary shock, of whatever cause, including killing, causes enlargement, with pooling of large quantities of blood. Bleeding an animal immediately after killing allows the spleen to partially deplete itself of blood.

Variable size indentations or earlike flaps may be present, particularly on the parietal surface of the head of the spleen. The splenic capsule consists of the outer, peritoneal lining, a collagenous/elastic layer containing numerous blood vessels and lymphatics, and an inner smooth muscle arranged in two layers.

There are numerous subcapsular and capsular

veins that receive blood and plasma directly from the red pulp (Krölling and Grau 1960). It is these veins containing blood that appear as small, reddish protrusions on the capsular surface. They were mistaken by Rooney (1970) for protrusions of red pulp through the capsule. The spleen of the horse is of storage type, containing a relatively small number of variable-sized splenic corpuscles (white pulp—usually not apparent grossly) and a large amount of red pulp (Trautmann and Fiebiger 1952). White pulp constitutes about 4%–5% of the volume of the spleen (Krölling and Grau 1960). The intrasplenic vascular system of the horse is simpler than that of many other species and is clearly illustrated and described by Krölling and Grau.

Aged horses often have splenic atrophy, with loss of red and white pulp and an apparent increase of connective tissue stroma. Histologically, the spleen contains numerous hemosiderophages, which increase in a nearly linear manner with age. This is of importance in the diagnosis of equine infectious anemia. Accessory splenic tissue may be found as discrete reddish nodules in the greater omentum and gastrosplenic ligament.

Acute splenitis

The spleen participates with the other lymphoid tissues in septicemias and viremias. Grossly, it is somewhat enlarged, darker, and softer than normal. There may be petechiae and ecchymoses on the capsular surfaces. With septicemia there is an increased amount of blood and an increase in the size of the splenic follicles, with clear, reactive centers. There may be activation—hypertrophy—of the reticular cells of the pulp sinusoids, with obvious phagocytosis. With viremias, specifically herpes-1, acute equine infectious anemia, and arteritis, the follicles have necrosis of lymphoid cells, with modest increases in immature lymphoid elements. With toxemia, for example, gastrointestinal malpositions, there is necrosis of the centers of the splenic follicles.

Specific infections such as tuberculosis and tumors such as lymphosarcomas may affect the spleen as well as other organs.

Abscess of the splenic lymph nodes

This is uncommon and usually caused by *Rhodococcus equi* in debilitated, cachectic individuals, whether the result of advanced age or debilitating disease, such as chronic equine infectious anemia, chronic fibrinopurulent pleuritis, and so forth. In all cases only the splenic lymph nodes are involved, with splenic enlargement secondary to impairment of the venous outflow. The prerequisite for this abscess, as for abscesses in the external iliac lymph nodes, is exhaustion of the immune system. There may be concomitant heavy infestations with ascarids and *A. perfoliata* as further evidence for the disabling of the immune system.

Rupture of the spleen

This is infrequent (Lukes 1901/02) and, when seen, almost always the result of **acute hemorrhagic infarction**. The rupture occurs on the parietal surface, the splitting open of an area of hemorrhagic infarction. The cause of the infarction, in all of our cases, has been thrombosis of the cecal artery in its extrasplenic and/or intrasplenic course by *S. vulgaris*, as already observed by Wiart (1875) cited by Cadeac (1896).

Mares kicking foals do not, as a rule, cause rupture of the spleen but, rather, rupture of the liver with or without fractures of the ribs. Piot-Bey (1912) reported a convincing case of rupture of the spleen in a young horse as a result of running into a pole.

Infectious diseases

Infectious anemia

Equine infectious anemia has been recognized as a significant cause of morbidity and mortality since the middle of the 19th century. Lignee (1843) cited by Ishii (1963) attributed the disease to nutrition. Anginiard (1861) cited by Ishii recognized the infectious nature of the disease. It has many synonyms, such as *Kreigsseuchen Anamie* and *Wechselfieber* [Ziegler (1925) cited by Cohrs (1961)]. The disease affects equids throughout the world. The association with arthropod-infested swampy areas provided a widely used synonym, *swamp fever* (Ishii 1963). With the development of an immunodiagnostic test and control measures, the disease appears to be less prevalent than in 1970 when Konno and Yamamoto considered it the most important infectious disease of equids.

The disease is caused by infection with a retrovirus of the subfamily, lentiviruses. It is antigenically and structurally related to other retroviruses, including human immunodeficiency viruses I and II, ovine visna virus, and caprine arthritis-encephalitis virus. A number of discrete strains with unique surface proteins are recognized and associated with certain geographical areas. Equine infectious anemia virus infects fixed and circulating monocyte and macrophage cells, and some strains of the virus are adapted for growth in tissue cultures of equine monocytes, kidney cells, and fibroblasts (Malmquist et al. 1973; Kono and Yoshino 1974).

Recent studies, with polymerase chain reaction techniques, have shown proviral DNA sequences in circulating monocytes of infected horses, suggesting these cells survive viral infection (O'Rourke et al. 1991). The virus buds from the cell membranes of infected cells, as do some other retroviruses (Gonda et al. 1978). Most common disinfectants, such as hypochlorite and chlorhexidine, kill the virus (Shen et al. 1977). Physical and chemical agents effecting viral viability were studied by Stein et al. (1944). The virus can be inactivated in serum by heating to 58°C for 30 minutes (Barnett 1972).

The virus is mechanically transferred from animal to animal by the bites of hematophagus flies such as horse flies and deer flies. Fomites, such as contaminated needles and syringes and grooming equipment, can also transfer the infection. Transmission is more fully discussed below.

The clinical and pathological aspects of infectious anemia have been studied since the early 1900s. There are extensive reviews of the early work: Ishii (1963) and Konno and Yamamoto (1970).

Three clinical forms are recognized: acute, subacute, and chronic. The chronic form is the most common (Issel and Coggins 1979). Classifications based on gross and microscopic pathology have been proposed (Konno and Yamamoto 1970), but they are of little practical value to either pathologist or clinician. The clinical signs depend on a number of factors: host resistance and immunity, viral virulence, environment and weather, transport, type of work or exercise, and intercurrent disease. The characteristic clinical signs associated with all forms of the disease are recurrent fever and anemia (Issel and Coggins 1979).

Acute

Diphasic or fluctuating fever and anemia appear within 7–20 days of infection (Konno and Yamamoto 1970). Horses with the acute form of the disease may die within 2–4 weeks. Issel and Coggins (1979) note that previously unexposed horses are most likely to die with the acute form of the disease. Viral replication in, and destruction of, monocytes occurs within 14 days of infection, together with progressive decrease in the number of red and white cells and platelets (Konno and Yamamoto 1970). Sideroleukocytes, neutrophils containing hemosiderin, appear in the circulation within 14 days of onset.

Gross lesions characteristic of the acute equine form of infectious anemia were described in 14 experimental cases by Konno and Yamamoto (1970). Subcutaneous edema and petechial hemorrhages were common. Enlargement of the spleen, liver, kidneys, heart, and lymph nodes occurred in most horses. Petechial hemorrhages were present on the diffusely congested lungs and in the endocardium, epicardium, and myocardium. There was diffuse congestion of lymph nodes.

Microscopically, there was extensive necrosis of lymphoid elements in the spleen and lymph nodes. There was diffuse and moderately severe hepatocytic necrosis, fatty vacuolation of hepatocytes, and degeneration of Kupffer cells and sinusoidal endothelium. Coagulation necrosis, sloughing of renal tubular epithelium, and interstitial hemorrhage were seen in the kidneys of acutely ill horses. There were foci of myocardial degeneration, moderately severe serofibrinous necrotizing pneumonitis, and focal petechial hemorrhage and necrosis of the adrenal cortex.

Subacute

Gross and microscopic lesions seen in the subacute form of the disease are similar to the acute cases but less severe. There is characteristic fever and progressive anemia. These animals may survive for months.

There is enlargement of spleen, lymph nodes, liver and kidneys (Konno and Yamamoto 1970), with petechial hemorrhages in the lung and heart. Necrosis of lymphoid elements in the spleen and lymph nodes and degeneration of epithelial cells in the liver, kidney, and adrenal cortex are common.

Animals surviving the initial phase of tissue necrosis frequently show activation of lymphoid germinal centers in the spleen and lymph nodes. Aggregates of macrophages and lymphocytes localize around areas of necrotic debris in the liver, kidney, heart, lungs, and adrenal glands (Konno and Yamamoto 1970).

Chronic

Chronic or **relapsing** equine infectious anemia is the most common form of the disease. Some of these animals are inapparent, asymptomatic carriers.

Periodic fever and coincident episodic anemia, at biweekly intervals, are characteristic of the chronic cases (Kono 1976). About 90% of such episodes occurred in the first year of infection. There is evidence to suggest that periodic exacerbations of clinical signs are associated with the appearance and proliferation of antigenic variants or exposure to such variants by reinfection (Kono et al. 1973). Work, intercurrent disease, or exposure to corticosteroids may cause acute exacerbations in chronically infected horses (Kono et al. 1976; Issel and Coggins 1979).

Gross and microscopic lesions in chronic cases of equine infectious anemia have been meticulously described in 47 experimental horses by Konno and Yamamoto (1970).

Gross lesions reflect activation of the reticuloendothelial system by prolonged contact with the virus. The affected horses are thin or emaciated. The spleen and lymph nodes are enlarged because of hyperplasia of lymphoid germinal centers. The architecture of the hepatic lobules may be distorted by necrosis, scarring, and nodular hyperplasia. There may be diffuse or dependent subcutaneous edema and petechial or ecchymotic hemorrhages (Henson and McGuire 1971).

Microscopic lesions include diffuse lymphoid hyperplasia, immune-complex glomerulonephritis, hepatocytic nodular hyperplasia, Kupffer cell hyperplasia and siderosis, and perivascular lymphocytic infiltration (Issel and Coggins 1979).

The cause of anemia has been debated, and it is apparent that several factors are responsible. McGuire et al. (1969a) found decreased red cell life span and both intravascular and extravascular hemolysis. Ferrokinetic studies in experimental ponies showed marked decreases in serum iron concentration and decreased saturation of transferrin during febrile/hemolytic periods. There was decreased plasma iron turnover and iron utilization, indicating impairment of erythrocyte production and bone marrow responsiveness. It is uncommon to find immature erythrocytic cells, such as reticulocytes or normoblasts, in severely anemic horses. Sentsui and Kono (1988) found a high percentage of erythrocytes containing virus during febrile episodes. Such erythrocytes adsorbed complement and were prone to phagocytosis by neutrophils because of the presence of viral hemagglutinins. There is little evidence that lysis of erythrocytes is mediated by antibody-dependent mechanisms, since few antibody-coated erythrocytes are found in the circulation during febrile, hemolytic episodes (Sentsui and Kono 1988).

Viral-induced thrombocytopenia, one cause of hemorrhage during the disease, was studied in experimental animals by Clabough et al. (1991). They found decreased numbers of platelets and an increase in platelet-associated immunoglobulins G and M during febrile episodes. Although not definitive, their results suggested binding of viral antigen—antibody complexes on the surface of platelets. Such platelets are targeted for phagocytosis by Kupffer cells and splenic macrophages. They were unable to find virus in association with megakaryocytes and did not find a decreased number of megakaryocytes. Thrombocytopenia was probably not caused by a failure of platelet production in the bone marrow.

The mechanism(s) of viral persistence in infected animals and the failure of the immune system to eliminate the virus have been studied. Banks et al. (1978) found that the immune system responds to the virus and produces neutralizing antibodies. Kono et al. (1978) found depressed responses to phytohemagglutinin and pokeweed mitogen by T- and B-lymphocytes of infected horses. They proposed that the activity of specific, sensitized lymphocytes might be inhibited either by a direct viral effect or by a cytokine secreted in response to viral infection. A similar hypothesis by Shively et al. (1982) was based on deficits in specific and nonspecific immune responsiveness. Fujimiya et al. (1979) found increased immunoglobulin G(T) and proposed that this "suppressor antibody" was a factor in immune hyporesponsiveness. Valpotic et al. (1989) found no defect in the ability of peripheral blood T-lymphocytes to form E-rosettes. In fact, they found more rosettes in infected horses. Valpotic and others concluded that persistent viral infection was caused by a combination of factors, including potentially immunosuppressive antibodies and cytokines, sequestration of virus within macrophages, and evolution of viral antigenic variants, as perhaps yet undefined factors.

Salinovich et al. (1986) demonstrated rapid evolution of alterations in surface glycoproteins, such as gp45 and gp90, in sequential episodes of viremia. They concluded that these alterations made the virus less susceptible to immune attack since antigenic variation made the virus less visible to immunocyte surveillance.

Although clinical signs are sufficient for the provisional diagnosis of infectious anemia, a definitive diagnosis requires the Coggins agar gel immunodiffusion test. This test detects antiviral antibody in the serum of infected horses. Other tests such as horse inoculation, complement fixation inhibition, and several other immunoassays have been used to detect the disease. Tests for antiviral antibody are not able to detect the disease in horses prior to antibody production or in animals with low titers (Issel and Coggins 1979). A number of early investigators found increased serum enzyme values in infected horses, including lactate dehydrogenase, leukocyte alkaline phosphatase, γ-glutamyltransferase, creatine phosphokinase, pyruvate kinase, and aldolase (Palomba et al. 1976).

As noted above, the common means of transmission is by hematophagus insects, which feed on viremic animals and bite susceptible hosts. Hawkins et al. (1973) noted that horse flies (*Tabanus fuscicostatus*) could transmit the infection from acutely infected ponies to susceptible ponies, but did not transmit the infection from chronically infected to susceptible animals. Stable flies (*Stomoxys calcitrans*) did not transmit infection from either acute or chronic ponies to susceptible ones.

It appears that transmission of the virus by horse flies is mechanical and not biological. The infection can also be transmitted from infected mares to foals, as noted below. Transmission on contaminated fomites such as grooming equipment and syringes and needles is well known (Issel and Coggins 1979). Major outbreaks in the past were associated with contaminated needles and syringes.

Several early investigators proposed that the virus of infectious anemia could be transmitted by endoparasites. Luhrs (1919) cited by Stein et al. (1939) reported transmission of the disease by subcutaneous injections of *Gasterophilus* larval extracts or suspensions of ova and larva of *Setaria equina*. A number of other investigators were unable to duplicate his work. Stein et al. (1939) reported successful transmission of the virus by subcutaneous injection of a saline extract of adult strongyles. Their results have not been confirmed. Attempts by Stein and coworkers to transmit the virus with strongyle larva or bot extracts were unsuccessful.

Transplacental transmission of equine infectious anemia was confirmed in a series of experiments by Stein and Mott (1942) and by observations of Kemen and Coggins (1972). Blood obtained from the newborn foal of an infected mare, prior to suckling, contained sufficient virus to infect a susceptible horse. Other experiments established the presence of virus in milk and semen, although transmission during coitus was not observed. Transmission of infection during nursing likewise was not observed by Stein and Mott, but was reported by Kemen and Coggins. Infectious anemia is said to cause late abortion in some mares.

Inapparent carriers are a risk for uninfected horses. Studies by Stein et al. (1955) showed that horses could remain carriers for up to 20 years. Carriers of the virus may have been responsible for epizootics of equine infectious anemia recorded in New England in 1947, South Africa in 1920–23, and Japan in the early decades of the century.

Carriers may resist infection with other viral strains. Stein et al. (1955) showed that some animals may be considered recovered carriers. Clinical observation and research over the past 40 years, however, indicates that once infected, a horse is always a potential carrier.

Kono (1973) reported the development of avirulent viral strains in tissue culture. Neither these strains nor other strategies have resulted in a successful vaccine.

Granulocytic ehrlichiosis

Two forms of ehrlichiosis are recognized in equids. Equine ehrlichial colitis, or **Potomac horse fever**, is discussed with the gastrointestinal system (see Chapter 3). A second form, found in the western United States and in tropical and subtropical areas around the world, is an infection primarily of granulocytic leukocytes (Gribble 1969; Oladosu and Olufemi 1992).

Granulocytic ehrlichiosis, or horse tick-borne fever, has been studied in natural and experimental infections. It is caused by the rickettsia *Ehrlichia equi* carried by the tick *Rhipicephalus evertsi*. The disease was first reported in a small number of horses in the vicinity of Sacramento, California, in the early 1960s. Since then the cosmopolitan nature of the disease has become apparent.

Affected animals show fever, anorexia, depression, and prominent limb edema. Blue-gray pleomorphic, intracytoplasmic inclusions are found in the neutrophils and eosinophils of infected horses (Gribble 1969). Horses, sheep, dogs, and goats inoculated with the blood of infected horses developed the disease, while cattle did not. Experimental horses developed fluctuating fever within 9 days of inoculation and several days before appearance of other clinical signs. Depression, neutropenia, and thrombocytopenia were seen. Subcutaneous edema, especially of the legs, developed within 1–15 days of infection. Hemorrhages in the subcutis and musculature at the time edema developed were the result of thrombocytopenia and proliferative, necrotizing vasculitis of small arteries and veins. Gribble noted that vascular lesions were most common in the small arteries of the subcutis of the legs, ovaries, and testes, and around nerves in the legs. Some horses also had increased amounts of peritoneal or pericardial fluid. Approximately 10% of experimental horses developed severe secondary bacterial infections. Younger horses seemed more resistant to the effects of infection. The similarity of the vascular lesions and clinical signs with those of equine viral arteritis, piroplasmosis, and infectious anemia have been noted by several authors.

Previously infected horses resisted reinfection (Gribble 1969). Mares infected during pregnancy did not abort. The disease was less severe in younger horses.

Oladosu and Olufemi (1992) reported that concurrent infection with *Babesia equi* decreased the severity of either infection, presumably by stimulation of the immune response.

Piroplasmosis

This disease, characterized by varying degrees of hemolytic anemia, fever, and icterus, is caused by infection with *Babesia equi* and *Babesia caballi* (Soulsby 1968). It has been called *tick-borne fever*, *biliary fever*, *anthrax fever*, *equine malaria*, and *equine babesiosis* [Theiler (1905), cited in De Waal and Potgieter (1987); and De Kock (1918) cited by De Waal and Potgieter (1987)].

Piroplasmosis is a cosmopolitan disease of the

tropics and subtropics, although it occurs regularly in more temperate areas such as the southern United States (Knowles et al. 1980). Barnett (1974) disputed the presence of the disease in British horses. In many tropical and subtropical areas, such as Puerto Rico and the Republic of South Africa, the disease is endemic and the rate of infection may approach 95% (Knowles et al. 1980; Tenter and Friedhoff 1986). The parasite is an hemoprotozooan, spread by ticks of the genera *Dermacentor*, *Hyalomma*, and *Rhipicephalus* (Soulsby 1968). *Babesia* sp. can be transmitted transovarially in ticks (Roby and Anthony 1963), between various maturational stages (Theiler 1906; De Waal and Potgieter 1987), and also by in utero infection in mares (Du Pleissis and Basson 1966). Transmission with infected syringes and needles has been documented at least once.

Piroplasmosis has been intensively studied in horses, ponies, and mules. Infection is induced by injection of red cells carrying the parasite. Parasitemia occurs in a biphasic manner, with a first peak 5–6 days and a second 10–12 days after infection. Fever, 106°/107°F, may coincide with or slightly precede parasitemia. Decreases in packed cell volume of approximately 25% may occur with the first phase of parasitemia in some horses and may exceed 50% following the second phase. The anemia of piroplasmosis is typically normocytic and normochromic (Allen et al. 1975). Infected animals are weak, listless, and anorectic. In some infections with *B. caballi* horses may develop paresis of the rear legs (Soulsby 1968). Horses with marked parasitemia and anemia are most likely to die. Some infections are peracute, deaths occurring 1–2 days after infection (Allen et al. 1973). Loss of erythrocytes coincides with twofold to threefold increases in free bilirubin in serum. In severe infections with *B. equi* there may be hemoglobinuria. Wide variations in leukocytic responses have been recorded in field and experimental cases (Rudolph et al. 1975). Transient leukopenia and lymphopenia may give way to leukocytosis. In at least one study (Rudolph et al. 1975), monocytosis and eosinopenia were seen. De Waal et al. (1987) reported thrombocytopenia.

Mortality is variable, depending at least upon the age of the horse. Older horses have a higher mortality rate than younger ones (Soulsby 1968). Infection and recovery appear to confer temporary immunity of roughly 1–2 years' duration, although De Waal et al. (1987) were able to cross-infect *B. equi* infected horses with *B. caballi* within 60 days of primary infection.

Horses succumbing to piroplasmosis have a variety of gross and microscopic lesions. The severity and distribution of lesions will depend on the species of parasite causing the infection (*B. equi* is considered more pathogenic than *B. caballi*), peak parasitemia and degree of anemia, duration of infection, and age of infected animal. Grossly, there may be marked subcutaneous edema and icterus. There are pleural edema and petechial hemorrhages of the pleura. The liver may be enlarged and discolored, and the spleen is typically enlarged and markedly congested. Petechial hemorrhages, a consequence of thrombocytopenia, are found throughout the body.

Microscopic lesions include erythrophagocytosis and pigment deposition in the liver, spleen, and lymph nodes; centrilobular hepatocytic necrosis; acute, multifocal hepatitis; and hypoxic centrilobular cloudy swelling of hepatocytes. Kupffer cell hyperplasia occurs. Foamy macrophages and erythrocyte-containing macrophages may be found in the vessels of the lung.

Diagnosis of equine piroplasmosis has depended on detecting typical clinical signs, finding the parasite in blood smears, and through serological means such as complement-fixation testing or indirect immunofluorescence. Both complement-fixation and immunofluorescent tests are recommended since each has a moderate rate of false reactions (Tenter and Friedhoff 1986). Posnett et al. (1991) developed a DNA probe assay with a higher rate of detection, and this promises to become the standard method of testing either alone or in combination with polymerase chain reaction detection.

Epizootic lymphangitis

This is a worldwide endemic disease of equids caused by *Histoplasma farciminosum*. It is a serious cause of debility (Gabal and Khalifa 1983). The primary lesions are fistulous tracts on the limbs with several horses in a group similarly affected. The infection may progress along the lymphatic vessels to the regional lymph nodes. Swollen lymph nodes and lymphatics can rupture, discharging creamy purulent material. Secondary bacterial infection occurs, and lesions may persist for months or years. Invasion of the respiratory tract is uncommon and has an unfavorable prognosis (Hutyra et al. 1926). The disease is to be differentiated, by culture and examination of exudates, from ulcerative lymphangitis caused by infection with *Corynebacterium pseudotuberculosis*. The latter is a more common cause of lymphangitis in temperate zones and discussed with the skin (see Chapter 15, "Integument").

Sporotrichosis

Sporotrichosis, caused by infection of horses with the fungus *Sporotrichum schenckii*, produces a condition known commonly as **ulcerative lymphangitis**. Members of the genus *Sporotrichum* are common plant saprophytes; of the 40 or so members of the genus, only *S. schenckii* is pathogenic (Alexandropoulos and Mims 1979). The fungus was first described by Schenk in 1898, as cited by Burdon and Williams (1968). While few organisms are generally seen in lesions, it grows readily in culture, producing cream and black leathery colonies (Burdon and Williams 1968).

Infection is acquired through cutaneous puncture wounds, with inoculation of the fungus into the subcutis (Bridges 1972). A pulmonary form, with infection by inhalation, has been documented in humans, but not in horses (Bridges 1972). The organism has a preference for growth in lymphoid tissue and lymphatics, and colonizes these structures after infection (Fig. 18.1). The pyogranulomatous inflammatory response to the presence of organisms leads to the development of nodular masses within lymphatics and nodes. Nodules may rupture and ulcerate the overlying skin. A protracted clinical course has been described, with rupture and healing of some nodules and formation of new ones along lymphatic channels (Bridges 1972). A red-brown, thin discharge may issue from rupturing nodules. In a few animals, the fungus may disseminate widely to viscera and tissues of the central nervous system.

Immune-mediated hemolytic anemia

Several cases of immune-mediated hemolytic anemia have been recorded, but it is rare in horses.

Autoimmune hemolytic anemia was diagnosed in 8 horses by direct and indirect Coombs' tests (Mair et al. 1990b). Five of the 8 cases were 10–20 years of age, the others ranging from 4 to 7 years. There were 2 ponies and 6 Thoroughbred or hunter-type horses. The clinical signs included depression, dullness, lethargy, pyrexia, icterus, and hemoglobinuria. Seven of the 8 animals were anemic, with decreased packed cell volume (8%–25%), red cell count, and hemoglobin. Anisocytosis was seen in 6 horses, and nucleated red cells were found in the peripheral circulation of 2. Red cells from 6 autoagglutinated spontaneously. One horse had thrombocytopenia. Four horses had malignancies, and 1 animal developed autoimmune hemolytic anemia 1 week after injection of an unspecified material. The cause of the hemolytic anemia could not be determined in 3 cases. Therapy with transfusions, corticosteroids, fluids, electrolytes, and antibiotics was successful in 4 animals, while the others either died or were killed.

An unusual case of primary immune-mediated hemolytic anemia and thrombocytopenia in a 3-week-old foal was reported by Sockett et al. (1987). The foal had epistaxis within 14 days of birth, and this continued for 2 weeks. The foal became markedly anemic with a red cell count of 4.33 million cells per μL and packed cell volume of 13%. Petechial hemorrhages were present on mucous membranes. A direct Coombs' test was positive, and there was severe thrombocytopenia: platelet count of 6,000/mm^3. Red cells autoagglutinated. High levels of serum bilirubin indicated that antibody-coated erythrocytes were being destroyed. Treatment with several corticosteroids and antibiotics resulted in improvement of clinical signs and hemogram. No cause was found.

Lokhorst and Breukink (1975) described two cases of autoimmune hemolytic anemia with cold agglutinins in a 6-month-old Dutch Standardbred colt and a 9-year-old Friesian mare. Hemoglobinuria was present in the colt but not the mare. No cause was found.

Reef (1983) described a case of possible

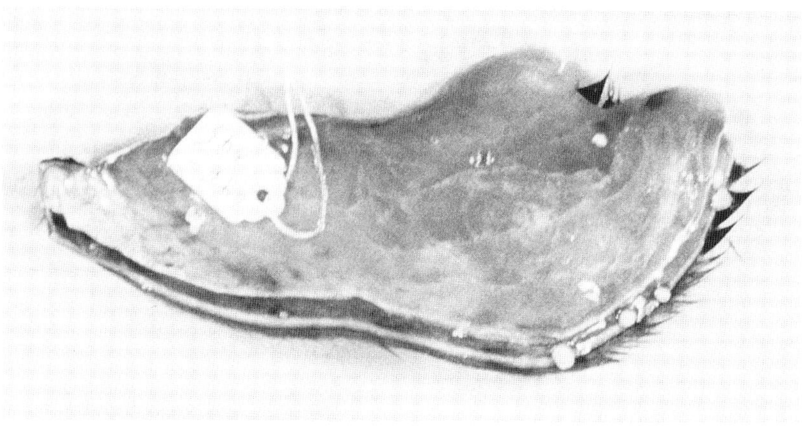

18.1. Lymphangitis associated with infection by *Sporotrichum* sp.

autoimmune hemolytic anemia in a horse with *Clostridium perfringens* cellulitis and enterotoxemia. The 10-year-old Quarter horse mare developed a deep pectoral cellulitis and dermal slough following infection of an injection site. The animal subsequently developed cold hemagglutinins and intravascular hemolysis: low packed cell volume (7%–12%), icterus, and hemoglobinuria, anisocytosis, poikilocytosis, and neutrophilia. The horse received multiple transfusions, which may have caused autosensitization to erythrocyte antigens. Despite therapy the horse died of renal and hepatic failure. Few cases of this type have been reported in horses, possibly because infection with *Clostridium perfringens* is uncommon. Three Shetland ponies inoculated with *Cl. perfringens* Type A enterotoxin did not develop hemolytic anemia (Ochoa and Kern 1980).

Immune-mediated hemolytic anemia following high-dose **penicillin therapy** was reported in 3 horses by Blue et al. (1987). All 3 had acute hemolytic crisis and icterus. There was a positive direct antiglobulin test and high levels of antipenicillin immunoglobulin G antibodies that agglutinated penicillin-coated equine erythrocytes. There were no autoantibodies against erythrocyte antigens. Two of the horses had immune-mediated thrombocytopenia. All 3 animals recovered once penicillin therapy was stopped.

Blood transfusions

Blood transfusions are used in treating neonatal isoerythrolysis and acute blood loss. The incidence of potential graft-versus-host reactions is rare. Horses receiving blood transfusions may develop alloantibodies, which decrease the life span of the transfused erythrocytes or which may induce anaphylactoid reactions on subsequent transfusions (Kallfelz et al. 1978). Blood group antigens Aa, Ae, Db, and Dc are most likely to sensitize horses, with Aa sensitization being most probable with blood transfusion (Wong et al. 1986). Sensitization following a single transfusion may persist for years.

Maternal colostral alloantibodies against foal erythrocyte antigens cause neonatal isoerythrolysis (see Chapter 12, "Neonate"). Maternal alloantibodies are said to interfere with conception and pregnancy, although this is poorly defined (Wong et al. 1986).

Three conditions in which vasoactive phenomena and hemolysis lead to debility and death are **purpura hemorrhagica, idiopathic thrombocytopenic purpura**, and **anaphylactoid purpura.**

Purpura hemorrhagica

Biggers and Ingram (1948) have provided a unique historical review of this condition, which was apparently first definitively described and given the name, *purpura hemorrhagica*, by Field in 1843.

The disease is largely sporadic, often occurring after outbreaks of respiratory disease or strangles. Frequency data from Moscow, 1893–1901 (Hutyra and Marek 1920), indicated that 0.4% of horses in that clinic were treated for purpura. Wirth (1985) found purpura hemorrhagica (morbus maculosus) in 1.3% of over 3000 postmortems. She also showed that the frequency in the autopsy population in Hannover dropped dramatically from 1933–1942 to 1973–1983, particularly between the periods 1933–1942 and 1943–1952. We have seen only a dozen cases of purpura hemorrhagica in over 10,000 postmortems. The clinical incidence is somewhat higher. Sorensen (1972) indicated that 1%–10% of animals will develop purpura within 2 to 4 weeks after an outbreak of respiratory disease or strangles. An occasional case has no such history.

Bryans et al. (1974) observed that purpura is particularly associated with streptococcal infections. The secondary invading streptococci (usually, *Streptococcus zooepidemicus*) in outbreaks of respiratory disease are the probable inciting agents for purpura rather than virus disease per se. Bryans recorded urticarial reactions in horses given experimental *S. equi* vaccines, as well as full-blown purpura in animals vaccinated more frequently than recommended. O'Dea (1969) made similar observations. The evidence indicates that sensitization to streptococcal antigens and subsequent immune-complex–mediated vasculitis is the basis for the disease.

Galan and Timoney (1985b) found streptococcal M antigen and immunoglobulin A in immune complexes of horses with lesions. It is of comparative interest that only horses and humans seem to react with immune-mediated vasculitis and hemolysis following infection with streptococci. The characteristic lesion in humans is poststreptococcal glomerulonephritis, while horses develop purpura hemorrhagica.

Sorensen (1972) has provided a thorough clinical description of the disease. There are hemorrhages in the skin and mucosae and bloody edema of subcutaneous and submucosal tissues. The mucosae of the nose, pharynx, and larynx are preferentially affected. The more distal portions of the respiratory tract are less often involved. There may be hemorrhages in the mucosa, muscularis, and serosa of the stomach and small intestine, less often more distal portions of the intestinal tract. The earliest clinical sign is petechiation of the nasal mucosa, followed by urticarial plaques in the skin and/or more generalized edema of the subcutaneous tissues. Yellowish edema fluid infiltrates the intermuscular connective tissue. The muscles undergo parenchymatous and fatty degeneration and are gray-brown or yellowish-brown and softened with streaks of punctate hemorrhages (King 1949). Inflammatory cell infiltration may occur later in the course of the disease. In an occasional case there may be hyalin or fibrinoid degeneration of the media of small muscular arteries/arterioles, but this seems to be exceptional. No defects in coagulation have been reported (Biggers et al. 1949) and platelet counts are normal.

Anaphylactoid purpura

A morphological variant of purpura hemorrhagica, consistent with Henoch-Schönlein anaphylactoid purpura in the human, was described by Gunson and Rooney (1977). An 8-year-old Thoroughbred gelding developed acute dyspnea and intractable colic following several weeks of chronic coughing. Laparotomy revealed numerous petechial and edematous nodules and wheals on the small and large intestine, and the animal was killed. A focus of β-hemolytic streptococcal infection in one lung lobe was found at postmortem, as well as diffuse, severe pulmonary hemorrhage, laryngeal mucosal hemorrhage, foci of muscle degeneration, and discrete hemorrhagic and necrotic foci on the serosa of the small and large intestine. There was pronounced multifocal and severe acute leukocytoclastic vasculitis, resembling the lesions of Henoch-Schönlein anaphylactoid purpura in humans. There were no renal lesions. Red cell and platelet counts were within normal limits. The authors proposed an immunological basis for the lesions in this horse. Anaphylactoid purpura in humans is associated with deposition of immunoglobulin A, immunoglobulin G, and complement in vessels, but this could not be investigated in this case.

Idiopathic thrombocytopenic purpura

This condition, rare in horses, appears when platelet numbers decrease and hemorrhaging occurs. The few cases reported have had epistaxis, melena, hematuria, and hemorrhages in the mucous membranes and gingiva (Meyers et al. 1987). In one case (Sorensen 1972) the horse had normal hemoglobin concentration and packed cell volume, but a platelet count of 33,000 per mm^3 and prolonged bleeding time. Hemoglobin progressively decreased, perhaps because of hemorrhage and sequestration in soft tissues.

Treatment with corticosteroids was beneficial. A similar case was reported by Smith (1978). Larson et al. (1983) reported two cases. Both Thoroughbred mares had epistaxis and platelet counts less than 5000/mm^3. Treatment with dexamethasone helped to resolve the condition, and circulating platelets increased to more than 50,000/mm^3 within a few days.

A case of idiopathic thrombocytopenic purpura in a 10-year-old Thoroughbred gelding initially responded to corticosteroids, but relapsed periodically (Morris and Whitlock 1983).

Meyers et al. (1987) consider idiopathic thrombocytopenic purpura a diagnosis of exclusion; it remains when other diseases such as drug reaction and neoplasia have been eliminated. Immune-mediated destruction of platelets has been observed in humans, but not the horse.

Congenital and developmental disorders

Immunodeficiency

Immune dysfunction in the human and horse has many similarities, including similar reactions to a number of pathogens. Both are prone to streptococcal infections of the upper respiratory tract, and are the two species that develop immune-mediated glomerulonephritis following streptococcal infection. Both human and horse are afflicted by immunodeficiency, and much has been learned of the genetic risk factors for combined immunodeficiency in the two species.

Perryman and Crawford (1979) proposed four disorders leading to failure or deficiency of the equine immune system. These included failure of passive transfer of colostral antibody, severe combined immunodeficiency, agammaglobulinemia, and selective deficiency of one or more antibody classes such as IgM. Failure of passive transfer of colostral antibody and severe combined immunodeficiency were considered the most important for morbidity, mortality, and economic loss.

Failure of passive transfer of antibody

Investigations by Jeffcott (1972) and Jeffcott and Jeffcott (1974) and McGuire et al. (1977) clearly established the importance of early passive immunity in foals. While the immune system is anatomically mature and competent before birth, resistance to pathogens is largely dependent on absorption of maternal colostral antibodies in the first 12–24 hours of life. The foal can absorb large immunoglobulin molecules through the intestinal mucosa up to, but not beyond, 24 hours.

McGuire et al. (1977) found, in 87 Thoroughbred foals and mares, that colostral antibody levels were directly proportional to those of serum antibodies. There was no preferential sequestration of antibodies in colostrum. Mares with low circulating antibody levels had low colostral antibody (<400 mg/100 mL; normal levels, 1100–8900 mg/100 mL) and were more likely to have foals that suffered from failure of passive antibody transfer. Failure to suckle colostrum, or delayed letdown of colostrum, while important, was uncommon. Kita et al. (1985) found that 5.3% of Arabian foals in Poland had failure of passive transfer, probably representative of horses in general.

Foals with serum immunoglobulin G levels less than 400 mg/100 ml at 24 hours of age were considered to have partial or complete failure of passive antibody transfer (McGuire et al. 1977). In a population of 87 foals, 7 of 9 with complete failure of passive transfer and immunoglobulin G levels less than 200 mg/100 mL of serum developed respiratory or gastrointestinal infections within the first weeks of life. Only 3 of 12 foals with partial failure, serum immunoglobulin levels of 200–400 mg/100 mL of serum at 24 hours, acquired infections. Sixty-six foals with normal passive transfer did not become infected. Six of 11 foals dying of infections within 2 weeks of birth had complete failure of passive antibody transfer, and 4 of the 11 had partial failure of transfer.

Combined immunodeficiency

McGuire et al. (1974b) described fatal combined immunodeficiency in Arabian foals. Extending earlier observations made by Johnston and Hutchins (1967) and McChesney et al. (1970), they defined immunodeficiency as the reason for the high rate of adenoviral infections in these foals. Systematic observations of 30 diseased and 78 normal Arabian foals showed that 10 of 30 sick, and 2 of 78 normal, foals lacked adequate circulating lymphocytes and had impaired ability to make one or more immunoglobulins. Lymphocyte counts less that 1000 cell/mm^3 (normal 4200 cell/mm^3) were typical of diseased foals. No immunoglobulin M was present in the sera of 75% of the diseased foals, and immunoglobulin A was missing in 25%. Unlike normal foals in which production of immunoglobulins starts between 16 and 24 days postpartum, immunodeficient foals did not produce antibodies and became susceptible to pathogens once maternal colostral antibodies were depleted by catabolism.

The immunodeficient foals did not have delayed hypersensitivity reactions to dinitrochlorobenzene or phytohemagglutinin A, indicating lack of T-lymphocyte function (McGuire et al. 1975; Hodgin et al. 1978). An in vitro rosette inhibition assay showed decreased production of a thymus-derived hormone, facteur thymique serique, which may play a role in T-cell development (Splitter et al. 1979). Lew et al. (1980), using immunofluorescent microscopy and the erythrocyte–antibody-complement rosette assay, showed that there were few or no circulating B-lymphocytes. While they found some T-lymphocytes in the blood with nonesterified esterase staining, these were severely hypofunctional. Immunodeficient foals were unable to reject xenograft skin effectively (Lew et al. 1980). Perryman in Felsburg et al. (1992) proposed that immunodeficient foals have a population of circulating immature T-lymphocytes and may also have natural killer (NK) cells since they could resist herpes virus infection.

Magnuson et al. (1980) reported that endogenous production of corticosteroids in normal and immunodeficient foals is similar, indicating that defective immunity was not the result of excessive endogenous or maternal corticosteroids during gestation or the postnatal period.

Studdert (1978) described the characteristic gross lesions. These included plum-red discoloration of the cranioventral portions of the lungs, pulmonary emphysema, cream-colored bronchial exudates, pulmonary abscesses caused by *Corynebacterium (Rhodococcus) equi*, and small or absent thymus glands. Mair et al. (1990b) isolated *Streptococcus zooepidemicus* from the lung abscesses of one immunodeficient foal, but *Rhodococcus equi* is by far the most common pathogen.

Histologically, there was marked thymic hypoplasia and absence of germinal centers in spleen and lymph nodes. Immunodeficient foals may also have purulent rhinitis, conjunctivitis, and tracheobronchitis. Adenoviral inclusions are easily found in hyperplastic bronchiolar epithelium (Studdert 1978). Johnston and Hutchins (1967) and McGuire et al. (1975) found that affected Arabian foals frequently succumbed to adenovirus pneumonia and suppurative bronchopneumonia early in life. Perryman and Crawford (1979) proposed that deficient production of equine interferon gamma might explain the enhanced susceptibility to certain viral infections. Other causes of death included hepatic failure and enteritis (Studdert 1978). Snyder et al. (1978) found infections with *Cryptosporidium parvum*. Mair et al. (1990a) saw simultaneous infection of the gastrointestinal tract with coronavirus and cryptosporidia in one immunodeficient foal.

Thompson et al. (1975) and Poppie and McGuire (1977) found that the genetic defect of combined immunodeficiency in Arabian foals was an autosomal recessive, non-sex-linked gene. They reported a 2.3% incidence in 257 Arabian foals and estimated that approximately 26% of adult Arabians carried the defect. The defect was not found in other breeds. A 3-year prospective breeding study with Arabians carrying the defect confirmed the mode of inheritance (Perryman and Torbeck 1980).

Selective immunoglobulin deficiency and agammaglobulinemia

Several cases of complete agammaglobulinemia have been reported in horses (Banks et al. 1976). The animals developed lethal infections as maternal antibody was catabolized. In one animal, the absence of B-lymphocytes suggested a variant of combined immunodeficiency.

Weldon et al. (1992) described a Standardbred colt with a selective deficiency of immunoglobulin M. The 3-month-old animal had a respiratory infection, together with peripheral lymphadenopathy for 3 weeks. It was marginally anemic with an elevated total white blood cell count, neutrophilia, and normal lymphocyte count. The colt was hypoalbuminemic, but not hyperglobulinemic, with high levels of immunoglobulin G, normal levels of immunoglobulin A, and no detectable immunoglobulin M. Although normal numbers of B-lymphocytes were present in the circulation, the cells failed to respond adequately to bacterial lipopolysaccharide, a selective B-cell mitogen. Circulating T-lymphocytes numbers were below normal.

At autopsy, there was a pulmonary abscess, *Rhodococcus equi*, diffuse lymphadenopathy, and diffuse bronchopneumonia. Weldon et al. postulated that the selective deficiency of immunoglobulin M compromised this colt in two ways. First, without synthesis of adequate levels of immunoglobulin M, there was no rapid response to pathogens. Second, because immunoglobulin M is the major antigen receptor on the cell surface of B-lymphocytes, these cells would not be able to bind antigens effectively or to respond by activation and transformation.

Hemophilia A

A congenital deficiency of clotting factor VIII causes hemophilia in horses (Hutchins et al. 1967; Archer and Allen 1972; Feldman and Giacopuzzi 1982). The disease has been recorded in Arabian, Thoroughbred, and Standardbred horses and is a sex-linked, recessive defect (Feldman and Giacopuzzi 1982).

Feldman and Giacopuzzi (1982) described a case in a 3-day-old Quarter horse colt. The animal was presented with markedly swollen joints in all four legs. It received plasma transfusions, but the packed cell volume and plasma protein levels decreased, and large areas of hemorrhage appeared over a hip area. Activated partial thromboplastin time was prolonged, but the prothrombin time was within normal limits. The animal died and, at autopsy, had multiple hemorrhagic foci in the lumbar musculature, myocardium, subcutis, joints, and large bowel serosa. An analysis of clotting factors showed that factor VIII levels were less than 5% of normal adult values.

Congenital prekallikrein deficiency

Deficiency of plasma prekallikrein was found in two Miniature horses. There was defective surface-initiated coagulation (prolonged activated partial thromboplastin time). The deficiency was an incidental finding during a routine examination for musculoskeletal problems when a blood sample failed to clot (Turrentine et al. 1986). Analysis of the pedigree of several affected animals indicated heterozygosity in the lineage. All horses were asymptomatic as in the comparable condition in humans.

Nutritional and metabolic disorders

Hyperlipemia

Hyperlipemia in ponies and horses was first reported by Schotman and Wagenaar (1969). While more often seen in ponies, especially Shetland pony mares, it has been recognized in undernourished and chronically diseased horses (Naylor et al. 1980).

Schotman and Wagenaar studied 138 naturally occurring cases, the majority in Shetland pony mares, in foal or recently foaled or aborted. Most were obese. Obese Shetland pony mares also predominated in a study of hyperlipemia by Watson et al. (1992a). Typical clinical signs included dullness, anorexia, transient colic or diarrhea, pasty feces, and icterus. While Dutch cases were most common in the spring, this was not the case in Scotland (Watson et al. 1992a). Despite therapy, including insulin supplementation and heparin, mortality is high, ranging from 20%–90% (Schotman and Wagenaar 1969; Naylor et al. 1980; Watson et al. 1992b).

Serum biochemical profiles were remarkable. Schotman and Wagenaar reported twofold to sevenfold increases in total serum lipids. There were significant increases in total and free cholesterol, phospholipids, neutral lipids, fatty acid esters, and free fatty acids. Lipase values were decreased. In a companion study Wensing et al. (1973) showed that hyperlipidemic ponies were markedly acidotic (pH < 7.3), had low base excess and pCO_2, and elevated levels of lactate dehydrogenase, γ-glutamyltransferase, and sorbitol dehydrogenase. These alterations were roughly predictive of clinical course, animals with marked acidosis and high enzyme levels being less likely to survive. Watson et al. (1992b) observed similar increases in cholesterol, triglycerides, and very low density lipoproteins. The increase in fraction 1 very low density lipoproteins accounted for the total increase in this fraction since this lipoprotein component was not detected in the sera of controls. A shift in the ratio of apolipoprotein substituents of very low density lipoproteins was detected by ultracentrifugation and electrophoresis. Watson et al. (1992b) also detected increased lipoprotein lipase and hepatic lipase activity, as well as an increase in plasma free fatty acids.

There were increases in serum alkaline phosphatase, γ-glutamyltransferase, bilirubin, urea nitrogen, and creatinine (Schotman and Wagenaar 1969; Watson et al. 1992b), indicating parenchymal damage or dysfunction of the liver and kidneys. Similar alterations in serum/plasma biochemical parameters were noted by Naylor et al. (1980), in horses with hyperlipidemia caused by underfeeding, and in several horses with renal disease. The genetics of the condition have not been well investigated. At least one case of congenital hyperlipemia has been reported Gilbert (1986). Preliminary studies of serum lipoprotein profiles in healthy Thoroughbred and Morgan horses and Shetland ponies have shown breed differences (Robie et al. 1975a,b).

The pathogenesis involves undernutrition, intercurrent disease, parturition, and alterations in lipid metabolism. It has been hypothesized that undernutrition fosters fat mobilization from tissue depots and overproduction of triglycerides by the liver (Watson et al. 1992b). Naylor et al. (1980) suggested that the removal of triglycerides from the circulation was blocked in animals with azotemia.

Ponies and horses with hyperlipidemia have fatty infiltration of parenchymatous organs at autopsy. The liver may be enlarged and friable, with hepatic rupture as a common cause of death in affected Shetlands (Schotman and Wagenaar 1969). Fatty change also occurs in kidneys and lungs. In one congenital case Gilbert (1986) reported thymic, splenic, and lymphoid hypoplasia, and pulmonary and cerebrospinal edema. Naylor et al. (1980) saw several variants of glomerulopathy and fibrosing tubulointerstitial nephritis in hyperlipemic horses, ponies, and a donkey.

Toxic disorders

Lead poisoning

Since the early 1900s numerous episodes of lead poisoning have been reported in horses exposed to forage and water contaminated by smelting and mining operations.

Knight and Burau (1973) described sudden death and debility in groups of horses pastured near a lead smelting operation in California. Soil and forage lead levels were very high, calculations indicating horses were ingesting approximately 6.4 mg/kg lead daily. This exceeded the 2.4 mg/kg/day known to cause signs of lead toxicity following chronic exposure (Hammond and Aronson 1964). Some horses died suddenly, while others had clinical signs of depression and disorientation, poor haircoat, malnourishment, and upper respiratory dysfunction. Basophilic stippling of red cells and a few metarubricytes indicated lead poisoning.

Dollahite et al. (1978) exposed horses to lead acetate in the diet for 6–8 months. They found that horses were more resistant than cattle to acute lead toxicity, tolerating in excess of 6.25 mg/kg for over 100 days. The sensitivity of individual animals varied markedly, however, and there was no dose-response relationship at the higher levels of lead. There were few gross or histopathological changes in these chronically exposed horses. Only one horse which had received 29.8 mg/kg lead acetate for 57 days had hepatocellular degeneration and purulent pneumonia. Ischemic changes were seen in nerve tissues, and inclusions were found in renal and hepatic epithelium, as well as in red cells. The marrow in long bones was bright red and gelatinous.

Burrows and Borchard (1982) compared the effect of forage contaminated with lead and cadmium from mining and smelting operations with that of lead acetate only in noncontaminated forage. After 11 weeks of feeding lead- and cadmium-contaminated forage, experimental ponies developed severe clinical signs including incoordination, depression, areflexia, weight loss, anorexia, and muscle tremors. Terminal aspiration pneumonia was seen in 2 of 4 animals.

Decreased packed cell volume, Howell-Jolly bodies, and nucleated red cells were indications of hemolytic anemia. The ponies fed lead acetate in noncontaminated forage had similar changes, which took longer to appear. The investigators concluded that synergism between lead and other contaminant heavy metals like cadmium and silver might determine susceptibility of horses and ponies to lead in the environment.

Heparin-induced erythrocyte agglutination

High-dose heparin therapy is used in the treatment of laminitis, prevention of disseminated intravascular coagulation, and as an adjunct to colic surgery for preventing fibrin polymerization (Mahaffey and Moore 1986). Duncan et al. (1983) reported that such therapy caused a decrease of red blood cell mass and an increase of bilirubin excretion, and concluded that heparin was inducing extravascular hemolysis. In a study of three horses on high-dose heparin following colic surgery, Mahaffey and Moore showed that heparin was not causing hemolysis, but, rather, microagglutination of erythrocytes. They proposed that previous observations of heparin toxicity were, in fact, laboratory artifacts since automated cell counters did not count aggregated erythrocytes. They offered convincing evidence by recounting trypsinized samples and showing that heparin did not induce cell loss, only agglutination.

Red maple toxicity

The ingestion of dried or wilted leaves of red maple trees (*Acer rubrum*) by horses causes a depletion of erythrocyte glutathione reductase and an increase in red cell fragility. Studies by George et al. (1982) in a group of 23 experimental horses and ponies showed that ingestion of dried leaves at 3 mg/kg/day for 3 days was sufficient to kill the animals. Both intravascular and extravascular hemolysis, with high levels of methemoglobin, were seen in naturally occurring and experimental cases. Oxidation of erythrocyte hemoglobin leads to the formation of Heinz bodies within 3–5 days of exposure to toxins in the leaves. The animals may die peracutely or may show profound cyanosis, tachycardia, dyspnea, icterus, and/or lassitude (George et al. 1982). High levels of hemoglobin breakdown products and methemoglobin turn both blood and urine brown. Urine may also contain significant levels of protein, bilirubin, and urobilinogen. In a comprehensive experimental study, George et al. (1982) found that, in spite of high levels of free hemoglobin and hemoglobin casts in distal convoluted tubules, the animals did not become azotemic or die in renal failure.

At autopsy there are lesions in liver, kidneys, spleen, and adrenals. The spleen may be enlarged and engorged with blood and macrophages containing erythrocyte fragments. The kidneys may be discolored dark brown or blue, with hemoglobin casts in distal convoluted tubules and scattered necrotic epithelial cells. Mucous membranes and the intima of large vessels are icteric. Centrilobular hepatocytic fatty vacuolation, Kupffer cell hemosiderin accumulation, and erythrophagocytosis are manifestations of hepatic hypoxemia. Pulmonary edema and adrenal cortical hemorrhages may occur, both features of anoxemia and circulatory failure.

Experimental work has shown that fresh red maple leaves either contain little toxin, or that it is in an inactive form. There is an accumulation of toxin in the late summer and autumn. Clinical observation indicates that dried leaves from blow downs or cut trees at any time in the summer are most toxic. Oxidative damage to hemoglobin and erythrocyte membrane sulfhydryl groups, following loss of glutathione reductase activity, is the primary pathogenetic event. Subsequent tissue changes are primarily anoxic or free radical mediated. The toxin has not been identified or chemically characterized.

Endotoxemia

Hematological and hemodynamic alterations caused by endotoxins are common in adult horses suffering acute abdominal crises and foals with neonatal septicemia (Ewert et al. 1985; Lavoie et al. 1990). There is transient depression of blood glucose and hyperinsulinemia, acidosis, neutropenia, anoxic tissue damage from hypoperfusion and hypotension, and disseminated intravascular coagulation (Ewert et al. 1985; Lavoie et al. 1990).

Endotoxin shock has been studied in horses using infusions of *E. coli* and *Salmonella typhimurium* endotoxins. Fessler et al. (1982) reported increased serum levels of creatine phosphokinase, lactate dehydrogenase, and intestinal phosphatase in ponies given *E. coli* endotoxin. There were decreases in venous pH and increased blood lactate levels within 1 hour of infusion. Ponies had increased packed cell volume, attributed to splenic contraction mediated by catecholamines. Bottoms et al. (1982) saw increases in thromboxane A_2 and prostacyclin levels following endotoxin infusion. They attributed the hypotension in endotoxemia to the presence of these vasodilators. Ewert et al. (1985) noted similar effects and found decreased numbers of platelets. Therapeutic mediators of the inflammatory response, such as flunixin meglumate, prednisone, and dexamethasone, partially corrected some of these abnormalities (Ewert et al. 1985).

Septicemic foals with endotoxemia may show clinical signs of depression, weakness, inability to suckle, circulatory collapse, pulmonary failure, and coma (Koterba et al. 1990). Lavoie et al. (1990) infused normal foals with low doses of *S. typhimurium* lipopolysaccharide endotoxin and reproduced some of these signs. Within 6–24 hours of exposure, foals became depressed and anorectic. A transient leukopenia was followed by leukocytosis.

Platelet counts decreased, but the change from pretreatment values was not significant. Increases in prothrombin time and activated partial thromboplastin time were noted. Pulmonary arterial pressure and pulmonary and systemic vascular resistance increased. The rectal temperature was elevated. Alterations in plasma amino acid concentrations were also seen in septicemic foals (Zicker et al. 1991). Morris and Moore (1991) showed significantly increased levels of tumor necrosis factor in septicemic foals and correlated high levels with poor survival. They noted that the production of tumor necrosis factor is stimulated by exposure of macrophages to endotoxin lipopolysaccharides.

There have been no convincing studies showing that endotoxin alone is a major factor in diseases of foals and horses. Experimental studies with reasonably purified endotoxins do not produce disease of the severity of naturally occurring bacterial disease or twisted intestines, for example. In the 1960s Doll, Bryans, and Rooney (unpublished) gave horses *E. coli* endotoxin intravenously and produced mild, nonlethal disease. Similar quantities of a bacteria-free filtrate of ingesta from normal horses produced much more severe clinical signs and lesions, at least resembling those of exhaustion shock. Endotoxins undoubtedly play some role in severe, life-threatening disease, but it is but one of many factors involved in the collapse of homeostasis in the severely compromised animal.

Diseases of unknown or unclassified etiology

Pancytopenia and aplastic anemia

There have been a few reports of pancytopenia and aplastic anemia in the horse for which no cause was found. Space-occupying bone marrow neoplasms, viral and bacterial infections, congenital or developmental stem cell maturation defects, bone marrow toxins such as chloramphenicol, and immune-mediated destruction can cause aplastic anemia (Berggren 1981; Rappeport and Nathan 1982; Camitta et al. 1982; Lavoie et al. 1987). Camitta et al. observed that no cause could be found for over 90% of the cases of pancytopenia. Angel et al. (1991) described a case of pancytopenia in a 10-year-old pony mare caused by **myelofibrosis**. The mare had refractory anemia, pale mucous membranes, and recurrent colic, neutropenia, and thrombocytopenia. Marrow aspirates were hypocellular. Despite therapy, the mare deteriorated and was killed 3 months after presentation. Postmortem findings included diffuse, severe myelofibrosis, multiple sites of extramedullary hematopoiesis, and renal cortical hemorrhages. The cause of the myelofibrosis was not determined.

Pancytopenia was reported in a 4-year-old Quarter horse with a positive direct Coombs' test for immunoglobulin-G coating of erythrocytes. There was anemia, thrombocytopenia, and neutropenia. The bone was hypocellular. Treatment with antibiotics, antipyretics, anabolic steroids, compatible whole blood transfusions, and corticosteroids produced clinical and clinicopathological improvement over 4 weeks. The therapeutic response and conversion to negative direct Coombs' test were considered compatible with immune-mediated pancytopenia.

Disseminated intravascular coagulation

Disseminated intravascular coagulation is an uncommon disorder of hemostasis in which an excessive amount of thrombin is present in the circulatory system, leading to the formation of fibrin thrombi and production of tissue anoxia (Morris and Beech 1983). This is frequently associated with consumption of plasma coagulant proteins and thrombocytes. In various species this phenomena has been associated with neoplasms, intestinal catastrophes, obstetrical complications, sepsis, and uremia.

Morris and Beech described six presumptive cases of disseminated intravascular coagulation in Thoroughbred and Standardbred horses from 9 months to 14 years of age. Pulmonary infections and abscesses, renal failure, colic, and cholangiocarcinoma were the primary disease processes. Clinical signs suggestive of hemostatic defects included epistaxis or prolonged bleeding from venipuncture sites. Thrombocytopenia (platelet count of less than 100,000/mm^3), prothrombin time greater than 13.5 seconds, activated partial thromboplastin time greater than 64 seconds, and excessive fibrin degradation products (>40 μg/mL) were considered indicative of disseminated intravascular coagulation.

A variety of lesions were seen grossly and microscopically. Gross lesions included hemorrhages on mucosal and serosal surfaces, foci of hepatic necrosis, thrombosis of the jugular vein, hemorrhagic enterocolitis, and renal discoloration indicative of renal infarction and tubular necrosis. Morris and Beech did not convincingly demonstrate microscopic fibrin thrombi in capillaries or arterioles, a putative hallmark of the condition.

Disseminated intravascular coagulation as a complication of colic was also reported in 23 horses by Welch et al. (1992). It has been produced in ponies with experimental strangulation of the intestine (McClure et al. 1979).

In addition to the criteria proposed by Morris and Beech (1983) for the diagnosis of disseminated intravascular coagulation, Welch and coworkers measured **antithrombin III** in cases of colic with hemostatic defects. This serine protease inhibitor is the most important modulator of thrombin formation in hypercoagulable states. Darien et al. (1991) found decreased levels of antithrombin III in colic and found that horses that developed disseminated intravascular coagulation and did not survive the colic episode had only 60% of normal levels of antithrombin III. Within hours of surgery, 11 of 14 horses with intestinal strangulation or infarction developed hemorrhagic diatheses, with decreased antithrombin III and increased circulating levels of fibrin degradation products. McClure et al. (1979) found hemostatic defects within 6 hours of the experimental induction of intestinal strangulation. They proposed that intestinal strangulation liberated tissue thromboplastin into the circulation, initiating the coagulopathy. Some horses with enterocolitis had increased levels of fibrin degradation products in the circulation, as well as thrombocytopenia (Welch et al. 1992). This indicated that not all episodes of disseminated intravascular coagulation developed in the same manner, although 89% of horses in this study did have decreased levels of antithrombin III.

In a retrospective study of 1487 colic cases over 5 years, Welch et al. (1992) found disseminated intravascular coagulation in 1.5%. They also found that the rate was nearly 4% in horses undergoing surgery. Survival rates following colic, colic surgery, and acute episodes of disseminated intravascular coagulation varied between 33% and 67%. No histopathological evidence of microthrombus formation was provided.

There is little doubt that disseminated intravascular coagulation, as defined clinicopathologically, occurs with some frequency in equine colic. It is not clear, however, how one defines the condition at postmortem or under the microscope. Sludging of blood, platelets, and so forth, after death is routine and difficult or impossible to distinguish from so-called "fibrin" thrombi. Hemorrhages, petechial and otherwise, are an inevitable accompaniment of terminal anoxia and in no way pathognomonic of disseminated intravascular coagulation. At present, disseminated intravascular coagulation is a disorder of clinical, and not morphological, pathology. Whether it has a significant relationship to the pathogenesis of any disease process is an open question.

Thrombasthenia

Thrombasthenia is a condition in which hemorrhage is caused by a defect in the function of platelets. It has rarely been diagnosed in horses (Miura et al. 1987; Sutherland et al. 1989). It may be associated with epistaxis or bruising, absence of clot retraction, and a lack of normal platelet aggregation in the presence of adenosine diphosphate or collagen. Miura described a case in a 6-month-old Thoroughbred foal that had hematomas, hemarthroses, mucosal hemorrhages, and melena and bleeding from puncture sites. There were similar findings in a 4-year-old Standardbred gelding with a 3 1/2-year history of episodic bleeding. Both horses had abnormal platelet activity in a variety of tests. The mode of inheritance was not studied in either horse and a cause not found. One horse was killed; no significant lesions were found at autopsy (Sutherland et al. 1989).

Neoplasia

Lymphosarcoma

Neoplastic disease of the hemolymphatic system is not common in horses. Neufeld (1973) reviewed about 100 cases of lymphosarcoma. No cases were reported in a large collection of animal neoplasms in South Africa (Jackson 1936). Neufeld reported that the disease is more common in horses aged 4–9 years. No breed predisposition was found. No viral agent has yet been found.

A variety of clinical signs are seen, including lameness, emaciation and anorexia, colic, enlargement of lymph nodes, cough, and cutaneous edema.

Typical cases have elevated absolute numbers of lymphocytes in the circulation, but leukemia is only seen in slightly more than half of the cases. Some horses are leukopenic. Farrelly et al. (1966) reported hemolytic anemia in one case and thrombocytopenia has been seen in others. McConnell et al. (1982) noted that the hemolytic anemia in some cases of lymphosarcoma can resemble that seen in equine infectious anemia. Conboy and Powers (1971) reported marked hemoconcentration and lymphopenia in a 22-year-old Arabian horse with lymphosarcoma. Perryman et al. (1984) and Furr et al. (1991) described lymphosarcoma in horses with clinical and clinicopathologic signs of immune deficiency, possibly caused by the suppressor activity of neoplastic cells.

Neoplastic infiltration and proliferation in soft tissues such as lymph nodes, liver, spleen, gut, and kidney occur in at least one-quarter of cases (Neufeld 1973). Nearly two-thirds had enlarged lymph nodes. Five cases of alimentary lymphosarcoma were described by Wiseman et al. (1974) and Roberts and Pinsent (1975). In our experience the alimentary form is somewhat more common in younger animals, with the ileum being most commonly affected.

Leukemia

Leukemia, per se, is rare. As noted above, Neufeld observed that less than half of all cases of lymphosarcoma have circulating neoplastic cells. Lymphoid leukemia, in the absence of a solid primary tumor, is very rare (Roberts 1977). One case in a 7-year-old Thoroughbred was described in detail (Roberts 1977). The animal had a 3- to 4-month history of weight loss, lassitude, and, in later stages, limb and pectoral edema. The white blood cell count was normal, but there was marked anemia, neutropenia, and thrombocytopenia. Almost all the circulating leukocytes were neoplastic lymphoblasts. At autopsy, there was replacement of bone marrow with neoplastic blast cells, as well as infiltration of hepatic and mesenteric lymph nodes, spleen, kidney, heart, and lungs. Similar signs were seen in a 4-year-old Thoroughbred in Japan with acute myelomonocytic leukemia (Mori et al. 1991). Ascites and pleural effusion were present. The primary site of neoplastic proliferation was the bone marrow.

Buechner-Maxwell et al. (1994) described myeloblastic leukemia in a horse with neoplastic infiltration of the gut, stomach, and lungs accompanied by secondary fungal growth, as in the case of Blue et al. (1987). Several investigators have reported intravascular leukostasis in cases of leukemia (Mori et al. 1991; Buechner-Maxwell et al. 1994).

Multiple myeloma

A number of cases of multiple myeloma have been published (Cornelius et al. 1959; Schalm et al. 1974; Markel and Dorr 1986; MacAllister et al. 1987; Henry et al. 1989). Most cases were old horses, but one was a 3-month-old foal (Henry et al. 1989). Horses with myeloma may have a nonspecific history of anorexia and lethargy. Several affected horses have initially presented with clinical lameness. Myeloma cells in human are known to secrete osteoclast activating factor, causing lysis of bone (Oken 1984), and this may be the cause of skeletal lesions in equine myeloma. The primary site of neoplastic cell proliferation is the bone marrow. Replacement of normal bone marrow with neoplastic cells may cause anemia, thrombocytopenia, and leukopenia. Serum monoclonal gammopathies are common in multiple myeloma, as are light chain aggregates (Bence-Jones proteins) in the urine. A foal and several horses with myeloma have had hemorrhagic diatheses caused by thrombocytopenia, and interference with the function of clotting factors and platelets (Henry et al. 1989). Myeloma has a poor prognosis, most horses dying or being killed within 3 months of diagnosis (Cornelius et al. 1959; Drew and Greatorex 1974; Schalm et al. 1974; Jacobs et al. 1983; Markel and Dorr 1986; MacAllister et al. 1987; Henry et al. 1989). At autopsy there are neoplastic plasmacytic infiltrates of various organs and the bone marrow.

Monoclonal gammopathies

Monoclonal gammopathies have been found in horses with multiple or solitary myeloma and lymphosarcoma (Markel and Dorr 1986; Schalm 1981). Transient monoclonal gammopathies have also been reported in 3 horses without neoplastic disease (Kent and Roberts 1990). In 2 of the 3 cases, the primary clinical signs were lethargy and loss of condition. α_2- and β_1-globulins were elevated. Antibiotics and anthelmintics apparently helped the animals with resolution of the gammopathy over a period of months, suggesting hyperresponsiveness or defective control of immunoglobulin synthesis as the basis of the gammopathy.

Myeloproliferative disease

Brumbaugh et al. (1982) described severe anemia and thrombocytopenia in a 5-year-old Quarter horse with myeloproliferative disease. They defined this bone marrow dysplasia as proliferation of one cell line in the marrow exceeding that of others, causing eventual exclusion of the other myeloid, thrombocytoid, or erythroid precursors. Clinical signs included depression, weight loss, and genital edema developing over 3 weeks. Therapy failed, and the animal developed progressive anemia, petechial hemorrhages on the oropharyngeal and nasal mucosa, and ulcerations of the oral mucosa. It is not clear if whole blood transfusions may have induced an hemolytic reaction. It was notable that prothrombin and partial thromboplastin times were within normal limits, indicating reasonably normal activity of the coagulation system. A myeloid to erythroid ratio of 30.5:1 was seen in the bone marrow. Serum lysozyme (muramidase), a marker of neutrophil bactericidal activity, was elevated. *Actinobacillus equuli* was cultured from the blood, probably because of immunosuppression.

At postmortem there were focal hemorrhages at sites of biopsy and bone marrow aspiration. There were petechial hemorrhages on the serosal surfaces of the abdominal organs, heart, larynx, and trachea. There were renal infarcts. Numerous lymph nodes were enlarged and reddish. Large numbers of myeloblastlike cells infiltrated organs such as the spleen, liver, kidneys, adrenal cortex, lymph nodes, bone marrow, and lungs.

CHAPTER 19

Autopsy Method

Beginning

The method is German (Dobberstein 1957), modified and extended, particularly with regard to the locomotor system. Throughout this chapter *left, right, dorsal, ventral, cranial,* and *caudal* refer to the carcass itself, the animal's left, right, dorsal, and so on. Since this chapter is concerned with technique per se, there will not be iteration and reiteration of the need to examine tissues as the dissection proceeds. The dissection is to facilitate careful, thorough examination and is not, necessarily, an art form.

The animal is placed in dorsal recumbency either on a special table with the aid of an electrical or mechanical hoist, or on the ground. In the latter case the prosector and assistant roll the animal onto the back, and the assistant steadies it in this position as the prosector cuts down the legs. A simple pipe rack may be used to advantage, but is not essential.

On the ground, cut down both rear legs by incising the skin, severing the medial muscles of the thigh, opening the hip joint, and transecting the round and accessory ligaments. The fore leg opposite the assistant is laid down by incising the skin, pectoral muscles, and the vessels and nerves in the axillary space. The second fore leg is laid down in the same manner and the assistant no longer required. Without the pipe rack support, the carcass will tip somewhat to one side. Pulling the head and neck around to the left will cause the carcass to tip somewhat to the right, the side from which the abdominal viscera will be removed.

With the animal on the table, the hip joint is not opened at this time. The rear legs remain cocked up, which will facilitate opening the pelvis. In case of peripheral nerve paralyses of the fore leg, the prosector may preserve the vessels and nerves of the axillary space, not cutting the leg all the way down until after dissection and examination of the brachial plexus.

Reflect the skin from the ventral surfaces of the head, neck, trunk, and the medial surfaces of the legs to the coronary band. Examine the subcutaneous tissues. The mammary glands, prepuce, scrotum, anus, and vulva are not skinned. Dissect the udder from the ventral body wall, cranial to caudal, including the superficial inguinal lymph nodes with the udder.

In the male, incise the scrotal skin and bluntly dissect the tunica vaginalis parietalis from the skin. Free the tunica to the external inguinal ring. Open the tunica to determine the position of the testis. Dissect the penis and sheath from the ventral body wall caudad to the ischial arch. Transect the crura of the penis as the penis curves around the ischial arch.

Standing on the animal's left, open the peritoneal cavity by an incision just caudal to the xiphoid cartilage (Fig. 19.1). The incision extends to the retroperitoneal fat. Break through this fat and the immediately subjacent peritoneum with the fingers. In the fresh carcass the pressure within the abdomen is below ambient, and air will rush in, ballooning out and loosening the abdominal wall. With postmortem gaseous distension the distended cecum and/or colon will bulge outward. One may think to puncture the viscus to relieve the distension and facilitate dissection. This is best not done since fluid ingesta will escape and interfere with the dissection and examination.

Carry the incision caudad along the midline to the pubis, with the knife point outward in order to avoid puncturing the viscera. In the foal, the incision should be carried around the umbilicus on each side, maintaining the continuity of umbilicus, urachus, and urinary bladder.

Continue the incision laterally along the cranial border of the pubis on both sides. In the male incise the flank to and into the inguinal canal, freeing the ductus, vessels, and testis, so that continuity is maintained.

Reflect the left abdominal wall by continuing from the cranial end of the midline incision parallel to the curve of the last rib. This should not be

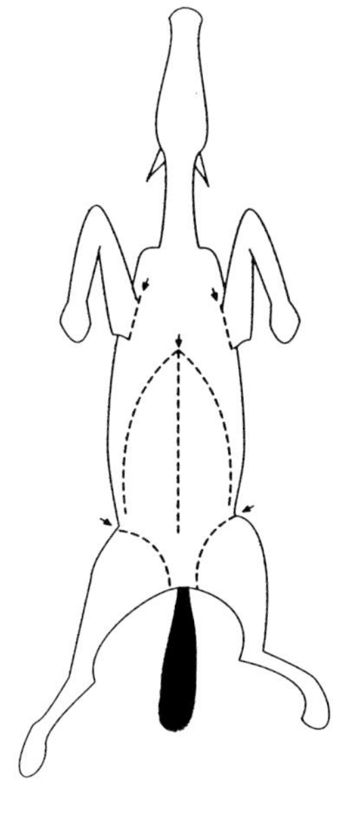

19.1. Schematic of carcass in dorsal recumbency. Lines of incision indicated.

carried so far that viscera spill out on the left side.

The prosector moves to the right side and reflects the right abdominal wall in the same manner. Examine the topography of the abdominal viscera, including manual displacement in order to see the liver, spleen, stomach, and genital tract (Fig. 19.2). Many malpositions of the gut are to be worked out at this time before artifactual displacement.

Allow and assist the cecum and ascending colon to roll out on the right side onto the viscera table or the ground. This may be accomplished by grasping the pelvic flexure and rolling, not lifting, the left colon somewhat cranially and to the left. When laid out on the right, the neurovascular complexes of the ascending colon should be uppermost (Fig. 19.3).

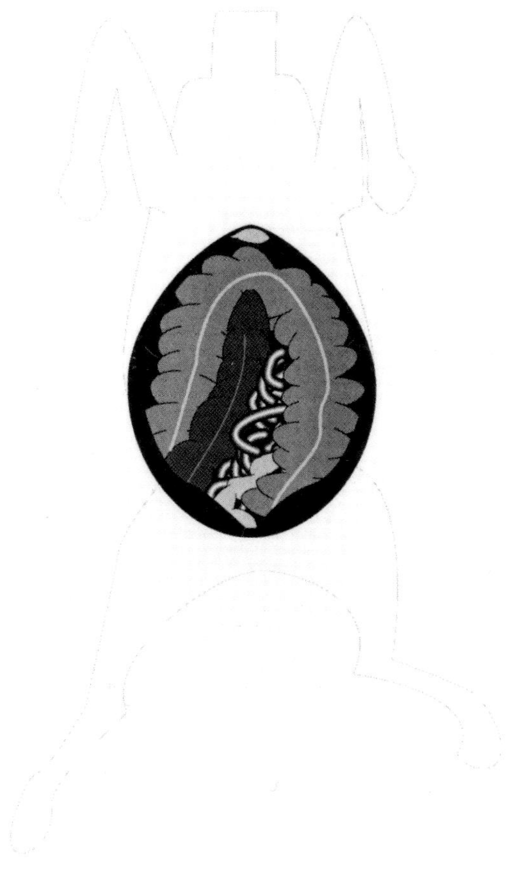

19.2. Schematic of the abdomen opened with viscera undisturbed.

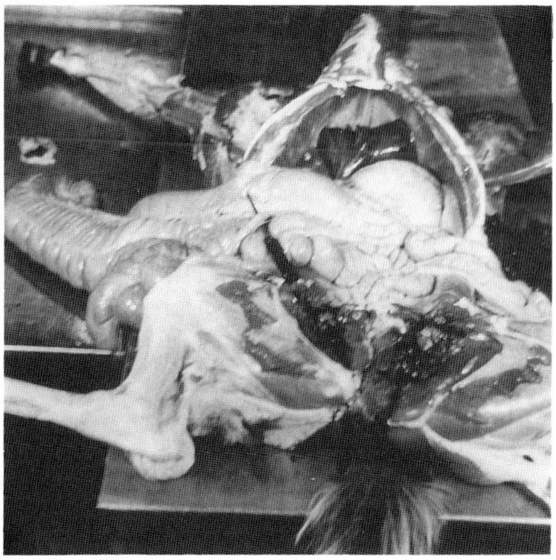

19.3. Large intestine laid out to the *right*, descending colon on the *left*.

Removal of small intestine

The descending colon is displaced out the left side and the small intestine drawn out on the right. Normally, there is a variable quantity of clear yellow peritoneal fluid. Identify the duodenocolic ligament, between the ascending duodenum and the transverse colon, and break it down by blunt dissection. This ligament is the anatomical junction between the ascending duodenum and the jejunum. Bluntly dissect the ascending duodenum to the caudal flexure, the anatomical junction with the descending duodenum. Transect the duodenum at the caudal flexure. Anatomical landmarks should be recognized, noted, and remembered for eventual localization of lesions.

Strip the intestine from the mesentery with the knife. Having the intestine hanging out on the right side tenses the mesentery and facilitates removal. Whenever cutting any tissue, tension facilitates the cutting. Whenever the knife is not being used, it should be fully plunged into the nearest skeletal muscle, for example, medial thigh muscles. It is easily found without unpleasant surprises.

Approaching the thick-walled ileum, identify the ileocecal fold and transect the ileum just proximal to that fold, leaving about 12 cm of the ileum with the cecum (Fig. 19.4).

With the small intestine removed, gather up the great mesentery in one hand. Identify the lymph

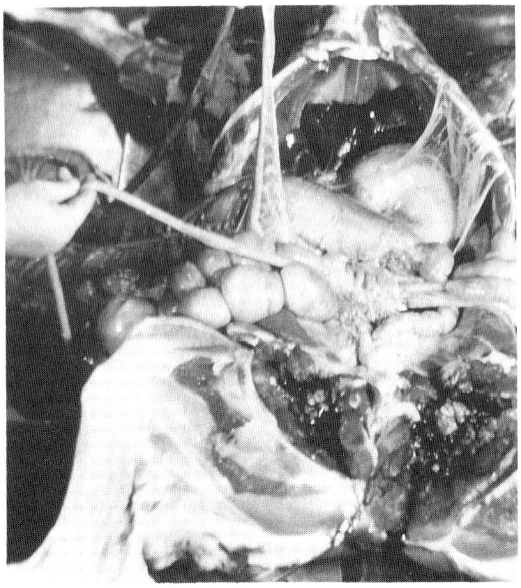

19.4. The small intestine stripped out. The descending duodenum is in the prosector's *right hand* and the ileum with the ileocecal fold extends *upward.*

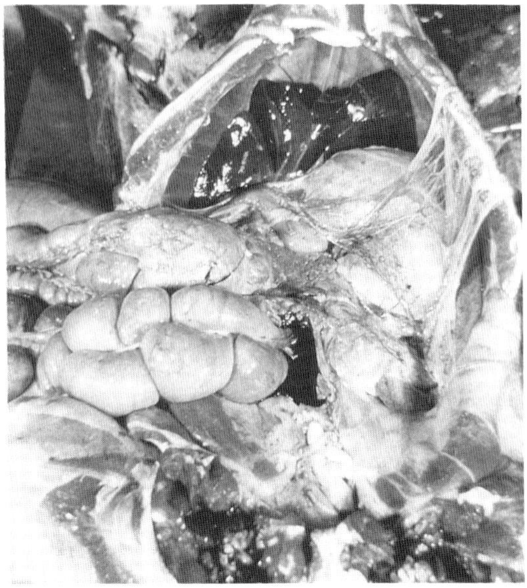

19.5. Omentum reflected and left lobe of pancreas visible.

nodes near the root; transect the root of the mesentery dorsal to the nodes and remove it.

Removal of large intestine

Isolate and examine the caudal mesenteric artery, ganglia, and nerves by bluntly peeling away half of the mesocolon and the fat surrounding the artery and neural tissue.

Transect the descending colon at its junction with the rectum, approximately the pelvic inlet. Pull the descending colon to the right and cut it free from the mesocolon, continuing proximally to the origin of the descending colon from the transverse colon.

Pick up the greater omentum, noting its attachments along the transverse colon. Bluntly dissect the omentum from those attachments and lay it over the stomach (Fig. 19.5).

Exerting steady even traction with one hand, bluntly dissect the transverse and right dorsal colon from the left lobe and body of the pancreas (Fig. 19.6). This requires care and patience, particularly in the decomposed carcass.

Dissection of cranial mesenteric artery

The cranial mesenteric artery is palpated as a firm, knobby cord just caudal to the pancreas and to the right of the midline. Bluntly dissect around the artery until it is isolated in the hand. Strip distally along the artery to isolate and identify the first 8–10 cm of the branches of the ileocecocolic artery: medial and lateral cecal arteries, and dorsal and ventral colic arteries. The small middle colic artery, which runs along the transverse colon to the descending colon, may also be isolated. It is usually snapped apart when the transverse colon is dissected from the pancreas.

Transect the cranial mesenteric artery as close to the aorta as possible, so that it remains with the large intestine as the latter is removed. This cut cannot be well visualized. Laying the knife flat and as far dorsally as reasonable will suffice for a clean cut.

The large intestine is now held in place only by the strong connective tissues between the head of the cecum and the sublumbar area. With steady traction, bluntly dissect through this tissue and roll the large intestine out of the abdomen. The descending duodenum is attached by its mesoduode-

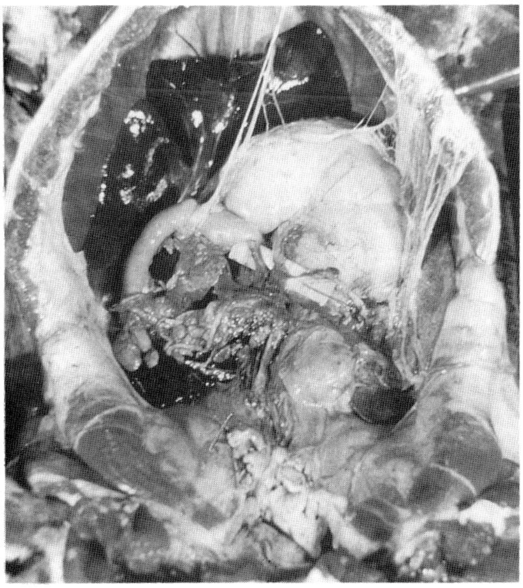

19.6. Large intestine removed. Lobes of pancreas freed. Three branches of celiac artery isolated (*center, in front of card*).

num to the right dorsal colon. Break down this attachment as the colon is removed, leaving the duodenum in situ.

Dissection of pancreas

With the hand as a spade, carefully bluntly dissect the left lobe of the pancreas from the sublumbar attachments, beginning at the left end and working to the right toward the body of the pancreas. Locate the shorter right lobe of the pancreas and bluntly dissect it from the sublumbar attachments. The two lobes are now free with the body still attached to the duodenum (Fig. 19.4).

The pancreas forms a ring around the portal vein. Break the thin dorsal strip. Many branches of the portal vein have already been seen. Their confluence into the major trunk is now clearly visible.

Tensing the tissues between the body of the pancreas and the duodenum, the pancreatic ducts can be appreciated. Tension between the duodenum and liver reveals the bile duct. They can be examined after evisceration.

Dissection of celiac artery

Examine the V-shaped space between the caudal edge of the left lobe of the pancreas and the duodenum ventral to the caudal vena cava, which is just dorsal to the portal vein. The hepatic branch of the celiac artery is palpable and visible. Isolate this artery to the portal area of the liver and transect. Moving the hand to the left, pick up the left gastric branch of the celiac artery before it fans out on the visceral surface of the stomach. Isolate and transect (Fig. 19.6).

Continuing to the left, pick up the large splenic artery in the space between the stomach, left kidney, and spleen. Isolate and transect. Since the liver, spleen, and stomach are removed separately, the dissection differs from that of the cranial mesenteric artery. The isolation and transection is done, so that possible thrombi are not blindly dislodged and lost.

Removal of spleen

Pull the tail of the spleen to the right and locate the splenorenal ligament. This space is an important site of displacement of the ascending colon. Sever the ligament and, drawing the spleen to the right, cut the gastrosplenic ligament. Remove the spleen, gastrosplenic ligament, and omentum as a unit.

Removal of stomach

Draw the stomach and duodenum caudad and identify the lesser omentum between stomach, duodenum, and liver. Bluntly break through the omentum from the dorsal side. Palpate the pylorus and transect the duodenum just distal to the pylorus. Continuing to draw the stomach caudad and to the right, isolate and transect the intraabdominal portion of the esophagus. Break down the gastrophrenic ligament and loose areolar tissue between the dorsal part of the greater curvature of the stomach and the crura of the diaphragm by blunt dissection and remove the stomach.

Removal of liver, pancreas, and descending duodenum

Sever the right lateral ligament of the liver for about 8 cm, tensing the ligament by lifting the right lobe of the liver toward the left. Insert the left hand under, dorsal to, the right lobe of the liver to the midline, palpating the short hepatorenal ligament between the caudate process of the liver and the right kidney. At the midline a small pocket is encountered. Punch several fingers firmly into the pocket, tearing the hepatorenal ligament. If no pocket is present, simply tear into the ligament near the midline. The fingers will show between the caudate process of the liver and the right kidney. Tear out the ligament to join the initial incision in the right lateral ligament. This may have to be repeated to free the caudate process completely from the right kidney.

Pull the left lobe of the liver to the right and incise the left lateral ligament to or near the midline. Draw the entire liver caudad and to the right and incise the falciform ligament, close to the liver and into, but not through, the caudal vena cava. Nick the wall of the vena cava and with two fingers tear open the left side of its wall as far caudally as reasonable.

Insert a finger into the large orifice of the hepatic vein of the left lobe and draw the liver out on the right side. Incise the right part of the wall of the vena cava, freeing the liver. If properly done, the dorsal half of the vena cava remains in the carcass and the ventral half comes out with the liver. The liver is unavoidably torn slightly as it is pulled out. Transect the vena cava as necessary to allow removal of the liver, duodenum, and pancreas en bloc.

Removal of urogenital tract

Remove the muscle from the ventral surface of the pelvis and remove a central block of bone by sagittal, parallel saw cuts through the pubis, obturator foramina, and ischium. Saw the pubis, first, into the foramen and then the ischium, on each side. Set the saw perpendicular to the bone; that is, the saw should be directed somewhat dorsomedially. On the table or in a pipe support, only one cut on the left or right may suffice. By sharply, briskly, snapping the two rear legs downward, the pelvis usually opens sufficiently as the ventral sacroiliac ligaments are torn. In the foal the cartilaginous symphysis pubis is readily split with the knife.

In the male the penis is freed from the symphysis and ischial arch. Free the anus and penis or vulva by a semicircular incision in the perineum. Lay the testes, ducts, and vessels into the pelvic cavity.

Incise the peritoneum cranial to the left kidney and adrenal gland, continuing the incision parallel and lateral to the lateral border of the kidney, ureter, and uterine horn to the pelvic inlet. Repeat on the right. In order to avoid puncturing the diaphragm, bluntly dissect the right kidney and adrenal from their sublumbar attachments and then incise the peritoneum to the pelvic inlet as on the left.

Transect the aorta just cranial to the celiac artery. Gathering both kidneys in one hand with one finger in the aorta, draw caudad and, with the knife flat in the frontal plane, free the entire mass of sublumbar viscera: kidneys, adrenals, aorta, vena cava, ureters, and reproductive organs. Continue through the pelvic cavity, including the testes and its attachments. Pulling back through the pelvic cavity, pull to one side and cut, then the other side and cut.

Locate and examine the external and internal iliac arteries. They were transected at the pelvic inlet during the above evisceration.

Slice and examine the iliopsoas muscles. Remove them, exposing the ventrocaudal aspect of the sacroiliac joints. These joints are lateral to, and approximately in the same transverse plane as, the prominent bump of the lumbosacral joint. If the pelvis was "sprung open," as described, one or both joints will be opened by tearing of the ventral ligaments. If sufficient force was used, there may also be a fracture of the tuber sacrale. Since spontaneous luxation of the sacroiliac joint can, also, be accompanied by such a fracture, careful interpretation is required. The sacroiliac joints may be examined at this time or with the dissection of the rear legs.

Dissection of diaphragm

Examine the diaphragm. The presence of air or fluids in the pleural cavity should be determined now. Pneumothorax is uncommon and only detected before the pleural cavities are opened. Usually air in the cavities is the result of an inadvertent knife stab in the thoracic wall. Incise the diaphragm on the right side along the costal insertion. Air enters the right pleural cavity. The loose caudal mediastinum shifts to the left, with air entering the area of the left pleural cavity but not the cavity itself. In some horses the caudal mediastinum is fenestrated, and air immediately enters both cavities.

Continue the incision in the diaphragm to the left. Pulling back on the diaphragm, tear loose the caudal mediastinum and transect the caudal vena cava and phrenic nerves. Free the thoracic esophagus and aorta from their respective hiatuses and lay the diaphragm down in the abdominal cavity.

Run the hand forward, alongside the heart, to the cranial mediastinum. Break that down and draw the hand strongly up and back, tearing the pericardium loose from its sternal attachments.

Removal of heart and lungs

Skin the ventral surface of the head and neck if not already done. Slice on either side of the larynx, carrying the incisions boldly and deeply forward just inside the rami of the mandible. Unite the two incisions transversely in the *angulus mentalis.*

Draw the tongue caudad out of the mandibular space. Transect the soft palate and free the dorsal wall of the pharynx by traction on the tongue, removing the pharyngeal ring intact. Palpate the stylohyoids (great cornua) and keratohyoids (small cornua) and insert the knife, edge forward, into the angle between them. Resting the tip of the knife on the hard palate or against the inside of the mandible, sever each articulation with a levering motion.

If a band saw is available, we prefer the following procedure. Rather than removing the pharynx and larynx, the trachea is transected just distal to the larynx. The head is removed as described below and is sawn on the midline after sawing off the premaxilla and mandible with the incisor teeth. The pharynx, larynx, guttural pouches and associated structures, specifically muscles, vessels, and nerves, can, then, be dissected on each half of the head. This is the method of choice particularly for investigating possible obstruction of the upper airways: ethmoidal hematoma, soft palate paralysis, epiglottic entrapment, guttural pouch tympanitis, and so forth, and, we think, the method of choice in all cases when a band saw is available.

With either method the jugular veins, carotid arteries, and vagus and recurrent nerves are best left in situ for examination. Transect the trachea and esophagus in the midcervical region. With a handhold incised between two tracheal rings, cut the vessels and nerves on both sides of the thoracic inlet and introduce the distal cut ends of the trachea and esophagus into the thoracic cavity. Within the cavity, grasp those cut ends and steadily pull the thoracic viscera out of the chest. The aorta will kink and needs to be bluntly dissected to avoid tearing it in half.

Removal of head

The head is removed by exerting strong dorsiflexion over the edge of the table or some other fulcrum, and transecting the rectus capitus ventralis muscle as it widens over the atlantooccipital joint. Cut into the spinal canal, transect the spinal cord, and disarticulate the atlantooccipital joints.

Dissection of fore leg

After overall examination, stand square to the bottom of the hoof and transect the flexor tendons and suspensory ligament just proximal to the proximal sesamoid bones. Open the digital synovial sheath by sliding the knife distad inside the sheath and cutting out through the medial insertion of the superficial flexor tendon. There is a well-developed, normal, mesotendon running from the deep face of the deep flexor tendon to the parietal wall of the digital synovial sheath. It contains vessels, nerves, and lymphatics. The superficial flexor may detach slips of tendon, which surround the deep flexor tendon. They are similar to, but more variable and less obvious than, the ring around the deep flexor at the fetlock.

Grasp the deep flexor tendon with a paper towel and pull it strongly distad to dorsiflex the coffin joint. Cut into the fibrous tissue to open the proximal palmar portion of the coffin joint. Insert the tip of the knife into the coffin joint and, using it as a fulcrum, lever the knife abaxially, severing the medial collateral ligament of the coffin joint. Continue around the dorsum, keeping the tip of the knife always in the joint, cutting the fascia, common extensor tendon, and lateral collateral ligament of the coffin joint. The latter is more readily severed from inside the joint. This dissection is not difficult in the foal but is more difficult and dangerous in older animals. The knife tip should always be in the joint, cutting by levering the knife, and the hands and knife handle should be dry and free of synovial fluid.

Place the hoof on a table. The tip of the knife is used to sever all the attachments, not unlike coring an apple, so that the navicular bone can be removed for examination.

Further routine examination of the hoof is difficult. Postmortem radiographs may be helpful.

Sagittal band saw section(s) can be employed. Piecemeal dissection and maceration are employed in special cases. The following method, described by Sack (1991), does work, but is tedious and often damages the laminae. The knife is run around the coronary band. Two saw cuts are placed from coronary band to bearing surface at the toe, about 2–3 cm apart. The strip of horn is pulled loose with nippers, and each half of the hoof wall is gradually pulled away with nippers. It has been said that boiling, followed by a sharp blow of the foot on a hard surface, will free the hoof wall, but we have never been successful. If histological material can be foregone, the digit may be left in a bucket of water for about a week. The hoof wall is easily removed (Heusser 1928), although the smell is daunting.

Pressing down on the distal end of the middle phalanx, transect the insertion of the straight sesamoidean ligament on the complementary fibrocartilage of the middle phalanx. Transect the medial collateral ligament and open the pastern joint.

Press down on the distal end of the proximal phalanx and sever the medial collateral ligament. Slide the knife proximally between the metacarpal and proximal sesamoid bones and cut outward, transecting the medial collateral sesamoid ligament. Open the dorsal pouch of the fetlock joint capsule. Slice the palmar ligament (intersesamoidean ligament).

After inspection and palpation, insert the knife between the suspensory and the flexor tendons and cut proximally to open the carpal synovial sheath. Continue proximally through and above the carpus to expose the check ligament of the superficial flexor tendon. Avoid transecting this ligament before it is examined.

Use sharp and blunt dissection to isolate and examine the two flexor tendons and the check ligament of the deep flexor tendon. The interosseus should be examined either now or later by careful dissection. If avulsion of the proximal end is suspected, the specimen should be saved for careful, fine dissection and sectioning.

Pressing down on the distal end of the third metacarpal (Mc3), flex the carpus slightly and transect the medial collateral ligament to open the radiocarpal joint. Cut the overhanging flaps of joint capsule on the dorsal surface in order to expose all the joint surfaces. Open the intracarpal joint, again being careful to cut and reflect the flaps of joint capsule. The carpometacarpal joint is difficult to open routinely. Lesions are rare. It should be examined if clinical findings or palpation indicate. A quick method is to separate the leg through the intracarpal joint, leaving the distal row of carpal bones with Mc3. A sharp, well-directed blow on the edge of a table, all the impact delivered to the dorsal face of the distal row of carpal bones, will spring open the carpometacarpal joint.

Press down on the distal end of the radius and transect the medial collateral ligament of the elbow, continuing the incision until the joint is widely exposed. The pectoral muscle may be removed to facilitate opening the joint.

Press down on the distal end of the humerus and open the shoulder joint by transecting the tendon of the *m. subscapularis.* If the cut is widely laid, the tendon of the *m. biceps brachii* will also be transected. Open the bicipital bursa widely. Slice and examine the muscles of the fore leg.

Specific directions for routine examination of blood vessels and nerves have not been given. It is understood that they are examined and dissected as necessary as the dissection proceeds.

This method provides a reasonably thorough examination of the major sites of lesions of the leg. Obviously, the clinical history or postmortem findings may dictate further and/or additional study. The muscles and fascia of the lateral surface of the leg, for example, have not been seen. The leg may be detached and rolled over with the structures on the lateral side still reasonably intact. The individual muscles and the lateral courses of such nerves as the radial may be examined. The fascial sheaths of the muscles should be slit open and reflected for appropriate examination of muscles. The deep fascia on the lateral aspect of the leg provides not only ensheathment for the muscles but, also, strong tensile resistance to laterally convex bending of the fore leg. This is readily appreciated by bending the leg in this manner.

Dissection of rear leg

The dissection from hoof to tarsus is as the fore leg. The tarsal synovial sheath is opened. There is no check ligament of the superficial flexor, the tendon having functionally comparable attachments to the tuber calcis. The check ligament of the deep flexor is much thinner than in the fore leg and may be absent.

Pressing down on the distal end of metatarsal (Mt3), transect the medial collateral ligament and the tendons of the *mm. peroneus tertius and tibialis cranialis* to open the tarsocrural joint widely. Examine the plantar tarsal ligament.

The intratarsal and tarsometatarsal joints are difficult to open routinely. A rapid method is to disarticulate through the tarsocrural joint, saw partially across the proximal end of Mt3, and, then, lay a frontal saw cut through the tarsal bones to join that initial cut at a right angle. Arthrosis (spavin) appears as brownish-yellow discoloration of the otherwise white articular cartilage. Further exposure with the knife is considerably easier once these saw cuts have been made.

Press down on the distal end of the tibia and sever the medial collateral ligament of the stifle. Continue the incision forward to the border of the medial patellar ligament. Slide the knife proximally along the medial ridge of the femoral trochlea, parallel to the medial patellar ligament. Cut outward, transecting the medial patellar ligament. Transect the insertions of the *m. quadriceps femoris* on the patella and reflect the patella laterally.

Insert the tip of the knife between the condyles of the femur and stab in to transect the cruciate ligaments after a preliminary examination of the area for possible cruciate avulsion. The stifle should fall open. The ligaments of the menisci may be severed to allow examination of the menisci and the tibial articular surfaces.

Open the coxal joint if not already done. The sacroiliac joints are examined now if not already done. As with the fore leg the lateral aspect of the rear leg has not yet been examined. This is more easily done by rolling the carcass to one side and then the other, rather than cutting off the rear leg. The trochanteric bursa and the muscles are examined.

Head and vertebral column

After overall examination, the skin is removed, and the salivary glands, lymph nodes, and muscles sliced and examined. The eyes are removed and fixed before dissection if indicated (see Chapter 5, "Eyes and Ears").

For routine examination the incisor teeth are removed by a transverse band saw cut behind the bodies of the premaxilla and mandible. The head is sawn in half on the midline on the band saw. This may already have been done as described earlier. The two halves of the brain are removed for examination. Frontal saw cuts are made to open the maxillary sinuses. All saw cuts are placed to avoid teeth. If the history suggests a lesion of the brain, the brain may be removed *en toto* after the usual removal of the calvarium with saw and chisel.

Examination of the teeth is facilitated by sawing through the ramus of the mandible and separating the mandibular and maxillary arcades. The temporomandibular joint is opened and examined at this time.

Examination of the vertebral column is tedious; there is no simple, rapid technique. After removing legs and ribs, the muscle is examined as it is removed from the vertebral column. After palpation the cervical part is removed by disarticulation at C7-T1. The remainder is sawn into convenient lengths. Each of these segments is, then, sawn sagittally just lateral to the spinal cord, opening the spinal canal on one side. The cord is removed, and the bony structures further examined, including maceration if necessary. In a given case it may be appropriate to remove the dorsal arches by saw and chisel work; for example, for examination of the lumbar spinal cord and cauda equina in suspected cases of neuritis of the cauda equina.

When ataxia is the presenting clinical sign, the cervical vertebral column may be disarticulated, keeping the spinal cord intact for eventual correlation of skeletal and cord lesions. Cervical nerves 1 and 2 are first severed with scissors or a long, thin-bladed knife within the spinal canal. Cervical vertebrae 2 and 3 are disarticulated as follows. Open both intervertebral articulations on the dorsal surface and cut away the ligamenta flava. The spinal cord is visible within the dura. The specimen is turned over, and the intervertebral disk is located by dorsiflexing the specimen. Insert the knife into the disk and cut as much as possible without entering the spinal canal. Continue cutting from the disk on each side to join the previous cuts in the capsules of the intervertebral joints. Try to disarticulate by ventroflexion over the edge of the table. A quick, sharp bend is necessary; if unsuccessful, repeat the cuts somewhat more deeply. Eventually, vertebrae 1 and 2 will separate as a unit and can be slipped off the spinal cord.

Sever the nerves leaving the spinal cord at the cervical 2–3 junction within the spinal canal as before. Disarticulate vertebrae 3–4 and slip vertebra 3 off the spinal cord. Continue. In this manner, the cervical spinal cord will be recovered intact within its dura, and the chondro-osseous lesions of stenotic myelopathy readily visualized. This technique is not difficult once learned, but does require practice.

Examination of viscera

The procedures for examination of the viscera are standard and not described in detail. An exception is the dissection of the heart and lungs. This method is more difficult to learn than the standard blood flow method, but permits a more thorough anatomical exploration.

Separate the aorta from the mediastinum by blunt dissection. Place the heart and lungs upside down with the ventral surfaces uppermost and the trachea pointing to the prosector's left, and the apex of the heart pointing at the prosector. Slice the pleural connection between the accessory lobe of the right lung and the left lung, continuing to open the pericardium to the apex. Tuck the pericardium under the heart (Fig. 19.7).

Open the left atrium from the cranial border, carrying the incision through the atrium and out into the major pulmonary veins coming from the lungs. Palpate the left atrioventricular orifice. Direct the knife through the atrioventricular orifice to the apex of the left ventricle close to and parallel to the right longitudinal groove. Cut out, opening the ventricle. Examine the left ventricle and palpate the aortic orifice (Fig. 19.8).

Spin the entire specimen around, *without lifting it,* so that the trachea is pointing to the right. Tip the apex of the heart toward the prosector. The pericardium may now be completely removed. Open the right atrium, continuing caudally to open the coronary sinus and the caudal vena cava and cranially to open the cranial vena cava. Examine the foramen ovale or its remnant. Palpate the right atrioventricular orifice. Direct the knife through the atrium and orifice, parallel and as close as possible to the right longitudinal groove, to the apex of the right ventricle and cut, opening the ventricle (Fig. 19.9). Redirect the knife from the apex parallel and close to the left longitudinal groove and cut. Now tip the apex of the heart away from the prosector. The origin and course of the pulmonary artery are clearly displayed. Continue the cut in the ventricle into the pulmonary artery and its major branches to the left and right lungs. Note that this last cut destroys the large pulmonary veins seen earlier (Fig. 19.10).

The connections between heart and lungs have been seen, and the organs are now separated for further, standard examination.

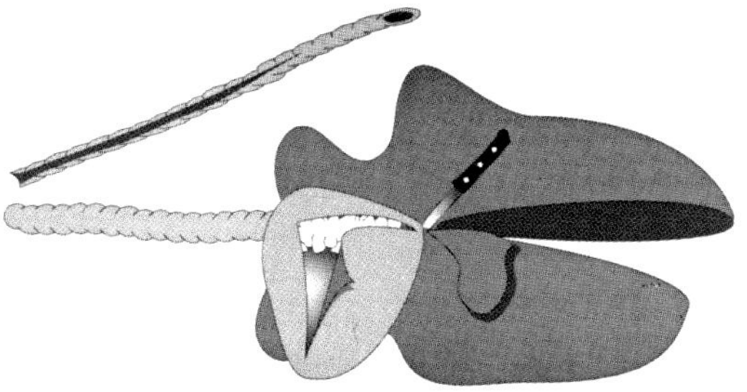

19.7. Schematic of steps in the examination of heart and lungs. Left side of heart, pericardium opened.

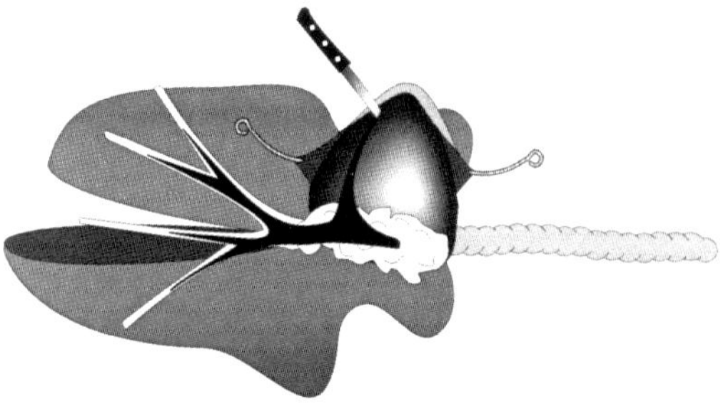

19.8. Schematic of pulmonary veins opened into left atrium, continuing into left ventricle.

The examination of the urogenital block begins with the specimen oriented dorsal side up. The aorta is opened and its branches to the several organs examined. The specimen may, then, be turned as required to examine all the organs, including the ureters, without complete separation of any organ from the parent specimen.

In the cervical region the jugular veins and carotid arteries are opened with scissors. This is useful in certain forensic cases. There is medial calcification in the carotid artery at the division into external, internal, and occipital arteries of many young Thoroughbred and Standardbred foals. It apparently disappears with age or at least is not routinely found in older animals and is of no clinical significance. The recurrent nerves and vagus

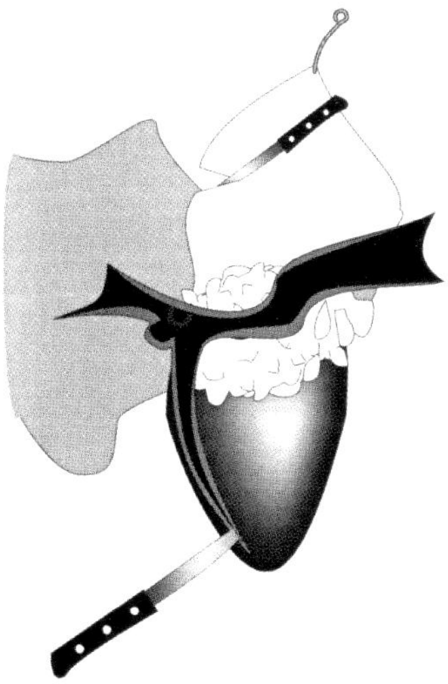

19.9. Schematic of right side with vena cava, right atrium, and right ventricle opened to apex.

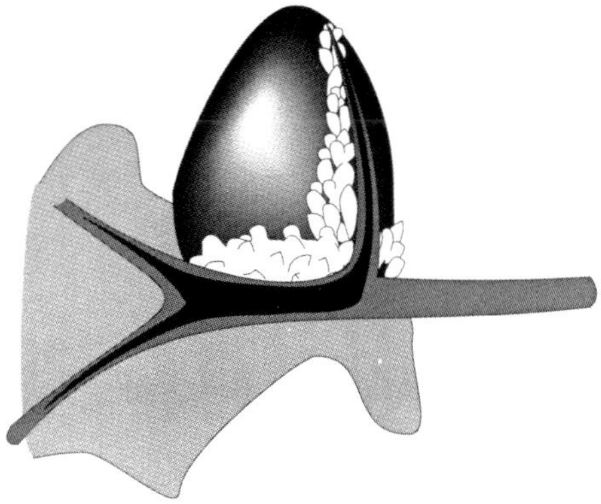

19.10. Schematic of heart flipped away as incision in right ventricle is continued out through the pulmonary artery.

nerves are readily available for examination.

The remaining viscera are opened, sliced, and examined in the standard manner. The pancreatic ducts and bile duct may be found by appropriate tension on the liver, pancreas, and duodenum. The cranial mesenteric artery is opened into the major branches. The examination is continued throughout the length of the branches in the event of infarction or displacements of the colon and/or cecum.

Miscellaneous

An example of body composition, including the heart weight as a percentage of body weight, is shown in Table 19-1.

Table 19-1. Body composition and heart weight of a 1110-lb horse

Body composition (%)[a]	
Muscles and tendons	45.0
Bones	12.4
Skin	6.02
Blood	5.9
Abdominal viscera	5.49
Thoracic viscera	1.6
Heart weight (%)[b]	
Schrittpferde	0.6
Vollblutpferde	1.04

[a]Source: Smith (1917).

[b]Source: Ellenberger and Baum (1910).

Note: In general, the light horse breeds (*Vollblutpferde*: Thoroughbred) will approximate 1.04%, while the heavier breeds (*Schrittpferde:* horses working at slower speeds, walk) approximate 0.6%.

CHAPTER 20

Forensics

Introduction

Unlike human forensic pathology, which is primarily concerned with the criminal cause of death, equine forensic pathology is usually concerned with civil liability in tort or under contracts, including insurance policies and sales agreements; in short, with money. Less often, but with distressing frequency, animals dead of neglect and/or maltreatment are presented for postmortem with eventual legal action in mind.

The pathologist should consider every case, fetus, foal, and adult, forensic until shown to be otherwise. Legal action may not be taken or brought to the pathologist's attention for several years after the fact. There is, in principle, no difference between a proper, thorough forensic autopsy and any other autopsy. The written records, the basis for virtually all legal proceedings, must be scrupulously kept, contain all relevant information and observations, and not contain speculations that the prosector would be reluctant to argue. This can be unfortunate, since speculations, hypotheses, and ideas of potential value to another pathologist at a later time might be lost. We first consider the pathologist as a witness, and then discuss some aspects of the forensic postmortem examination.

Witness, usual

The pathologist may be a witness either because of direct involvement with the postmortem examination and interpretation, or as an expert asked to review a case and give an opinion. We consider direct involvement first, recognizing that there are many areas of overlap. The experience given here is with the American legal system; we have had only limited exposure to equine legal matters in other venues.

The pathologist need, in principle, only confirm that the written record is the proper record and contains all the information available on the particular case. In other words, the pathologist is a witness to the facts found at postmortem and in subsequent examinations. The diagnoses do constitute opinion, in whole or in part, but they are in the written record, and the pathologist may choose not to elaborate. Courts often consider the pathologist as an expert, whether qualified by legal procedure or not, and attorneys will use that to seek elaboration of the opinions given in the autopsy report.

Of first importance, the pathologist will often be required to give a deposition, at which time attorneys can freely ask questions that may or may not appear in a court proceeding, including questions of opinion about the case. Under the federal rules of civil procedure, and in most states, experts should not be deposed except under extraordinary circumstances. In practice, however, attorneys almost always agree to deposing each other's experts. Since money is usually the issue, the attorneys are having a "trial by combat" of their expert witnesses in hopes of settlement before reaching trial.

Since the majority of suits are settled without coming to trial, the process of deposition is important.

While the deposition may seem less official than an appearance in court, it is not. The pathologist should prepare as carefully for a deposition as for an appearance in court. The casual nature of the deposition process, lawyers bantering, having coffee, and so on, should not lull one into a false sense of ease or casual speculation, on or off the record.

The deposition is part of the process of discovery and means just that; the attorneys are trying to learn as much as they can about the case, what you know and are willing to say, and what kind of witness you might be before a judge and/or jury. In many ways it is like an audition for a part in a play. Invariably, you will have been called or subpoenaed by one side, and the attorney or attorneys for that side will discuss your role, what type of questions they will ask, and what you may expect from the attorneys of the other side. It is important, however difficult, to keep in mind that you are a disinterested party whose task is to provide the court with information that will permit a proper and informed judgment to be rendered. This is as true of the deposition as the trial; the better informed the attorneys are, the better they can do their job of advocacy, and it is the pathologist's task, as a witness to fact, to see that they clearly understand the postmortem findings and report.

Even though you are appearing as a witness only with regard to the postmortem findings, attorneys will usually ask questions beyond that limited purview. They are not interested in the pathology per se; they are interested in what that pathology says about who did what, when, why, and did they do it correctly or incorrectly. An example is fatal peritonitis as a result of a torn rectum. You can answer the question, how was the rectum torn, by listing the possible causes and giving probability. It is most likely it was done during rectal examination. Then, you will be asked if that occurred in this particular case. Your answer is that you do not know; you can only state that to be the most likely possibility. To say that is what happened in this case is to give an opinion. With the first answer you may not be asked to appear at trial. With the second answer you almost certainly will be asked to appear and support that opinion under direct and cross-examination.

The findings in the autopsy report may be questioned. The attorney, in this case, has had another expert examine your report, perhaps including the microscopic slides. The opinion of that pathologist does not agree with yours, and the attorney's questions will be designed to find out if you are truly competent, and have interpreted the lesions appropriately and according to accepted standards. You should have been made aware of this adversarial report and should have a copy of it for consideration before the deposition. If such a report is alluded to in questioning, and you have not seen it, state that you have not seen it and cannot comment until you have. It is not proper, and your attorney will see to it, that you be taken by surprise by reports of other experts.

Every answer, every statement, that you make on the record during a deposition can be used, verbatim or otherwise, during trial. Be careful to think through the reply or statement that you make, and be certain that it is precisely what you want to say. If you are in any doubt of the question, ask for restatement or rephrasing. If you do not know the answer, say so. Do not hesitate to say that you believe yourself unqualified to give an opinion. Anything recorded during the deposition can appear in court. It will often appear in court after you have been asked and have answered a question. If your answer does not agree with the one you gave to the same or a similar question during the deposition, your testimony is seriously impaired, and you may, in fact, be impeached. The opposing attorney will have studied your deposition in detail and developed his questions in order to dilute, impair, or completely discredit you as a witness.

Nothing of what has been said should be construed to mean that one refuses to cooperate in either answering questions or the discovery process; this is not the case. Many pathologists, many people, do not wish to be involved in legal proceedings in any way. Involvement with horses assures that the pathologist will some day become involved, like it or not. It is by far better to accept the inevitable and be as cooperative as possible, even cheerful, when dealing with attorneys. They have their job to do and be assured that they will do it. A surly, monosyllabic manner will not make your job or their job any easier.

You will usually be asked to bring to the deposition all materials in your possession that are relevant to the case; certain items may be specified. If your appearance is as the result of a subpoena *duces tecum,* you are legally required to provide everything asked for and relevant, if it exists. This raises difficult questions. If you have notes made during the postmortem, while reading slides, or reviewing the literature, this material is covered by subpoena. You may well not wish to have your random thoughts, jargon, and shorthand subjected to adversarial scrutiny. One answer, of course, is to destroy such notes as they are made, so that they do not exist on paper, computer disk, or elsewhere when the subpoena arrives. Such materials are easily misinterpreted, or your opinion may have changed since the notes were made. Since you are not on trial, it is your best judgment of the facts that should be available, and not random notes, which may have been part of your thinking processes as you developed that judgment. As a point of law, however, such materials are covered by subpoena if they exist. Obviously, one can destroy the materials after being subpoenaed. Attorneys know that happens, and, even with exquisitely careful wording, may indicate that might be a good idea. In fact, it is illegal.

You may well have supplementary notes and materials, which you do not wish to destroy, either in fact or in appearance. It may be material, for example, which will eventually be published as a case report, compilation of cases, and so forth. Discuss this possibility with your attorney. He or she, and only he or she, can request the court to rule that the documents and materials in question are protected from discovery.

Do not bring notes, other than as discussed above, or have notes with you to remind you of anything. This is true of both deposition and trial. You must do your preparation beforehand and have the material essentially memorized. Any printed or written material, including reprints, books, and drawings, can become part of the official record if you bring them to deposition or trial. These admonitions are not intended to deny proper information to the attorneys. Your thought processes as you developed your report, or your opinion, in the case of an expert witness, is simply none of their business. They are to have your best, final judgment and are not to be parties to your thinking as you proceeded to that judgment. Attorneys, needless to say, feel differently about that.

Attorneys use three basic approaches in their questioning: (a) apparently neutral, just the facts and nothing but the facts; (b) friendly, we're just good, old boys chatting; and/or (c) frankly aggressive, adversarial—I know you're lying and you know it, too, and I'm going to see to it that everybody knows it. No matter what the approach, your responses should be clear, concise, and neutral. No matter how relaxed or angry you might be, it is imperative that your state of mind remain your own. Sulky, defensive, offended replies indicate to the questioner that further questioning might provoke an outburst useful in discrediting you as a reliable witness or in eliciting potentially useful information. You are responsible for providing factual evidence and expert opinion and should do so in a dispassionate manner. The attorney is not involved with you as a personality. He or she neither likes you nor dislikes you; you are simply part of his or her work. Often enough, after a thorough grilling, the proceedings go off the record, and your tormentor will say something like, "sorry, just part of my job. Like some coffee?" One of the authors was once grilled unmercifully for over 6 hours by an attorney who was a friend before that and after that.

Some attorneys use all three approaches, seemingly at random. Do not ever believe that an attorney is doing anything at random. It is almost always true that they have done more homework on the case than you have. You feel somewhat secure in your training and experience. They know they don't know, and they work hard to become expert, and will often surprise you with the breadth, if not depth, of their knowledge.

Be very careful when you cite literature in discussion with attorneys and, particularly, during deposition or trial. They will read that citation and, if a book, the whole book. It is routine and proper, once having established in court that you are relying in any measure on information from a book, to ask you questions about any other matter included in that book. The book has become a measure of your expertise. If you must cite a book, be certain you know it from cover to cover. In the best case do not cite books but the journal articles from which the material in the book was derived. If your experience coincides with text material, even if your knowledge initially came from the text, cite your experience and knowledge, not the book.

It is essential that preparation for answering specific questions from literature references be flawless; such articles should be committed to memory. If, for example, it is your opinion that some percentage of equine melanomas have malignant biological behavior, references may be cited. It is not necessary to argue that many are benign or to argue in refutation of other opinions, which may say that all, for example, are benign.

You will usually be advised to take your time with answers, to request clarification if necessary, to answer as fully as you like. The latter is important. Under no circumstances are you required to answer yes or no. If badgered to do so, simply state that you cannot answer or that you can answer, but that qualification is necessary, and proceed immediately with the qualifying statements. Only a poor attorney will try to interrupt, and will immediately be reprimanded by the judge. The good attorney will listen carefully, looking for his or her next question in your qualifying statements. The yes or no demand of television courtrooms is grossly inaccurate and not allowed in the real world.

Expert witness

What has been said above concerns the pathologist directly involved with a given case. You may be asked to be an expert witness; you are asked to review and give opinions on a matter or case in which you were not directly involved. It is your choice to become an expert witness. You cannot be subpoenaed as an expert because you were not directly involved. Remember, though, that involvement with the case could involve such things as reviewing slides for another pathologist, discussing it on the telephone, and so on. If asked to be an expert witness, be certain that you have not been involved with the matter in any way whatsoever. If in doubt, explain the situation to the attorney requesting your services. There are numerous texts on being an expert witness, but the best source of information is the attorney for whom you choose to work.

As an expert witness you will be asked to give opinions as to cause, responsibility for actions, behavior of principals in the case, and so on. It is obvious, perhaps, that lines of distinction are often unclear. A pathological diagnosis may be purely factual—the femur was broken. The opinion comes when you are asked if it could have been repaired or if the fracture occurred because of negligent care of fences by farm personnel. Always your opinion will be wanted for matters extending beyond the strictly pathological. The pathological diagnoses are usually accepted as such; the attorney wants to go beyond that to the causes and the actions of humans, which may have led to the pathological diagnosis. As already discussed, however, your gross and microscopic findings may come in question when another expert has given contrary views. You will have seen the contrary report and should be prepared to counter. The opposing attorney would like to discredit you as a pathologist on factual grounds such as this. That is a certain way to dispose of you as a witness. He or she knows, however, that it is technically more difficult to do so. Being a pathologist of experience, board certified, and so on does not mean that every effort will not be made to discredit you on any and all grounds. That's what the process is all about, and, as already emphasized, it has nothing to do with you personally.

One becomes an expert witness by choice, not by subpoena, and there are a number of reasons to do so. The first is simply the conviction that one's expertise should be made available in the interests of fairness and justice. One may feel an obligation to appear on behalf of professional colleagues in liability cases, while not appearing in opposition to such colleagues. That is your judgment. If agreeing to serve for a colleague, however, the case should stand on its factual merits. If you feel your colleague was at fault, do not serve as a witness to falsehood.

It is a fact that some veterinarians (and others) appear as expert witnesses primarily for money. On average such work pays very well; one charges per hour at least what is charged by attorneys in the area. If one's motivation is money, we have little more to say. Beware, however, the appellation, quickly earned among attorneys, that you are a hired gun. The attorney who asks you to be an expert witness will check, or has already checked, your past record because his or her case, in part, stands or falls upon your credibility. Be assured that the opposing attorney will be even more thorough. There are companies that specialize in providing information about expert witnesses for attorneys. Be completely honest about previous litigation experience; the attorneys will find out or already know.

There are as many ways for an expert and attorney to work together as there are attorneys and experts. The general approach is that the expert should be brought in early and contribute to the development of the case, providing information and expertise that the attorney does not possess. This approach is not only more satisfying for the expert, but usually leads to more effective presentation of the case, abandonment of an untenable position, or perhaps abandonment of the case entirely.

You will be asked to provide the attorney with a report on materials which he or she has provided. Even though this may be a preliminary report, which is modified as new information is discovered, it should be carefully thought out and worded since it may well appear at either deposition or trial. Even if you prepare a second or third report, which are superseding, those original reports may still be brought out during discovery. If a later report does not agree with an earlier report, the reasons for the change should be carefully delineated. Keep only copies of reports that you actually submit. Drafts, notes, and preparatory scribblings are best destroyed as soon as the report is prepared.

The type of case to avoid, at all times, is that presented to you with the statement that the case is going to trial, and an expert is needed to support the case in court. That is, purely and entirely, hired gun. Even if you could support the case, which was developed without your assistance, it is rarely advisable to do so. Attorneys vary in capability and experience, and one cannot hope to assure oneself of their competence if you meet them for the first time outside the courtroom. One of the authors did that once, and the attorney, totally and miserably unprepared, made fools of both of us with inept questioning. You cannot present your expert opinion in court by yourself. Legal procedure requires that the attorney question you in order to bring out facts and opinion. That must be carefully and thoroughly discussed and rehearsed beforehand.

As an expert witness the tendency is almost overwhelming to become an advocate for those for whom you are working. No one likes to lose. As best possible, maintain your objectivity and role as provider of expert information. Here, as for all legal matters, do not talk about a case with anyone other than the attorney who retained you unless he or she agrees or asks that you do so. The amount of money involved in a litigation, for example, even the outcome of the litigation, is not the expert's business. Do not become involved with the litigants in any way, however slight, before or after you have appeared. Be polite but do not engage in small talk, or accept an invitation to lunch or a ride to the airport. Your dealings are entirely with the attorney who has retained you. If in doubt, ask for advice.

Your attorney may request that you remain, after you have testified, in order to advise about cross-examination of opposition witnesses. Do not remain in the courtroom unless asked to do so. You do not have an interest in the outcome of the case. Some courts permit experts to hear the testimony of opposing experts, while others do not. Your attorney will know the rules of the court. If in doubt, ask what you are to do.

Before agreeing to be an expert witness, be certain that you have the time to fulfill your responsibility; a considerable amount may be required. Be certain, as well, that you have no personal agenda coloring your approach to the case. Years ago one of the authors was an expert witness in a matter involving a horse that suffered a massive failure of the carpus during a race after many intraarticular injections of steroids. He informed the attorney that one reason for my involvement was my opposition to steroid abuse in racehorses. Gently and effectively, he taught me that the litigation was not to decide principle, but to determine liability in the specific case. If one wishes to argue a principle, do not try to do it as an expert witness.

As an expert witness at a trial, not in the deposition, you must be qualified through questioning by your attorney. You will be asked your training, experience, and so forth. The attorney for the other side may try to disqualify you. He or she may read a definition of pathology from a dictionary and ask if that is correct, hoping, with your agreement, to indicate to the court that you are not qualified to give an opinion about anything other than postmortem findings. If your testimony, indeed, does extend beyond that, your answer should be of the nature, "yes, that is correct, but I also consult with practicing veterinarians, conduct a private practice of my own, have additional training in neurology," or whatever is appropriate to indicate to the court your qualifications to give an opinion in the case. Usually your attorney should qualify you as a veterinarian first and, then, as a pathologist within that profession. As a veterinarian, first, you are qualified to give an opinion about clinical matters.

If you are considering becoming an expert witness, for whatever reason, remember that appearing at deposition or in court is, essentially, a performance, akin to a dissertation defense or a talk at a meeting. Your appearance and manner, your presentation of yourself, is as important, in the final analysis, as the factual expertise you may possess. An attorney came to the waiting room to bring me into court to testify, saying "Hey, hey, it's showtime!" However frivolous that may sound, it is true. Good trial lawyers and expert witnesses realize and accept that. If you freeze up giving a toast, or sweat for weeks over a 10-minute talk to the Rotary Club, expert witnessing is probably not for you.

You should, with great care, decide if you are indeed an expert. Recognize your limitations. It is a devastating experience to have your limits overreached in open court.

When testifying, the witness is to direct answers to the jury, not to the attorney asking the questions. Clear, concise, nontechnical answers should be given and repeated, in modified form, if the jury does not seem to comprehend. Analogies, similes, and metaphors are useful tools for getting the message across, but must be used with great care and only if discussed with your attorney in advance. They can be as much of a trap on cross-examination as they seemed useful on direct examination. It is often difficult to translate technical matters into homey, everyday language, but that is part of the task of the expert witness, working and rehearsing with the attorney. Juries will appreciate that you are trying to inform them; they will not appreciate professional arrogance and "talking down." Serving time as a juror is excellent preparation for serving as a witness.

It is uncommon for a pathologist to become a defendant in a litigation. Under such circumstances (and, happily, the authors have no experience of that) one takes the advice of the physician not to treat oneself. Obtain an attorney experienced in medicolegal matters and suggest experts who can support your case.

Veterinarians with malpractice insurance are often disconcerted when the insurance carrier agrees to settle the case without going to trial. They want a trial at law to clear their names, vindicate judgment, and so on. While perfectly natural, and even laudable, remember that the insurance company is taking the financial risk. Their concern is not with your reputation, but with their bottom line. They will settle if they feel that is the financially sound thing to do. If you do not want that to happen, you will have to self-insure.

Reports

The necessity for complete, accurate reports is well known, if often observed only in the breach. We shall note here only those matters that are peculiar to the forensic aspect of horse postmortems.

The pathologist must realize that the quality of his or her interpretation may depend on data provided by the referring veterinarian. A written history may suggest approaches or tests that might otherwise not be used. Fluids and ingesta may be collected and saved if the history suggests poisoning even though tissue changes are not present. Antemortem observations, radiographs, clinical pathology data, and other material should be reviewed when available. While you cannot be "caught off-guard" in court by such data, failure to include comment in the postmortem report might be detrimental to the case.

The basic autopsy report, containing gross, microscopic, and laboratory findings and the interpretation of the case, is submitted to the attending veterinarian with a summary report to the owner, manager, or insurance representative. If requested by the owner, manager, or insurance representative, the basic autopsy report is provided to them with the notation that the interpretation of the report should be taken with the attending veterinarian. There is little purpose in withholding the basic report since, in the event of legal action, it will be subpoenaed. As already discussed the pathologist may feel that comments or observations should be recorded for future research purposes, but should not be available to laypersons. One is, then, on the horns of a dilemma. Separate records may be kept as one's personal files. In the event of legal action the pathologist will be asked if such notes or files exist. The honest answer will eventuate in a subpoena. A not honest answer is . . . a not honest answer. As noted previously your attorney can request the court to protect certain materials from discovery, but that is only a possibility and not a guarantee. It is undoubtedly best that all records should be so clear, noncontradictory, and brilliant that there is no problem about their appearance in public, however unlikely that may be.

Specific forensic matters

By far the most difficult cases, in every sense, are those animals that die suddenly, with few or no clinical signs and little relevant history. Most, but far from all, occur on the racetrack. Rarely can the postmortem be undertaken in a timely manner. The history, if any, is usually vague, if not palpably deceptive. It is possible that there is nothing relevant, but often enough there is an air of doubt and suspicion. The presence of an insurance adjuster, unless a wise and experienced one, can compound obfuscation.

The insurance adjuster is employed to collect and examine the facts in a case in order to determine if the terms of a policy have been met, and whether a valid claim is being made. Adjusters always require a copy of the postmortem report and may request that they attend the postmortem. Try to cooperate fully with them, even the inexperienced know-it-alls; encourage them to attend the postmortem, respond fully to their questions, and allow photographs if they wish. As a rule adjusters are thorough and professional and respond to respect shown for the job that they have to do. On occasion the adjuster can provide the pathologist with information not made available by farm or racetrack personnel. The role of the adjuster vis-à-vis the veterinary pathologist is akin to that of the investigating detective and the forensic medical pathologist.

Encourage attendance at a postmortem by the veterinarian(s), owners, and managers. Discuss the case openly and frankly with them, show them the lesions, and respond to their questions. Make it a point to summarize the findings and interpretations when the postmortem has been completed, what more is to be done, and so forth. There are far fewer complaints and far fewer frivolous legal proceedings with an open-door policy.

Sudden death on the racetrack

There are two cases: the animal dies during training or racing or dies in the stall. In the first case an obvious cause of death may be found, such as massive hemorrhaging into the lungs. Microscopic and cultural studies should be done. While massive pulmonary hemorrhage may be the result of asphyxia, in some cases there is an acute bacterial pneumonia (*Streptococcus zooepidemicus*) not suspected before the animal entered the race or work. Sections of the nasal mucosa may provide evidence of viral infection as the primary disease. It is not unusual for horses to experience viral respiratory infection on the racetrack, and quite usual for trainers to return them to training and racing before full biological recovery.

All too often no cause of death can be found. Platt (1982), for example, found a cause of death in only about 50% of such cases. The heart is usually suspected and rarely implicated, even with intensive follow-up studies. Stroke, cerebrovascular accident, is the second suspected cause, but is virtually unknown in horses.

The animal dying suddenly in the stall will have no clinical history or one describing terminal asphyxial convulsions. The postmortem is almost always negative, with only an enlarged spleen and petechial hemorrhages in the respiratory system to suggest primary shock.

The pathologist is on the spot in these cases. There is no result less satisfactory to all concerned than no result. The suspicions raised by the sudden death are compounded and rarely can be resolved. It is obvious that toxicological studies should be undertaken, and equally obvious that they rarely are because of the costs involved in a blind search. The owner of an insured horse is responsible, under the terms of most insurance policies, for having the postmortem performed, including follow-up studies. They are rarely willing to agree to such costs, and the insurance underwriters usually stand on the terms of the policy and will not agree to assume the cost.

In any event toxicological studies are probably of little use unless there are clinical signs and lesions that can be correlated with the findings. Most horses in racing, and other performance events as well, at least in North America, are given a variety of compounds and drugs. Forensic chemists of experience realize this. They further realize that they are limited by time and cost in attempting to characterize the variety of foreign materials, which may be found in the urine and blood of horses, much less determining if those materials are biologically active in the quantities present.

Horses are feloniously killed, usually in order to collect insurance. A profession has apparently developed to do such things by contract. Various methods have been used, including curarelike drugs with plastic bag asphyxiation. Despite one's best efforts and the collaboration of experienced investigators and adjustors, more escape prosecution than are caught.

This gloomy picture can be somewhat mitigated by the following. During a postmortem on a case of sudden and/or suspicious death, care should be particularly directed to finding injection sites. Bleeding around the jugular veins is easily found. Injection sites in the subcutaneous tissues and muscle of the neck and rear leg require careful skinning, not restricted to the usual sites of injection. If found, such injection sites should be removed en bloc and saved in an appropriately sealed and labeled container. Often the material injected leaks into the perijugular tissues, or is present in the tissues in fairly high concentration in subcutaneous and intramuscular injection sites. Obviously the chemist has a better opportunity to identify the material injected. Even when the history indicates that therapy was given, these sites should be saved for eventual chemical study.

If materials are saved for toxicological analysis, it is of primary importance that the containers be sealed, dated, and stored, so that continuous control and possession—chain of custody—of the material can be established. If it can be shown that there was any period when the material could have been tampered with after collection, the toxicological evidence is worthless. It is peculiar that evidence of uninterrupted control is meticulously examined for toxicological materials, but not for histological specimens and sections. In fact, a chain of custody is required for all, and, in any given case, an attorney may bring continuous control of histological materials into question.

When bleeding around the jugular veins is found, with or without a history of an injection having been given, particular attention should be directed to the source of the blood. It may be from either the vein or the carotid artery. Careful dissection, including opening the vessels, usually reveals the injection site. Not all intravenous injections are given by veterinarians, and inadvertent carotid puncture is frequent enough even when given by an experienced individual. Almost any material given by intracarotid injection can kill a horse. This is not to imply criminal intent, only that a cause of death can be found if the carotid has been punctured. It may be noted that "successful" intracarotid injection must be done with a syringe. Attempts to infuse fluid by gravity into the carotid fail because of the pressure within the artery.

Sudden death elsewhere

Although broken down in this manner, it is apparent that no absolute restriction of causes to venues is implied. Two general cases may be considered: an animal found dead in the field or paddock without premonitory signs, or death immediately or within minutes after injection of a drug or compound.

In the latter case there will be no lesions except those of primary shock. Intracarotid injection should be looked for. A history of repeated, particularly intravenous, injections of a given agent suggests the possibility of an **allergic drug reaction**. This has been seen with intravenous penicillins and injectable vitamin mixtures. While one might hope to find lesions of anaphylactic shock, in fact none have been seen in such cases, only in experimental cases of sensitization to foreign proteins, as discussed in the chapter on shock (see Chapter 17).

Often there is no history of repeated injections, and one is left with a presumptive diagnosis, **untoward drug reaction**, which cannot be confirmed. Untoward drug reactions seem to be more common in individuals in a high state of training, but there is no hard data. There is firm anecdotal evidence that highly trained horses react unfavorably, though rarely fatally, to various vaccinations at a higher rate than animals not in a high state of training.

In the case of the animal found dead, there are several possibilities. Lightning strike, acute gastric dilatation with or without rupture, torsion of the ascending colon, exhaustion shock, and Theiler's disease are all prospects, and all can occur when the animal has not been observed, for example, during the night, on weekends, or during sales with most personnel off the farm. Unattended foaling mares may have delayed delivery with a dead foal with lesions of neonatal asphyxia. An artery may rupture during foaling and the mare found dead. Rupture of the ovarian artery can occur in older mares long before foaling.

Lightning strike can be difficult. If the characteristic arborizing singeing of hair is present, the diagnosis is established. In most cases the lightning strikes the withers and the arborizing pattern can be followed to the coronary band of one or, rarely, both front feet. While opinions differ widely, our experience is that such arborizations are found in about 50% of deaths caused by lightning strike. In its absence, the acutely engorged spleen, history of thunderstorm, and absence of other lesions are strongly suggestive. If there is fracture of the thoracic vertebrae, as well, we consider the diagnosis established. The immediate cause of death is primary shock the result of the electrical charge causing irreversible fibrillation of the heart. Fibrillation occurs in all fatal electrical shock in horses whatever the source of the electricity.

Horses are killed by lightning if they are struck directly, skin singeing being present, or if, in general, they are within 300 m of the strike, the electricity coursing through the ground and into the horse through the feet. In these cases, of course, no skin lesions are seen. Horses near the edge of the 300-m zone may show no disease or illness as such, but they can behave strangely: fearful, easily frightened, off feed, and somewhat ataxic for up to 24–36 hours after the strike. Although speculative, it is possible that these animals received enough electricity to elicit the signs observed, but not enough to cause cardiac fibrillation and death.

Intestinal clostridiosis (Weirup 1977) may be suggested as a cause of death, but it is not yet clear that this is, indeed, a specific disease entity (see Chapter 17, "Shock").

Bee stinging, as a cause of sudden death, has been suggested since Aristotle (Balme 1991). We have seen no example or reports of lesions.

Anesthetic deaths

These are thorny problems for the practicing veterinarian. With the exception of academic clinics and large surgical practices, a qualified anesthesiologist may not be available and adequate control of the anesthetized animal not achieved. This is particularly true, as is well known, of old, obese, or debilitated animals. It also seems to be the case with individuals in a high state of training and may be associated with the untoward drug reactions discussed earlier.

The postmortem examination is principally directed to finding a reason for the animal not being able to withstand anesthesia: cirrhosis of the liver, renal disease, heart disease, and so on. Such contributing lesions are only occasionally found. It is certainly incumbent upon the surgeon and/or anesthesiologist to routinely screen for such problems when time permits.

A rare cause of death under anesthesia occurs with attempts to repair fractures of large long bones. Embolization of fatty tissue from the marrow cavity has been found in the brain and in the lungs, with significant hemorrhage, in a few cases.

In the absence of contributory lesions the pathologist is left with a diagnosis of shock under anesthesia, speculating about untoward drug reactions and such. Repeated exposure to fluothane has been implicated in anesthetic deaths in humans, but there has been no definite implication of fluothane in the horse. During a period in which methoxyfluothane was used in one clinic, there were several anesthetic deaths with striking pulmonary edema. No further deaths, with such pulmonary edema, were seen when use of that agent was discontinued. No further studies were done.

An animal may survive anesthesia, only to die unexpectedly during recovery. Such deaths were more common in earlier days of surgery under general anesthesia, either intravenous or inhalation, than today. The principal finding in those cases, apart from trauma inflicted during recovery, was severe dehydration. This was so severe that the tissues fairly crunched when handled, serous membranes adhering to each other and to the prosector. With the recognition of the heavy fluid loss during prolonged surgery, and in colic cases the already existing depletion of fluid, and adequate fluid replacement before and during surgery, such cases are less often seen.

Neurological disease and chronic locomotor disease

Insurance policies are written to cover death from natural causes and destruction on humane grounds. They are not written to cover loss of use. And thereby hangs a tale. We shall take as the paradigmatic case that of the yearling horse with ataxia as a result of cervical stenotic myelopathy. The problems presented in this case can be generalized to other chronic conditions that prevent the horse from working or racing.

With the diagnosis of wobbler established and agreed to by all concerned, the question is one of destruction. The animal has no useful future but is obviously not suffering acute, unmanageable pain. Insurance adjusters and underwriters are notoriously inconsistent in their response to the opinion that the horse should be put down on humane grounds. Some always agree, others never agree, and many apparently make a judgment based on the value of the trainer and/or owner as a buyer of insurance. My criterion, as an expert in neurology (the problem rarely arises for the pathologist), is that if the horse is or would be unable to care for itself and live a normal life (for a horse) in a natural setting, it should be put down. It is well to state that opinion and forget the case.

The pathologist may become involved when asked to give an opinion whether the damage found at postmortem was sufficient to justify destruction. The consistent reply is that such a determination has to be made by the attending and consulting clinical veterinarians. The pathologist cannot second-guess the clinical opinion in such a matter, unless, of course, he or she also gave a clinical opinion. The pathologist certainly can, and should, second-guess the clinical *diagnosis*, but not matters of judgment about humane destruction.

Starvation, abuse, mistreatment, and shooting

The lesions of cachexia, inanition, are well known and the same as in other species. In most cases the cause—chronic disease, parasitism, old age, and/or neglected teeth—is evident. Neglect does occur. Animals may be abandoned, pastures be disastrously overgrazed, wells go dry. Such cases are often referred by officials of humane organizations and legal action can be expected. The pathologist tries to determine if criminal activity or stupidity has caused the death of an animal. In many localities, there is a fine line between misdemeanor charges for animal neglect and prosecution for felonious animal cruelty. The pathological evidence may not resolve the matter, but evidence of severe trauma, fractures, or gunshot wounds should be carefully described and documented by photographs and/or radiographs as evidence of possible felony.

One may encounter an animal with strong evidence of mistreatment, neglect, or cruel treatment without clinical history for such mistreatment or involvement of humane or police officials. It is the duty of a veterinarian, pathologist in this case, to report such matters to proper authorities. Remember it is not your task to indict or prosecute. Present your opinion and supporting data as requested by the authorities. Further action on your side is not appropriate unless officially requested.

In addition to dehydration, drastic weight loss, and serous atrophy of fat, there is starvation anemia. Cohrs (1961) pointed out the need for differentiating the anemia of starvation and equine infectious anemia. This can be particularly troublesome with chronic, recurring infectious anemia where cachexia and inanition are common. In both cases there will be hemosiderosis of spleen and liver. With equine infectious anemia there is proliferation of lymphoid tissue, while with starvation the lymphoid tissue is atrophic. Serological tests for infectious anemia are, of course, available if sera was saved before death.

Horses are shot. When legitimate, the shot is to the forehead. With virtually any caliber, .22 and above, the bullet goes through the cranium to lodge in the neck in the vicinity of the pharyngeal soft tissues and larynx. Larger calibers may do astonishing exit damage to the ventral cranium.

Felonious, malevolent, and accidental shooting does occur, though infrequently in our experience. Patient examination is necessary to determine the point of entry, path, exit, and organs damaged. If the missile can be recovered, it should be handled like a toxicological specimen as eventual material evidence.

Bibliography

Abbott A C and Prendergast J 1934 Histological variations in animals thyroids in Western Canada *Canadian Medical Association Journal* 31: 465-473

Ackerman N, Johnson J H, and Dorn C R 1977 Navicular disease in the horse: risk factors, radiographic changes, and response to therapy *Journal of the American Veterinary Medical Association* 170: 182-87

Ackermann R 1939 Über die Damfigkeit zugrunde liegenden Lungenveränderungen beim Pferde. *Dissertation*, Leipzig

Acland H M and Kenney R M 1983 Lesions of contagious equine metritis in mares. *Veterinary Pathology* 20: 330-41

Acland H M, Gunson D E, Gillette D M 1983 Ulcerative duodenitis in foals *Veterinary Pathology* 20: 653-661

Acland H M, Mann P C, Robertson J L, Divers T J, Lichtensteiger C 1984 Toxic hepatopathy in neonatal foals *Veterinary Pathology* 21: 3-9

Adams L G, Dollahite J W, Romane W M, Bullard T L, and Bridges C H 1969 Cystitis and ataxia associated with sorghum ingestion by horses *Journal of the American Veterinary Medical Association* 155: 518-524

Adams O R 1961 Fibrotic myopathy and ossifying myopathy in the hindlegs of horses *Journal of the American Veterinary Medical Association* 139: 1089

Adams O R 1966 *Lameness in Horses* 2nd Ed. Philadelphia, Lea and Febiger

Adams R, Calderwood-Mays M B, and Peyton L C 1988a Malignant lymphoma in three horses with ulcerative pharyngitis *Journal of the American Veterinary Medical Association* 191: 674-676

Adams R, Koterba M, Cudd T C, and Baker W A 1988b Exploratory celiotomy for suspected urinary tract disruption in neonatal foals: A review of 18 cases *Equine Veterinary Journal* 20: 13-17

Adams S B, Steckel R, and Blevins W 1985 Diskospondylitis in 5 horses *Journal of the American Veterinary Medical Association* 186: 270-72

Aho R 1987 Mycological studies of *Microsporum equinum* isolated in Finland, Sweden, and Norway *Journal of Medical and Veterinary Mycology* 25: 255-260

Ainsworth G C and Austwick P K C 1959 Fungal diseases of animals, Farnham Royal Commonwealth Agriculture Bureau Review Series, No. 6, p 148ff

Akashi H, Konishi S, and Ogata M 1975 Studies on equine viral arteritis II. A serological survey of equine viral arteritis in horses imported in 1973/74 *Japanese Journal of Veterinary Science* 38: 71-73

Akerblom A 1930 *Hufmechanismus des Pferdes* Hannover

Akerblom A 1934 Über die Etiologie und Pathogenese der Hufrehe beim Pferde *Skandinavisk Archiv Physiologie* (Suppl) 68

Albert the Great 1987 *Man and the Beasts*. Scanlon J J (Trans) Binghamton New York, Medieval and Renaissance Texts and Studies

Alexander D J 1982 Ecological aspects of influenza A viruses in animals and their relationship to human influenza: a review *Journal of the Royal Society of Medicine* 75: 799-810

Alexander F 1909 Über die Entzundung der Kronbeinbeugesehne am Vorderfuss des Pferdes *Monatschrift Tierheilkunde* 20: 193-223

Alexander F 1946 The rate of passage of food residues through the digestive tract of the horse *Journal of Comparative Pathology Therapeutics* 56: 266-68

Alexander F 1950 A radiological study of the digestive tract of the foal *Quarterly Journal of Experimental Physiology* 36: 213-17

Alexander F 1952a Some functions of the large intestine of the horse *Quarterly Journal of Experimental Physiology* 37: 205-14

Alexander F 1952b The effects of some humoral agents on the horse ileum *British Journal of Pharmacology* 7: 25-32

Alexander F 1962 The concentration of certain electrolytes in the digestive tract of the horse and pig *Research Veterinary Science* 3: 78-84

Alexander F and Benzie D 1951 A radiological study of the digestive tract of the foal *Quarterly Journal of Experimental Physiology* 36: 213-217

Alexander J T and Rooney J R 1972 The biomechanics, surgery, and prognosis of equine fractures 1967-71 *Proceedings American Association of Equine Practitioners* 18: 219-26

Alexander R A and Nietz W O 1935 The transmission of louping ill by ticks (Rhipicephalus appendiculatus) *Veterinary Journal* 89: 320-323

Alexander R McN 1989 On the synchronization of breathing with running in wallabies (Macropus spp.) and horses (Equus caballus) *Journal of Zoology London* 218: 69-85

Alexander R McN 1990 Elastic mechanisms in the locomotion of vertebrates *Netherlands Journal of Zoology* 40: 93-105

Alexander R McN and Bennet-Clark H C 1977 Storage of elastic strain energy in muscle and other tissues *Nature* 265: 114-17

Alexopoulos C J and Mims C W 1979 *Introductory Mycology* (3rd edition) New York, John Wiley and Sons

Alfaro A A and Mendoza L 1990 Four cases of equine bone lesions caused by *Pythium insidiosum Equine Veterinary Journal* 22: 295-297

Al-Kafawi AA, Al-Ani F K, Al-Bassam L S, and Youkob A

Y 1977 Haematological changes in Arabian horses infected with glanders *Veterinary Record* 101: 427

Allam N M and Lemcke R M 1975 Mycoplasmas isolated from the respiratory tract of horses *Journal of Hygiene* 74: 385-407

Allen B and Archer R K 1971 Haptoglobins in the horse *Veterinary Record* 89: 106-109

Allen D A, Clark E S, Moore J N, and Prasse K W 1990 Evaluation of equine digital Starling forces and hemodynamics during early laminitis *American Journal of Veterinary Research* 151: 1930-1934

Allen G R and Bryans J T 1986 Molecular epizootiology, pathogenesis, and prophylaxis of equine herpesvirus-1 infections *Progress Veterinary Microbiology Immunology* 2: 78-144

Allen P C, Frerichs W M, and Holbrook A A 1975 Experimental acute *Babesia caballi* infections I. Red blood cell dynamics *Experimental Parasitology* 37: 67-77

Alms M 1961 Fracture mechanics *Journal of Bone Joint Surgery* 43B: 162

Alstad A D and Berg I E 1979 Disseminated *Micronema deletrix* infection in the horse *Journal of the American Veterinary Medical Association* 174: 264-266

Altera D and Clark L 1970 Equine cutaneous mastocytosis *Path Vet* 7: 43-55

Amis T C, Pascoe J R, and Hornof W 1984 Topographic distribution of pulmonary ventilation and perfusion in the horse *American Journal of Veterinary Research* 45: 1597-1601

Amman E 1987 Strukturveränderungen im Strahlbein beim gesunder und lähmer Pferde *Dissertation*, Berne

Amman K and Fackelman G E 1971 *Wiener Tierärztliche Monatschrift* 58: 151-53

Ammann K 1939 Das Lungenemphsem des Pferdes und Rindes *Archiv Tierheilkunde* 74: 348-401

Amoss M S, Hood D M, Miller W G, Hightower D, McGrath J P, McMullan W C, and Scrutchfield L 1979 Equine laminitis: II. Elevation in serum testosterone associated with induced and naturally occurring laminitis *Journal of Equine Medicine Surgery* 3: 171-175

Amoss M S, Hood D M, Williams J D, Stephens K A, Gremmel S M, Grosenbaugh D A, and Olivier A 1988 Concentrations of plasma catecholamines, serum aldosterone and plasma renin activity following induced laminitis in the horse *Southwestern Veterinarian* 38: 16-25

Amtmann E, Muller H, and Sauer G 1980 Equine connective tissue tumors contain unintegrated bovine papilloma virus DNA *Journal of Virology* 35(3): 962-964

Andersen A C and Hart G H 1943 Histological changes in the retina of the vitamin A deficient horse *American Journal of Veterinary Research* 4: 307-17

Anderson C A and Divers T J 1983 Systemic granulomatous inflammation in a horse grazing hairy vetch *Journal of the American Veterinary Medical Association* 183: 569-570

Anderson G A, Mount M E, Vrins A A, and Ziemer E L 1983 Fatal acorn poisoning in a horse: pathological findings and diagnostic considerations *Journal of the American Veterinary Medical Association* 182: 1105-10

Anderson J K 1961 *Ancient Greek Horsemanship* Berkeley University California Press

Anderson W A and King J M 1988 Subclinical lumbar polyradiculopathy in multiple aged mammalian species *Cornell Veterinarian* 78: 185-189

Anderson W I, LaHunta A de, Vesely K R, Tucker G W 1990a Infarction of the pons and medulla oblongata caused by arteriolar thrombosis in a horse *Cornell Veterinarian* 80: 285-289

Anderson W I, Scott D W, and Crameri F M 1990b Two rare cutaneous neoplasms in horses: apocrine gland adenocarcinoma and carcinosarcoma *Cornell Veterinarian* 80: 339-345

Andrews E J 1971 Oxalate nephropathy in a horse *Journal of the American Veterinary Medical Association* 159: 49-52

Andrews F M, Rosol T J, Kohn C W, Reed S M, and Dibartola S P 1986 Bilateral renal hypoplasia in four young horses *Journal of American Medical Association* 189: 209-212

Angel K L, Spano J S, Schumacher J, and Kwapien R P 1991 Myelophthisic pancytopenia in a pony mare *Journal of the American Veterinary Medical Association* 198: 1039-1042

Angelos J, Oppenheim Y, Rebhun W, Mohammed, H, and Antczak D F 1988 Evaluation of breed as a risk factor for sarcoid and uveitis in horses *Animal Genetics* 19: 417-425

Anon. 1892/93 Retention cyst upon the epiglottis *American Veterinary Revue* 16: 464

Anon. 1940 Equine encephalomyelitis, 1935-1939 *Journal of the American Veterinary Medical Association* 96: 559-560

Antal R, Szabo I, Antal V, Vadja G, Polner A, Totth B, Szollar I, and Stipkovits L 1988 Respiratory disease of horses associated with mycoplasma infection *Journal of Veterinary Medicine* 35: 264-270

Antal A, Szabo I, Vadja G, Antal V D, Polner A, Totth B, Szollar I, and Stipkovits L 1989a Immunoglobulin concentration in the blood serum of foals suffering from pneumonia associated with mycoplasm infection *Archiv Experimental Veterinar Medizin* 43: 747-750

Antal V, Antal T, Szabo I, Vadja G, Polner A, Szollar I, Totth B, Laber G, and Stipkovits L 1989b Epizootiological examination of a respiratory disease associated with mycoplasma infection in horse *Archiv Experimental Veterinar Medizin* 43: 751-754

Anzai T, Kamada M, Kanemaru T, and Oikawa M 1989 Isolation of *Mycobacterium avium* complex from the thoroughbred racehorse with fatal pneumonia *Bulletin Equine Research Institute* 26: 73-7

Archer R K and Allen B S 1972 True hemophilia in horses *Veterinary Record* 91: 655-56

Aref S 1982 A random walk model for the migration of Strongylus vulgaris in the intestinal arteries of the horse *Cornell Veterinarian* 72: 64-75

Argenzio R A 1975 Functions of the equine large intestine

and their interrelationship in disease *Cornell Veterinarian* 65: 303-30

Argenzio R A, Lowe J E, Pickard D W, and Stevens C E 1974 Digesta passage and water exchange in the equine large intestine *American Journal of Physiology* 226: 1035-42

Arndt H J 1928 Bemerkungen zur Leberamyloidose bei russischen Pferden *Münchener Tierärztliche Wochenschrift* 79: 321-3

Arndt H J 1931 Über die Amyloidose der Serumpferde *Archiv wissenprakttierhlkunde* 63: 1-11

Asmundsson T, Gunnarsson E, and Johannsson T 1983 Haysickness in Icelandic horses: Precipitin tests and other studies *Equine Veterinary Journal* 15: 229-232

Attenburrow D P, Donnelly J J, and Soulsby E J L 1983 Periodic ophthalmia (recurrent uveitis) of horses: An evaluation of the aetiological role of microfilariae of *Onchocerca cervicalis* and the clinical management of the condition *Equine Veterinary Journal* 2 (supplement): 48-56

Auer J A, Watkins J P, White N A, Taylor T S, and Rooney J R 1986 Slab fractures of the fourth and intermediate carpal bones in five horses *Journal of the American Veterinary Medical Association* 188: 595-601

Aulage 1891/2 Lipoma *American Veterinary Revue* 15 Abstract from *Recueil Médecine Vétérinare.*

Austin R J and Dies K H 1981 *Klossiella equi* in the kidneys of a horse *Canadian Veterinary Journal* 22: 159-161

Averons M 1896/7 Biliary calculi *American Veterinary Revue* 20: 531-32

Awad F I, Amin M M, Salama S A, and Aly M M 1981 The incidence of African horsesickness antibodies in animals of various species in Egypt *Bulletin Animal Health Producers Africa* 29: 285

Axe J W 1906 *The horse and its treatment in health and disease* IV. Gresham, London

Badiali L, Abou-Youssef M H, Radwan A I, Hamdy F M, and Hildebrandt P K 1968 Moldy corn poisoning as the major cause of an encephalomalacia syndrome in Egyptian equidae *American Journal of Veterinary Research* 29: 2029-2035

Bailey G D and Love D N 1991 Oral associated bacterial infection in horses: studies on the normal anaerobic flora from the pharyngeal tonsillar surface and its association with lower respiratory tract and paraoral infections *Veterinary Microbiology* 367-379

Bain A M 1963 *Corynebacterium equi* infection in the equine *Australian Veterinary Journal 39: 116-121*

Bain A M 1966 The role of infestion in infertility in the Thoroughbred mare *Veterinary Record* 78: 168-173

Bain A M, Rofe J C, Hotson I K, and Murphy S 1969 *Habronema megastoma* larvae associated with pulmonary abscesses in a foal *Australian Veterinary Journal* 45: 101-102

Baird A N and Frelier P F 1990 Squamous cell carcinoma originating from an epithelial scar in a horse *Journal of the American Veterinary Medical Association* 196: 1999-2000

Baird J D 1971 Lactation tetany (eclampsia) in a Shetland pony mare *Australian Veterinary Journal* 47: 402-404

Baird J D 1974 Cerebellar hypoplasia and degeneration in part-Arab horses *Australian Veterinary Journal* 50: 25-28

Baird J D and Mackenzie C D 1974 Cerebellar hypoplasia and degeneration in part-Arab horses *Australian Veterinary J* 50(1): 25-28

Baker D and Kreeger J 1987 Infiltrative lipoma in the heart of a horse *Cornell Veterinarian* 77: 258-262

Baker G J 1970 Some aspects of equine dental disease *Equine Veterinary Journal* 2: 105-10

Baker G J 1974 Some aspects of equine dental decay *Equine Veterinary Journal* 6: 127-30

Baker G J 1979 A study of dental disease in the horse *Dissertation*, Glasgow

Baker H J and Lindsey J R 1968 Equine goiter due to excess dietary iodide *Journal of the American Veterinary Medical Association* 153: 1618-25

Baker J R 1973 A case of generalized avian tuberculosis in a horse *Veterinary Record* 93: 105-6

Baker J R and Ellis C E 1981a A survey of post mortem findings in 480 horses 1958 to 1980: (1) Causes of death *Equine Veterinary Journal* 13(1): 43-46

Baker J R and Ellis C E 1981b A survey of post mortem findings in 480 horses 1958 to 1980: (2) Disease processes not directly related to the cause of death *Equine Veterinary Journal* 13(1): 47-50

Baker J R and Leyland A 1973 Diarrhoea in the horse associated with stress and tetracycline therapy *Veterinary Record* 93: 583-4

Baker J R and Leyland A 1975 Histological survey of tumours of the horse, with particular reference to those of the skin *Veterinary Record* 96: 419-422

Baker J R and Ritchie H E 1974 Diabetes mellitus in the horse: a case report and review of the literature *Equine Veterinary Journal* 6: 7-11

Baker K P and Quinn P J 1978 A report on clinical aspects and histopathology of sweet itch *Equine Veterinary Journal* 10: 243-248

Balme D M (trans) 1991 *Aristotle History of Animals.* Books VII-X. Cambridge, Loeb Classical Library, Harvard University Press

Balozet L and Chainet L 1937 Epithelioma primitif du pancreas chez un cheval *Bulletin Academie Vétérinaire France* 10: 301-4

Banham G G 1882 Stringhalt in horses *Veterinary Journal* 15: 73-91

Banks K L 1979 Anti-glomerular basement membrane antibody in horses *American Journal of Pathology* 94: 443-446

Banks K L, Henson J B, and McGuire T C 1972a Immunologically mediated glomerulitis of horses I. Pathogenesis in persistent infection by equine infectious anemia virus *Laboratory Investigation* 26: 701-707

Banks K L, Henson J B, and McGuire T C 1972b Immunologically mediated glomerulitis of horses II. Antiglomerular basement membrane antibody and other mechanisms in spontaneous disease *Laboratory*

Investigation 26: 708-715

Banks K L, McGuire T C, and Jerrells T R 1976 Absence of B lymphocytes in a horse with primary agammaglobulinemia *Clinical Immunology and Immunopathology* 5(2): 282-290

Banks K L, Crawford T B, and McGuire T C 1978 Cellular immune mechanisms in the immunopathogenesis of equine infectious anemia *Journal of Equine Medicine and Surgery Supplement* 1: 359-362

Barakat S E D M and Ford E J H 1988 Further studies on the diagnostic value of γ-glutamyl transpeptidase and 5′-nucleotidase in cattle, sheep and horses *Research Veterinary Science* 44: 354-360

Barclay W P and LaHunta A de 1979 Cryptococcal meningitis in a horse *Journal of the American Veterinary Medical Association* 174: 1236-1238

Barclay W, Foerner J J, and Phillips T 1987 Osteochondral fragmentation of the plantar aspect of the proximal phalanx as a cause of lameness in horses: 19 cases (1981-85) *Journal of the American Veterinary Medical Association* 191: 855-57

Barker I K and Dreumel A A van 1985 The alimentary system. In Jubb and Kennedy *The Pathology of Domestic Animals* Orlando, Academic Press

Barkley J E 1982 Equine loss trends *Modern Veterinary Practice*: 405-406

Barlow R M 1969 Neuropathological observations in grass sickness of horses *Journal of Comparative Pathology* 79: 407-411

Barnes J E 1938 "Dry sweating" of horses in Colombo *Veterinary Record* 50: 977-979

Barnett D 1972 Heat inactivation of equine infectious anemia virus in equine serum *Proceedings of the U S Animal Health Association* 76: 231-236

Barnett K C and Platt H 1990 Intraocular melanomata in the horse *Equine Veterinary Journal* 10 (supplement): 76-82

Barnett K C, Rossdale P D, Wade J F 1983 Equine ophthalmology *Equine Veterinary Journal* (Suppl 2): November

Barnett K C, Rossdale P D, Wade J F 1990 Equine ophthalmology II *Equine Veterinary Journal* (Suppl 10), September

Barnett S F 1974 Babesia of horses in Britain *Veterinary Record* 95: 346-347

Barone R and Ruet L 1955 Recherches experimentales sur les corps strie des solipedes *Bulletin Societe Vétérinaire Lyon* 3: 141-59

Bartels J E and Vaughan J T 1969 Persistent right aortic arch in the horse *Journal of the American Veterinary Medical Association* 154: 406-409

Bartke 1900 Kriegs chirurgie und Statistik. In *Bayer-Fröhner Handbuch der tierärztlichen chirurgie und Geburtshilfe.* Vol 4 Vienna, Braumuller

Barton M D and Embury D H 1987 Studies on the pathogenesis of *Rhodococcus equi* infection in foals *Australian Veterinary Journal* 64: 332-339

Barton M D and Knight I 1972 Cryptococcal meningitis of a horse *Australian Veterinary Journal* 48: 534

Bartsch A R C, McConnell E E, Imes G D, and Schmidt J M 1977 A review of exertional rhabdomyolysis in wild and domestic animals and man *Veterinary Pathology* 14: 314-24

Bastianello S S 1982 A survey of neoplasia in domestic species over a 40-year period from 1935 to 1974 in the Republic of South Africa. I. Tumours occurring in cattle *Onderstepoort Journal of Veterinary Research* 49: 195-204

Batte E G and Miller W S 1953 Ringworm in horses and its control *Journal of the American Veterinary Medical Association* 123: 111-114

Bauer J E, Meyer D J, Campbell M, and McMurphy R 1990 Serum lipid and lipoprotein changes in ponies with experimentally induced liver disease *American Journal of Veterinary Research* 51: 1380-1384

Baumann R 1957 Die Geshwurige Lymphgefassentzundung der Einhufer (Lymphangitis ulcerosa) *Wiener Tierärztliche Monatschrift* 44: 292-96

Baumann R and Gratzl E 1931 Paratyphus-Breslau-Erkrankungen beim Pferd *Wiener Tierärztliche Monatschrift* 18: 322,353

Baxter G M 1986 Equine laminitis caused by distal displacement of the distal phalanx: 12 cases (1976-1985) *Journal of the American Veterinary Medical Association* 189: 326-329

Baxter G M, Laskey R E, Tackett R L, Moore J N, and Allen D 1989a In vitro reactivity of digital arteries and veins to vaso constrictive mediators in healthy horses and in horses with early laminitis *American Journal of Veterinary Research* 50: 508-517

Baxter G M, Tackett R L, and Moore J N 1989b Reactivity of equine palmar digital arteries and veins to vasodilating agents *Veterinary Surgery* 18: 221-226

Baxter G M, Moore J N, and Tackett R L 1991 In vitro responses of equine digital vessels to dopamine and fenoldopam *Equine Veterinary Journal* 23: 48-52

Bayer J 1878 Threadworms in the eye *Ost Viertel Wiss Vet* 49: 113-116

Bayly W M and Robertson J T 1982 Epistaxis caused by foreign body penetration of a guttural pouch *Journal of the American Veterinary Medical Association* 180: 1232-1234

Bayly W M, Paradis M R, and Reed S M 1980 Equine renal biopsy: indications, technic, interpretation and complications *Modern Veterinary Practice*: 763-768

Bayly W M, Reed S M, Leathers C W, Brown C M, Traub J L, Paradis M R, and Palmer G H 1982 Multiple congenital heart anomalies in five Arabian foals *Journal of the American Veterinary Medical Association* 181: 684-689

Bayly W M, Brobst D F, and Elfers R S 1986a Serum and urinary biochemistry and enzyme changes in ponies with acute renal failure *Cornell Veterinarian* 76: 306-316

Bayly W M, Elfers R S, Liggitt H D, Brobst D F, Gavin P R, and Reed S M 1986b A reproducible means of studying acute renal failure in the horse *Cornell Veterinarian* 76: 287-298

Bayly W M, Liggitt H D, Huston L J, and Laegreid W W 1986c Stress and its effect on equine pulmonary mucosal defenses *Proceedings American Association Equine Practitioners* 32: 253-262

Becht J L and Page E H 1979 Neonatal isoerythrolysis in the foal: an evaluation of predictive and diagnostic field tests *Proceedings American Association Equine Practioners* 25: 247-259

Becht J L, Thacker H L, and Page E H 1979 Malignant seminoma in a stallion *Journal of the American Veterinary Medical Association* 175: 292-293

Becht J L, Page E H, Morter R L, Boon G D, and Thacker H L 1983 Experimental productions of neonatal isoerythrolysis in the foal *Cornell Veterinarian* 73: 380-389

Becker J 1970 Zähne. Vol 5 *Joest's Handbuch der Speziellen pathologischen Anatomie der Haustiere* 3rd Ed. Berlin, Parey

Beckmann O 1936 Über veränderungen des Gleichbeinapparates am Fesselgelenke des Pferdes *Deutsche Tierärztliche Wochenschrift* 44: 234

Beech J 1975 Cytology of tracheobronchial aspirates in horses *Veterinary Pathology* 12: 157-164

Beech J 1979 Diseases of the lung *Veterinary Clinics North America: Large Animal Practice* 1: 149-169

Beech J 1984 Neuroaxonal dystrophy of the accessory cuncate nucleus in horses *Veterinary Pathology* 21: 384-393

Beech J 1991 Chronic obstructive pulmonary disease *Veterinary Clinics of North America: Equine Practice* 7: 79-91

Beech J and Dodd D C 1974 Toxoplasma-like encephalomyelitis in the horse *Veterinary Pathology* 11: 87-96

Beech J and Haskins M 1987 Genetic studies of neuraxonal dystrophy in the Morgan *American Journal of Veterinary Research* 48: 109-113

Beech J, Dubielzig R, and Bester R 1977 Portal vein anomaly and hepatic encephalopathy in a horse *Journal of American Medical Association* 170: 164-166

Beech J, Sweeney C R, and Irby N 1983 Keratomycoses in 11 horses *Equine Veterinary Journal* 2 (supplement): 39-44

Beech J, Aguirre G, and Gross S 1984a Congential nuclear cataracts in the Morgan horse *Journal of the American Veterinary Medical Association* 184: 1363-1365

Beech J, Bloom J C, and Hodge T G 1984b Erythrocytosis in a horse *Journal of American Veterinary Medical Association* 184: 986-989

Behr M J, Hackett R P, Bentinck-Smith J, Hillman R B, King J M, and Tennant B C 1981 Metabolic abnormalities associated with rupture of the urinary bladder in neonatal foals *Journal of the American Veterinary Medical Association* 178: 263-266

Belin M 1946 La listerellose equine *Bulletin Academie France* 19: 176-181

Belknap J K and Moore J N 1989 Evaluation of heparin for prophylaxis of equine laminitis: 71 cases (1980-1986) *Journal of the American Veterinary Medical Association* 195: 505-507

Belknap J, Arden W, and Yamini B 1988 Septic periorchitis in a horse *Journal of the American Veterinary Medical Association* 192: 363-364

Berge E 1928 Vergleichende Betrachtung der Speicheldrusenerkrankung bei Pferd, Rind, und Hund *Tierärztliche Rundschau* 34: 926

Berge E 1933 Über die lokale Malazie der Sesambein am Fesselgelenke des Pferdes, ein Beitrag zur Pathologie und Klinik der "Gleichbeinlähme" *Berliner Tierärztliche Wochenschrift* 49: 629-33,645-49

Berge E 1936 Über du Arthritis deformans beim Fohlen *Berliner Tierärztliche Wochenschrift* 52: 645-49

Berge P, Pomeau Y, and Vidal C 1984 *Order Within Chaos* New York, Wiley

Bergen W C, Gier H T, Marion G B, and Coffman J R 1970 A developmental concept of equine cryptorchism *Biology of Reproduction* 3: 82-92

Berger G and Eigendorf B 1976 *Tierzucht* 30: 227-29

Berggren P C 1981 Aplastic anemia in a horse *journal of the American Veterinary Medical Association* 179(12): 1400-1402

Bergmann V, Dietz O, Gangel H, Schutzler H, and Kle B 1990 Zur Klinik und Pathomorphologie der equinen Parese *Monatschrift Veterinärmedicin* 45: 310-14

Berkeland R and Haakenstad L H 1968 Intracapsular bony fragments of the distal tibia of the horse *Journal of the American Veterinary Medical Association* 152: 1526

Bernard W, Reef V B, Clark E S, Vaala W, and Ehnen S J 1990 Pericarditis in horses: six cases (1982-1986) *Journal of the American Veterinary Medical Association* 196: 468-471

Berrocal A and Ingh T S G A M van den 1987 Pathology of equine phycomycosis *Veterinary Quarterly* 9: 180-184

Berry C R, Merritt A M, Burrows C F, and Campbell M 1986 Evaluation of the myoelectrical activity of the equine ileum infected with *Strongylus vulgaris* larvae *American Journal of Veterinary Research* 47: 27-30

Berthelsen H and Eriksson K 1935 Epitheliogenesis imperfecta neonatorum in a foal, possibly of a herditary nature *Journal of Comparative Pathology Therapeutics* 48: 285-97

Bertone J J and Dill S G 1985 Traumatic gastropericarditis in a horse *Journal of the American Veterinary Medical Association* 187: 742-743

Besch E D and Griffiths H J 1956 Demonstration of a Demodex equi (Raillet, 1895) from a horse in Minnesota *Journal of the American Veterinary Medical Association* 128: 82-83

Beurgelt C D, Hines S A, Cantor G, Stirk A, and Wilson J H 1986 A retrospective study of proliferative interstitial lung disease of horses in Florida *Veterinary Pathology* 23: 750-56

Beurgelt C D, Green S L, Mayhew I G, Wilson J H, and Merritt A M 1988 Avian mycobacteriosis in three horses *Cornell Veterinarian* 78: 365-80

Beveridge W I B 1977 *Influenza—The Last Great Plague* Heinemann, London

Beveridge W I B, Mahaffey L W, and Rose M A 1965 Influenza in horses *Veterinary Record* 77: 57-59

Bibrack B 1963 Über die formale und kausale Genese der Zehenarterienobliterationen beim Pferde *Zentrablatt Veterinärmedicin* 10: 67

Bickmeier K 1963 Über Polydaktylie beim Pferd *Deutsche Tierärztliche Wochenschrift* 47: 161-67

Bierer B W 1969 Electrophoretic analysis of blood serum and plasma proteins of normal horses *American Journal of Veterinary Research* 30: 2237-2240

Bierling 1914 *Münchener Tierärztliche Wochenschrift*: 1041

Biggers J D and Ingram P L 1948 Studies on equine purpura haemorrhagica—a review of the literature *British Veterinary Journal* 104: 214-20

Biggers J D, Ingram PL, and Murray C B 1949 Studies on equine purpura haemorrhagica IV. Haematology *British Veterinary Journal* 105: 191-200

Binninger C E and Piper R C 1968 Hyperplastic dermatitis of the equine ear *Journal of the American Veterinary Medical Association* 153: 69-75

Birks E K and Hultgren B D 1988 Pericardial haemangiosarcoma in a horse *Journal of Comparative Pathology* 99: 105-107

Bishop A E, Hodson N P, Major J H, Probert L, and Yeats J 1984 The regulatory peptide system of the large bowel in equine grass sickness *Experientia* 40: 801-6

Bishop M W H, David J S E, and Messervy A 1964 Some observations on cryptorchidism in the horse *Veterinary Record* 76: 1041-1048

Bishop S P, Cole C R, and Smetzer D L 1966 Functional and morphological pathology of equine aortic insufficiency *Veterinary Pathology* 3: 137-58

Bitsch V 1972 Cases of equine coital exanthema in Denmark: 281-283

Bitsch V and Dam A 1971 Nervous disturbances in horses in relation to infection with equine rhinopneumonitis virus *Acta Veterinaria Scandinavia* 12: 134-136

Bittner H 1927 Beitrag zur Mechanik der Brustwirbelkette des Pferdes *Archiv Wissenprakt Tierheilk* 156: 236

Björck G and Nilsson G 1971 Chronic progressive pododermatitis in the horse *Equine Veterinary Journal* 3: 65-7

Björck G, Everz K E, Hansen H-J, and Henricson B 1973 Congenital cerebellar ataxia in the Gotland pony breed *Zentralblatt Veterinärmedicine* 20A: 341-54

Blackford J 1984 Superficial and deep mycoses in horses *Veterinary Clinics of North America: Large Animal Practice* 6: 47-58

Blackwell N J 1973 Colitis in equines associated with strongyle larvae *Veterinary Record* 93: 401-2

Blackwell R B and White II N A 1982 Duodenitis-jejunitis in the horse *Equine Colic Research Symposium University* Athens, Georgia

Blakeslee J R, Olsen R G, McAllister E S, Fassbender J, and Dennis R 1975 Evidence of respiratory tract infection induced by equine herpesvirus, type 2, in the horse *Canadian Journal of Microbiology* 21: 1940-1946

Blanchard T L, Varner D D, Hurtgen J P, Love C C, Cummings M R, Strezmienski, Benson C, Kenney R M 1988 Bilateral seminal vesiculitis and ampullitis in a stallion *Journal of the American Veterinary Medical Association* 192: 525-526

Blanchard T L, Schumacher J, Edwards J F, Varner D D, Lewis R D, Everett K, and Joyce J R 1991 Priapism in a stallion with generalized malignant melanoma *Journal of the American Veterinary Medical Association* 198: 1043-1044

Blaney B J, Garnter R J W, and McKensie R A 1981 The effects of oxalate in some tropical grasses on the availability to horses of calcium, phosphorus, and magnesium *Journal of Agricultural Science, Cambridge* 97: 507

Blaskovic D, Szanto J, Kapitancik B, Lesso J, Lackovic V, and Skarda R 1966 Experimental pathogenesis of A/equi 1 influenza virus infection in horses *Acta Virologia* 10: 513-520

Blaskovic D, Kaptiancik B, Sabo A, Styk B, Vrtiak O, and Kaplan M 1969a Experimental infection of horses with A/equi 2/Miami/1/63 and human A2/Hong Kong/1/68 influenza viruses I. The course of infection and virus recovery *Acta Virologia* 13: 499-506

Blaskovic D, Kaptiancik B, Sabo A, Styk B, Vrtiak O, and Kaplan M 1969b Experimental infection of horses with A/equi 2/Miami/1/63 and human A2/Hong Kong/1/68 influenza viruses II. Antibody response to the infection *Acta Virologia* 13: 507-514

Blasse 1909 Untersuchungen über die Arthrosis des Kiefergelenkes beim Pferde *Monatshefte Tierheilkunde* 20: 519-58

Blogg J R, Barton M D, Graydon R, and Cust R E 1983 Blindness caused by *Rhodococcus equi* infection in a foal *Equine Veterinary Journal* 2 (supplement): 25-26

Blood D C and Henderson J A 1963 *Veterinary Medicine* 2nd Ed Baltimore, Williams and Wilkins

Blue M G 1979 *Equine Veterinary Journal* 11: 76-84

Blum H 1967 *A transformation for extracting new descriptors of shape* Cambridge, MIT Press

Blythe L L, Cardinet G H, Meagher D, Brown M, and Wheat JD 1983 Palatal myositis in horses with dorsal displacement of the soft palate *Journal of the American Veterinary Medical Association* 183: 781-85

Blythe L L, Watrous B J, Pearson E G, and Walker L L 1990 Otitis media/interna in the horse- a cause of head shaking and skull fractures *Proceedings Annual Conference American Association Equine Practitioners*

Blythe L L, Craig A M, Lassen E D, Rowe K E, and Appell L H 1991a Serially determined plasma α-tocopherol concentrations and results of oral vitamin E absorption tests in clinically normal horses and horses with degenerative myeloencephalopathy *American Journal of Veterinary Research* 52: 908-11

Blythe L L, Hultgren B D, Craig A M, Appell L H, Lassen E D, Mattson D E, and Duffield D 1991b Clinical, viral, and genetic evaluation of equine degenerative myeloencephalopathy in a family of Appaloosas *Journal of the American Veterinary Medical Association* 198:

1005-1013

Bogdaschew N 1937 Anatomischer-histologischer Bau der Metacarpalknochen und zum teil der Metatarsalknochen einiger Pferderassen im Zusammenhang miit Ihre Funktion *Anatomischer Anzeiger* 83: 103-21

Bogert A J van den 1989 Computer simulation of locomotion in the horse *Dissertation*, Utrecht

Bohanon T C, Beard W L, and Robertson J T 1990 Laryngeal Hemiplegia in draft horses: A review of 27 cases *Veterinary Surgery* 19: 456-459

Bohm H 1959 Schilddrusenkrebs bei einem Pferd *Tierärztliche Umschau* 14: 351-3

Böhm R 1954 Untersuchungen über den Einfluss der intrauterinen Lage auf de Gleidmassenstellungen bei Fohlen und deren Wandlusfähigkeit besonders im Hinblick auf den angeborenen Sehnenstelzfuss *Dissertation*, Hannover

Bolbol A E and Saleh A S 1987 Survey on equine hoof infection in Upper Egypt *Journal of Egyptian Veterinary Medical Association* 47: 545-553

Boles C L, Raker C W, and Wheat J D 1978 Epiglottic entrapment by arytenoepiglottic folds in the horse *Journal of the American Veterinary Medical Association* 172: 338-42

Bolliger C 1991 *The equine hoof* Basel, Hoffmann-LaRoche

Bollinger O 1869 Über eigentumliche Korperchen in den feinen Arterien des intestinaltraktus beim Pferde *Virchows Archiv* 47: 89-95

Bollwein A and Hänichen T 1989 Altersabhängige Veränderungen an den Zwishcehnwirbelscheiben der Halswirbelsaule des Pferdes *Tierärztliche Praxis* 17: 73-6

Bolton J R, Lees M J, Robinson W F, Thomas J B, and Klein K T 1990 Ocular neoplasms of vascular origin in the horse *Equine Veterinary Journal* 10 (supplement): 73-75

Bonagura J D 1985 Equine heart disease an overview *Veterinary Clinics of North America: Equine Practice* 1: 267-274

Boomker J, Coetzer J A W, and Scott D B 1976 Black grain mycetoma (maduromycosis) in horses *Onderstepoort Journal of Veterinary Research* 44: 249-252

Borst G H A 1978 Tetralogie van Fallot bij een koudbloed veulen *Tijdschrift voor Diergeneeskunde* 103: 968-970

Bottoms G D, Fessler J F, Roesel O F, Moore A B, and Frauenfelder H C 1981 Endotoxin-induced hemodynamic changes in ponies: effects of flunixin meglumine *American Journal of Veterinary Research* 42: 1514-1518

Bottoms G D, Templeton C B, Fessler J F, Johnson M A, Roesel O F, Ewert K M, and Adams S B 1982 Thromboxane, prostaglandin I_2 (epoprostenol), and the hemodynamic changes in equine endotoxin shock *American Journal of Veterinary Research* 42: 999-1002

Boudinot F D, Funderburg E D, and Moore J N 1991 Effects of pasture grass estrogen concentrations on the incidence of colon distension and torsion in broodmares *4th Equine Colic Research Symposium* Athens, Georgia

Bourdin P 1978 African horsesickness in Senegal: serological tests and vaccination In Bryans J T and Gerber H (eds) *Equine Infectious Diseases IV*, Princeton, Vet Publications

Bowman K F, Vaughn J T, Quick C B, Hankes G H, Reddin R W 1978 Megaesophagus in a colt *Journal of the American Veterinary Medical Association* 172: 334-37

Boy M G, Galligan D T, and Divers T J 1990 Protozoal encephalomyelitis in horses: 82 cases (1972-1986) *Journal of the American Veterinary Medical Association* 196: 632-634

Boyd W L and Bishop L M 1937 Pyelonephritis of cattle and horses *Journal of the American Veterinary Medical Association* 90: 154-159

Boyle M 1990 Immune related infertility in stallions *Equine Veterinary Journal* 22: 67-72

Bracher V 1987 Zur Erfassung der Dunkelziffer COPD-kranker Pferde *Dissertation* Zurich

Bracher V, Fellenberg R von, Winder C N, Gruenig G, Hermann M, and Kraehmann A 1991 An investigation of the incidence of chronic obstructive pulmonary disease (COPD) in random populations of Swiss horses *Equine Veterinary Journal* 23: 136-141

Braekman W L 1986 *Of Hawks and Horses* Brussels Scripta

Bramble D M and Carrier D R 1983 Running and breathing in mammals *Science* 219(4582: 251-256

Bramlage L R, Gabel A A, and Hackett R P 1980 Avulsion fractures of the origin of the suspensory ligament in the horse *Journal of the American Veterinary Medical Association* 176: 1004-10

Brandt A J 1940 Über Hypophysenadenome bei Hund und Pferd *Skandinavisk Veterinärtidskrift* 59: 875-917

Braverman Y 1988 Preferred landing sites of *Culicoides* species (Diptera: Ceratopogonidae) on a horse in Israel and its relevance to summer seasonal recurrent dermatitis (sweet itch) *Equine Veterinary Journal* 20: 426-429

Breeze R G, Brown C M and Turk M A M 1984a 3-methylindole as a model of equine obstructive lung disease *Equine Veterinary Journal* 16: 108-112

Breeze R G, Laegrid W W, Bayly W M, and Wilson B J 1984b Perilla ketone toxicity: A chemical model for the study of equine restrictive lung disease *Equine Veterinary Journal* 16: 180-184

Brendecke 1926 Morphologie des Ovars vom Pferd *Dissertation*, Hannover

Bridges C H 1972 Mycotic diseases In *Equine Medicine and Surgery* 2nd Ed Wheaton, American Veterinary Publications

Bridges C H and Harris E D 1988 Experimentally induced cartilaginous fractures (osteochondritis dissencans) in foals fed low-copper diets *Journal of the American Veterinary Medical Association* 193: 215-21

Bridges C H and Moffitt P G 1990 Influence of variable content of dietary zinc on copper metabolism of weanling foals *American Journal of Veterinary Research* 51: 275-80

Bridges C H, Womack J E, Harris E D, and Scrutchfield W L 1984 Consideration of copper metabolism in osteochondrosis of suckling foals *Journal of the American Veterinary Medical Association* 185: 173-78

Brion P, Fontaine M, Fontaine M-P, and Moraillon R 1966 Grippe du cheval. Enzooties en 1965 en France *Recueil de Medecine Veterinaire* 142: 269-279

Britton J W 1939 Trichostrongylosis in equines *Cornell Veterinarian* 29: 322-30

Brobst D F, Carroll R J, and Bayly W M 1986 Urinary enzyme concentrations in healthy horses *Cornell Veterinarian* 76: 299-305

Brocq-Rousseu, Urbain A, and Barotte J 1927 Etude des teignes du cheval et de l'immunite dans les teignes experimentales *Annales Institute Pasteur* 41: 513-553

Brostrom H, Larsson A, and Troedsson M 1987 Allergic dermatitis (sweet itch) of Icelandic horses in Sweden: An epidemiological study *Equine Veterinary Journal* 19: 229-236

Brostrom H, Fahlbrink E, Dubath M L, and Lazary S 1988 Association between equine leucocyte antigens (ELA) and equine sarcoid tumors in the population of Swedish Halfbreds and some of their families *Veterinary Immunology and Immunopathology* 19: 215-223

Brostrom H, Paulie S, and Perlmann P 1989 Surface antigens on equine sarcoid cells and normal dermal fibroblasts as assessed by xenogeneic antisera *Research Veterinary Science* 46: 172-179

Brostrom J, Bredeberg-Raden U, England J, Obel N, Perlmann V 1979 Cell-mediated immunity in horses with sarcoid tumors against sarcoid cells *in vitro American Journal of Veterinary Research* 40: 1701-1706

Brown C C, McClure J J, Triche P, and Crowder C 1988 Use of immunohistochemical methods for diagnosis of equine pythiosis *American Journal of Veterinary Research* 49: 1866-1868

Brown C M 1985 Acquired cardiovascular disease *Veterinary Clinics of North America: Equine Practice* 1: 371-382

Brown C M, Bell T G, Paradis M R, and Breeze R G 1983 Rupture of mitral chordae tendineae in two horses *Journal of the American Veterinary Medical Association* 182: 281-283

Brown M P and McCallum F J 1976 Observations on growth plates in foals *Veterinary Record* 98: 443-46

Brown P J, Holt P E 1985 Primary renal cell carcinoma in four horses *Equine Veterinary Journal* 17: 473-477

Brown T T and Patton C S 1977 Protozoal encephalomyelitis in horses *Journal of the American Veterinary Medical Association* 171: 492

Brownie C F, Cullen J 1987 Characterization of experimentally induced equine leukoencephalomalacia (ELEM) in ponies (Equus Caballus): Preliminary report *Veterinary Human Toxicology* 29: 34-38

Brumbaugh G W, Stitzel K A, Zinkl J G, and Feldman B F 1982 Myelomonocytic myeloproliferative disease in a horse *Journal of the American Veterinary Medical Association* 180: 313-316

Brunemann J 1941 Beiträg zure Histologie des Hufkrebses *Deutsche Tierärztliche Wochenschrift* 49: 480-1

Bruner J 1941 Beobachtungen über unregalmassige Abkauung an den Zähnen rezentger und fossiler Equiden *Palaebiologica* 7: 273-81

Bryans J T 1968 The herpesviruses in disease of the horse *Proceedings American Association Equine Practitioners*: 119-125

Bryans J T 1972a Leptospirosis. In *Equine Medicine and Surgery* 2nd Ed. Wheaton, American Veterinary Publications

Bryans J T 1972b Salmonellosis. In *Equine Medicine and Surgery* 2nd Ed. Wheaton, American Veterinary Publications

Bryans J T and Prickett M E 1972 A consideration of the pathogenesis of abortigenic disease caused by equine herpesvirus-1 *Proceedings 3rd International Conference Equine Infectious Disease*: 34-40

Bryans J T, Doll E R, and Shephard B P 1964 The etiology of strangles *Cornell Veterinarian* 54: 198-205

Buck W B, Haliburton J C, Thilsted J P, Lock T F, and Vesonder R F 1979 Equine encephalomalacia: Comparative pathology of naturally occurring and experimental cases *American Association of Veterinary Laboratory Diagnosticians 22nd Annual Proceedings*: 239-258

Buckley S S and MacCallum N G 1901/02 Acute haemorrhagic encephalitis prevalent among horses in Maryland *American Veterinary Revue* 25: 99-102

Budras K D, Hullinger R L, and Sack W O 1989 Light and electron microscopy of keratinization in the laminar epidermis of the equine hoof with reference to laminitis *American Journal of Veterinary Research* 50: 1150-1160

Buechner-Maxwell V, Zhang C, Robertson J L, Jain N C, Antczak D, Feldman B F, Murray M J 1994 Intravascular leukostasis and systemic aspergillosis in a horse with subacute subleukemic myelomonocytic leukemia *Journal of Veterinary Internal Medicine* 8: 258-263

Buergelt C D, Cooley A J, Hines S A, and Pipers F S 1985 *Veterinary Pathology* 22: 333-337

Buergelt C D, Hines S A, Cantor G, Stirk A, and Wilson J H 1986 A retrospective study of proliferative interstitial lung disease in horses in Florida *Veterinary Pathology* 23: 750-756

Bugh G R 1988 *The Horsemen of Athens* Princeton, Princeton University Press

Buhler 1936 *Dissertation*, Leipzig

Bullen J J 1951 Epizootic lymphangitis *Journal of the Royal Army Veterinary Corps* 22: 8-11

Buntain B, Greig W A, and Thompson H 1979 Chronic nephritis in a pony *Veterinary Record* 104: 307-309

Burdon K L, Williams R P, 1968 *Microbiology* (6th edition) New York, The MacMillan Company

Burgess E C and Mattison M 1987 Encephalitis associated with *Borrelia burgdorferi* infection in a horse *Journal of the American Veterinary Medical Association* 191: 1457-1458

Burgess E C, Gillette D, and Pickett J P 1986 Arthritis and panuveitis as manifestations of *Borrelia burgdorferi* infection in a Wisconsin pony *Journal of the American Veterinary Medical Association* 189: 1340-42

Burgess E C, Gendron-Fitzpatrick A, and Mattison M 1988

Foal mortality associated with natural infection of pregnant mares with *Borrelia burgdorferi.* In Powell, D.G. (Ed) *Equine Infectious Diseases V* Lexington, University Press of Kentucky

Burgi 1910 Canker of the horse's foot and grease Abstract from *Schweizer Archiv Tierheilkunde* 52

Burns G A 1992 The teniae of the equine intestinal tract *Cornell Veterinarian* 82: 187-212

Burns K F and Matumoto M 1949a Japanese equine encephalomyelitis. Review of the literature *Journal of the American Veterinary Medical Association* 115: 112-115

Burns K F and Matumoto M 1949b Japanese equine encephalomyelitis: 1947 epizootic 1. Epizootiology *Journal of the American Veterinary Medical Association* 115: 167-170

Burns K F, Tigertt W D, and Matumoto M 1949 Japanese equine encephalomyelitis: 1947 epizootic II. Serological and etiological studies *American Journal of Hygiene* 50: 27-45

Burrell M H 1985 Endoscopic and virological observations on respiratory disease in a group of young Thoroughbred horses in training *Equine Veterinary Journal* 17: 99-103

Burrell M H, Mackintosh M E, and Taylor C E D 1986 Isolation of *Streptococcus pneumoniae* from the respiratory tract of horses *Equine Veterinary Journal* 18: 183-186

Burrows G E and Borchard R E 1982 Experimental lead toxicosis in ponies: Comparison of the effects of smelter effluent-contaminated hay and lead acetate *American Journal of Veterinary Research* 43: 2129-2133

Burrows R 1969 Equine rhinoviruses In Bryans J T and Gerber H (eds) *Proceedings 2nd International Conference Equine Infectious Diseases* Basel, Karger 154-165

Burrows R and Goodridge R 1984 Studies of persistent and latent equine herpesvirus-1 and herpesvirus-3 infections in the Pirbright pony herd In Wittman *Latent Herpesvirus Infections in Veterinary Medicine* Nijhoff Boston 307-319

Burrows R, Goodridge D, Denyer M, Hutchings G, and Frank C J 1982 Equine influenza infections in Great Britain, 1979 *Veterinary Record* 110: 494-497

Burson W M 1912 Azoturia in work oxen *American Veterinary Revue* 41: 218-20

Butler I V and Armbruster B 1984 Struktur und abgangsursachen bei schlachtpferden *Deutsche tierarztliche Wochenschrift* 91: 330-331

Button C, Gross D R, Albert J A, and Kitzman J V 1978 Tricuspid atresia in a foal *Journal of the American Veterinary Medical Association* 172: 825-830

Button C, Scrutchfield W L, Clark R G, Knauer K W, Schmitz D G 1980 Multiple atrial dysrhythmias in a horse *Journal of the American Veterinary Medical Association* 177: 714-719

Byars T D 1984 Allergic skin diseases in the horse *Veterinary Clinics of North America: Large Animal Practice* 6: 87-90

Byars T D and Becht J L 1991 Pleuropneumonia *Veterinary Clinics of North America: Equine Practice* 7: 63-78

Byars T D and Greene C E 1982 Idiopathic thrombocytopenic purpura in the horse *Journal of the American Veterinary Medical Association* 180: 1422-1424

Bynum D, Ledbetter W B, Boyd C L, and Ray D R 1971 Flexural properties of the equine metacarpus *Journal of Biomedical Materials Research* 5: 63

Byrne R J 1972 The control of Eastern and Western arboviral encephalomyelitis of horses In *Proceedings of the 3rd International Conference on Equine Infectious Diseases*, Karger, Basel 115-123

Byrne R J, Hetrick F M, Scanlon J E, Hastings A W, and Locke L N 1961 Observations on Eastern equine encephalitis in Maryland in 1959 *Journal of the American Veterinary Medical Association* 139: 661-664

Cadeac C 1893 *Pathologie generale et anatomie pathologique generale des animaux domestiques* Paris, Bailliere

Cadeac C 1896 *Pathologie interne des animaux domestiques Maladies du appareil digestif, intestin, liver, peritoneum, nose and sinuses* Vols 1,2,3 Paris, Bailliere

Cadeac C 1897a *Pathologie des animaux domestiques. Respiratoire* Vol 4 Paris, Bailliere

Cadeac C 1897b *Pathologie interne des animaux domestiques Maladies du vaisseaux* Vol 5 Paris, Bailliere

Cadeac C 1899a *Pathologie interne des animaux domestiques Maladies du sang, generales, et l'appareil urinaire* Vol 6 Paris, Bailliere

Cadeac C 1899b *Pathologie interne des animaux domestiques Maladies du peau* Vol 7 Paris, Bailliere

Cadeac C 1899c *Pathologie interne des animaux domestiques Maladies du system nerveaux* Vol 8 Paris, Bailliere

Cadeac C 1905 *Pathologie chirurgicale de la peau et les vaisseaux* Paris, Bailliere

Cadeac C 1907 *Pathologie chirurgicale des articulations* Paris, Bailliere

Cadeac C 1908 *Pathologie interne. Bouche, Pharynx, Estomac* Paris, Bailliere

Cadeac C 1909 *Pathologie chirurgicale des articulations, Arthrites* Paris, Bailliere

Cadiot P J 1910 Kranheiten der Nase. In *Bayer-Fröhner Handbuch der tierärztlichen chirurgie und Geburtshilfe.* Vol 3 Vienna, Braumuller

Cadore J L 1987 Les affections chroniques de l'appareil respiratoire superior du cheval. *Pratique Vétérinaire Equine* 19: 23-30

Cahill J and Goulden B E 1986 Equine laryngeal hemiplegia *New Zealand Veterinary Journal* 34: 161-93

Cahill J I and Goulden B E 1987 The pathogenesis of equine laryngeal hemiplegia A review *New Zealand Veterinary Journal* 35: 82-90

Cahill J I and Goulden B E 1989 Further evidence for a CNS component in equine laryngeal hemiplegia *New Zealand Veterinary Journal* 37: 89-90

Cahill J I, Goulden B E, and Pearce HG 1985 A review and some observations on stringhalt *New Zealand Veterinary Journal* 133: 101-4

Cahill J I, Goulden B E, and Jolly R D 1986 Stringhalt in horses: A distal axonopathy *Neuropathology and Applied Neurobiology* 12: 459-475

Callender G R and Kelser R A 1938 Degenerative Arthritis—a comparison of the pathological changes in man and equine *American Journal of Pathology* 14: 253-72

Campbell C K 1990 Pythiosis *Equine Veterinary Journal* 22: 227-228

Campbell E, Gumbrell R C, and Murfitt C G 1971 The occurrence of *Dictyocaulus arnfieldi* in the lungs of horses *New Zealand Veterinary Journal* 19: 217-219

Campbell M I, Colahan P T, Brown M P, Grandstedt M E, and Peyton, L C 1984 Cecal impaction in the horse. *Journal of the American Veterinary Medical Association* 184: 950-52

Cannon W B 1911 *The Mechanical Factors of Digestion* New York, Longmans

Capen C C 1985 The Endocrine Glands In Jubb K, Kennedy P and Palmer N *The Pathology of Domestic Animals* 3rd Ed New York, Academic Press

Carlens O 1927 Beitrag zur Kenntnis der embryonalen Entwicklung des Extremitätenskeletts beim Pferd und Rind. I. Die Entwicklung des knorpeligen Extremitätenskeletts *Gegenbauer's Morphoologisches Jahrbuch* 58: 153-196

Carlson G P and O'Brien M A 1990 Anaerobic bacterial pneumonia with septicemia in two racehorses *Journal of the American Veterinary Medical Association* 196: 941-943

Carlström B 1926/27 Experimentelle Untersuchungen und Klinische Beobachtungen über Veränderungen der Lage des Bauchorgane in Zusammenhang mit Magenüberfullung beim Pferd *Archiv Tierheilkunde* 55: 361-92

Carlström B 1930a Über die Aetiologie und Pathogenese der Kreuzlähme des Pferdes. *Skandinavisk Archiv Physiologie* 61: 161-/62: 1-69

Carlström B 1930b *Über die Aetiologie und Pathogenese der Kreuzlähme des Pferdes* Berlin, de Gruyter

Carlström B 1931/32 cited in Innes JRM and Saunders L Z 1962 in *Comparative Neuropathology* New York Academic Press

Carnine B L, Schneider G, Cook J E, Leipold H W 1977 Pericardial mesothelioma in a horse *Veterinary Pathology* 14: 513-515

Carter D R and Hayes W C 1977 Compact bone fatigue damage *Clinical Orthopaedics Related Research* 127: 265-74

Carter EI, Valli VE, McSherry BJ, Milne F J, Robinson G A, and Lumsden J H 1974 The kinetics of hematopoiesis in the light horse. I. The lifespan of peripheral blood cells in the normal horse *Canadian Journal of Comparative Medicine and Veterinary Science* 38(3): 303-313

Cattabiania F, Cabassi E, Allodi C, Gianelli F 1976 Bacterial flora of the conjunctival sac of the horse (in Italian) *Ann Sclavo* 18(1): 91-119

Cello R M 1971 Ocular onchocercihiasis in the horse (Onchocerca cervicalis) *Equine Veterinary Journal* 3(4): 148-154

Chaffin M K, Fuenteable I C, Welch R D, and Edwards J F 1991 Retrospective study: idiopathic muscular hypertrophy of the equine small intestine (1980-90) *4th Equine Colic Research Symposium* Athens, Georgia

Chaffin M K, Fuenteable I C, Schumacher J, Welch R D, and Edwards J F 1992 Idiopathic muscular hypertrophy of the equine small intestine: 11 cases (1980-91) *Equine Veterinary Journal* 24: 372-78

Chan C W and Collins E A 1985 Case of angiosarcoma of the nasal passage of the horse *Equine Veterinary Journal* 17: 214-8

Charlton K M, Mitchell D, Girard A, and Corner A H 1976 Meningoencephalomyelitis in horses associated with equine herpersvirus I infection *Veterinary Pathology* 13: 59-68

Chavatte P, Brown G, Ousey J C, Silver M, Cottrill C, Fowden A L, McGladdery A J, and Rossdale P D 1991 Studies of bone marrow and leucocyte counts in peripheral blood in fetal and newborn foals *Journal of Reproduction and Fertility* 44: 603-608

Cheevers W P, Roberson S M, Brassfield A L, Davis W C, and Crawford T B 1982 Isolation of a retrovirus from cultured equine sarcoid tumor cells *American Journal of Veterinary Research* 43: 804-806

Cheville N F 1983 *Cell Pathology* 2nd Ed Ames, Iowa State University Press

Chiaravalle A M and Aramburu H G 1944 Bile secretion in horses with biliary fistulas *Veterinary Bulletin* 14: 66

Chiejina S N and Mason J A 1977 Immature stages of Trichonema spp as a cause of diarrhoea in adult horses in spring *Veterinary Record* 100: 360-1

Chladek D W and Ruth G R 1976 Isolation of *Actinobacillus lignieresi* from an epidural abcess in a horse with progressive paralysis *Journal of the American Veterinary Medical Association* 168: 64-66

Cho S N, Collins M T, Reif J S, and McChesney A E 1983 Experimental infections of horses with *Legionella pneumophila American Journal of Veterinary Research* 44: 662-668

Church S, West H J, and Baker J R 1987 Two cases of pancreatic adenocarcinoma in horses *Equine Veterinary Journal* 19: 77-9

Cimprich R E 1974 Equine granulomatous enteritis *Veterinary Pathology* 11: 535-47

Cimprich R E 1981 Granulomatous enteritis of horses: clinical and postmortem findings. *Compendium Continuing Education Practicing Veterinarian* 3: s437-s440

Clabough D L, Gebhard D, Flaherty M T, Whetter L E, Perry S T, Coggins L, and Fuller F J 1991 Immune-mediated thrombocytopenia in horses infected with equine infectious anemia *Journal of Virology* 65: 6242-6251

Clara M 1956 *Die Arterio-venosen Anastomosen* Vienna, Springer-Verlag

Clark E G, Turner A S, Boysen B G, and Rouse B T 1978 Listeriosis in an Arabian foal with combined immunodeficiency *Journal of the American Veterinary Medical Association* 172: 363-66

Clarke A F 1985 Review of exercise induced pulmonary haemorrhage and its possible relationship with mechanical stress *Equine Veterinary Journal* 17: 166-172

Clarke A F 1987a A review of environmental and host factors in relation to equine respiratory disease *Equine Veterinary Journal* 19: 435-441

Clarke A F 1987b Chronic pulmonary disease—A multifaceted disease complex in the horse *Irish Veterinary Journal* 41: 258-264

Clarke L L, Garner H E, and Hatfield D 1982 Plasma volume, electrolyte, and endocrine changes during onset of laminitis hypertension in horses *American Journal of Veterinary Research* 43: 1551-1555

Clarke L L, Roberts M C, and Argenzio R A 1990 Feeding and digestive problems in horses: physiological responses to a concentrated meal *Veterinary Clinics North America* 6: 433-50

Clayton H M 1991 *Conditioning Sport Horses* Saskatoon, Sport Horse Publications

Clayton H M and Duncan J L 1981 Natural infection with *Dictyocaulus arnfieldi* in pony and donkey foals *Research Veterinary Science* 31: 278-280

Cline J M, Schlafer D W, Callihan D R, Vanderwall D, and Drazek F J 1991 Abortion and granulomatous colitis due to *Mycobacterium avium* complex infection in a horse *Veterinary Pathology* 28: 89-91

Clutton-Brock J 1992 *Horse Power* Cambridge Harvard University Press

Codazza D and Sampieri G 1973 Su alcuni aspetti epizoologici delle affezioni genitali da *Klebsiella pneumoniae* negli equini *Folia veterinaria latina* 3: 424-437

Code C F and Hester H E 1939 The blood histamine during anaphylactic shock in the horse and calf *American Journal of Physiology* 127: 71-7

Coffman J R 1973 Refractory laminitis *Veterinary Clinics of North America* 3: 291-301

Coffman J R and Carlson K L 1971 Verminous arteritis in horses *Journal of the American Veterinary Medical Association* 158: 1358-1360

Coffman J R and Garner H E 1972 Acute laminitis *Journal of the American Veterinary Medical Association* 161: 1280-1283

Coffman J R, Mussman H C, and Cawley L P 1969 Lactic dehydrogenase isoenzymes in equine infectious anemia *Cornell Veterinarian* 59: 397-404

Coggins L 1975 Viral respiratory infections of horses: Host resistance and immunity *Journal of the American Veterinary Medical Association* 166: 78-80

Coggins L 1979 Viral respiratory disease *Veterinary Clinics North America: Large Animal Practice* 1: 59-72

Coggins L and Kemen M J 1975 Viral respiratory infections of horses: Some specific viruses affecting the horse *Journal of the American Veterinary Medical Association* 166: 80-83

Cohen C and Sivan D 1983 The Ugaritic hippiatric texts: a critical edition *American Oriental Series* Essay 9

Cohrs P 1941a Aussprache *Deutsche Tierärztliche Wochenschrift* 49: 111

Cohrs P 1941b Die Erschopfung des Pferdes *Deutsche Tierärztliche Wochenschrift* 49: 277-81

Cohrs P 1941c Die infektiosen Katarrhe der Atmungsorgane des Pferdes *Berliner Münchener Tierärztliche Wochenschrift* 57: 218-20

Cohrs P 1961 In *Nieberle und Cohrs Lehrbuch der Speziellen Pathologie der Haustiere* Berlin, Parey

Cohrs P and Messow C 1929 Vol 1 Gelenke In Dobberstein J, Pallaske G, and Stünzi H (Eds) *Joest's Handbuch der Speziellen Pathologischen Anatomie der Haustiere*, 3rd Ed Berlin, Parey

Cohrs P and Streich W 1943 Verknocherungen der rechten Herzvorkammer beim Pferde *Deutsche Tierärztliche Wochenschrift* 51: 92-5

Coignoul F L, Cheville N F 1984 Pathology of maternal genital tract, placenta, and fetus in equine viral arteritis *Veterinary Pathology* 21(3): 333-340

Cole C R 1946 Changes in the equine larynx associated with laryngeal hemiplegia *American Journal of Veterinary Research* 7: 69

Cole H H, Guilbert H R, and Goss H 1932 Further considerations of properties of gonad-stimulating principle of mare serum *American Journal of Physiology* 102: 227-232

Cole J R, Hall R F, Gosser H S, Hendricks J B, Pursell A R, Senne D A, Pearson J E, Gipson G A 1986 Transmissibility and abortigenic effect of equine viral arteritis in mares *Journal of the American Veterinary Medical Association* 189(7): 769-771

Coles B M, Stevens D R, and Hunter R L 1978 Equine nodular dermatitis associated with *Alternaria tenuis* infection *Veterinary Pathology* 15: 779-780

Colin G 1886/88 *Traite de Physiologie Comparee des Animaux* Paris, Bailliere

Collatos C, Clark E S, Reef V B, and Morris D D 1990 Septicemia, atrial fibrillation, cardiomegaly, left atrial mass, and *Rhodococcus equi* septic osteoarthritis in a foal *Journal of the American Veterinary Medical Association* 197: 1039-1042

Colles C M 1991 Laminitis research *Equine Veterinary Journal* 23: 237-238

Colles C M and Hickman J 1977 The arterial supply of the navicular bone and its variations in navicular disease *Equine Veterinary Journal* 9: 150-154

Colles C M, Garner H E, and Coffman J R 1980 The blood supply of the horse's foot: chronic lameness, laminitis, pedal osteitis *Proceedings of the American Association of Equine Practitioners* 25: 385-97

Collins D H 1950 *Pathology of Articular and Spinal Disease* Baltimore Williams and Wilkins

Collins J D, Kelly W R, Twomey T, Farrelly B T, and Whitty B T 1971 Brucella-associated vertebral osteomyelitis in a thoroughbred mare *Veterinary Record* 88(13): 321-26

Collins M T, Cho S N, and Reif J S 1982 Prevalence of antibodies to *Legionella pneumophila* in animal populations *Journal of Clinical Microbiology* 15: 130-136

Conboy H S and Powers R D 1971 Equine malignant

lymphoma *Journal of the American Veterinary Medical Association* 159: 53-54

Conboy H S, Rezabek G B, and Rooney J R 1991 *Unpublished observations*

Conner M, Gillespie J, Schiff E, Holmes D, Frey M, and Quick S 1984 Experimental infection of horses and ponies by oral and intranasal routes with the New York State reovirus type 3 and German reovirus types 1 and 3 equine isolates *Zentralblatte Veterinarmedizin B* 31: 707-717

Conner M E and Darlington R W 1980 Rotavirus infection in foals *American Journal of Veterinary Research* 41(10: 1699-1703

Connole M D 1973 Equine phycomycosis *Australian Veterinary Journal* 49: 214-215

Cook C S, Peiffer R L, and Harling D E 1983 Equine recurrent uveitis *Equine Veterinary Journal* 2 (supplement): 57-60

Cook W R 1966 Observations on the aetiology of epistaxis and cranial nerve paralysis in the horse *Veterinary Record* 78: 396-407

Cook W R 1970 Skeletal radiology of the equine head *Veterinary Radiology* 11: 35-55

Cook W R 1973 Diarrhoea in the horse associated with stress and tetracycline therapy *Veterinary Record* 93: 15-16

Cook W R 1974 Some observations on disease of the ear, nose, and throat in the horse *Veterinary Record* 94: 533-41

Cook W R 1976 Chronic bronchitis and alveolar emphysema in the horse *Veterinary Record* 99: 448-451

Cook W R and Littlewort M C G 1974 Progressive hematoma of the ethmoid region in the horse *Equine Veterinary Journal* 6: 101-8

Cook W R, Campbell R S F, and Dawson C 1968 The pathology and etiology of guttural pouch mycosis in the horse *Veterinary Record* 3: 422

Cooley A J, Reinhard M K, Gross T L, Fadok V A, and Levy M 1987 Molluscum contagiosum in a horse with granulomatous enteritis *Journal of Comparative Pathology* 97: 29-34

Coombs R R A, Crowhurst R C, Day F T, Heard D H, Hinde I T, Hoogstraten J, Parry H B 1948 Haemolytic disease of newborn foals due to iso-immunization of pregnancy *J Hyg* 46: 403-418

Cordy D R 1954 Nigropallidal encephalomalacia in horses associated with ingestion of yellow star thistle *Journal of Neuropathology and Experimental Neurology* 13: 330-342

Cordy, D R 1984 Pathomorphology and pathogenesis of bacterial meningoventriculitis of neonatal ungulates *Veterinary Pathology* 21: 587-591

Corke M J 1981 An outbreak of sulphur poisoning in horses *Veterinary Record* 109: 212-213

Cornelius C E, Goodbary R F, and Kennedy P C 1959 Plasma-cell myelomatosis in a horse *Cornell Veterinarian* 49: 479-483

Cornick J L 1990 Diagnosis and treatment of pulmonary histoplasmosis in a horse *Cornell Veterinarian* 80: 97-103

Correa W M and Calderin G G 1966 Anhidrosis, dry coat syndrome in the Thoroughbred *Journal of the American Veterinary Medical Association* 149: 1556-1560

Cotchin E 1960 Tumours of farm animals: A survey of tumors examined at the Royal Veterinary College, London, during 1950-60 *Veterinary Record* 72: 816-823

Cotchin E A 1977 A general survey of tumors in the horse *Equine Veterinary Journal* 9: 16-21

Cotton W E 1927 The causal agent of vesicular stomatitis proved to be a filter-passing virus *Journal of the American Veterinary Medical Association* 70: 168-184

Cox J E, Williams J H, Rowe P H, and Smith J A 1973 Testosterone in normal, cryptorchid, and castrated male horses *Equine Veterinary Journal* 5: 85-90

Cox J E, Edwards G B, and Neal PA 1979 An analysis of 500 cases of equine cryptorchidism *Equine Veterinary Journal* 11: 113-116

Cox J H, DeBowes R M, and Leipold H W 1989 Congenital malignant melanoma in two foals *Journal of the American Veterinary Medical Association* 194: 945-947

Craig J F and Kehoe D 1921 Horse pox and coital exanthema *Journal of Comparative Pathology and Therapeutics* 34: 126-129

Cranley J J 1982 Hydatidosis *Equine Veterinary Journal* 14: 153-7

Cranley J J 1983 Focal medial calcification of the pulmonary artery: a survey of 1066 horses *Equine Veterinary Journal* 15: 278-80

Cranley J J and McCullagh K G 1981 Ischemic myocardial fibrosis and aortic strongylosis in the horse *Equine Veterinary Journal* 13: 35-52

Crawford T B and Archer B G 1978 Demonstration of RNA-dependent DNA polymerase in EIA virus *Journal of Equine Medicine and Surgery Suppl* 1: 395-399

Crawford T B and Henson J B 1971 Viral arteritis of horses *Advances in Experimental Medicine Biology* 22: 175-183

Crew F A E 1922 A histological study of the undescended testicle of the horse *Journal of Comparative Pathology and Therapeutics* 35: 62-69

Crinion R A P and O'Connor J P 1978 Selenium intoxication in horses *Irish Veterinary Journal* 32(5): 81-86

Critchley K L 1976 An interventricular septal defect, pulmonary stenosis and bicuspid pulmonary valve in a Welsch pony foal *Equine Veterinary Journal* 8: 176-178

Cross R S 1966 Equine periodic ophthalmia *Veterinary Record* 78: 8-17

Crouch R F, Atherton G, and Platt H 1972 Venereal transmission of *Klebsiella aerogenes* in a thoroughbred stud from a persistently infected stallion *Veterinary Record* 90: 21-24

Crowe M W and Swerczek T W 1985 Equine congenital defects *American Journal of Veterinary Research* 46: 353-58

Crowhurst F A, Dickinson G, and Burrows R 1981 An outbreak of paresis in mares and geldings associated with equine herpesvirus 1 *Veterinary Record* 190(24): 527-528

Cullen J M, Whiteside J, Umstead J A, and Whitacre M D 1987 A mixed germ cell-sex cord-stromal neoplasm of the testis in a stallion *Veterinary Pathology* 24: 575-577

Cummings J F, Lahunta A de, Fuhrer, G L, Valentine B A, and Cooper B J 1990 Equine motor neuron disease: a preliminary report *Cornell Veterinarian* 80: 357-9

Cummings J F, Lahunta A de, Mohammed H O, Divers T J 1991 Equine motor neuron disease: a new neurological disorder *Equine Practice* 13: 15-18

Cusick P K, Sells D M, Hamilton D P, and Hardenbrook H J 1974 Toxoplasmosis in two horses *Journal of the American Veterinary Medical Association* 164: 77-80

Cymbaluk N F, Fretz P B, and Loew F M 1978 Amprolium-induced thiamine deficiency in horses: Clinical features *American Journal of Veterinary Research* 39: 255-261

Daels P F, Starr M, Kindahl H, Fredriksson G, Hughes J P and Stabenfeldt G H 1987 Effect of *Salmonella typhimurium* endotoxin on PGF-2α release and fetal death in the mare *Journal Reproduction Fertility* 35 (Supplement): 485-492

Dahme E and Schebitz H 1970 Zur Pathogenese der spinalen Ataxie des Pferdes unter Zugrundelegung neuerer Befunde *Zentrablatt Veterinärmedicine.A* 17: 120-43

Dakyns H G 1897 *The Works of Xenophon* Vol. 3 New York, Macmillan

Dalin G and Jeffcott L B 1986 Sacroiliac joint of the horse I Gross morphology *Anatomie Histologie Embryologie* 15: 80-94,99-107

Dämmrich K 1985 Vol 4 Entwicklungsstörungen des Skeletts In Dobberstein J, Pallaske G, and Stünzi H (Eds) *Joest's Handbuch der Speziellen Pathologischen Anatomie der Haustiere* 3rd Ed Berlin, Parey.

Damodaran S and Ramachandran P V 1975 A survey of neoplasms of equidae *Indian Veterinary Journal* 52: 531-534

Darbyshire J H and Pereira H G 1964 An adenovirus precipitating antibody present in some sera of different animal species and its association with bovine respiratory disease *Nature* 201: 895-897

Darien B J and Feldman B F 1992 Hemostasis in the newborn foal *Current Therapy in Equine Medicine* 3: 427-428

Darien B J, Belknap J, and Nietfeld J 1988 Cerebrospinal fluid changes in two horses with central nervous system nematodiasis (*Micronema deletrix*) *Journal of Veterinary Internal Medicine* 2: 201-205

Darien B J, Potempa J, Moore J N, and Travis J 1991 Antithrombin III activity in horses with colic: an analysis of 46 cases *Equine Veterinary Journal* 23: 211-214

Darmstaedter L, du Bois-Reymond R, and Schaefer C 1908 *Handbuch der Geschichte der Nfaturwissenschaften und der Technik* 2nd Ed Berlin, Springer

Dart A J, Snyder J R, Julian D, and Hinds D M 1991a Microvascular circulation of the cecum in horses *American Journal of Veterinary Research* 52: 1545-50

Dart A J, Snyder J R, Pascoe J R, Farver T B, and Galuppo L D 1991b Disorders of the equine descending colon: 102 cases (1979-89) *4th Equine Colic Research Symposium* Athens, Georgia

Datta S C A 1933 The etiology of bursatti *Indian Journal of Veterinary Science* 3: 217-236

Daubney R 1967 Viral encephalitis of equine and domestic ruminants in the Near East: Part II *Advances in Veterinary Science* 8: 419-439

Daubney R and Mahlau E A 1957 Near-eastern equine encephalomyelitis *Nature* 179: 584-585

Daubney R and Mahlau E A 1967 Viral encephalomyelitis of equines and domestic ruminants in the Near East: Part I *Advances in Veterinary Science* 8: 375-397

David J S E and McCullagh K G 1978 A case of spermatic arteriovenous anastomosis in the horse *Equine Veterinary Journal* 10: 94-96

Davidson H J, Blanchard G L, Wheeler C A, and Render J A 1991 Anterior uveal melanoma, with secondary keratitis, cataract, and glaucoma in a horse *Journal of the American Veterinary Medical Association* 199: 1049-1050

Davis S W, Daft B N, and Dubey J P 1991 *Sarcocytis neurona* cultured in vitro from a horse with equine protozoal myelitis *Equine Veterinary Journal* 23: 315-317

Day M J and Penhale W J 1986 Immunodiagnosis of autoimmune skin disease in the dog, cat and horse *Australian Veterinary Journal* 63: 65-68

DeBowes R M, Leipold H W, and Turner-Beatty M 1987 Cerebellar abiotrophy *Veterinary Clinics of North America: Equine practice* 3: 345-352

Debrade M 1892/93 Granulosa cell tumor (abstract) *American Veterinary Revue* 16: 640

Deegan E 1972 Die prognostische Bedeutung des "Hegglin-Syndroms" bei der Hyperlipamie der Ponys *Deutsche Tierärtzliche Wochenschrift* 79: 289-312

Deegan E 1976 Diagnostik und Bedeutung von Reizbildungsstorungen beim Pferd *Deutsche Tierärtzliche Wochenscrift* 83: 361-367

Deegan E and Klein H J 1987 Rostrale Verlagerung des Arcus palatopharyngicus beim Pferd *Pferdheilkunde* 3: 303-8

Deegan E, Freytag K, and Hertsch B 1976 Diagnose der Schlunderkrankungen beim Pferde *Tierärztliche Praxis* 4: 207-21

Deem D A and Fregin G F 1982 Atrial fibrillation in horses: A review of 106 clinical cases, with consideration of prevalence, clinical signs, and prognosis *Journal of the American Veterinary Medical Association* 180: 261-265

Deem D A and Harrington D D 1980 *Nocardia brasiliensis* in a horse with pneumonia and pleuritis *Cornell Veterinarian* 70: 321-328

DeJong D A 1917 The relationship between contagious pustular dermatitis of the horse, equine variola, and vaccinia *Journal of Comparative Pathology Therapeutics* 30: 242-62

Delius Ch 1982 Pathomorpholgische und röntgenologische Veränderungen am isolierten Strahlbein beim Pferd *Dissertation*, Hannover

DeMoor A, Verschooten F, Desmet P, and Steenhaut M 1972 Osteochondritis dissecans of the tibiotarsal joint of the horse *Equine Veterinary Journal* 4: 139

Denny H R 1973 A review of brucellosis *Equine Veterinary Journal* 5: 121-5

Deorani V P S 1966 Studies on pathological lesions due to

Strongylus vulgaris infection in an Indian pony *Indian Veterinary Journal* 43: 865-868

Derksen F J and Robinson N E 1980 Esophageal and intrapleural pressures in the healthy, conscious pony. *American Journal of Veterinary Research* 41: 1756

Derksen F J, Reed S M, and Hall C C 1981 Aneurysm of aortic arch and bicarotid trunk in a horse *Journal of the American Veterinary Medical Association* 179: 692-694

Derksen F J, Robinson N E, and Slocombe R F 1982 3-methylindole-induced pulmonary toxicosis in ponies *American Journal of Veterinary Research* 43: 603-607

Derksen F J, Scott J S, Slocombe R F, and Robinson N E 1987 *Micropolyspora faeni* causes airway inflammation but not hyperresponsiveness in sensitized ponies *Journal Applied Physiology* 62: 1398-1404

Derksen F J, Robinson N E, Scott J S, and Stick J A 1988 Aerosolized *Micropolyspora faeni* antigen as a cause of pulmonary dysfunction in ponies with recurrent airway obstruction (heaves) *American Journal of Veterinary Research* 49: 933-938

Desbrosse F, Dodin A, and Galimand M 1978 La pseudo-morve ou melioidose: Maladie due au bacille de Whitmore, mise en evidence dans la region Ouest-Parisienne *Bulletin Societe Veterinare Practice de France* 62: 657-672

Detilleux P G, Cheville N F, and Sheahan B J 1989 Ultrastructure and lectin histiochemistry of equine cutaneous histiolymphocytic lymphosarcomas *Veterinary Pathology* 26: 409-419

Detweiler D K, Patterson D F, Luginbuhl H 1972 Observations on naturally occurring fibrosis and necrosis in dogs *Recent Advances and Studies in Cardiac Structure and Metabolism* 1: 574-578

Deubel 1932 Beobachtung an Pferden mit enzootischer Haemogloinamie *Tierärtzliche Rundschau* 38: 414-16

Devas M B 1961 Compression stress fractures in man and greyhounds *Journal Bone Joint Surg* 43B: 540

Devries G A and Josephus Jitta C R 1973 An epizootic in horses in the Netherlands caused by *Trichophyton equinum* var. *Equinum Sabouraudia* 11: 137-139

Devriese L A and Haesebrouck F 1992 *Streptococcus suis* infections in horses and cats *Veterinary Record* 130: 380

Devriese L A, Vlaminick K, Nuytten J, and De Keersmaecker P 1983 *Staphylococcus hyicus* in skin lesions of horses *Equine Veterinary Journal* 15: 263-265

Devriese L A, Nzuambe D, and Godard C 1984/85 Identification and characteristics of staphylococci isolated from lesions and normal skin of horses *Veterinary Microbiology* 10: 269-277

De Waal D T and Potgieter F T 1987 The transstadial transmission of *Babesia caballi* by *Rhipicephalus evertsi Onderstepoort Journal of Veterinary Research* 54: 655-656

De Waal D T, Van Heerden J, and Potgieter F T 1987 An investigation into the clinical pathological changes and serological response in horses experimentally infected with *Babesia equi* and *Babesia caballi Onderstepoort Journal of Veterinary Research* 54: 561-568

Dewes H F 1982 The onset and consequences of tarsal bone fractures in foals *New Zealand Veterinary Journal* 30: 129-35

Dewes H F 1989 The association between weather, frenzied behaviour, percutaneous invasion by *Strongyloides westeri* larvae and *Rhodococcus* equi disease in foals *New Zealand Veterinary Journal* 37(2): 69-73

Dice P F and Cooley P L 1990 Peripheral corneal ulcers in the horse *Equine Veterinary Journal* 10 (supplement): 18-21

Dickerson J W T, Southgate D A T, and King J M 1967 The origin and development of hippomanes in the horse and zebra 2. The chemical composition of the foetal fluids and hippomanes *Journal Anatomy* 101: 285-93

Dieckerhoff 1888 *Lehrbuch der Speziellen Pathologies und Therapie*. Berlin

Dieckerhoff 1890 Über die Diagnose des Kehlkopfpfeifens *Berliner Thierärztliche Wochenschrift* 43: 337-40

Dihlmann 1922 Über Osteome *Berliner Tierärtzliche Wochenscrift* 38: 267-8

Dill S G, Simoncini D C, Bolton G R, Rendano V T, Crissman J W, King J M, and Tennant B C 1982 Fibrinous pericarditis in the horse *Journal of the American Veterinary Medical Association* 180: 266-271

Dill S G, Kallfelz F A, Lahunta A de, and Waldron C H 1989a Serum vitamin E and blood glutathione peroxidase values of horses with degenerative myeloencephalopathy *Americal Journal of Veterinary Research* 50: 166-168

Dill S G, Hintz H A, Lahunta A de, and Waldron C H 1989b Plasma and liver copper values in horses with equine degenerative myeloencephalopathy *Canadian Journal of Veterinary Research* 53: 29-32

Dill S G, Correa M T, Erb H N, Lahunta A de, Kallfelz F A, and Waldron C 1990 Factors associated with the development of equine degenerative myeloencephalopathy *American Journal of Veterinary Research* 51: 1300-1305

Dimery N J, Alexander R McN, and Ker R F 1986 Elastic extension of the leg tendons in the locomotion of horses (Equus caballus) *Journal Zoology, London* 210: 415-25

Dimock W W 1931 *Corynebacterium equi* in pneumonia in foals *Journal of the American Veterinary Medical Association* 79: 809-812

Dimock W W and Edwards P R 1927 Genital infection in mares by an organism of the *Encapsulatus* group *Journal of the American Veterinary Medical Association* 70: 469-480

Dimock W W and Edwards P R 1928 Pathology and bacteriology of the reproductive organs of mares in relation to sterility *Kentucky Agricultural Experiment Station Bulletin* 86.

Dimock W W and Edwards P R 1932 Infections of fetuses and foals *Kentucky Agricultural Experiment Station Bulletin* 333

Dimock W W and Edwards P R 1933 Is there a filterable virus of abortion of mares? *Kentucky Agricultural Experiment Station Bulletin* 333.

Dimock W W, Westerfield C, and Doll E R 1944 The equine thyroid in health and disease *Journal of the*

American Veterinary Medical Association 104: 313-17

Dimock W W, Edwards P R, and Bruner D W 1947 Infections of fetuses and foals *Kentucky Agricultural Experiment Station Bulletin* 509

Divers T J, George L W, and George J W 1982 Hemolytic anemia in horses after ingestion of red maple leaves *Journal of the American Veterinary Medical Association* 180: 300-2

Divers T J, Byars T D, Leitch M, and Crowell W A 1987 Acute renal failure in six horses resulting from haemodynamic causes *Equine Veterinary Journal* 19: 178-184

Dixon P M, McPherson E A, and Muir A 1977 Familial methaemoglobinaemia and haemolytic anaemia in the horse associated with decreased erythrocytic glutathione reductase and glutathione *Equine Veterinary Journal* 9: 198-201

Dixon P M, McGorum B C, Long K J, and Else R W 1992 Acute eosinophilic interstitial pulmonary disease in a pony *Veterinary Record* 130: 367-372

Dixon R J, Hartley W J, Hutchins D R, Lepherd E E, Feilen C, Jones R F, Love D N, Sabine M, and Wells A L 1978 Perinatal foal mortality associated with a herpesvirus *Australian Veterinary Journal* 54: 103-105

Dobberstein J 1926 Über einen Fall von Leberkoller des Pferdes und die dabei gefundenen Gehirnveränderungen *Deutsch Tierärztliche Wochenschrift* 34: 501-10

Dobberstein J 1938 Der Sektionbefund in der gerichtlichen tierheilkunde I Die chronische Kolik des Pferdes *Berliner Münchener Tierärztliche Wochenshcrift* 493-9

Dobberstein J 1950 Zur Statitik der Kolik *Nordiska Veterinärmedicin* 2: 707-720

Dobberstein J 1957 *Richtlinien für die Sektion der Haustiere* Berlin, Paul Parey

Dobberstein J and Dinter W 1942 Beitrage zur Sektionsstatistik der Kolik des Pferdes *Archiv wissenschaftlige Prakt Tierheilkunde* 76: 256

Dobberstein J and Hartmann H 1932 Über die Anastosenbildung im Bereich der Blind- und Grimmdarmarterien des Pferdes und ihre Bedeutung für die Enstehung der Embolilschen Kolik *Berliner Tierärztliche Wochenschrift* 397-402

Dobberstein J and Tamaschke Ch 1969 Vol.1 Metastatische Geschwulste des Knochens In Dobberstein J, Pallaske G, and Stünzi H (Eds) *Joest's Handbuch der Speziellen Pathologischen Anatomie der Haustiere* 3rd Ed Berlin, Parey

Dobin M A Endokarditis beim Pferd *Monatsh Veterinarmed* 23(16): 630-633

Dobos-Kovacs M 1981 Idult, difuz membranoproliferativ glomerulonefritisz es szovodmenyei loban *Magyar Allatorvosok Lapja* 36: 533-535

Doby P B, Schnurrenburger P R, Martin R J, Hanson L E, Sherick G W, and Schoenholz W K 1966 Western encephalitis in Illinois horses and ponies *Journal of the American Veterinary Medical Association* 148: 422-427

Dodd D C, Blakeley A A, Thornbury R S, and Dewes H F 1960 Muscle degeneration and yellow fat disease in foals *New Zealand Veterinary Journal* 8: 45-58

Doll E R 1952 Observations on the clinical features and pathology of hemolytic icterus of newborn foals *Mer J Vet Res* 13: 504-508

Doll E R 1961 Influenza of horses *Annual Review Respiratory Disease* 83: 48-50

Doll E R 1972 Viral Rhinopneumonitis In *Equine Medicine and Surgery* 2nd Ed Illinois, American Veterinary Publications

Doll E R and Bryans J T 1963 Epizootiology of equine viral rhinopneumonitis *Journal of the American Veterinary Medical Association* 142: 31-37

Doll E R, Bryans J T, McCollum W H, Crowe M E W 1957a Isolation of a filterable agent causing arteritis of horses and abortion by mares. Its differentiation from the equine abortion (influenza) virus *Cornell Veterinarian* 47: 3

Doll E R, Knappenberger R E, and Bryans J T 1957b An outbreak of abortion caused by the equine arteritis virus *Cornell Veterinarian* 47: 69

Dollahite J W, Younger R L, Crookshank H R, Jones L P, and Peterson H D 1978 Chronic lead poisoning in horses *American Journal of Veterinary Research* 39: 961-964

Dollar J A W 1920 *Regional Veterinary Surgery and Operative Technique*, Chicago, Alex Eger

Donaldson R S 1973 Eversion of the bladder in a mare *Veterinary Record* 104: 408-410

Doran R E and Collins L G 1986 Mastocytoma in a horse *Equine Veterinary Journal* 18: 500-502

Dorn C R, Garner H E, Coffman J R, Hahn A W, and Tritschler L G 1975 Castration and other factors affecting the risk of equine laminitis *Cornell Veterinarian* 65: 57-64

Dorr T E, Higgins R J, Dangler C A, Madigan, J E, and Witham C L 1984 Protozoal myeloencephalitis in horses in California *Journal of the American Veterinary Medical Association* 185: 801-802

Dow S M, Leendertz J A, Silver I A, and Goodship A E 1991 Identification of subclinical tendon injury from ground reaction force analysis *Equine Veterinary Journal* 23(4): 266-72

Drahn F 1921 Die Polydactylie des Pferdes *Berliner Tierärztliche Wochenschrift* 37: 75

Drechsler O von 1958 Neue Gedanken über die Atiologie der Langsachsendrehung des grossen Colon beim Pferd *Deutscher Tierärztliche Wochenschrift* 65: 298-303

Dreesen D W 1991 Association of colonic distension, displacement, and volvulus with pasture grasses *4th Equine Colic Research Symposium* Athens, Georgia

Drew B, Barber W P, and Williams D G 1975 The effect of excess dietary iodine on pregnant mares and foals *Veterinary Record* 97: 93

Drew R A and Greatorex J C 1974 Vertebral plasma cell myeloma causing posterior paralysis in a horse *Equine Veterinary Journal* 6(3): 131-134

Driscoll J, Hintz H E, and Schryver H F 1978 Goiter in foals caused by excessive iodine *Journal of the American Veterinary Medical Association* 173: 838

Drommer W 1966 Über Blitzschaden bei Tieren *Deutscher Tierärztliche Wochenschrift* 73: 596-603

Drudge J H 1985 *Parasites, Pests, and Predators* In Gaafer S M, Howard W E, and Marsh R E (Eds) Amsterdam, Elsevier

Drudge J H 1986 Large strongyles *Veterinary Clinics North America* 2: 263-80

Drudge J H and Lyons E T 1986 *Internal parasites of Equids with emphasis on treatment and control* Somerville, New Jersey, Hoechst-Roussel

Dubey J P, Davis S W, Speer C A, Bowman D D, Lahunta A de, Granstrom D E, and Topper M J 1991 *Journal Parasitology* 77: 212-18

Dudan F, Rossi G L, and Luginbuhl H 1984 *Schweizer Archiv Tierheilkunde* 126: 527-38

Dudan F, Rossi G L, and Luginbuhl H 1985 *Schweizer Archiv Tierheilkunde* 127: 319-38,369-78

Duff H M 1933 *Journal of Comparative Pathology Therapeutics* 46: 42-6

Dugan S J, Roberts S M, Curtis C R, and Severin G A 1991 Prognostic factors and survival of horses with ocular/adnexal squamous cell carcinoma: 147 cases (1978-1988) *Journal of the American Veterinary Medical Association* 198: 298-303

Dukes H H 1942 *The Phyiology of Domestic Animals* Ithaca, Comstock

Duncan C S 1961 Oak leaf poisoning in two horses *Cornell Veterinarian* 51: 159-62

Duncan I D and Brook D 1985 Bilateral laryngeal paralysis in the horse *Equine Veterinary Journal* 17: 228-233

Duncan I D and Schneider R K 1985 Equine suprascapular neuropathy (sweeney): clinical and pathological observations *Proceedings American Association Equine Practitioners*

Duncan I D, Griffiths I R, McQueen A, Baker G O 1974 The pathology of equine laryngeal hemiplegia *Acta Neuropathologica* 27: 337-48

Duncan I D, Griffiths I R, and Madrid R E 1978 A light and electron microscopic study of the neuropathy of equine idiopathic laryngeal hemiplegia *Neuropathology and Applied Neurobiology* 4: 483-501

Duncan I D, Schneider R K, and Hammang J P 1987 Subclinical entrapment neuropathy of the equine suprascapular nerve *Acta Neuropathologica* 74: 53-61

Duncan S G, Meyers K M, and Reed S M 1983 Reduction of the red blood cell mass of horses: Toxic effect of heparin anticoagulant therapy *American Journal of Veterinary Research* 44: 2271-2276

Dungworth D L and Fowler M E 1966 Cerebellar hypoplasia and degeneration in a foal *Cornell Veterinarian* 56: 17-24

Du Pleissis J L and Basson P A 1966 Babesiosis in aborted equine foetuses: A report on two cases in South Africa *Journal of the South African Veterinary Medical Association* 37: 271-275

Dutta S K, Penney B E, Myrup A C, Robl M G, Rice R M 1988 Disease features in horses with induced equine monocytic ehrlichiosis (Potomac horse fever) *American Journal of Veterinary Research* 49: 1747-1751

Dyce K M, Hartman W, and Aalfs R H G 1976 A cinefluoroscopic study of the caecal base of the horse *Research Veterinary Science* 20: 40-6

Dyce K M, Sack W O, Wensing C J G 1987 *Textbook of Veterinary Anatomy*, Philadelphia, WB Saunders

Dye V, Robertson J L, Aclund H, and Hong C B 1993 Morphologic characteristics of equine melanomas and relationship to biological behavior (in preparation)

Dyson S 1990 Musculoskeletal injuries of the equine athlete: are these sports related? *Proceedings International Conference Equine Sport Medicine*, Stockholm

Dyson S 1991 Lameness due to pain associated with the distal interphalangeal joint: 45 cases *Equine Veterinary Journal* 23: 128-35

Dyson S and Platt H 1985 Panniculitis in an aged pony resembling Weber-Christian disease in man *Equine Veterinary Journal* 17: 145-147

Dziezyc J, Kern T J, and Wolf E D 1983 Microphthalmia in a foal *Equine Veterinary Journal* 2 (supplement): 15-17

Dziezyc J, Samuelson D A, and Merideh R 1990 Ciliary cysts in three ponies *Equine Veterinary Journal* 10 (supplement): 22-25

Dziezyc J, Millichamp N J, and Keller C B 1991 Use of phacofragmentation for cataract removal in horses: 12 cases (1985-1989) *Journal of the American Veterinary Medical Association* 198: 1774-1778

Eamens G J, MacAdam J F, and Laing E A 1984 Skeletal abnormalities in young horses associated with zinc toxicity and hypocuprosis *Australian Veterinary Journal* 61: 205-7

Easley J R 1985 Erythrogram and red cell distribution width of equidae with experimentally induced anemia *American Journal of Veterinary Research* 46: 2378-2384

Easley K J 1988 Diagnosis and treatment of vesicovaginal reflux in the mare *Veterinary Clinics of North America: Equine Practice* 4: 407-416

Eastwood B J 1969 Mycotic flora of the apparently normal equine eye MS Thesis, Iowa State University

Eberbeck E and Hemmert-Halswick A 1943 Zur Pathogenese der Spatschaden des ansteckenden Katarrhs der Luftwege bzw. der Druse des Pferdes *Archiv fur wissenschaftliche und praktische Tierheilkunde* 78: 334-351

Edington N, Wright J A, Patel J R, Edwards G B, and Griffiths L 1984 Equine adenovirus 1 isolated from cauda equina neuritis *Research Veterinary Science* 37: 252-254

Edington N, Bridges C G, and Patel J R 1986 Endothelial cell infection and thrombosis in paralysis caused by equid herpevirus-I: equine stroke *Archives Virology* 90: 111-24

Edwards F G 1923 Sprains of the flexor tendons *Veterinary Record* 3: 113-6

Edwards G V J 1931 Care and management of colliery horses *Veterinary Record* 11: 1069-72

Eeckhout A V 1905/06 Laryngeal ecchondrosis in a horse that had stridulent laryngitis *American Veterinary Revue* 29: 604-5

Ehnen S J, Divers T J, Gillette D, and Reef V B 1990 Obstructive nephrolithiasis and ureterolithiasis associated with chronic renal failure in horses: eight cases (1981-

1987) *Journal American Medical Association* 197: 249-253

Eisenmenger E, Kreisel A, Schonbauer M, and Freiler I 1986 Filarien (Onchocerca reticulata) als Ursache von granulomatosen Wundheilungsstörungen an den Extremitäten von Pferd. *Wiener Tierärztliche Monatsschrift* 73: 244-47

Ek N 1981 Concentration of serum transferrin in sick horses and its relationship to serum albumin content *Acta Veterinaria Scandanavia* 22: 260-271

Ekfalck A 1990 Amino acids in different layers of the matrix of the normal equine hoof *Journal of Veterinary Medicine* 37: 1-8

Ekfalck A, Jones B and Obel N 1991 Possible importance for laminitis research of recent studies on substances influencing the differentiation of cultured keratinocytes *Journal of Veterinary Medicine* 38: 721-727

Ekfalck A, Rodriguez H, and Obel N 1992 Histopathology in post-surgical laminitis with a peracute course in a horse *Equine Veterinary Journal* 24: 321-324

Ekman S 1990 Ataxia in Swedish warmblood and Standardbred horses *Journal of Veterinary Medicine* 37: 379-391

Elfers R S, Bayly W M, Brobst D F, Reed S M, Liggitt H D, Hawker C D, and Baylink D J 1986 Alterations in calcium, phosphorous and C-terminal parathyroid hormone levels in equine acute renal disease *Cornell Veterinarian* 76: 317-329

El Shorafa W M, Feaster J P, and Ott E A 1979 Horse metacarpal bone: age, ash content, cortical area, and failure stress interrelationships *Journal Animal Science* 49: 979-982

Elias H 1946 The tonsils of the horse *American Journal of Veterinary Research* 7: 343-49

Elias H 1948 Growth of the adrenal cortex in domestic ungulata *American Journal of Veterinary Research* 9: 173-89

Elinder C G, Stenstrom T, Piscator M, Linnman L, and Jonsson L 1980 Water hardness in relation to cadmium accumulation and microscopic signs of cardiovascular disease in horses *Archives of Environmental Health* 35: 81-84

Ellenberger W 1917 Kann Rohrzucker die Ursache des Kelfkopfpfeifens sein? *Zeitschrift Veterinärkunde* 29: 109-13

Ellenberger W and Scheunert A 1910 *Vergleichende Physiologie der Haustiere* Berlin, Paul Parey

Elliot H B 1899/90 Pulmonary filariasis in a mule *American Veterinary Revue* 23: 435-6

Ellis D R 1979 Fractures of the proximal sesamoid bones in Thoroughbred foals *Equine Veterinary Journal* 11: 48

Ellis W A and O'Brien J J 1988 Leptospirosis in horses In Powell D G (Ed) *Equine Infectious Disease V* Lexington, University Press of Kentucky

Ellis W A, Bryson D G, O'Brien J J, and Neill S D 1983 Leptospiral infection in aborted equine foetuses *Equine Veterinary Journal* 15: 317-24

Else R W and Holmes J R 1972a Cardiac pathology in the horse (1) Gross pathology *Equine Veterinary Journal* 4: 1-8

Else R W and Holmes J R 1972b Cardiac pathology in the horse (2) Microscopic pathology *Equine Veterinary Journal* 4: 57-62

Else R W and Holmes J R 1972c Cardiac pathology in the horse (3) Clinical correlations *Equine Veterinary Journal* 4: 195-196

Else R W and Holmes J R 1972d Pathological changes in atrial fibrillation in the horse *Equine Veterinary Journal* 4: 56-64

Emerson F G and Jarvis A A 1968 Listeriosis in ponies *Journal of the American Veterinary Medical Association* 152: 1645-1646

Emmons R W, Woodie J D, Laub R L, and Oshiro L S 1983 Main Drain virus as a cause of equine encephalomyelitis *Journal of the American Veterinary Medical Association* 183: 555-558

England J J, Watson R E, and Larson K A 1973 Virus-like particles in an equine sarcoid cell line *American Journal of Veterinary Research* 34: 1601-1603

Enigk K 1950 Zur Entwicklung von *Strongylus vulgaris* (Nematodes) in Wirstiere *Zeitschrift Tropenmedicine Parasitology* 2: 287-306

Enigk K 1951a Pathogenese der thrombotischembolischen Kolik des Pferdes *Monatschrift praktische Tierheilkunde* 3: 65

Enigk K 1951b Weitere Untersuchungen zur Biolgie von *Strongylus vulgaris* (Nematodies) im Wirtstiere *Zeitschrift Tropenmedicine Parasitologie* 2: 523-35

Enigk K 1970 Development of the three species of Strongyles of the horse during the prepatent period In Bryans J T and Gerber H (Eds) *2nd International Congress Equine Infectious Diseases* Basel, Karger

Epstein V 1984 Relationship between potassium administration, hyperkalemia and the electrocardiogram: An experimental study *Equine Veterinary Journal* 16: 453-456

Erasmus B J 1978 A new approach to polyvalent immunization against African horsesickness In Bryans J T and Gerber H (Eds) *4th International Congress Equine Infectious Diseases* Basel, Karger

Erasmus B J, Young E, Pieterse L M, and Boshoff S T 1978 The susceptibility of zebra and elephants to African horsesickness virus In Bryans J T and Gerber H (Eds) *4th International Congress Equine Infectious Diseases* Basel, Karger

Erbsloh J K E 1975 Babesiosis in the newborn foal *Journal Reproduction Fertility* 23 (Supplement): 725-726

Eriksson K 1955 Hereditary aniridia with secondary cataract in horses *Nordiska Veterinärmedicine* 7: 773-93

Estes P C and Cheville N F 1970 The ultrastructure of vascular lesions in equine viral arteritis *American Journal Pathology* 58: 235-253

Evans C L 1957 Sweating in relation to sympathetic innervation *British Medical Bulletin* 134: 197-201

Evans C L, Nisbet A M and Ross K A 1957a A histological study of the sweat glands of normal and dry-coated horses *Journal of Comparative Pathology* 67: 397-405

Evans C L, Smith D F G, Ross K A, and Weil-Malherbe H 1957b Physiologic factors in the condition of "dry coat" in horses *Journal of Physiology* 135(2): 41P-42P

Evans E T R, Evans W C, and Roberts H E 1951 Studies on bracken poisoning in the horse *British Veterinary Journal* 107: 364-73; 399-411

Evans J H and Barbenel J C 1975 Structure and mechanical properties of tendon related to function *Equine Veterinary Journal* 7: 1-8

Eveleth D F and Gifford R 1943 Johne's disease in farm animals *Journal of the American Veterinary Medical Association* 102: 27-34

Ewert K M, Fessler J F, Templeton C B, Bottoms G D, Latshaw H S, and Johnson M A 1985 Endotoxin-induced hematologic and blood chemical changes in ponies: Effects of flunixin meglumine, dexamethasone, and prednisolone *American Journal of Veterinary Research* 46: 24-30

Eyre P 1982 Corticosteroids potentiate vasoconstriction in the equine hoof: A possible pharmacological basis for laminitis *American Association Equine Practitioners Newsletter* 2: 141-142

Eyre P and Elmes P J 1980 Corticosteroid-induced laminitis? Further observations on the isolated, perfused hoof *Veterinary Research Communication* 4: 139-143

Eyre P and Lewis A J 1973 Acute systemic anaphylaxis in the horse *British Journal Pharmacology* 48: 426-37

Eyre P, Elmes P J, and Strickland S 1979 Corticosteroid-potentiated vascular responses of the equine digit: a possible pharmacologic basis for laminitis *American Journal of Veterinary Research* 40: 135-138

Fadok V A 1984 Parasitic skin diseases of large animals *Veterinary Clinics of North America: Large Animal Practice* 6: 3-26

Fadok V A and Greiner E C 1990 Equine insect hypersensitivity: skin test and biopsy results correlated with clinical data *Equine Veterinary Journal* 22: 236-240

Fairman S and Cutshall C S 1953 *Mechanics of Materials* New York, Wiley

Fankhauser R 1968 Entzundliche Gefässveränderungen als Grunlage von Ruckenmarksläsionen beim Pferd *Schweizer Archiv Tierheilkunde* 110: 171-179

Fankhauser R and Gerber H 1970 Zerebrale Vaskulitis beim Pferd *Archives Experimental Veterinary Medicine* 24: 61-71

Fankhauser R, Luginbuhl H, and McGrath J T 1974 Tumours of the nervous system: domestic animals *Bulletin WHO* 50: 53-69

Fankhauser R, Gerber H, Cravero G C, and Straub R 1975 Klinik und Pathologie der Neuritis caudae equina *Schweiz Archiv Tierheilkunde* 117: 675-99

Farrell R K, Sande R D, and Lincoln S D 1971 Nigropallidal encephalomalacia in a horse *Journal of the American Veterinary Medical Association*

Farrelly B T 1954 The pathogenesis and significance of parasitic endarteritis and thrombosis in the ascending aorta of the horse *Veterinary Record* 66: 53-61

Farrelly B T, Collins J D, and Collins S M 1966 Autoimmune haemolytic anaemia (AHA) in the horse *Irish Veterinary Journal* 20: 42-45

Farris H E, Fraunfelder F T, and Mason C T 1976 Cryotherapy of equine sarcoid and other lesions *Veterinary Medicine/Small Animal Clinician* 71: 325-29

Fatemi-Nainie S, Anderson L W, and Cheevers W P 1984 Culture characteristics and tumorigenicity of the equine sarcoid-derived MC-1 cell line *American Journal of Veterinary Research* 45: 1105-1108

Fawi M T 1971 *Histoplasma farciminosum*, the aetiological agent of equine cryptococcal pneumonia *Sabouraudia* 9: 123-125

Fayer R and Dubey J P 1982 Development of Sarcocytis fayeri in the equine *Journal Parasitology* 68(5): 856-880

Fayer R, Mayhew I G, Baird J D, et al. 1990 Epidemiology of equine protozoal myeloencephalitis in North America based on histologically confirmed cases: a report *Journal Veterinary Internal Medicine* 4(2): 54-57

Feldman B F and Giacopuzzi R L 1982 Hemophilia A (Factor VIII deficiency) in a colt *Equine Practice* 4: 24-30

Fellenberg G von 1987 Proteasen und Proteaseninhibitoren von moglicher klinischer Relevanz bei der COPD des Pferdes *Tierärtzliche Praxis* 15: 399-407

Felsburg P J, Somberg R L, and Perryman L E 1992 Domestic animal models of severe combined immunodeficiency: canine x-linked severe combined immunodeficiency and severe combined immunodeficiency in horses *Immunodeficiency Reviews* 3: 277-303

Ferris D H, Badiali L, Abou-Youssef M, and Beamer P D 1968 A note on experimental rabies in the donkey *Cornell Veterinarian* 58: 270-277

Fessler J F, Bottoms G D, Roesel O F, Moore A B, Frauenfelder H C, and Boon G D 1982 Endotoxin-induced change in hemograms, plasma enzymes, and blood chemical values in anesthetized ponies: effects of flunixin meglumine *American Journal of Veterinary Research* 43: 141-144

Field J R and Jeffcott L B 1989 Equine laminitis- another hypothesis for pathogenesis *Medical Hypotheses* 30: 203-210

Fincher M G and Olafson P 1934 Chronic diffuse glomerulonephritis in a horse *Cornell Veterinarian* 24: 356-360

Firth E C 1976 Dissecting hematoma of corpus spongiosum and urinary bladder rupture in a stallion *Journal of the American Veterinary Medical Association* 169: 800-801

Firth E C 1977 Vestibular disease, and its relationship to facial paralysis in the horse; a clinical study of 7 cases *Australian Veterinary Journal* 53(12): 560-565

Firth E C 1983 Current concepts of infectious arthritis in foals *Equine Veterinary Journal* 15: 5-9

Fischer A T, Spier S, Carlson G P, and Hackett R P 1985 Neoplasia of the equine urinary bladder as a cause of hematuria *Journal of the American Veterinary Medical Association* 186: 1294-1296

Fjeldborg J 1987 Radiographische Festellung der Epiglottislange bei Pferden mit Entrapment der Epiglottis

Pferdheilkunde 3: 9-13

Fleming G. 1882 Laryngismus paralytica ("Roaring") *Veterinary Journal* 14: 1-12;81-96

Fletcher J M 1937 Louping ill in the horse *Veterinary Record* 49: 17-18

Flores J M, Rodriguez M, Castano M, Gonzalez J L, and Gallego E 1984 Pulmonary complications of equine influenza *Medicina Veterinaria* 1: 21-23

Foerner J J 1967 The diagnosis and correction of false nostril noises *Proceedings Annual Convention American Association Equine Practitioners*

Foil L and Foil C 1986 Parasitic skin diseases *Veterinary Clinics of North America: Equine Practice* 2: 403-437

Folger A F 1909 Pathologie der Nebennieren bei den Haustieren *Monatschrift Tierheilkunde* 20: 145-92

Ford E J H and Gopinath C 1974 The excretion of phylloerythrin and bilirubin by the horse *Research Veterinary Science* 16: 186-198

Ford J and Lokai M D 1980 Complications of *Streptococcus equi* infection *Equine Practice* 4: 41-44

Ford T S, Freeman D E, Ross M W, Richardson D W, and Martin R B, and Madison J B 1990 Ileocecal intussusception in horses: 26 cases (1981-88) *Journal of the American Veterinary Medical Association* 196: 121-26

Foreman J H and Santschi E M 1989 Equine bacterial meningitis-Part II: Key facts *Compendium of Continuing Education in Veterinary Medicine* 11: 640-644

Foreman J H, Potter K A, Bayly W M, and Liggitt H D 1986 Generalized steatitis associated with selenium deficiency and normal vitamin E status in a foal *Journal of the American Veterinary Medical Association* 1891(1): 83-86

Foreman J H, Weidner J P, Parry B W, and Hargis A 1990 Pleural effusion secondary to thoracic metastatic mammary adenocarcinoma in a mare *Journal of the American Veterinary Medical Association* 197: 1193-1195

Forenbacher S 1952 Schachtelhalmvergiftung der Pferde—eine B1-Avitaminose *Schweizer Archiv Tierheilkunde* 94: 153-71

Forssell G 1914/15 Untersuchungen über die Wirkungsweise der Beugesehnen am Vorderfuss des Pferdes. Über die funktionelle Struktur der Sehnen. *Zeitschrift Tiermedicine* 18: 184-8,467-75

Forsyth A A 1941 Grass disease in a coal mine *British Veterinary Journal* 97: 26-28

Foss F R, Genetzky R M, Riedesel E A, and Graham C 1983 Cervical intervertebral disk protrusion in two horses *Canadian Veterinary Journal* 24: 188-91

Fowler M E 1965 Nigropallidal encephalomalacia in the horse *Journal of the American Veterinary Medical Association* 147(6): 607-616

Frame S R, Harrington D D, Fessler J, and Frame P F 1988 Hereditary junctional mechanobullous disease in a foal *Journal of the American Veterinary Medical Association* 193: 1420-24

Franco D A 1969 Thrombocytopenia and its relationship to sporadic idiopathic epistaxis in Thoroughbreds *Veterinary Medicine/Small Animal Clinician* December 64: 1071-1072

Frank E R 1935 Pyramidal disease *North American Veterinarian* 16: 34

Frauenfelder H C, Kazacos K R, and Lichtenfels J R 1980 Cerebrospinal nematodiasis caused by a filarid in a horse *Journal of the American Veterinary Medical Association* 177: 359-62

Frederick D 1990 (Letter) Excisions of melanomas in horses *Journal of the American Veterinary Medical Association* 196: 1201-1202

Freeman D E, Koch D B, and Boles C L 1979 Mesodiverticular bands as a cause of small intestinal strangulation and volvulus in the horse *Journal of the American Veterinary Medical Association* 175: 1089-94

Freeman D E, Cimprich R E, Richardson D W, Gentile D G, Orsini J A, Tulleners E P, and Fetrow J P 1988 Early mucosal healing and chronic changes in pony jejunum after various types of strangulation obstruction *American Journal of Veterinary Research* 49: 810-818

Freestone J F and Carlson G P 1991 Muscle disorders in the horse: a retrospective study *Equine Veterinary Journal* 23: 86-90

Freestone J F, Thomas W P, Carlson G P, and Brumbaugh G W 1987 Idiopathic effusive pericarditis with tamponade in the horse *Equine Veterinary Journal* 19: 38-42

Fregin G F 1982 The equine electrocardiogram with standardized body and limb positions *Cornell Veterinarian* 72(3): 304-324

Freudenberg F 1956 Beobactaungen uber Fructbarkett, Brucellose and Tuberculose bei Gemeinschaftswide von Jungrinden des mitteldeutschen Trockengebietes *Mh Vet Med* 11: 432-436

Fretz P B 1980 Angular limb deformities in foals *Veterinary Clinics North America* 2: 125-50

Fretz P B, Babiuk L A, and McLaughlin B 1979 Equine respiratory disease on Western Canada racetracks *Canadian Veterinary Journal* 20: 58-61

Fricker C H, Riek W, and Hugelshofer J 1980 Verschluss der Digitalareterien beim Pferd *Tierärztliche Praxis* 10: 81-90

Fricker C, Riek W, and Hugelshofer J 1981 Der Verschluss der Digitalarterien als Lahmheitsursache beim Pferd *Schweizer Archiv Tierheilkunde* 123: 235-240

Fricker C H, Riek W, and Hugelshofer J 1982 Occlusion of the digital arteries—A model for pathogenesis of navicular disease *Equine Veterinary Journal* 14: 203-207

Friedberger and Fröhner 1895 *Pathology and Therapeutics of Domestic Animals* Zuill, W.L. (trans) Philadelphia, Zuill

Frischbier 1928 Versuche über die Festigkeit, Dehnbarkeit und Elastizität der wichtigsten Streck- und Beugesehnene des Pferdes *Zeitschrift Veterinärkunde* 8: 273-304

Fröhner E 1905 *Allgemeine Chirurgie* Vienna, Braumuller

Frost R D I 1974 Sweet itch (correspondence) *Veterinary Record* 94: 28

Frothingham L 1902 A tumor-like lesion in the lung of a horse caused by *Blastomyces* (Torula) *Journal Medical Research* 3: 31-43

Fuchs G 1959 Über Veränderungen an den Nebennieren des Pferdes bei verschiedenen Kranheiten *Dissertation*, Leipzig

Fulton R E, Doane F W, and Macpherson L W 1970 The fine structure of equine papillomas and the equine papilloma virus *Journal Ultrastructure Research* 30: 328-343

Funkquist B 1992 Aspects of studies on the pathogenesis of equine laminitis *Equine Veterinary Journal* 24: 253-255

Furr M O, Anver M, and Wise M 1991 Intervertebral disk prolapse and diskspondylitis in a horse *Journal of the American Veterinary Medical Association* 198: 2095-96

Furr M O, Crisman M V, Robertson J L, Barta O, Swecker, W S 1992 Immunodeficiency associated with lymphosarcoma in a horse *Journal American Veterinary Medical Association* 201(32): 307-309

Gabal M A and Khalifa K 1983 Study on the immune response and serological diagnosis of equine histoplasmosis (epizootic lymphangitis) *Zentralblatte Veterinar Medizin* 30: 317-321

Gabbiani G and Majno G 1972 Dupuytren's contracture: fibroblast contraction? *American Journal Pathology* 66: 131-37

Gainer J H, Amster R L, Needham J W, and Schilling K F 1966 Altered serum lipoproteins in equine infectious anemia: comparisons of values among normal horses and horses infected with *Babesia caballi American Journal of Veterinary Research* 27: 1611-1621

Galan J E and Timoney J F 1985a Mucosal nasopharyngeal responses of horses to protein antigens of *Streptococcus equi Infection Immunology* 47: 623-628

Galan J E and Timoney J F 1985b Immune complexes in purpura hemorrhagica of the horse contain IgA and M antigen of *Streptococcus equi Journal of Immunology* 135: 3134-3137

Galey F D, Beasley V R, Schaeffer D J, and Davis L E 1989 Antagonism in isolated equine digital vessels of contraction induced by epinephrine in the presence of hydrocortisone and an aqueous extract of black walnut (*Juglans nigra*) *Journal of Veterinary Pharmacologic Therapeutics* 12: 411-420

Galey F D, Twardock A R, Goetz T E, Schaeffer D J, Hall J O, and Beasley V R 1990 Gamma scintigraphic analysis of the distribution of perfusion of blood in the equine foot during black walnut (*Juglans nigra*)- induced laminitis *American Journal of Veterinary Research* 151: 688-695

Galey F D, Whiteley H E, Goetz T E, Kuenstler A R, Davis C A, and Beasley, V R 1991 Black walnut (*Juglans nigra*) toxicosis: A model for equine laminitis *Journal of Comparative Pathology* 104: 313-326

Gard G P, Marshall, I D, Walker K H, Acland H M, and De Sarem W G 1977 Association of Australian arboviruses with nervous disease in horses *Australian Veterinary Journal* 53: 61-66

Gardiner M R 1964 Horse problems in the Kimberleys. A review of current horse disease and ill-thrift problems in the Kimberley region of Western Australia, with emphasis on the "Kimberley horse disease" *Journal Agriculture Western Australia* 5: 576-581

Gardner S Y, Reef V B, and Spencer P A 1991 Ultrasonographic evaluation of horses with thrombophlebitis of the jugular vein: 46 cases (1985-1988) *Journal of the American Veterinary Medical Association* 199: 370-373

Garma-Avina A, Valli V E, and Lumsden, J H 1981 Equine congenital cutaneous papillomatosis: A report of 5 cases *Equine Veterinary Journal* 13: 59-61

Garner H E 1975 Pathophysiology of equine laminitis *Proceedings American Association of Equine Practitioners* 21: 384-387

Garner H E 1982 Laminitis modeling *American Association of Equine Practioners Newsletter* 2: 116-119

Garner, H E, Coffman J R, Hahn A W, Ackerman N, and Johnson J H 1974 Clinical characterization of equine laminitis and associated hypertension *Journal of the American Veterinary Medical Association* 165: 727

Garner H E, Coffman J R, Hahn A W, Ackerman N, and Johnson J H 1975a Equine laminitis and associated hypertension: A review *Journal of the American Veterinary Medical Association* 166: 56-57

Garner H E, Coffman J R, Hahn A W, Hutcheson D P, and Tumbleson M E 1975b Equine laminitis of alimentary origin: An experimental model *American Journal of Veterinary Research* 36: 441-444

Garner H E, Coffman J R, Halliwell W H, and Brown, E M 1975c Clinical signs of acute alimentary laminitis correlated with cardiovascular and histopathologic alterations 20: 61-65

Garner H E, Moore J N, Johnson J H, Clark L, Amend J F, Tritschler L G, Coffman J R, Sprouse R F, Hutcheson D P, and Salem C A 1978 Changes in the caecal flora associated with the onset of laminitis *Equine Veterinary Journal* 10: 249-52

Garner H E, Sprouse R F, Moore J N, Coffman J R 1981 A mechanistic approach to prevention and treatment of acute equine laminitis *Proceedings of the American Association of Equine Practitioners* 1981 27: 489

Garner H E, Hahn A W, Salem C, Coffman J R, Hutcheson D P, and Johnson, J H 1977 Cardiac output, left ventricular ejection rate, plasma volume, and heart rate changes in equine laminitis-hypertension *American Journal of Veterinary Research* 38: 725-729

Gavard M 1890 Luxation tibio-astragalienne *Journal Medicine Veterinaire* 41: 410-11

Gay CC and Speirs V C 1978 Parastic arteritis and its consequences in horses *Australian Veterinary Journal* 54: 600-601

Gebauer M R, Pickett B W, Voss J L, and Swierstra E E 1974 Reproductive physiology of the stallion: daily sperm output and testicular measurements *Journal of the American Veterinary Medical Association* 165: 711-713

Geisel O, Boch E, and Bachmann P A 1977 Zum Vorkommen und zur Histogenese unterscheidlicher fetaler Pneumopathien beim Virusabort des Pferdes *Berliner und Münchener Tierärtzliche Wochenschrift* 90: 429-432

Geiser D R 1975 The azoturia tying-up syndrome *Veterinary Medicine/ Small Animal Clinician* June: 710-713

Geiser D R, Henton J R, and Held J P 1988 Tympanic bulla, petrous temporal bone, and hyoid apparatus diseases in horses *Compendium Continuing Education Practicing Veterinarian* 10: 740-55

Gelatt K N 1974 Pseudomonas ulcerative keratitis and abscess in a horse *VM SAC* 69(10): 1309-1310

Gelatt K N 1979 Neuroretinopathy in the horse *Journal of Equine Medicine and Surgery* 3: 91-94

Gelatt K N 1981 *Textbook of Veterinary Ophthalmology*, Philadelphia, Lea and Febiger

Gelatt K N 1982 The eye-diseases and diagnoses In Mansmann R A, McAllister E S, Pratt P W (eds) *Equine Medicine and Surgery,* 3rd ed, Santa Barbara, American Veterinary Publications

Gelatt K N, Leipold H W, and Coffman, J R 1969 Bilateral optic nerve hypoplasia in a colt *Journal of the American Veterinary Medical Association* 155: 627-631

Gelatt K N, Leipold, H W, Finocchio E J, and Coffman J R 1971 Optic disc astrocytoma in a horse *Canadian Veterinary Journal* 12: 53-55

Gelberg H B and McEntee K 1987 Equine testicular interstitial cell tumors *Veterinary Pathology* 24: 231-234

Gelberg H B, Zachary J F, Everitt J I et al. 1985 Sudden death in training and racing Thoroughbred horses *Journal of the American Veterinary Medical Association* 187: 1354-1356

Gelberg H B, Smetzer D L, and Foreman J H 1991 Pulmonary hypertension as a cause of atrial fibrillation in young horses: four cases (1980-1989) *Journal of the American Veterinary Medical Association* 198: 679-682

Gelderblom W C, Thiel P G, Jaskiewicz K, and Marasas W F 1986 Investigation on the carcinogenicity of fusarin C-a mutagenic metabolite of Fusarium moniliforme *Carcinogeneis* 7(11): 1899-1901

Gentry P A, Feldman B F, O'Neill S L, Madigan J E, and Zinkl J G 1992 Evaluation of the haemostatic profile in the pre- and post parturient mare, with particular focus on the perinatal period *Equine Veterinary Journal* 24: 33-36

Geor R J, Clark E G, Haines D M, and Napier P G 1990 Systemic lupus erythematosus in a filly *Journal of the American Veterinary Medical Association* 197: 1489-1492

Geor R J, Becker R L, Kanara E W, Hovda L R, Sweeney W H, Winter T F, Rorick J K, Ruth G R, Hope E, and Murphy M J 1992 Toxicosis in horses after ingestion of hoary alyssum *Journal of the American Veterinary Medical Association* 201: 63-67

Georg L K, Kaplan W, and Camp L B 1957 Equine ringworm with special reference to *Trichophyton equinum American Journal of Veterinary Research* 18: 798-810

George L W and White S L 1984 Autoimmune skin disease of large animals *Veterinary Clinics of North America: Large Animal Practice* 6: 79-86

George L W, Tanner M L, Roberson E L, and Burke T M 1981 Chronic respiratory disease in a horse infected with *Dictyocaulus arnfieldi Journal of the American Veterinary Medical Association* 179: 820-822

George L W, Divers T J, Mahaffey E A, and Suarez M J H 1982 Heinz body anemia and methemoglobinemia in ponies given red maple (*Acer rubrum L*) leaves *Veterinary Pathology* 19: 521-533

Georgi J R 1973 The Kikuchi-Enigk model of *Strongylus vulgaris* migration in horses *Cornell Veterinarian* 63: 220

Gerber H 1966 Influenza des Pferdes *Schweizer Archiv fur Tierheilkunde* 108: 167-189

Gerber H 1969a Klinik und Therapie Chronischer Lugenleiden des Pferdes *Deutsche Tierärtzliche Wochenscrift* 76: 234

Gerber H 1969b Clinical features, sequelae and epidemiology of equine influenza In Bryans J T and Gerber H (eds) *proceedings 2nd International Conference Equine Infectious Diseases* Basel, Karger 63-80

Gerber H 1973 Chronic pulmonary disease in the horse *Equine Veterinary Journal* 5: 26-33

Gerber H 1989 The genetic basis of some equine diseases *Equine Veterinary Journal* 21: 244-248

Gerlach F 1922 Serumkrankheit bei Rind und Pferd *Zeitschrift Immunitätsforschnung* 34: 75-94

Geyer H 1992 Hoof problems of Lipizzan horses and treatment with biotin *Seminar, Gluck Equine Research Center*

Gibbs E P J 1976 Equine viral encephalitis *Equine Veterinary Journal* 8: 66-71

Gibbs E P J, Roberts M C, and Morris J M 1972 Equine coital exanthema in the United Kingdom *Equine Veterinary Journal* 4: 74-80

Gibson K T and Alders R C 1987 Eosinophilic enterocolitis and dermatitis in two horses *Equine Veterinary Journal* 19: 247-52

Gilbert R O 1986 Congenital hyperlipaemia in a Shetland pony foal *Equine Veterinary Journal* 18: 498-500

Giles C J, Urquhart K A, and Longstaffe J A 1985 Larval cyathostomiasis (immature *Trichonema*-induced enteropathy): a report of 15 clinical cases *Equine Veterinary Journal* 17: 196-201

Gillespie J H and Timoney J F 1981 *Hagan and Bruner Infectious Diseases of Domestic Animals* 7th Ed Ithaca, Comstock

Gillespie J R 1975 Postnatal lung growth and function in the foal *Journal Reproductive Fertility* 23: 667-671

Gillespie J R 1976 External Respiration In Phillis J W (Ed) *Veterinary Physiology* Philadelphia, Saunders

Gilman A R 1952 Plasma protein changes in equine infectious anemia *American Journal of Veterinary Research* 13: 83-89

Gilmour J S 1973 Observations on neuronal changes in grass sickness of horses *Research in Veterinary Science* 15: 197-200

Gilmour J S and Fraser J A 1977 Ataxia in a Welsh Cob filly due to a venous malformation in the thoracic spinal cord *Equine Veterinary Journal* 9(1): 40-42

Giltner L T and Shahan M S 1933 The 1933 outbreak of infectious equine encephalomyelitis in the Eastern states *North American Veterinarian* 14: 25-27

Gilyard R T 1944 Chronic anhidrosis with lowered blood chlorides in race horses *Cornell Veterinarian* 34: 332-336

Ginther O J 1992 *Reproductive Biology of the Mare 2nd Ed.* Cross Plaines, Ginther

Girard A, Greig A S, and Mitchell D 1968 A virus associated with vulvitis and balanitis in the horse—A preliminary report *Canadian Journal of Comparative Medicine* 32: 603-604

Glastonbury P A and Day D G 1985 Degenerative optic neuropathy in a horse *Australian Veterinary Journal* 62: 243-244

Glaze M B 1983 Equine adnexal habronemiasis *Equine Veterinary Journal* 2 (supplement): 71-73

Glaze M B, Gossett K A, McCoy D J, and Kreeger J M 1990 A case of equine adnexal lymphosarcoma *Equine Veterinary Journal* 10 (supplement): 83-84

Gleiser C A, Gochenour W S Jr, Berge T O, and Tigertt W D 1962 The comparative pathology of experimental Venezuelan equine encephalomyelitis infection in different animal hosts *Journal of Infectious Diseases* 110: 80-97

Goad M E 1984 Pulmonary pythiosis in a horse *Veterinary Pathology* 21(2): 261-262

Godglück G 1967 Vol 6 Darm In Dobberstein J, Pallaske G, and Stünzi H (Eds) *Joest's Handbuch der Speziellen Pathologischen Anatomie der Haustiere* Berlin, Parey

Goetz T E, Ogilvie G K, Keegan K G, and Johnson P J 1990 Cimetidine for treatment of melanomas in three horses *Journal of the American Veterinary Medical Association* 196: 449-452

Goldberg S A 1918a Historical facts concerning the pathology of spavin *Journal of the American Veterinary Medical Association* 53: 745

Goldberg S A 1918b The pathology of spavin *Journal Medical Research* 38: 225

Goldspinck G 1980 Locomotion and the sliding filament mechanism In Elder H Y and Trueman E R (Eds) *Aspects of Animal Movement* New York, Cambridge

Goldstein K 1939 *The Organism* New York, The American Book Company

Golnik W, Michalska Z, and Michalak T 1981 Natural equine viral arteritis in foals *Schweizer Archiv Tierheilkunde* 123: 523-533

Golub B, Falk G, and Spine W W 1967 Lung abscess due to *Corynebacterium equi*. Report of first human infection *Annals Internal Medicine* 66: 1174-1177

Gonda M A, Charman H P, Walker J L, and Coggins L 1978 Scanning and transmission electron microscopic study of equine infectious anemia virus *American Journal of Veterinary Research* 39(5): 731-740

Gordon M B 1942 The hippiatric texts from Ugarit *Annals Medical History* 4: 406-08

Goret P, Michel C, and Toma B 1969 Clinical aspects of equine infectious anemia In Bryans J T and Gerber H (eds) *Proceedings 2nd International Conference Equine Infectious Diseases* Basel, Karger 166-171

Gorlin R J, Barron C N, Chuadry A P, and Clark J J 1959 The oral and pharyngeal pathology of domestic animals *American Journal of Veterinary Research* 20: 1032-61

Görnemann W 1939 Kehldeckelmissbildung als Ursache respiratorischen Kehlkopfpfeifens *Deutsche Tierärztliche Wochenschrift* 47: 38-9

Goto H, Shimizu, Abe T, and Kanamitsu M 1975 Sero-epidemiological study of equine influenza in Japan *Journal Clinical Microbiology* 2: 89-93

Gottlieb 1919 Rehbein *Wiener Tierärztliche Monatsschrift* 6: 250,283

Goubaux A 1886/1887 Memoire sur les deviations de la colonne vertebrale consideres dans la region dorso-lombaire, chex les animaux domestiques. *Recueil Médecine Vétérinaire* 63/4: 707-741

Goubeaud G J 1899/90 New theory of the etiology of shoe-boil *American Veterinary Revue* 23: 615-26

Gould D J, Byrne R J, and Hayes D E 1964 Experimental infection of horses with Japanese encephalitis virus by mosquito bite *American Journal of Tropical Medicine and Hygiene* 13: 742-746

Gould S J 1983 *Hen's Teeth and Horse's Toes.* New York, Norton.

Goulden B E, Anderson L J 1981 Equine laryngeal hemiplegia, part 1: physical characteristics of affected animals *New Zealand Veterinary Journal* 29: 150-153

Graham R 1936 Cornstalk disease investigations toxic encephalitis or non-virus encephalitis of horses *Veterinary Medicine* 31: 46-50

Granstrom D E, Giles R C, Tuttle P A, Williams N M, Poonacha K B, Petrites-Murray M B, Tramontin R R, Swerczek T W, Hong C B, Rezabek G B, Lyons E T, and Drudge J H 1991 Immunohistochemical diagnosis of protozoan parasites in lesions of equine protozoal myeloencephalitis *Journal of Veterinary Diagnostic Investigation* 3: 75-77

Grant B, Slatter D H, and Dunlap J S 1973 *Thelazia* sp. (nematoda) & dermoid cysts in a horse with torticollis *Veterinary Medicine/Small Animal Clinician* 68: 62-64

Grant B D and Tennant B 1973 Volvulus associated with Meckel's diverticulum in horse *Journal of the American Veterinary Medical Association* 162: 550-1

Grant R C, Basson P A, and Kidd A B 1985 Paralysis and lipofuscin-like pigmentation of farm stock caused by the plant, *Trachyandra laxa* var. *laxa* Onderstepoort Journal of Veterinary Research 52: 255-259

Gratzl E 1934a Die Pathogenese der Blinddarmverstofungen des Pferdes *Wiener Tierärztliche Monatsschrift* 21: 481-94,616-25

Gratzl E 1934b Untersuchungen über die Morphologie und Funktion der Luftsäcke am lebenden Pferd *Wiener Tierärztliche Monatsschrift* 21: 5-78,97-106

Gratzl E 1947 Die Pferdegrippe *Wiener Tierärztliche Monatsschrift* 34: 566-79

Gratzl E 1960 Eine durch Mangelfutterun (insbesondere thiaminmangel) bedingte Enzephaomyelopathie bei Pferden in Österreich *Wiener Tierärztliche Monatsschrift* 47: 51-66

Gravesen S, Lowenstein H, and Weeke B 1978 Demonstration, isolation and identification of culturable microfungi and bacteria in horse hair and dandruff *Allergy* 33: 89-92

Gray T de 1639 *The Compleat Horsemen and Expert Farrier* London, Harper

Greatorex J C 1977 Diagnosis and treatment of "verminous aneurysm" formation in the horse *Veterinary Record* 101: 184-187

Green D A 1961 Studies on growth rate in horses *British Veterinary Journal* 117: 181-91

Green D A 1969 Studies of growth rate in Thoroughbred foals *British Veterinary Journal* 125: 539-45

Green G M, Jakob G J, Low R B et al. 1977 Defense mechanisms of the respiratory membrane *American Review Respiratory Disease* 115: 479-514

Greenwood R E S and Simson A R B 1980 Clinical report of a paralytic syndrome affecting stallions, mares and foals on a Thoroughbred studfarm *Equine Veterinary Journal* 12: 113-117

Gribble D H 1969 Equine ehrlichiosis *Journal of the American Veterinary Medical Association* 155: 462-469

Gribble D H 1972 Ehrlichiosis In: Catcott E J (Ed) *Equine Medicine Surgery* 2nd Ed Illinois, American Veterinary Publications

Grieg J R 1928 Acute "grass sickness": an interpretation of the clinical symptoms *Veterinary Record* 8: 31-4

Grini O 1943 Listerella monocytogenes as the cause of septicaemia in foals *Norsk Vet Tidsskr* 55: 97-104

Gröndahl A M 1992 The incidence of bony fragments and osteochondrosis in the metacarpo- and metatarsophalangeal joints of Standardbred trotters *Journal of Equine Veterinary Science* 12: 81-5

Grosenbaugh D A, Amoss M S, Hood D M, Morgan S J, and Williams J D 1988 Epidermal growth factor-mediated effects on equine vascular smooth muscle cells *American Journal Physiology* 255: C447-C451

Grosenbaugh D A, Amoss M S, Hood D M, and Williams J D 1990 EGF receptor-binding activity in the urine of normal horses and horses affected by chronic laminitis *Domestic Animal Endocrinology* 7: 277-289

Grosenbaugh D A, Hood D M, Amoss M S Jr, and Williams J D 1991 Characterisation and distribution of epidermal growth factor receptors in equine hoof wall laminar tissue: comparison of normal horses and horses affected with chronic laminitis *Equine Veterinary Journal* 23: 201-206

Grossman B S, Brobst D F, Kramer J W, Bayly W M, and Reed S M 1982 Urinary indices for differentiation of prerenal azotemia and renal azotemia in horses *Journal of the American Veterinary Medical Association* 180: 284-288

Groth W 1968 Vol 3 Die Schildruse. Glandula thyroidea In Dobberstein J, Pallaske G, and Stünzi H (Eds) *Joest's Handbuch der Speziellen Pathologischen Anatomie der Haustiere* 3rd. Ed Berlin, Parey

Grünig G, von Fellenberg R, Maier R, and Corboz L 1986 Elastase-producing microorganisms in horse lung: Their possible role in the pathogenesis of chronic pulmonary disease in the horse *Equine Veterinary Journal* 18: 396-400

Gunson D E 1983 Renal papillary necrosis in horses *Journal of the American Veterinary Medical Association* 182: 263-266

Gunson D E and Rooney J R 1977 Anaphylactoid purpura in a horse *Veterinary Pathology* 14: 325-31

Gunson D E and Soma L R 1983 Renal papillary necrosis in horses after phenylbutazone and water depletion *Veterinary Pathology* 70: 603-10

Gunson D E, Kowalczyk D F, Shoop C R 1982 Environmental zinc and cadmium pollution associated with generalized osteochondrosis, osteoporosis, and nephrocalcinosis in horses *Journal of the American Veterinary Medical Association* 180: 295-99

Gunson D E, Halliwell E W, and Minor R R 1984 Dermal collagen degradation and phagocytosis *Archives Dermatology* 120: 599-604

Gunson D E, Sweeney C R, and Soma L R 1988 Sudden death attributable to exercise-induced pulmonary haemorrhage in racehorses: nine cases (1981-83) *Journal of the American Veterinary Medical Association* 193: 102-106

Guoth A G von 1927 Beinhautenzundung der dorsalen Wand des metacarpus und die transformation der Knochenstruktur bei Rennpferden *Archiv Wissenschäftliche Tierheilkunde* 56: 159-177

Guoth A G von 1940 Über Achropathie beim Pferde *Deutsche Tierzärztliche Wochenschrift* 48: 354-55

Guoth A G von 1941 Die Luxation der Kronbeinbeugesehne vom Sprungbeinhöcker beim Pferd *Deutsche Tierzärztliche Wochenschrift* 49: 373-6

Gupta B N, Keahey K K, and Ellis D J 1972 Cutaneous involvement of malignant lymphoma in a horse *Cornell Veterinarian* 62: 205-315

Gutmann W 1899 Vol 3 Krankheiten des Magens und Darmes In *Bayer-Fröhner Handbuch der Thierärztlichen Chirurgie und Geburtshilfe* Vienna, Braumuller

Gygax A P, Donawick W J, and Gledhill B L 1973 Haematocoele in a stallion and recovery of fertility following unilateral castration *Equine Veterinary Journal* 5: 128-130

Gygax A P, Ganjam V K, and Kenney R M 1979 Clinical, microbiological, and histological changes associated with uterine involution in the mare *Journal Reproduction Fertility* (Suppl)27: 571-78

Gylstorff I 1971 Vol 4 Pathologie der Gravidität In Dobberstein J, Pallaske G, and Stünzi H (Eds) *Joest's Handbuch der Speziellen Pathologischen Anatomie der Haustiere* 3rd Ed Berlin, Parey

Haakenstad L H 1953 Undersökelser över den patoligste hoftleddluksajon hos hest med hensyn til lidelsens vesen og etiolgiske forhold *Nordiska Veterinärmedicin* 5: 884-96

Haakenstad L H 1955 Undersökelser över ringfot hos hest *Nordiska Veterinärmedicin* 7: 3

Haakenstad L H 1969 Chronic bone and joint diseases in relationship to conformation in the horse *Equine Veterinary Journal* 1: 248-60

Haaland M A and Davidson J P 1983 Spontaneous left atrial rupture with associated chronic fibrotic myocarditis in a stallion *Veterinary Medicine/Small Animal Clinician*

August: 1284-1287

Haan J de and Hoogkamer L J 1903 Hypomycosis destruens equi. Bostartige Schimmelkrankheit des Pferdes *Archiv fur wissenshaftliche und praktische Tierheilkunde* 29: 395-410

Habel R E and Budras K-D 1992 Anatomy of the prepubic tendon in the horse, cow, sheep, goat and dog *American Journal of Veterinary Research* 53: 2183-95

Hach P, Borovansky J, and Duchon J 1973 Melanosomes of horse benign melanoma *Proceedings Czechoslovak Morphologists* 21: 275-277

Hadlow 1962 cited in Innes J R M and Saunders L Z 1962 in *Comparative Neuropathology* New York Academic Press

Hagler W M and Behlow R F 1981 Salivary syndrome in horses: identification of slaframine in red clover hay *Applied Environmental Microbiology* 42: 1067-73

Hale J H and Witherington D H 1953 Encephalitis in racehorses in Malaya *Journal of Comparative Pathology* 63: 195-198

Hale J H and Witherington D H 1954 A serological survey of antibodies to Japanese B encephalitis virus among horses in Malaya *Annals of Tropical Medicine and Parasitology* 48: 15-20

Haliburton J C, Vesonder R R, Lock T F, and Buck W B 1979 Equine leucoencephalomalacia (ELEM): a study of Fusarium moniliforme as an etiologic agent *Veterinary and Human Toxicology* 21(5): 348-351

Hall L W and Stark L E 1983 COPD—Or is it? *Equine Veterinary Journal* 15: 185-187

Halldordsottir S and Larsen H J 1991 An epidemiological study of summer eczema in Icelandic horses in Norway *Equine Veterinary Journal* 23: 296-299

Halliwell R E W, Fleischman J B, Mackay-Smith M, Beech J, And Gunson D 1979 The role of allergy in chronic pulmonary disease of horses *Journal of the American Veterinary Medical Association* 174: 277-281

Hallmich P 1939 Pathologisch-anatomische Untersuchungen über die rezidivierende Blinddarmverstoffung des Pferds und ihr forensischer Nachweis *Archiv Tierheilkunde* 74: 433-41

Hamada M and Itakura C 1990 Ultrastructural morphology of hypomelanosis in equine cutaneous papilloma *Journal of Comparative Pathology* 103: 199-213

Hamada M, Oyamada T, Yoshikawa H, Yoshikawa T, and Itakura C 1990 Histopathological development of equine cutaneous papillomas *Journal of Comparative Pathology* 102: 393-403

Hamilton D P and Byerly C S 1974 Congenital malignant melanoma in a foal *Journal of the American Veterinary Medical Association* 164(10): 1040-1041

Hammel E P and Raker C W 1972 Myotonia In Catcott E J and Smithcors J E (Eds) *Equine Medicine Surgery* 2nd Ed American Veterinary Publications

Hammond C J, Mason D K, and Watkins K L 1986 *Equine Veterinary Journal* 8: 284-7

Hammond P B and Aronson A L 1964 Lead poisoning of cattle and horses in the vicinity of a smelter *Annals of the New York Academy of Science* 111: 595-611

Hammond T, Severin G A, and Snyder S 1983 Equine ocular onchocerciasis: A case report *Equine Veterinary Journal* 2 (supplement): 74-75

Hamori D 1944 Contracture *Veterinary Bulletin* 14: 422-3

Hamori D 1983 *Constitutional Disorders and Hereditary Disease* Amsterdam, Elsevier

Hancar F 1956 *Das Pferd in prähistorischer und früher historischer Zeit* Vienna, Verlag Herold

Hansen H-J 1969 Vol 1 Erkrankung der Zwischenwirbelscheiben (Diskuserkrankungen) In Dobberstein J, Pallaske G, and Stünzi H. (Eds) *Joest's Handbuch der Speziellen Pathologischen Anatomie der Haustiere* 3rd Ed Berlin, Parey

Hansen M A, Fossum K, and Teige J 1971 *Salmonella typhimurium* infection in horses *Nordiska Veterinärmedicin* 23: 475-83

Hanson R P 1972a Vesicular Stomatitis In Catcott E J and Smithcors J E (Eds) *Equine Medicine Surgery* 2nd Ed Illinois, American Veterinary Publications

Hanson R P 1972b Virology and epidemiology of Eastern and Western arboviral encephalomyelitis of horses In Bryans J T and Gerber H (Eds) *Proceedings of the 3rd International Conference on Equine Infectious Disease* 100-113

Hardy J, Marcoux M, and Breton L 1987 Prevalence et description des fragments articulaires retrouves au boulet chez de cheval Standardbred *Pratique Vétérinaire Equine* 19: 27-32

Hardy J, Robertson J T, and Wilkie D A 1990 Ishemic optic neuropathy and blindness after arterial occlusion for treatment of guttural pouch mycosis in two horses *Journal of the American Veterinary Medical Association* 196: 1631-1634

Hargis A M and McElwain T F 1984 Vascular neoplasia in the skin of horses *Journal of the American Veterinary Medical Association* 9: 1121-1124

Harrington D D 1982 Acute vitamin D2 (ergocalciferol) toxicosis in horses: case report and experimental studies *Journal American Veterinary Medical Association* 180: 867-73

Harrington D D, Walsh J, and White V 1973 Clinical and pathological findings in horses fed zinc deficient diets *Proceedings 3rd Equine Nutrition Physiology Symposium*

Harrison I W 1988 Equine large intestinal volvulus: A review of 124 cases *Veterinary Surgery* 17: 77-81

Harrison I W 1989 Cecal torsion in a horse as a consequence of cecocolic fold hypoplasia *Cornell Veterinarian* 79: 315-317

Hartley W J and Dixon R J 1979 An outbreak of foal perinatal mortality due to equine herpes virus type I pathologic observations *Equine Veterinary Journal* 11: 215-18

Hartley W J and Dodd D C 1957 Muscular dystrophy in New Zealand livestock *New Zealand Veterinary Journal* 5: 61-6

Hartley W J and Gibson A J F 1971 Observations of *Swainsona galegifolia* poisoning in cattle in northern New

South Wales *Australian Veterinary Journal* 47: 300-305

Hartley W J, Kuberski T, LeGonidec G, and Daynes P 1982 The pathology of Gomen disease: A cerebellar disorder of horses in New Caledonia *Veterinary Pathology* 19: 399-405

Haschek W M, King J M, and Tennant B C 1981 Primary renal cell carcinoma in two horses *Journal of the American Veterinary Medical Association* 179: 992-994

Hawkins J A, Adams W V, Cook L, Wilson B H, and Roth E E 1973 Role of horse fly *(Tabanus fuscicostatus* Hine) and stable fly (*Stomxys calcitrans* L.) in transmission of equine infectious anemia to ponies in Louisiana *American Journal of Veterinary Research* 34: 1583-1586

Hayes H M 1974 Congenital umbilical and inguinal hernias in cattle, horses, swine, dogs, and cats: risk by breed and sex among hospital patients *American Journal of Veterinary Research* 35: 839-42

Hayes H M 1986 *Corynebacterium pseudotuberculosis* in the horse: Study of 117 clinical cases and considerations of etiopathogenesis *Equine Veterinary Journal* 18: 467-71

Haynes P F 1980 Diseases of the metacarpophalangeal joint and metacarpus *Veterinary Clinics North America* 2: 33-59

Haynes P F, Snider T G, McClure J R, and McClure J J 1980 Chronic chondritis of the equine arytenoid cartilage *Journal of the American Veterinary Medical Association* 177: 1135-42

Heath E, Aire T, and Fujiwara K 1985 Microtubular mass defect of spermatozoa in the stallion *American Journal of Veterinary Research* 46: 1121-1125

Heath S E, Bell R J, Clark E G, and Haines D M 1990 Idiopathic granulomatous disease involving the skin in a horse *Journal of the American Veterinary Medical Association* 197: 1033-1036

Heffner K A, White S D, Frevert C W, and Jakowski R 1988 *Corynebacterium* folliculitis in a horse *Journal of the American Veterinary Medical Association* 193: 89-90

Heffron C J and Baker G J 1979a Observations on the mechanism of functional obstruction of the nasopharyngeal airway in the horse *Equine Veterinary Journal* 11: 142-7

Heffron C J and Baker G J 1979b Endoscopic observations on the deglutition reflex in the horse *Equine Veterinary Journal* 11: 137-41

Heffron C J, Baker G J, and Lee R 1979 Fluoroscopic investigations of pharyngeal function in the horse *Equine Veterinary Journal* 11: 148-52

Hegreberg G A and Reed S M 1990 Skeletal muscle changes associated with equine myotonic dystrophy *Acta Neuropathologica* 80: 426-431

Heidrich K 1917 Verrenkung des Kreuzdarmbeingelenkes *Berlin Veterinär Wes Sachsen* 62: 95

Held J P and Geiser D 1983 Ataxia as the only clinical sign of cerebrospinal meningitis in a horse with equine infectious anemia *Journal of the American Veterinary Medical Association* 183: 324-325

Held J P, McGavin M D, and Geiser D 1983 Ataxia as the only clinical sign of cerebrospinal meningitis in a horse with equine infectious anemia *Journal of the American Veterinary Medical Association* 183(3): 324-325

Held J P, Wright B, and Henton J E 1986 Pyelonephritis associated with renal failure in a horse *Journal of the American Veterinary Medical Association* 189: 688-689

Held J P, Prater P, Toal R L, Blackford J T, and McCracken M 1989 Sperm granuloma in a stallion *Journal of the American Veterinary Medical Association* 194: 267-268

Held J P, Adair S, McGavin M D, Adams W H, Toal R, and Henton J 1990 Bacterial epididymitis in two stallions *Journal of the American Veterinary Medical Association* 197: 602-604

Hell 1900 Krankheiten der Muskeln, Facian, Nerven, und Gefässe. In *Bayer-Fröhner Handbuch der tierärztlichen chirurgie und Geburtshilfe* Vol 4 Vienna, Braumuller

Henry M and Vanderplassche M 1981 Pathology of the oviduct in mares *Vlaams Diergeneesk Tidjschrift* 50: 301-25

Henry M, Prasse K, and White S 1989 Hemorrhagic diathesis caused by multiple myeloma in a three-month-old foal *Journal of the American Veterinary Medical Association* 194: 392-394

Hensel C, Bisping W, and Schimmelpfennig H 1961 Aspergillus abort beim Pferd *Berliner Münchener Tierärztliche Wochenschrift* 74: 290-3

Henson J B And McGuire T C 1971 Immunopathology of equine infectious anemia *American Journal Clinical Pathology* 56: 306-314

Hermans W A 1970 A hereditary anomaly in Shetland ponies *Netherland Journal of Veterinary Science* 3: 55-63

Hertsch B 1981 Arteriographische Untersuchungen an den Extremitäten beim Pferd *Dissertation*, Hannover

Hertsch B 1990 Orthopädische probleme bei Fohlen—angeborene beugestellungen und durchtrittigkeit *Collegium Veterinarium* 21: 74-8

Hertsch B and Becker C 1986 Zum Vorkommen der aseptischen nekrose im ligamentum palmare bzw. plantare beim Pferd—ein Beitrag zum differenzierung der Gleichbeinerkrankungen *Deutsche Tierärztliche Wochenschrift* 93: 263-66

Hertsch B, Wissdorf H, and Zeller R 1982 Die sogenannten "Gefässlocher" des Strahlbeins und ihre Beziehung zum Hufgelenk *Tierärztliche Praxis* 10: 365-79

Hertzel H 1936 Die auf die Geschlectsorgane wirkenden Hormone und ihre therapeutische Anwendug *Wiener Tierärztliche Monatschrift* 23: 299-304

Heusser H 1928 Über den Bau und die Funktion des Pferdeshufes und ihre Beziehungen zur Hufknorpelverknocherung und zum Hufmechanismus *Schweizer Archiv Tierheilkunde* 165-82

Heymering H 1990 *On the Horse's Foot, Shoes, and Shoeing* Cascade, Maryland, St. Eloy

Hickman J 1964 *Veterinary Orthopaedics*. Edinburgh, Oliver & Boyd

Hickman J 1970 Glanders: a contribution to epidemiology *Equine Veterinary Journal* 2: 137-58

Higashi T and Harasawa R 1989 DNA restriction analysis of

equine adenovirus serotype I *Journal of Veterinary Medicine* 36: 473-476

Higgins R, Biberstein E L, Jang S S 1984 Nutritionally variant streptoccci from corneal ulcers in horses *Journal Clinical Microbiology* 20(6): 1130-1134

Hilbert B J, Rendano V T 1975 Venous aneurysm in a horse *Journal American Veterinary Medical Association* 167(5): 394-396

Hilbert B J, Huxtable C R, and Pawley S E 1980 Cryptococcal pneumonia in a horse *Australian Veterinary Journal* 56: 391-392

Hilledge C J 1986 Review of *Corynebacterium (Rhodococcus) equi* lung abscesses in foals: Pathogenesis, diagnosis and treatment *Veterinary Record* 119: 261-264

Hilledge C J 1987 Dum spiro spero, dum spero vivo— "Whilst I breathe I hope, whilst I hope I live" *Equine Veterinary Journal* 19: 375-376

Hilledge C J and Whitlock T W 1986 Sex variation in the prevalence of exercise induced pulmonary haemorrhage in horses *Research Veterinary Science* 40

Hilwig R W 1977 Cardiac arrhythmias in the horse *Journal of the American Veterinary Medical Association* 170: 153-163

Hinchcliff K W and Adams W M 1991 Critical pulmonary stenosis in a newborn foal *Equine Veterinary Journal* 23: 318-320

Hines M T 1984 Immunologically mediated ocular disease in the horse *Veterinary Clinics North America: Large Animal Practice* 6: 501-512

Hines M T, Jarpe A, Halliwell R E W 1992 Equine recurrent uveitis: Immunization of ponies with equine retinal S antigen *Progress Veterinary Comparative Ophthalmology* 2: 3-11

Hinton M, Jones D R E, Lewis I M, and Thomson P E 1977 A clotting defect in an Arab colt foal *Equine Veterinary Journal* 9: 1-3

Hintz H F 1990 Molds, Mycotoxins, and Mycotoxicosis *Veterinary Clinics of North America: Equine Practice* 6: 419-431

Hintz H F and Snyder J R 1992 In Robinson, N.E. (Ed) *Current Therapy in Equine Medicine* 3. Philadelphia, Saunders

Hintz H F, Hogue D E, Walker E F, Lowe J E, and Schryver M F 1971 Apparent digestion in various segments of the digestive tract of ponies fed diets with varying roughage-grain ratios *Journal Animal Science* 32: 245-48

Hintz H F, Schryver H F, and Lowe JE 1976 Delayed growth response and limb conformation in young horses *Proceedings Cornell Nutrition Conference*

Hippen F 1949 Erbbiologische Untersuchungen der Fohlensataxie im Oldenburger Zuchgebiet *Dissertation*, Hannover

Hjärre A and Carlström B 1933 Om levercirrhos hos häst in anslutning till utfodring med alsikerikt klöverhö *Skandinavisk Veterinärtidskrift* 23: 12-18

Hobmaier M 1922 *Berliner Tierärztliche Wochenschrift* 16: 181-84

Hodgkin E C, McGuire T C, Perryman L E, and Grant B D 1978 Evaluation of delayed hypersensitivity responses in normal horses and immunodeficient foals *American Journal of Veterinary Research* 39: 1161-1167

Hofer B, Steck F, Gerber H, Lohrer J, Nicolet J, and Paccaud M F 1973 An investigation of the etiology of viral respiratory disease in a remount depot In Bryans J T and Gerber H (Eds) *Proceedings 3rd International Conference Equine Infectious Diseases* Basel, Karger pp. 527-545

Hoff H E, Geddes L A, and McCrady J D 1966 The contributions of the horse to knowledge of the heart and circulation III. James MacKenzie, Thomas Lewis, and the nature of atrial fibrillation *Connecticut Medicine* 30: 43-48

Holland C J, Ristic M, Cole A I, Johnson P, Baker G, and Goetz T 1985 Isolation, experimental transmission, and characterization of causative agent of Potomac Horse Fever *Science* 227: 522-524

Holman H H, Gordon W S, and Pattison I H 1944 Observations on the pathology and histology of grass sickness in horses *Journal of Comparative Pathology* 54: 97-107

Holmes J R 1977 Prognosis of equine cardiac conditions *Equine Veterinary Journal* 9: 181-182

Holmes J R and Miller P J 1984 Three cases of ruptures mitral valve chordae in the horse *Equine Veterinary Journal* 16: 125-135

Holmes J R, Rezakhani A, and Else R W 1973 Rupture of a dissecting aortic aneurysm into the left pulmonary artery in a horse *Equine Veterinary Journal* 5: 65-70

Holmes J R, Henigan M, Williams R B, and Witherington D H 1986 Paroxysmal atrial fibrillation in racehorses *Equine Veterinary Journal* 18: 37-42

Holshuh H J and Howard E B 1982 Pineoblastoma, a primitive neuroectodermal tumor in the brain of the horse *Veterinary Pathology* 19: 567-569

Holt D E and Pearson H 1984 Urolithiasis in the horse- a review of 13 cases *Equine Veterinary Journal* 16

Holt P E and Mair T S 1990 Ten cases of bladder paralysis associated with sabulous urolithiasis in horses *Veterinary Record* 127: 108-110

Hood D M Current concepts of the physiopathology of laminitis 25: 13-20

Hood D M, Amoss M S, and Hightower D 1978 Equine laminitis I: Radioisotopic analysis of the hemodynamics of the foot during the acute disease *Journal of Equine Medicine and Surgery* 2: 439-44

Hood D M, Gremmel S M, Amoss M S, Button C, and Hightower D 1979 Equine laminitis III. Coagulation dysfunction in the developmental and acute disease *Journal of Equine Medicine and Surgery* 3: 355-360

Hood D M, Amoss M S, and Grosenbaugh D A 1990 Equine laminitis: A potential model of Raynaud's phenomena *Angiology* April: 270-277

Hooper P T 1968 Epizootic cystitis in horses *Australian Veterinary Journal* 44: 11-14

Hooper W D 1936 *Marcus Tertius Varro on Agriculture*

London, William Heinemann

Hope W D, Wilson J H, Garry M R, and Calderwood-Mays M B 1989 Chronic renal failure associated with bilateral nephroliths and ureteroliths in a two-year-old Thoroughbred colt *Equine Veterinary Journal* 21: 228-231

Horner G W 1980 Serological relationship between abortifacient and respiratory strains of equine herpesvirus type 1 in New Zealand *New Zealand Veterinary Journal* 29: 7-8

Hort W 1977 Myocardial hypertrophy. Light microscopic findings on the myocardium. Blood supply. Ventricular dilatation and heart failure *Basic Research Cardiology* 72: 203-208

Hosie B D, Gould D W, Hunter A R, Low J C, Munro R, and Wilson H C 1986 Acute myopathy in horses at grass in east and south east Scotland *Veterinary Record* 119: 444-449

Houttu J 1991 Arthroscopic removal of osteochondral fragments of the palmar/plantar aspect of the metacarpo-metatarsophalangeal joints *Equine Veterinary Journal* 23: 163-5

Hoven R van den and Franken P 1983 Clinical aspects of lymphosarcoma in the horse: A clinical report of 16 cases *Equine Veterinary Journal* 15: 49-53

Hoven R van den, Breukink H J, Wensing H J, Meijer A E F H, and Tigges A J 1986 Loosely coupled skeletal muscle mitochondria in exertional rhabdomylosis *Equine Veterinary Journal* 18: 418-21

Hoven R van den, Meijer A E F H, Breukink H J, and Wensing T 1988 Enzyme histochemistry on muscle biopsies as an aid in the diagnosis of diseases of the equine neuromuscular system: A study of six cases *Equine Veterinary Journal* 20: 46-53

Howarth S, Lucke V M, and Pearson H 1991 Squamous cell carcinoma of the equine external genitalia: a review and assessment of penile amputations and urethrostomy as a surgical treatment *Equine Veterinary Journal* 23: 53-58

Hsiung Ta-Shih 1930 A monograph on the protozoa of the large intestine of the horse *Iowa State College Journal Science* 4: 359-423

Hubbell J A E, Reed S M, Myer C W, and Muir W W 1988 Sequelae of myelography in the horse *Equine Veterinary Journal* 20: 438-440

Hug A 1937 Über chronische Atembeschwerden des Pferdes *Schweiz Archiv Tierheilkunde* 79: 251-80

Hughes D E and Pugh G W 1970 Isolation and description of a Moraxella from horses with conjunctivitis *American Journal of Veterinary Research* 31(3): 457-463

Hughes P E and Howard E B 1984 Endocardial fibroelastosis as a cause of sudden death in the horse *Equine Practice* 6: 23-26

Hulland T J 1985 Muscles and Tendons In Jubb K, Kennedy P C, and Palmer, N (Eds) *The Pathology of the Domestic Animals* 3rd Ed New York, Academic Press

Hultgren B D 1982 Ileocolonic aganglionosis in white progeny of overo spotted horses *Journal of the American Veterinary Medical Association* 180: 289-92

Hunt D A, Snyder J R, Morgan J P, and Pascoe J R 1990 Femoral capita physeal fractures in 25 foals *Veterinary Surgery* 19: 41-9

Hunt L D, Blythe L, and Holtan D W 1983 Ryegrass staggers in ponies fed processed ryegrass straw *Journal of the American Veterinary Medical Association* 182: 285-286

Hunt M and Rossdale P D 1963 A specific venereal disease of Thoroughbred mares *Veterinary Record* 75: 1092-1093

Hunt R J, Allen D, and Moore J N 1990a Effect of endotoxin administration on equine digital hemodynamics and Starling forces *American Journal of Veterinary Research* 151: 1703-1707

Hunt R J, Hay W, Collatos C, and Welles E 1990b Testicular seminoma associated with torsion of the spermatic cord in two cryptorchid stallions *Journal of the American Veterinary Medical Association* 197: 1484-1486

Hunt R J, Allen D, Baxter G M, Jackman B R, and Parks A H 1991 Mid-metacarpal deep digital flexor tenotomy in the management of refractory laminitis in horses *Veterinary Surgery* 20: 15-20

Huntington P J, Jeffcott L B, Friend S C E, Luff A R, Finkelstein D, and Flynn R 1989 Australian stringhalt-epidemiological, clinical, and neurological investigations *Equine Veterinary Journal* 21: 266-73

Huntington P J, Ellis P M, Forman A J, and Timoney P J 1990 Equine viral arteritis *Australian Veterinary Journal* 67: 429-431

Hupka E 1926a Zur Pathogenese des erworbenen Stelzfuss der Fohlen *Deutsch Tierärztliche Wochenschrift* 34: 73-8

Hupka E 1926b Über Flugstaubvergiftungen in der Umgebung von Metallhutten *Wiener Tierärztliche Monatschrift* 42: 763-75

Hurst E W 1950 Some observations on the pathogenesis of Eastern equine encephalomyelitis and louping-ill in young and old animals, with special reference to routes of entry of the viruses into the nervous system *Journal of Comparative Pathology* 60: 237-262

Huskamp B 1982 Equine Colic Research Symposium, Athens, Georgia

Huskamp B 1983 In Dietz, O.and Wiesner,E. (Eds) *Diseases of the Horse* Basel Karger

Huskamp B 1985 Diagnosis of gastroduodenitis and its surgical treatment by a temporary duodenocecostomy *Equine Veterinary Journal* 17: 314-16

Huskamp B and Kopf N 1980 Die Verlagerung des Colon ascendes in den Milznierenraum *Tierärztliche Praxis* 8: 327,495

Huskamp B and Nowak M 1988 Insertionsdesmopathien beim Pferde und einige ihrer Lokalisationen *Pferdeheilkunde* 4: 3-12

Hussain S T 1975 Evolutionary and functional anatomy of the pelvic limb in fossil and recent equidae (Perissodactyla, Mammalia) *Anatomia Histologia Embryologia* 4: 179-222

Huston R, Saperstein G, and Leipold H W 1977 Congenital defects in foals 1: 146-161

Hutchins D R, Lepherd E E, and Crook I G 1967 A case of

equine haemophilia *Australian Veterinary Journal* 43: 83-87

Hutt F B 1968 Genetic defects of bones and joints in domestic animals *Cornell Veterinarian* (Suppl) 58: 104

Hutyra F and Marek J 1920 *Spezielle Pathologie und Therapie der Haustiere* 5th Ed Jena, Gustav Fischer

Hutyra F and Marek J 1922 *Special Pathology and Therapeutics of Domestic Animals* Chicago, A Eger

Hutyra F and Marek J 1926 *Special Pathology and Therapeutics of Domestic Animals* Chicago, A Eger

Huxtable C R, Chapman H M, Main D C, Vass D, Pearse B H G, and Hilbert B J 1987 Neurological disease and lipofuscinosis in horses and sheep grazing *Trachyandra divaricata* (branched onion weed) in south Western Australia *Australian Veterinary Journal* 64: 105-108

Hyland A 1990 *Equus: The Horse in the Roman World* New Haven Yale University Press

Hyllseth B, Magnusson P, and Marusyk H 1969 Studies on equine arteritis virus In Bryans J T and Gerber H (eds) *Proceedings 2nd International Conference Equine Infectious Diseases* Basel, Karger 140-142

Hyslop N S G 1980 Dermatophilosis (streptothricosis) in animals and man *Comparative Immunology Microbiology Infectious Disease* 2: 389-404

Ihrke P J, Wong A, Stannard A A, Vivrette S L 1988 Cutaneous fungal flora in twenty horses free of skin or ocular disease *American Journal of Veterinary Research* 49: 770-772

Innes J R M 1949 *British Veterinary Journal* 107: 373-83

Innes J R M and Saunders L Z 1962 *Comparative Neuropathology*, New York Academic Press

Innes J R M, Shoho C, and Pillai C R 1952 Epizootic cerebro-spinal nematodiasis or setariasis focal encephalomyelomalacia in animals in the Orient caused by immature *Setaria digitata*: a disease which may occur in animals in other parts of the world *British Veterinary Journal* 108: 71-88

Irwin C F P and Rac R 1957 Cryptococcus infection in a horse *Australian Veterinary Journal* 33: 97-98

Irwin D H G and Howell D W 1980 Equine pyelonephritis and unilateral nephrectomy *Journal South African Veterinary Association* 51: 235-236

Ishihara R and Ueno H 1957a Studies on the summer mange ("Kasen" disease) of the horse in Japan. I. Genetical studies on predisposition to summer mange *Bulletin of the National Institute of Animal Health* 32: 179-200

Ishihara R and Ueno H 1957b Studies on the summer manage ("Kasen" disease) of the horse in Japan. IV. Etiology considered from prevention and treatment *Bulletin of the National Institute of Animal Health* 33: 129-143

Ishihara R and Ueno H 1958 Studies on the summer manage ("Kasen" disease) of the horse in Japan. VI. Etiological study of the nematodes of filaria, especially Onchocerca cervicalis *Bulletin of the National Institute of Animal Health* 35: 161-178

Ishii S 1963 Equine infectious anemia or swamp fever *Advances in Veterinary Science* 8: 263-298

Issel C J and Coggins L 1979 Equine infectious anemia: current knowledge *Journal of the American Veterinary Medical Association* 174: 727-733

Jackson C 1936 The incidence and pathology of tumours of domesticated animals in South Africa. A study of the Onderstepoort collection of neoplasms with special reference to their histopathology *Onderstepoort Journal of Veterinary Science and Animal Industry* 6: 9-460

Jackson T and Kendrick J W 1971 Paralysis of horses associated with equine herpesvirus 1 infection *Journal of the American Veterinary Medical Association* 158: 1351-1357

Jackson T A, Osburn B I, Cordy D R, and Kendrick J W 1977 Equine herpesvirus I infection of horses. Studies on the experimentally induced neurologic disease *American Journal of Veterinary Research* 38: 709-719

Jacobs R M, Kociba G J, and Ruoff W W 1983 Monoclonal gammopathy in a horse with defective hemostasis *Veterinary Pathology 20(5): 643-647*

Jacobshagen E 1937 Grundzuge des Innenreliefs vom Rumpfdarm der Wirbeltiere *Anatomischer Anzeiger* 83: 241-61

Jaeschke G and Rudolph R 1985 Die Leukose des Pferdes 1. Nomenklatur, Klinik und Patholgie (Ubersichtsreferat) *Berliner Münchener Tierärtzliche Wochenschrift* 98: 88-94

Jakob G J 1981 Mechanisms of virus-induced bacterial superinfections of the lung *Clinical Chest Medicine* 2: 59-68

Jakob W 1971 Spontaneous amyloidosis of mammals *Veterinary Pathology* 8: 292-306

Jakovljevic S, Gibbs C,and Yeats J J 1982 Traumatic fractures of the equine hock. A report of 13 cases *Equine Veterinary Journal* 14: 62

James V S 1968 A family tendency to equine sarcoids *Southwestern Veterinarian* Spring: 234-235

Janis C 1976 The evolutionary strategy of the equidae and the origins of rumen and cecal digestion *Evolution* 30: 757-74

Jarmai K 1938 Über eienem Fall von generaiserter Lipoidose beim Pferd *Archiv Tierheilkunde* 73: 115-33

Jasko D J and Roth L 1984 Granulomatous colitis associated with small strongyle larvae in a horse *Journal of the American Veterinary Medical Association* 185: 553-554

Jeffcott L B 1969 Haemolytic disease of the new born foal *Equine Veterinary Journal* 97: 165-170

Jeffcott L B 1972 Passive immunity and its transfer with special reference to the horse *Cambridge Phil Soc Rev* 47(4): 439-464

Jeffcott L B 1975 The diagnosis of diseases of the horse's back *Equine Veterinary Journal* 7: 69-78

Jeffcott L B 1980 *Equine Veterinary Journal* 12: 197-210

Jeffcott L B 1982 Pelvic lesions in the horse *Equine Practice* 4: 21-47

Jeffcott L B 1991 Osteochondrosis in the horse—searching for the key to pathogenesis *Equine Veterinary Journal* 23: 331-338

Jeffcott L B and Dalin G 1980 Natural rigidity of the horse's backbone *Equine Veterinary Journal* 12: 101-108

Jeffcott L B and Jeffcott T J 1974 Studies of passive immunity in the foal III. The characterization and significance of neonatal proteinuria *J Comp Path* 84: 455-465

Jeffcott L B and Whitwell K 1973 Twinning as a cause of foetal and neonatal loss in the thoroughbred mare *Journal of Comparative Pathology* 83: 91-106

Jeffcott L B, Rossdale P D, Freestone J, Frank C J, and Towers-Clark P F 1982 An assessment of wastage in thoroughbred racing from conception to four years of age *Equine Veterinary Journal* 14: 185-198

Jeffcott L B, Dalin G, Ekman S, and Olsson S-E 1985 Sacroiliac lesions as a cause of chronic poor performance in competitive horses *Equine Veterinary Journal* 17: 111-18

Jeleff W 1957 Beitrag zur fetalen Histopathologie des Virusabortes der Stute mit besonder Berucksichtigung der Differentialdiagnose *Archives Experimental Veterinary Medicine* 11: 906-20

Jenkinson D M, Montgomery I, Elder H Y, Mason D K, Collins E A, and Snow D H 1985 Ultrastructural variations in the sweat glands of anhidrotic horses *Equine Veterinary Journal* 17: 287-291

Joest E 1914/15 Untersuchungen über das Plexuscholesteatom des Pferdes *Zeitschrift Tiermedicin* 18: 241-70

Joest E 1920 Ein Fall von knotchen-formiger aspergillusmykose der lunge beim Pferde *Berlin Institut Tierärtzliche Hochschrift* 1919: 32-36

Joest E 1923 On arytenoid ulcer/chondritis *Spezielle pathologische Anatomie der Haustiere* Berlin, Schoetz

Joest E 1926 Über Spondylitis deformans beim Pferde *Berliner Tierärztliche Wochenschrift* 42: 505-7

Jogi P and Norberg I 1962 Malformation of the hip joint in a standardbred horse *Veterinary Record* 74: 421

Johnson B, Baldwin C, Timoney P, and Ely R 1991 Arteritis in equine fetuses aborted due to equine viral arteritis *Veterinary Pathology* 28: 248-250

Johnson E J, Scott D W, and Smith C A 1981 Pemphigus foliaceus in the horse *Equine Practice* 3: 40-45

Johnson G C, Kohn C W, Johnson C W, Garry F, Scott D, and Martin S 1988 Ultrastructure of junctional epidermolysis bullosa in Belgian foals *Journal of Comparative Pathology* 98: 329-336

Johnson J A, Prescott J F, and Markham R J F 1983 The pathology of experimental *Corynebacterium equi* infection in foals following intrabronchial challenge *Veterinary Pathology* 20: 440-449

Johnson K H and Johnson D W 1966 Granulomas associated with *Micronema deletrix* in the maxillae of a horse *Journal of the American Veterinary Medical Association* 149: 155-159

Johnson T J, Kenney R M, McGee W R, and Polk H C Jr 1980 *Pseudomonas* infection in a stallion: A case report *Proceedings American Association Equine Practitioners* 26: 111-116

Johnston J K and Morris D D 1987 Comparison of duodenitis/ proximal jejunitis and small intestinal obstruction in horses: 68 cases (1977-85) *Journal of the American Veterinary Medical Association* 191: 849-54

Johnston J K, Neely D P, and Latterman S A 1987 Hematuria caused by abdominal abscessation in a foal *Journal of the American Veterinary Medical Association* 191: 971-972

Johnston J K, Divers T J, and Reef V B 1989 Cholelithiasis in the horse: 10 cases (1982-86) *Journal of the American Veterinary Medical Association* 194: 405-409

Johnston K G and Hutchins D R 1967 Suspected adenovirus bronchitis in Arab foals *Australian Veterinary Journal* 43: 600-605

Johnstone A C 1987 Congenital vascular tumors in the skin of horses *Journal of Comparative Pathology* 97: 365-8

Johnstone I B and Blackwell T E 1984 Disseminated intravascular coagulation in a horse with postpartum ulcerative colitis and laminitis *Canadian Veterinary Journal* 25: 195-198

Johnstone I B and Crane S 1986 Hemostatic abnormalities in equine colic *American Journal of Veterinary Research* 47: 356-358

Jones T C 1942 Equine periodic opththalmia *American Journal of Veterinary Research* 3: 45-71

Jones T C and Maurer F D 1942 Heredity in periodic ophthalmia *Journal of the American Veterinary Medical Association* 101: 248-249

Jones T C, Doll E R, and Bryans J T 1957 The lesions of equine viral arteritis *Cornell Veterinarian* 47: 52

Jones W E 1979 Search for the lethal white horses, genetic diseases *Horse Rider* 11: 44-49

Jordan W H, Gaafar S M, and Carlton W W 1975 *Micronema deletrix* in the brain of a horse *Veterinary Medicine/Small Animal Clinician* 70: 707-709

Joyce J R 1983 Aniridia in a Quarterhorse *Equine Veterinary Journal* 2 (supplement): 21-22

Joyce J R, Hanselka D W, Boyd C L 1972 Treatment of habronemiasis of the adnexa of the equine eye *VM SAC 67(9): 1008-1009*

Joyce J R, Martin J E, Storts R W, and Skow L 1990 Iridial hypoplasia (aniridia) accompanied by limbic dermoids and cataracts in a group of related Quarterhorses *Equine Veterinary Journal* 10 (supplement): 26-28

Jubb K V F and Kennedy P C 1970 *Pathology of Domestic Animals, 2nd ed*, New York, Academic Press

Jubb K V F and Kennedy P C 1985 *Pathology of Domestic Animals*, Orlando, Academic Press

Jubb K V F, Kennedy P C, and Palmer N 1985a Bone disease of unknown cause. Hypertrophic osteopathy *The Pathology of Domestic Animals* 3rd Ed New York, Academic Press

Jubb K V F, Kennedy P C, and Palmer N 1985b Borna disease. *The Pathology of Domestic Animals* 3rd Ed New York, Academic Press

Kallfelz F A, Whitlock R H, and Schultz R D 1978 Survival of ^{58}Fe-labeled erythrocytes in cross-transfused equine blood *American Journal of Veterinary Research* 39: 617-620

Kameya T 1973 Clinical studies on laminitis in the racehorse *Experimental Reports Equine Health Laboratory* 10: 19-

40 (Japanese)

Kameya T 1980 Studies on laminitis in the racehorse: Clinical aspects and relationship between chemical composition and histopathological findings of affected hoofs *Journal of Veterinary Science* 42: 19-29

Kameya T, Kiryu K and Kaneko M 1980 Histopathogenesis of thickening of the hoof wall laminae in equine laminitis *Japanese Journal of Veterinary Science* 42: 361-371

Kaminjolo J S Jr and Winqvist G 1975 Histopathology of skin lesions in Uashin Gishu skin disease of horses *Journal of Comparative Pathology* 85: 391-395

Kanemaru T, Kaneko M, Oikawa M, Yoshihara T, and Tomioka Y 1985 Macroscopical examination of pulmonary lesions in foals *Bulletin Equine Research Institute* 22: 48-52

Kaneps A J, Shires G M H, and Watrous B J 1985 Cystic calculi in two horses *Journal of the American Veterinary Medical Association* 187: 737-739

Kaplan W, Chandler FW, Ajello L, Gauthier R, Higgins R, and Cayouette P 1975 Equine phaeohyphomycosis caused by *Drechslera spicifera Canadian Veterinary Journal* 16: 205-208

Karasszon D 1988 *A Concise History of Veterinary Medicine* Budapest, Akademiai Kiado

Karcher L F, Scott D W, Paradis M, and Anderson W I 1990 Sterile nodular panniculitis in five horses *Journal of the American Veterinary Medical Association* 196: 1823-6

Kasel J A, Byrne R J, and Harvey E W 1968 Experimental human B influenza virus infection in Chincoteague ponies *Nature* 219: 968-969

Katz J L 1980 The structure and biomechanics of bone *Symposium Society Experimental Biology* 34: 137-68

Kaup F J, Drommer W, and Deegen E 1990a Ultrastructural findings in horses with chronic obstructive pulmonary disease (COPD) I: Alterations of the larger conducting airways *Equine Veterinary Journal* 22: 343-348

Kaup F J, Drommer W, Damsch S, and Deegen E 1990b Ultrastructural findings in horses with chronic obstructive pulmonary disease II: pathomorphological changes of the terminal airways and the alveolar region *Equine Veterinary Journal* 22: 349-355

Keane D P, Little P B, Wilkie B N, Artsob H, and Thorsen J 1988 Agents of equine viral encephalomyelitis: Correlation of serum and cerebrospinal fluid antibodies *Canadian Journal of Veterinary Research* 52: 229-235

Keiper R and Houpt K 1984 Reproduction in feral horses: an eight year study *American Journal of Veterinary Research* 45: 991-5

Keller J 1957 Ein Beitrag zum Problem der Enterolithiasis beim Pferde *Dissertation*, Hannover

Keller S D and Horney F D 1985 Diseases of the equine small colon *Compendium Continuing Education Practicing Veterinarian* 7: 113-18

Kellerman T S, Marasas W F O, Thiel P F, Gelderblom W C A, Cawood M, and Coetzer J A W 1990 Leukoencephalomalacia in two horses induced by oral dosing of Fumonsin B1 *Onderstepoort Journal of Veterinary Research* 57: 269-75

Kelley D C and Knappenberger T E 1968 Cutaneous Streptothricosis (Equine Dermatophilosis) in Kansas horses *Veterinary Medicine/Small Animal Clinician*: 1055-1056

Kelly D F and Watson W J B 1976 Epidermoid cyst of the brain in the horse *Equine Veterinary Journal* 8: 110-112

Kelly W R 1985 The Liver and Biliary System In Jubb K, Kennedy P C, and Palmer N (Eds) *The Pathology of Domestic Animals* 3rd Ed Orlando, Academic Press

Kelser R A and Callender G R 1938 Equine degenerative arthritis *Veterinary Medicine* 33: 307-20

Kemen M J Jr 1978 Clinical aspects of viral respiratory infections in horses *Journal of the American Veterinary Medical Association* 166: 85-88

Kemen M J and Coggins L 1972 Equine infectious anemia: transmission from infected mares to foals *Journal of the American Veterinary Medical Association* 161: 496-499

Kenney R M 1978 Cyclic and pathological changes of the mare endometrium as detected by biopsy, with a note on early embryonic death *Journal of the American Veterinary Medical Association* 172: 241-62

Kent J E and Roberts C A 1990 Serum protein changes in four horses with monoclonal gammopathy *Equine Veterinary Journal* 22: 373-376

Kern T J, Brooks D E, and White M M 1983 Equine keratomycosis: Current concepts of diagnosis and therapy *Equine Veterinary Journal* 2 (supplement): 33-38

Kerr J F R 1971 Shrinkage necrosis: a distinct mode of cellular death *Journal Pathology* 105: 13-20

Kerr J F R 1987 Apoptosis In Kerr J F R, Searle J, Harmon B V, Bishop C J, and Potten C S (Eds) *Perspectives on Mammalian Cell Death* Oxford University Press

Kerr O M, Pearson G R, and Rice D A 1982 Pancreatic adenocarcinoma in a donkey *Equine Veterinary Journal* 14: 338-339

Kheng C S, Chee T K, Marchette N J, Garcia R, Rudnick A, and Coughlan R F 1968 Japanese B encephalitis in a horse *Australian Veterinary Journal* 44: 23-25

Kikkuli 1977 *The Kikkuli Text on the Training of Horses* Probst G F (Trans) Lexington, Kentucky, King Library Press

Kikuchi K 1928 Über Alterveränderungen am Gehirn des Pferdes *Archiv Tierheilkunde* 58: 541-73

Kimball A and Frank E R 1945 The isolation of *Actinomyces bovis* from fistulous withers and poll evil *American Journal of Veterinary Research* 6: 39-44

King A S 1949 Studies on equine purpura haemorrhagica, Article 3—morbid anatomy and histology *British Veterinary Journal* 105: 35-54

King J M 1967 The origin and development of hippomanes in the horse and zebra.I The location, morphology and histology of the hippomanes *Journal Anatomy* 101: 277-84

King J M, Roth L, and Haschek W M 1982 Myocardial necrosis secondary to neural lesions in domestic animals *Journal of the American Veterinary Medical Association* 180: 144-148

King J M, Flint T J, and Anderson W I 1988 Incomplete

subaortic stenotic rings in domestic animals-a newly described congenital anomaly *Cornell* Veterinarian 78(3): 263-271

King T C, Priehs D R, Gumm G G, and Miller T R 1991 Therapeutic management of ocular squamous cell carcinoma in the horse: 43 cases (1979-1989) *Equine Veterinary Journal* 23: 449-452

Kiper M L, MacAllister C, and Qualls C Jr 1988 Hematochezia attributable to cranial mesenteric arterial aneurysm with connecting tracts to cecum and ileum in a horse *Journal of the American Veterinary Medical Association* 193: 1278-1283

Kiper M L, Traub-Dargatz J, and Curtis C R 1990 Gastric rupture in horses: 50 cases (1979-87) *Journal of the American Veterinary Medical Association* 196: 333-6

Kirchhoff H 1982 Die Bedeutung der Mykoplasmen in den Genitalorganen von Rind, Pferd und Schwein *Berliner Munchener Tierarztliche Wochenschrift* 95: 121-125

Kirker-Head C A, Loeffler D, and Held J P 1985 Pelvic limb lameness due to malignant melanoma in a horse *Journal of the American Veterinary Medical Association* 186: 1215-1217

Kiryu K 1980 Cardiopathology of arrythymias in the horse *Proceedings American Association Equine Practitioners* 26: 457-468

Kiryu K, Kaneko M, Ariyama Y, and Satoh H 1968 Coronary aneurysm accompanied by rupture in a colt: Its formal pathogenesis *Experimental Reports Equine Health Laboratory* 5: 35-44

Kiryu K, Kaneko M, and Satoh H 1978 Cardiopathological observations on histopathogenesis of wandering pacemaker in horses *Japanese Journal of Veterinary Science* 40: 131-140

Kiryu K, Kaneko M, Kanemaru T, Yoshihara T, Hasegawa M, Tomioka Y 1985 Cardiopathology of sinoatrial block in horses *Japanese Journal of Veterinary Science* 47: 45-54

Kiryu K, Nakamura T, Kaneko M, Oikawa M, and Yoshihara T 1987 Cardiopathology of sudden cardiac death in the race horse *Heart Vessels* 2: 40-46

Kissling R E and Chamberlain R W 1967 Venezuelan equine encephalitis *Advances in Veterinary Science* 11: 65-84

Kissling R E and Rubin H 1951 Pathology of Eastern equine encephalitis *American Journal of Veterinary Research* 12: 100-105

Kissling R E, Chamberlain R W, Eidson M E, Sikes R K, and Bucca M A 1954 Studies on the North American arthropod-borne encephalitides II. Eastern equine encephalitis in horses *American Journal of Hygiene* 60: 237-250

Kita J, Frymus T, Crisman M V, and Perryman L E 1985 Survey of Arabian foals in Poland for immune system disorders *Equine Veterinary Science* 5: 290-292

Kitamura N, Yamada J, Calingasan N Y, and Yamashita T 1984 Immunochemical distribution of endocrine cells in the gastrointestinal tract of the horse *Equine Veterinary Journal* 16: 103-7

Kitt T 1900 *Lehrbuch der Pathologischen Anatomie der Haustiere* 2nd Ed Stuttgart, Enke

Kitt T 1923 *Lehrbuch der Pathologischen Anatomie der Haustiere* 5th Ed Stuttgart, Enke

Klaus H and Matthias D 1958 *Archiv Experimental Veterinary Medicine* 12: 151-72

Klein L 1990 Anesthetic complications in the horse *Veterinary Clinics North America* 6: 665-692

Klein W R, Bras G E, Misdorp W, et al. 1986 Equine sarcoid: BCG immunotherapy compared to cryosurgery in a prospective randomised clinical trial *Cancer Immunology Immunotherapy* 21: 133-140

Klyza J P 1983 Botulism syndromes: shaker foals and forage poisoning In *Current Therapy Equine Medicine.* Philadelphia, W.B. Saunders

Knight H D and Burau R G 1973 Chronic lead poisoning in horses *Journal of the American Veterinary Medical Association* 162: 781-786

Knight H D and Hietala S 1978 Transtracheal washings: bacteriological results from normal and diseased horses *Proceedings American College Veterinary Internal Medicine* pp. 120-131

Knight P R 1968 Equine cystitis and ataxia associated with grazing of pastures dominated by sorghum species *Australian Veterinary Journal* 44: 257

Knowles R C, Mathis R M, Bryant J E, and Willers K H 1966 Equine piroplasmosis *Journal of the American Veterinary Medical Association* 148: 407-409

Knowles R C, Hourrigan J L, and Holbrook A A 1980 Equine piroplasmosis *Equine Practice* 2: 10-14

Knudsen E 1959 Renal clearance studies on the horse I. Inulin, endogenous creatinine and urea *Acta Veterinaria Scandinavia* 1: 52-66

Koch P and Fischer H 1950 Einige seltenere Falle von Missbildungen *Tierärztliche Umschau* 5: 349-351

Koch P and Fischer H 1952a Die Oldenberger Fohlenataxie als Erbkrankheit *Tierärztliche Umschau* 7: 244

Koch P and Fischer H 1952b Erblich bedingte Blingeburten von Fohlen eines deutschen Zuchtgebietes *Tierärztliche Umschau* 7: 46-48

Koch S A, Cowles R R, Schmidt G R, Mayo J A, and Bowman R W 1978 Ocular disease in the newborn horse: A preliminary report *Journal of Equine Medicine and Surgery* 2: 167-170

Kochi O 1947 Pathologisch-anatomische und Bakteriologiskche Untersuchungen über das Wesen der Strahlfaule des Pferdes *Schweiz Archiv Tierheilkunde* 89: 338,384

Koehne G W, Herren C E, Gibson R B, and Northington W A 1981 An outbreak of *Bordetella bronchiseptica* respiratory disease in foals *Veterinary Medicine/Small Animal Clinician* April: 507-508

Köhler H 1951 Endarteritis obliterans der Zehnenarterien beim Pferd *Frankfurt Zeitschrift Pathologie* 62: 326-44

Köhler H 1968 In *Joest's Handbuch der Speziellen pathologischen Anatomie der Haustiere* 3rd Ed Berlin, Parey

Kohn CW and Chew D J 1987 Laboratory diagnosis and characterization of renal disease in horses *Veterinary Clinics of North America: Equine Practice* 3: 585-615

Kohn C W, Johnson G C, Garry F, Johnson C W, Martin S, and Scott, D W 1989 Mechanobullous disease in two Belgian foals *Equine Veterinary Journal* 21: 297-301

Konno S and Yamamoto H 1970 Pathology of equine infectious anemia. Proposed classification of pathologic types of disease *Cornell V*eterinarian 60: 393-449

Kono Y 1976 Viral antigen production in horse kidney cell cultures infected persistently with equine infectious anemia virus *National Institute Animal Health Quarterly* 16(10: 31-32

Kono Y and Yoshino T 1974 Propagation of equine infectious anemia virus in horse kidney cell culture *National Institute of Animal Health Quarterly* 14(4): 155-162

Kono Y, Kobayashi K, and Fukunaga Y 1971 Serological comparison among various strains of equine infectious anemia virus *Archiv Virusforschung* 34: 202-208

Kono Y, Kobayashi K, and Fukunaga Y 1973 Antigenic drift of equine infectious anemia virus in chronically infected horses *Archiv fur die gesamte Virusforschung* 41: 1-10

Kono Y, Sentsui H, and Murakami Y 1978 Lymphocyte responses to specific viral antigen and nonspecific mitogens in horses infected with equine infectious anemia virus *Journal of Equine Medicine and Surgery* (Suppl) 1: 363-373

Kopf N, Niebauer G W, and Rettenbacher G 1979 Innere Verletzungen als Ursache oder Folge von Ileus beim Pferd *Wiener Tierärztliche Monatschrift* 66: 233-47

Kostner M 1948 Die Mechanik des Abortus *Wiener Tierärztliche Monatschrift* 35: 263-275

Koterba A M 1990 *Equine Clinical Neonatology*, Philadelphia, Lea and Febiger

Koterba A M, Brewer B D, and Tarplee F A 1984 Clinical and clinicopathological characteristics of the septicaemic neonatal foal: Review of 38 cases *Equine Veterinary Journal* 16: 376-383

Kraft W, Mayer H, and Eikmeier H 1975 Diagnostische Bewertung verschiedener Blutbefunde beim Pferd *Tierarztliche Praxis* 3: 199-204

Krage P 1942 Zur Ätiologie der enzootischen leber-Gehirnkrankung bei Pferden. *Berliner Münchener Tierärztliche Wochenschrift* 58: 156-7

Krage P 1944 Listerella-infection bei fohlen *Berliner Münchener Tieräztliche Wochenschrift/Wiener Tieräarztliche Monatschrift* Jan 21: 30-31

Kral F 1960 Grundsatze der Behandlung der hautkrankheiten bie Haustieren *Kleintier Praxis* 5: 1-7

Krause C 1927 Pathologie der Blutgefässe der Tiere *Ergal Pathologie Pathologische Anatomie* 22: 350-431

Krause C 1930/31 Über sogenannte Zwerchfellhernien bei Haustieren nebst Nierenagenese des Pferdes *Archiv Tierheilkunde* 62: 567-601

Krogh P 1976 Mycotoxic nephropathy *Advances in Veterinary Science and Comparative Medicine* 20: 147-70

Krogsrud J and Onstadt O 1971 Exanthema coitale der Pferde (Equine coital exanthema. Isolation of a virus and transmission experiments) *Acta Veterinaria Scandinavia* 12: 1-14

Krölling O and Grau H 1960 *Lehrbuch der Histologie und Verleichenden Mimroskopischen Anatomie der Haustiere* 10th Ed Berlin, Parey

Kroneman J and Wensvoort P 1968 Muscular dystrophy and yellow fat disease in Shetland pony foals *Netherlands Journal of Veterinary Science* 1: 42-48

Krooke L 1969 Metabolic bone diseases of endocrine origin In Dobberstein J, Pallaske G, Stunzel H (eds) *Handbuch der Speziellen Pathologischen Anatomie der Haustiere*, Berlin, Parey

Krook L and Lowe J E 1964 Nutritional secondary hyperparathyroidism in the horse *Pathologica Veterinaria* (Suppl) 11

Krook L and Maylin G A 1989 *Race Horses at Risk* Downingtown, Pennsylvania, Racing Systems

Krook L, Wasserman R H, Shively J N, Tashjian A H Jr, Brokken T D, and Morton J F 1975 Hypercalcemia and calcinosis in Florida horses: implication of the shrub, *Cestrum diurnum*, as the causative agent *Cornell Veterinarian* 65: 26-56

Kroon H M and Plank G M van der 1931 Enkele Subletaalfactoren bij Huisdieren in Nederland *Tijdschrift Diergeneesk* 58: 681-94

Krüger 1938 Knochenbeinlagerungen im Sehnen-und Bandpapparat der Pferdezehe *Deutsche Tierärtzliche Wochenshrift* 49: 49-57

Kumanomido T, Kamada M, Wada R, Kenemaru T, Sugiura T, and Akiyama Y 1988 Pathogenicity for horses of original Sagiyama Virus, a member of the Getah Virus group *Veterinary Microbiology* 17: 367-373

Kunkle G A and Greiner E C 1982 Dermatitis in horses and man caused by the straw itch mite *Journal of the American Veterinary Medical Association* 181: 467-469

Ladds P W, Dennis S M, and Njoku C O 1974 Pathology of listeric infections in domestic animals *Veterinary Bulletin* 44(2): 67-74

Ladds P W, Thomas A D, and Potts B 1981 Meliodosis with acute meningoencephalomyelitis in a horse *Australian Veterinary Journal* 57(1): 36-38

Lahunta A de 1990 Abiotrophy in domestic animals: A review *Canadian Journal of Veterinary Research* 54: 65-76

Lamy P 1901/02 Osteoma of the gluteal aponeurosis of a horse *American Veterinary Revue* 25: 141

Lancaster W D and Olson C 1982 Animal papillomaviruses *Microbiology Reviews* 46(2): 191-207

Lane J G and Mair T S 1987 Observations on headshaking in the horse *Equine Veterinary Journal* 19: 331-336

Lane J G, Lonstaffe J A, and Gibbs C 1987 Equine paranasal cysts: A report of 15 cases *Equine Veterinary Journal* 19: 537-44

Langham R F and Hallman E T 1940 Some observations on nephritis in horses *American Journal of Veterinary Research* 1: 49-52

Langham R F and Hallman E T 1941 The incidence of glomerulonephritis in domesticated animals *Journal of American Veterinary Medical Association*

Lanzillotti-and Buonsanti N 1900 Krankheiten der Gelenke In

Bayer-Fröhner Handbuch der Tierärztlichen chirurgie und Geburtshilfe Vol 4 Vienna, Braumuller

Laplace J P 1972 Gastrointestinal motility in the pig: descriptive study by electromyography and nutritional correlations *Recueil Medicine Veterinarie* 148: 37-61

Larsen A B, Moon, H W, and Merkel R S 1972 Susceptibility of horses to *Mycobacterium paratuberculosis*. American Journal of Veterinary Research 33: 2185-89

Larson V L and Busch R H 1985 Equine tracheobronchial lavage: comparison of lavage cytologic and pulmonary histopathologic findings *American Journal of Veterinary Research* 46: 144-146

Larson V L, Perman V, and Stevens J B 1983 Idiopathic thrombocytopenic purpura in two horses *Journal of the American Veterinary Medical Association* 183: 328-330

Latimer C A, Wyman M, and Hamilton J 1983 An ophthalmic survey of the neonatal horse *Equine Veterinary Journal* 2 (supplement): 9-14

Latimer C A, Wyman M, and Diesem C D 1985 Radiographic and gross anatomy of the nasolacrimal duct of the horse *American Journal of Veterinary Research* 46: 451-458

Lavoie J P, Morris D D, Zinkl J G, Lloyd K, Divers T J 1987 Pancytopenia caused by bone marrow aplasia in a horse *Journal of the American Veterinary Medical Association* 191: 1462-1464

Lavoie J P, Madigan J E, Cullor J S, and Powell W E 1990 Haemodynamic, pathological, haematological and behavioural changes during endotoxin infusion in equine neonates *Equine Veterinary Journal* 22: 23-29

Lawrence R 1804 *An Inquiry into the Structure and Animal Economy of the Horse* London, Baldwin

Lazary S, Gerber H, Glatt P A, and Straub R 1985 Equine leucocyte antigens in sarcoid-affected horses *Equine Veterinary Journal* 17: 283-286

Leblanc P, Cadeac C, and Carougeau C 1902 *Pathologie chirurgicale generale* Paris, Bailliere

Leclainche E 1935 *Histoire de la Medecine Veterinarire* Toulouse, Office du Livre

Leclainche E 1936 L'anatomie de Ruini *Berl Tierartz Wochen* 52: 229-230

LeCouteur R A and Child G 1989 3rd Ed Diseases of the Spinal Cord In *Textbook of Veterinary Internal Medicine*

Lee C G and Ross A D 1977 Renal coccidiosis of the horse associated with *Klossiella equi Australian Veterinary Journal* 53: 287-288

Lees M J, Schuh J C L, Barber S M, and Farrow C S 1987 A congenital web defect in a quarterhorse filly *Equine Veterinary Journal* 19: 561-63

Lees P and Higgins A J 1985 Clinical pharmacology and therapeutic uses of non-steroidal anti-inflammatory drugs in the horse *Equine Veterinary Journal* 17: 83-96

LeGonidec G, Kuberski T, Daynes P, and Hartley W J 1981 A neurologic disease of horses in New Caledonia *Australian Veterinary Journal* 57: 194-195

Leith D E 1976 Comparative mammalian respiratory mechanics *Physiologist* 19: 485-510

Leland S E, Drudge J H, Wyant Z N, and Elam G W 1961 Studies on *Trichostrongylus axei* VII. Some quantitative and pathologic aspects of natural and experimental infection in the horse *American Journal of Veterinary Research* 22: 128-38

Leone N C, Shupe J L, Gardner E J, Millar E A, Olson A E, Phillips E C 1987 Hereditary multiple exostoses: a comparative human-equine epidemiologic study *J Hereditary* 78(3): 171-177

Leonhardt W 1923 Über die Herzzerresissung beim Pferde und ihre Therapie *Berlin Tierärztliche Wochenschrift* 39: 147-50

Lerner A B and Cage G W 1973 Melanomas in horses *Yale Journal of Biology and Medicine* 46(5): 646-649

Lerner D J and McCracken M D 1978 Hyperelastosis cutis in 2 horses *Journal of Equine Medicine and Surgery* 2: 350-352

LeRoux P L 1924 Helminths collected from equines in Edinburgh and in London *Journal Helminthology* 11: 111-34

Leslie I W and Davies D R T 1958 Tuberculosis of the horse caused by the avian type of tubercle bacillus *Veterinary Record* 70: 82-4

Leue G 1937 Kaubildkunde, ein neuer Weg tierärztliche Erkenntnis *Cited by Leue 1941*

Leue G 1941 Bezierhungen zwischen Zähneanomalien und Verdaungsstorungen beim Pferd unter Heranziehung von Daubildern. *Dissertation*, Hannover

Leuthold A 1943 Beitrag zur Kenntnis der Fohlengonitis *Festschrift Oskar Burg*, Oslo

Leuthold A 1975 Strahlbeinlamheit und Streckfortsatzfrakture am Hufbein *Schweiz Archiv Tierheilkunde* 117: 469-73

Levene A 1971 Equine melanotic disease *Tumori* 57: 133-168

Levene A 1979 Disseminated dermal melanocytosis terminating in melanoma *British Journal of Dermatology* 101: 197-205

Lew A M, Hosking C S, and Studdert M J 1980 Immunologic aspects of combined immunodeficiency disease in Arabian foals *American Journal of Veterinary Research* 41: 1161-1166

Lewis P F 1969 Epidemiology of major respiratory diseases of the horse *Australian Veterinary Journal* 45: 231-236

Liénard A 1928 Etude des oscillations entretenues *Revue Generale de L'Electricite* 23: 901-912

Lienaux 1909 Remarks on the nature of hypertrophying osteoarthropathy—a case in a tuberculous horse *American Veterinary Revue* 35: 464-5

Lienaux and Zwanenpoete 1910 Fracture of the neck of the femur *American Veterinary Revue* 37: 667-8

Liggett A D, Weiss R, and Blue J L 1987 Myospherulosis in the subcutis of a pony *Canadian Journal of Veterinary Research* 51: 150-151

Lilleengen K 1934 Hjärtmissbildningar hos djuren *Skandinaviska Veterinärtidskrift* 24: 493-555

Lindberg R 1984 Pathology of equine granulomatous enteritis *Journal of Comparative Pathology* 94: 233-47

Lindberg R, Persson S G B, Jones B Thoren-Tolling K, and

Ederoth M 1985 *Zablonski Veterinärmedicin* 32: 526-39

Lindholm A, Bjerneld H, and Saltin B 1974a Glycogen depletion pattern in muscle fibres of trotting horses *Acta Physiologica Scandinavia* 90: 475-84

Lindholm A, Johansson H E, and Kjaersgaard P 1974b Acute rhabdomylosis ("tying-up") in standardbred horses. A morphological and biochemical study *Acta Veterinaria Scandinavia* 15: 325-39

Lindley W H 1978 Acute pulmonary edema *Modern Veterinary Practice* 59: 64-65

Lindsay W A, McMartin R B, and McClure J R 1982 Management of slab fractures of the third tarsal bone in 5 horses *Equine Veterinary Journal* 14: 55-8

Lindt S 1970 Vol 5 Magen In Dobberstein J, Pallaske G, and Stünzi H (Eds) *Joest's Handbuch der Speziellen Pathologischen Anatomie der Haustiere* 3rd Ed Berlin, Parey

Little C and Hilbert B 1987 Pelvic fractures in horses *Journal of the American Veterinary Medical Association* 190: 1203-6

Little P B 1972 Cerebrospinal nematodiasis of horses *Journal of the American Veterinary Medical Association* 160: 1407-13

Little P B and Thorsen J 1976 Disseminated necrotizing myeloencephalitis: A herpes associated neurological disease of horses *Veterinary Pathology* 13(3): 161-171

Little P B, Thorsen J, Moore W, and Weninger N 1985 Powassan viral encephalitis: A review and experimental studies in the horse and rabbit *Veterinary Pathology* 22: 500-507

Little W L 1913 Periodontal disease in the horse *Journal of Comparative Pathology Therapeutics* 26: 240-49

Littlejohn A 1980 Studies on the physiopathology of chronic obstructive pulmonary disease in horses. I. Clinical signs *Onderstepoort Journal of Veterinary Research* 47: 159-162

Littlejohn A and Bowles F 1980 Studies on the physiopathology of chronic obstructive pulmonary disease in the horse. II. Right heart haemodynamics *Onderstepoort Journal of Veterinary Research* 47: 187-192

Littlejohn A and Bowles F 1982 Studies on the physiopathology of chronic obstructive pulmonary disease in the horse. VI. The alveolar dead space *Onderstepoort Journal of Veterinary Research* 49: 71-72

Liu I K M, Jang S, Johnson G C, Knight H D, Hawkins D 1977 Abortion associated with generalized Corynebacterium pseudotuberculosis infection in a mare *Journal of the American Veterinary Medical Association* 170(10): 1086-1087

Liu I K M, Lantz K C, Schlafke S, Bowers J M, and Enders A C 1990 Clinical observations of oviductal masses in the mare *Proceedings Annual Conference American Association Equine Practitioners*

Liu S K, Dolensek E P, Adams C R, Tappe J P 1983 Myelopathy and vitamin E deficiency in six Mongolian wild horses *Journal of the American Veterinary Medical Association* 183: 1266-1268

Livesey M A, Keane D P, and Sarmiento J 1984 Epistaxis in a Standardbred weanling caused by fibrous dysplasia *Equine Veterinary Journal* 16: 144-146

Lloyd K, Hintz H F, Wheat J D, and Schryver H 1987 Enteroliths in horses *Cornell Veterinarian* 77: 172-86

Lloyd K C, Peterson P R, Wheat J D, Ryan A E, and Clark J H 1988 Keratomas in horses: Seven cases (1975-1986) *Journal of the American Veterinary Medical Association* 193: 967-970

Lloyd K C K, Wheat J D, Ryan A M, and Matthews M 1989 Ulceration in the proximal portion of the urethra as a cause of hematuria in horses: Four cases (1978-1985) *Journal American Veterinary Medical Association* 194: 1324-1326

Lloyd S and Soulsby E J L 1978 Survey of infection with Onchocerca cervicalis, a filarial nematode in horse, 1 mule and 1 donkey in eastern United States *American Journal of Veterinary Research* 39(12): 1962-1963

Lockley M R and Wise R 1984 Pneumococcal infections *British Medical Journal* 288: 1179-1180

Loeven K 1987 Overo crosses and aganglionosis *Journal of Equine Veterinary Science* 7: 249-50

Löhrer A 1981 Statische Untersuchungen über die Strahlbeinlahmheit im Schweizerischen Kavalleriebestand von 1952-1972 *Dissertation*, Berne

Lokhorst H M and Breukink H J 1975 Auto-immune hemolytic anemia in two horses *Tijdschrift voor Diergeneeskunde* 100: 752-757

Lombard C W, Scarratt W K, and Buergelt C D 1983 Ventricular septal defects in the horse *Journal of the American Veterinary Medical Association* 183: 562-565

Long J R and Mitchell L 1971 Pulmonary aspergillosis in a mare *Canadian Veterinary Journal* 12: 16-18

Looser F 1929 Über die Ossifikationsstorungen bei Kretinismus *Verhandlung Deutsch Pathologishe Gesellshaft* 24: 352-60

Lowe J E 1976 Sex, breed, and age incidence of navicular disease *Proceedings Annual Conference American Association Equine Practitioners*

Lowe J E, Baldwin B H, Foote R H, Hillman R B, and Kallefelz F A 1975 Semen characteristics in thyroidectomized stallions *Journal of Reproduction and Fertility* (Suppl) 23: 81-86

Lowell F C 1964 Observations on heaves. An asthma-like syndrome in the horse *Journal of Allergy* 35: 322-330

Lubroth J 1987 African horsesickness and the epizootic in Spain, 1987 *Proceedings American Association Equine Practitioners* 33: 871-877

Luginbuhl H 1963 Comparative aspects of tumors of the nervous system *Annals New York Academy Sciences* 108: 702-721

Lukes H 1901/2 Ruptured spleen *American Veterinary Revue* 25: 225-6

Lumsden J H, Valli V E, McSherry B J, Robinson G A, Claxton M J 1975 The kinetics of hematopoiesis in the light horse II. The hematological response to hemorrhagic anemia *Canadian Journal of Comparitive Medicine* 39: 324-331

Lundvall R L 1967 The bacterial and mycotic flora of the normal conjunctival sac in the horse *Proceedings of the American Association of Equine Practice* 13: 101-106

Lutz W H and Gabel A A 1969 Spavin in standardbred racehorses: diagnosis and treatment *Modern Veterinary Practice* 50: 38

Lyons E 1992 Personal communication

Lyons E T 1991 Unpublished observation: *Eleaphora bohmi*

Lyons E T, Drudge J H, Tolliver S C 1980a Age distribution of horses in Kentucky infected with the eye worm Thelazia lacrimalis *Journal of the American Veterinary Medical Association* 176(3): 221-223

Lyons E T, Drudge J H, Tolliver S C 1980b Experimental infections of Thelazia lacrimalis: maturation of third-stage larvae from face flies (Musca autumnalis) in eyes of ponies *Journal Parasitology* 66(1): 181-182

Lyons E T, Drudge J H, Tolliver S C, Swerczek T W, and Crowe M W 1984 Prevalence of *Anoplocephala perfoliata* and lesions of *Draschia megastoma* in thoroughbreds in Kentucky at necropsy *American Journal of Veterinary Research* 45: 996-9

Lyons E T, Tolliver S C, Drudge J H, Swerczek T W, and Crowe M W 1985 Parasites in lungs of dead equids in Kentucky: Emphasis on *Dictyocaulus arnfieldi American Journal of Veterinary Research* 46: 924-927

Lyons E T, Tolliver S C, Drudge J H, Swerczek T W, and Crowe M W 1986 *Onchocerca spp.*: frequency in throughbreds at necropsy in Kentucky *American Journal of Veterinary Research* 47: 880-2

Lysholt B and Sonnichsen H V 1969 Senestylefod hos fol og plage *Nordiska Veterinärmedicin* 21: 601

MacAllister C G 1983 Effects of toxic doses of phenylbutazone in ponies *American Journal of Veterinary Research* 44: 2277-2279

MacAllister C, Qualls C, Tyler R, and Root C R 1987 Multiple myeloma in a horse *Journal of the American Veterinary Medical Assoication* 191(3): 337-339

MacCallum W G and Buckley S S 1904 Acute epizootic leucoencephalitis in horses *Journal of Experimental Medicine* 6: 56-74

MacDonald A A, Fowden A L, Silver I M, Ousey J, and Rossdale P D 1988 The foramen ovale of the foetal and neonatal foal *Equine Veterinary Journal* 20: 255-60

MacDougall, D F and Ricketts S W 1987 Progress in equine nephrology [editorial] *Equine Veterinary Journal* 16: 172-173

MacFadden B J 1992 *Fossil Horses*. New York, Cambridge

Machida N, Yasuda J, and Too K 1989 Three cases of paroxysmal atrial fibrillation in the Thoroughbred newborn foal *Equine Veterinary Journal* 21: 66-68

MacKay R J and Urquhart K A 1979 An outbreak of eosinophilic bronchitis in horses possibly associated with *Dictyocaulus arnfieldi* infection *Equine Veterinary Journal* 11: 110-112

Mackay-Smith M P, Cushing L S, and Leslie J A 1972 "carpal-canal" syndrome in horses *Journal of the American Veterinary Medical Association* 160: 993-7

Madewell B R and Munn R J 1989 Tubuloreticular inclusions in equine connective tissue neoplasms *Journal of Comparative Pathology* 100: 449-452

Madewell B R, Priester W A, Gillette E L, and Snyder S P 1976 Neoplasms of the nasal passages and paranasal sinuses in domestic animals as reported by 13 veterinary schools *American Journal of Veterinary Research* 37: 851-6

Madigan J E and Gribble D 1987a Equine ehrlichiosis in northern California: 49 cases (1968-81) *Journal of the American Veterinary Medical Association* 190: 445-8

Madigan J E and Higgins R J 1987b Equine protozoal myeloencephalitis *Veterinary Clinics of North America: Equine Practice* 3: 397-403

Maede Y, Inaba M, Amano Y, Murase T, Goto I, Itakura C 1991 Cryoglobulinemia in a horse *Journal of Veterinary Medical Science* 53: 379-383

Magnuson N S, Perryman L E, Grant B, and Estergreen V L 1980 Total plasma corticosteroid concentrations in horses with combined immunodeficiency *American Journal of Veterinary Research* 41: 826-828

Magnussen H 1938 Pyemia in foals caused by *Corynebacterium equi Veterinary Record* 50: 1459-1468

Magnusson H 1923 Spezifische infektiose Pneumonie beim Fohlen. Ein neuer Eitererreger beim Pferd *Archiv Wissenschaft Praktik-Tierheilkunde* 50: 22

Mahaffey E A and Moore J N 1986 Erythrocyte agglutination associated with heparin treatment in three horses *Journal of the American Veterinary Medical Association* 189: 1478-1480

Mahaffey L W 1958 Fenestration of the aortic and pulmonary semilunar valves in the horse *Veterinary Record* 70: 415-8

Mahaffey L W 1959 Ganglionic lesions in grass sickness of horses *Veterinary Record* 71: 170-1

Mair T S 1987 The value of tracheal aspirates in the diagnosis of chronic pulmonary diseases in the horse *Equine Veterinary Journal* 19: 463-465

Mair T S and Lane J G 1989 Pneumonia, lung abscesses and pleuritis in adult horses: a review of 51 cases *Equine Veterinary Journal* 21: 175-180

Mair T S and Wills J M 1992 *Chlamydia psittaci* infection in horses: results of a prevalence survey and experimental challenge *Veterinary Record* 130: 417-419

Mair T S and Yeo S P 1987 Equine pleuropneumonia: The importance of anaerobic bacteria and the potential value of metronidazole in treatment *Veterinary Record* 121: 109-110

Mair T S, Taylor F G R, Gibbs C, and Lucke V M 1986 Generalized avian tuberculosis in horses *Equine Veterinary Journal* 18: 220

Mair T S, Stokes C R, and Bourne F J 1987a Cellular content of secretions obtained by lavage from different levels of the equine respiratory tract *Equine Veterinary Journal* 19: 458-462

Mair T S, Stokes C R, and Bourne F J 1987b Quantification of immunoglobulins in respiratory tract secretions of the horse *Veterinary Immunology Immunopathology* 14: 197-203

Mair T S, Stokes C R, and Bourne F J 1988 Increased local IgA production in chronic obstructive pulmonary disease *Equine Veterinary Journal* 20: 214-216

Mair T S, Taylor F G R, Harbour D A, and Pearson G R 1990a Concurrent cryptosporidium and coronavirus infections in an Arabian foal with combined immunodeficiency syndrome *Veterinary Record* 126: 127-130

Mair T S, Taylor F G R, and Hillyer M H 1990b Autoimmune haemolytic anaemia in eight horses *Veterinary Record* 126: 51-53

Mair T S, Yeo S P, and Lucke V M 1990c Hypercalcaemia and soft tissue mineralisation associated with lymphosarcoma in two horses *Veterinary Record* 126: 99-101

Malark J L, Nixon A J, Houghland M A, and Brown M P 1992 Equine coxofemoral luxation: 17 cases (1975-90) *Cornell Veterinarian* 82: 79-90

Malmquist W A, Barnett D, and Becvar C S 1973 Production of equine infectious anemia agent in a persistently infected cell line *Arch Gesamt Virusforsch* 42(6): 361-370

Mammoli R 1960 Nova tecnia operatoria nel trattamentodella parilisi della falsa norice nel cavallo *Veterinaria* 62: 144-148

Mangrulkar M Y 1944 Melanomata in domesticated animals *Indian Journal of Veterinary Science* 14: 178-185

Manning J P and Gosser H S 1973 Neuritis of the cauda equina in horses *Veterinary Medicine/Small Animal Clinician* 60: 1162-1165

Manninger R and Csontos J 1941 Virusabortus der Stuten *Deutsch Tierärztliche Wochenschrift* 49: 105-8

Manninger R and Mocsy J 1959 In *Hutyra, Marek, Manninger, Mocsy Spezielle Pathologie und Therapie der Haustiere* Jena, Fischer

Mansmann R A 1983 The stages of equine pleuropneumonia *Proceedings American Association Equine Practitioners* 29: 61-63

Marasas W F O, Kellerman T S, Pienaar J G, and Naude T W 1976 Leukoencephalomalacia: A mycotoxicosis of equidae caused by *Fusarium moniliforme* Sheldon *Onderstepoort Journal of Veterinary Research* 43: 113-122

Marasas W F O, Kellerman T S, Gelderblom W C A, Coetzer J A W, Thiel P G and Van der Lugt 1988 Leukoencephalomalacia in a horse induced by fumonisin B1 isolated from *Fusarium moniliforme Onderstepoort Journal of Veterinary Research* 55: 197-203

Marcato P S and Simoni P 1982 Pigmentation of renal cortical tubules in horses: 572

Marcilese N A, Fraga A H, and Figueiras H D 1964 Iron content in the blood of horses (in Spanish) *Gac Veterinarian* 26: 81-83

Marcus L C and Ross J M Jr 1967 Microscopic lesions in the hearts of aged horses and mules *Veterinary Pathology* 4: 162-85

Mariat F, Destombes P, and Segretain G 1977 The mycetomas: clinical features, pathology, etiology, and epidemiology *Contributions to Microbiology Immunology* 4: 1-39

Markel M D And Dorr T E 1986 Multiple myeloma in a horse *Journal of the American Veterinary Medical Association* 188(6): 621-623

Markel M D, Dyer R M, and Hattel A L 1984 Acute renal failure associated with application of a mercuric blister in a horse *Journal of the American Veterinary Medical Association* 185: 92-94

Markel M D, Wheat J D, and Jang S S 1986 Cellulitis associated with coagulase-positive staphylococci in racehorses: nine cases (1975-1984) *Journal of the American Veterinary Medical Association* 189: 1600-1603

Markel M D, Wheat J D, and Jones K 1988 Genital neoplasms treated by en bloc resection and penile retroversion in horses: 10 cases (1977-1986) *Journal of the American Veterinary Medical Association* 192: 396-400

Markham G 1660 *The Perfect Horse-man* London, Humphrey Moseley

Marks D, Mackay-Smith M P, Cushing L S, and Leslie J A 1970 Etiology and diagnosis of laryngeal hemiplegia in horses *Journal of the American Veterinary Medical Association* 157: 429-436

Marks V G and Budras K D 1987 Licht-und elektronenmikroskopische Untersuchungen uber die akute Hufrehe des Pferdes *Berliner Munchener Tierärztliche Wochenschrift* 100: 82-88

Marolt J, Pajtl M, Geres V, and Adrasic N 1962 Uber aseptische Frakturen des normalen and veranderten Strahlbeines beim Pferde *Deutsch Tierärztliche Wochenschrift* 69: 133-135

Martens R J, Fiske R A, and Renshaw H W 1982 Experimental subacute foal pneumonia induced by aerosol administration of *Corynebacterium equi Equine Veterinary Journal* 14: 111-116

Marti E, Gerber H, Essich G, Oulehla J, and Lazary S 1991 The genetic basis of equine allergic diseases 1. Chronic hypersensitivity bronchitis *Equine Veterinary Journal* 23: 457-460

Martin L, Kaswan R, and Chapman W 1986 *Equine Veterinary Journal* 18: 133-7

Martin W J 1899/1900 Rupture of the internal iliac artery *American Veterinary Revue* 23: 114-16

Martin W J 1900/01 Spavin: its etiology and treatment *American Veterinary Revue* 24: 464-74

Marx M B, Jones M B, Kimberlin D S, Furcolow M L 1972 Survey of histoplasmin and blastomycin test reactors among Thoroughbred horses in central Kentucky *American Journal of Veterinary Research* 33(8): 1701-1705

Mason B J E 1973 Laryngeal hemiplegia: a further look at Haslam's anomaly of the left recurrent nerve *Equine Veterinary Journal* 5: 150-155

Mason D K, Collins E A, and Watkins K L 1984 Effect of bedding on the incidence of exercise induced pulmonary haemorrhage in racehorses in Hong Kong *Veterinary Record* 115: 268-269

Mason D K, Watkins K L, McNie J T, and Luk C M 1990 Haematological measurements as an aid to early diagnosis and prognosis of respiratory viral infections in thoroughbred horses *Veterinary Record* 126: 359-363

Mason J H and Robinson E M 1938 The isolation of *Clostridium welchii*, type B, from foals affected with dysentery *Onderstepoort Journal of Veterinary Science* 11: 333-7

Mason T A and McLean A A 1977 Ostechondritis dissecans of the head of the humerus in two foals *Equine Veterinary Journal* 9: 189

Masri M D, Olcott B M, Nicholson S S, McClure J J, Schmidt S P, Freestone J F and Kornagay W R 1987 Clinical, epidemiologic and pathologic evaluation of an outbreak of mycotoxic encephalomalacia in South Louisiana horses *Proceedings of the American Association of Equine Practitioners* 367-374

Matthew W D and Chubb S H No Date 7th Ed *Evolution of the Horse* American Museum Natural History No. 36

Matthews A G 1979 Identification and characterisation of the major antiproteases in equine serum and an investigation of their role in the onset of chronic obstructive pulmonary disease (COPD) *Equine Veterinary Journal* 11: 177-182

Matthews A G and Crispin S M 1987 Diseases of the equine iris *Veterinary Annual* 27: 156-172

Matthews A G and Handscombe M C 1983a Uveitis in the horse: a review of the aetiological and immunopathological aspects of the disease *Equine Veterinary Journal* 2 (supplement): 61-64

Matthews A G and Handscombe M C 1983b Bilateral cataract formation and subluxation of the lenses in a foal *Equine Veterinary Journal* 2 (supplement): 23-24

Matthews A G and Handscombe M C 1983c Superficial keratitis in the horse: Treatment with the antiviral drug idoxuridine *Equine Veterinary Journal* 2 (supplement): 29-31

Matthews A G, Crispin S M, and Parker J 1990a The equine fundus. II. Normal variants and colobomata *Equine Veterinary Journal* 10 (supplement): 50-54

Matthews A G, Crispin S M, and Parker J 1990b The equine fundus. III. Pathological variants *Equine Veterinary Journal* 10 (supplement): 55-61

Mathias C J 1992 In Wingate D L and Bannister R (Eds) *Autonomic Failure* New York, Oxford

Matthias D 1968 Die Nebennieren Vol 3 In Dobberstein J, Pallaske G, and Stünzi H (Eds) *Joest's Handbuch der Speziellen Pathologischen Anatomie der Haustiere* 3rd Ed Berlin, Parey

Matsuda H, Koyama H, Oikawa M, Yoshihara T, and Kaneko M 1991 Nerve growth factor-like activity detected in equine periperal blood after running exercise *Journal of Veterinary Medicine* 38: 557-559

Matumoto M, Ishizaki R, and Shimuzu T 1965 Serological survey of equine rhinopneumonitis virus infection among horses in various countries *Archiv Gesellschaft Virusforschungen* 50: 609-623

Mauderer H 1938 Erbfehler in der Pferdzucht *Deutsch Tierärztliche Wochenschrift* 46: 649

Maurer F D 1962 Equine piroplasmosis- another emerging disease *Journal of the American Veterinary Medical Association* 141: 699-702

Maurer F D and McCully R M 1963 African horse-sickness—with emphasis on pathology *American Journal of Veterinary Research* 24: 235

Maxie M G 1985 In Jubb K, Kennedy P C, and Palmer N *The Pathology of Domestic Animals* 3rd Ed Orlando, Academic Press

Maxie M G and Physick-Sheard P W 1985 Aortic-iliac thrombosis in horses *Veterinary Pathology* 22: 238-49

Mayer H, Kinzler M, and Sickel E 1976 Listeriose in einem Reitpferdbestand *Berlin München Tierärztliche Wochenschrift* 89: 209-11

Mayfield M A and Martin M T 1979 Corynebacterium pseudotuberculosis in Texas horses *S W Vet* 32(2): 133-136

Mayhew I G 1982 Observations on vascular accidents in the central nervous system of neonatal foals *Journal Reproduction Fertility* 32 (Supplement): 569-575

Mayhew I G and Ferguson H O 1987 Clinical, clinicopathologic, and epidemiologic features of anhidrosis in central Florida Thoroughbred horses *Journal of Veterinary Internal Medicine* 1: 136-141

Mayhew I G and Kryger M D 1975 Aortic-Iliac-Femoral thrombosis in a horse *Veterinary Medicine/Small Animal Clinician*: 1281-1284

Mayhew I G and MacKay R J 1982 The Nervous System In Mansmann R A and McAllister G S (Eds) *Equine Medicine and Surgery* 3rd Ed Wheaton, American Veterinary Publications

Mayhew I G, Lahunta A de, Whitlock R H, and Geary J C 1977 Equine degenerative myeloencephalopathy *Journal of the American Veterinary Medical Association* 170: 195-201

Mayhew I G, Watson A G, and Heissan J A 1978 Congenital occipitoatlantoaxial malformations in the horse *Equine Veterinary Journal* 10: 103

Mayhew I G, Lichtenfels J R, Greiner E C, MacKay R J and Enloe C W 1982 Migration of a spiruroid nematode through the brain of a horse *Journal of the American Veterinary Medical Association* 180: 1306-1311

Mayhew I G, Brown C M, Stowe H D, Trapp A L, Derksen F J, and Clement, S F 1987 Equine degenerative myeloencephalopathy: A vitamin E deficiency that may be familial *Journal of Veterinary Internal Medicine* 1: 45-50

McCaig J 1973 A survey to establish the incidence of sweet itch in ponies in the United Kingdom *Veterinary Record* 93: 444-446

McCausland I P and Milestone B A 1976 Diffuse mesangioproliferative glomerulonephritis in a horse *New Zealand Veterinary Journal* 24: 239-241

McChesney A E 1975a Viral respiratory infections of horses: Structure and function of lungs in relation to viral infection *Journal of the American Veterinary Medical Association* 166: 76-77

McChesney A E 1975b Viral respiratory infections of horses:

Pathogenesis *Journal of the American Veterinary Medical Association* 166: 77-78

McChesney A E 1982 Adenoviral infection in Arabian foals In Mansmann R A and McAllister G S (Eds) *Equine Medicine and Surgery* 3rd Ed Wheaton, American Veterinary Publications

McChesney A E, England J J, Adcock J L, Stackhouse L L, and Chow T L 1970 Adenoviral infection in suckling Arabian foals *Pathologia Veterinaria (Veterinary Pathology)* 7: 547-565

McChesney A E, England J J, and Rich L J 1973 Adenoviral infection in foals *Journal of the American Veterinary Medical Association* 162: 545-9

McClay C B, Weiss D J, Smith C M, Gordon B 1992 Evaluation of hemorheologic variables as implications for exercise-induced pulmonary hemorrhage in racing Thoroughbreds *American Journal of Veterinary Research* 53: 1380-1385

McClure J J, Lindsay W A, Taylor W, Ochoa R, Issel C J, and Coulter S J 1982 Ataxia in four horses with equine infectious anemia *Journal of the American Veterinary Medical Association* 180: 279-283

McClure J J, Koch C, Powell M, and McClure J R 1988 *Animal Genetics* 19: 427-33

McClure J R, McClure J J, and Usenik E A 1979 Disseminated intravascular coagulation in ponies with surgically induced strangulation obstruction of the small intestine *Veterinary Surgery* 8: 78-83

McCollum W H, Prickett M E, and Bryans J T 1971 Temporal distribution of equine arteritis virus in respiratory mucosa, tissues and body fluids of horses infected by inhalation *Research Veterinary Science* 12: 459-464

McConnell S, Katada M, Fiske R A, and Martens J G 1982 Equine lymphosarcoma diagnosed as equine infectious anaemia in a young horse *Equine Veterinary Journal* 14: 160-162

McCraw B M and Slocombe J O D 1974 Early development of and pathology associated with *Strongylus edentatus* *Canadian Journal of Comparative Medicine* 38: 124-38

McCraw B M and Slocombe J O D 1985 *Strongylus equinus*: development and pathological effects in the equine host *Canadian Journal of Comparative Medicine* 49: 372-83

McCue P M 1989 Equine leukoencephalomalacia *Compendium of Continuing Education for Veterinarians* 11: 646-651

McCue P M and Wilson W D 1989 Equine mastitis—a review of 28 cases *Equine Veterinary Journal* 21: 351-353

McCue P M, Freeman D E, and Donawick W J 1989 Guttural pouch tympany: 15 cases (1977-86) *Journal of the American Veterinary Medical Association* 194: 1761-63

McCully R M and Neitz W O 1971 Clinicopathological study on experimental *Trypanosoma brucei* infection in horses. Part 2. Histopathological findings in the nervous system and other organs of treated and untreated horses reacting to nagana *Onderstepoort Journal of Veterinary Research* 38: 141-176

McDonald D R and Cleary D J 1970 Toxoplasmosis in the equine *Southwestern Veterinarian* Spring: 213-214

McEntee K 1985 Vol 4 Pathology of the Female Reproductive System In Dobberstein J, Pallaske G, and Stünzi H (Eds) *Joest's Handbuch der Speziellen Pathologischen Anatomie der Haustiere* 3rd Ed Berlin, Parey

McEntee K 1990 *Reproductive Pathology of Domestic Animals* New York, Academic Press

McEntee M 1987 Eumycotic mycetoma: Review and report of a cutaneous lesion caused by *Pseudallescheria boydii* in a horse *Journal of the American Veterinary Medical Association* 191: 1459-1461

McEntee M, Summers B A, Lahunta A de, and Cummings J 1987 Meningocerebral hemangiomatosis resembling Sturge-Weber disease in a horse *Acta Neuropathologica* 74: 405-410

McEntee M F 1991 Equine cutaneous mastocytoma: morphology, biological behaviour and evolution of the lesion *Journal of Comparative Pathology* 104: 171-178

McEwen S A and Hulland T J 1986 Histochemical and morphometric evaluation of skeletal muscle from horses with exertional rhabdomylosis (tying-up) *Veterinary Pathology* 23: 400-10

McFadyean J 1933 Equine melanomatosis *Journal of Comparative Pathology* 46: 186-204

McGavin M D and Fadok V A 1984 Factors limiting the usefulness of histopathologic examination of skin biopsies in the diagnosis of large animal dermatoses *Veterinary Clinic of North America: Large Animal Practice* 6: 203-213

McGee W R 1969a Clinical aspects of disease caused by equine herpesvirus 1 In Bryans J T and Gerber H (Eds) *Proceedings of the 2nd International Conference on Equine Infectious Disease*, Basel, Karger 13-17

McGee W R 1969b The clinical aspects of streptococcal infections of the horse In Bryans J T and Gerber H (Eds) *Proceedings of the 2nd International Conference on Equine Infectious Disease*, Basel, Karger 227-230

McGraw B M and Slocombe J O D 1978 *Strongylus edentatus*: development and lesions from ten weeks postinfection to patency *Canadian Journal of Comparative Medicine* 42: 339-56

McGuire T C, Henson J B, and Quist S E 1969a Impaired bone marrow response in equine infectious anemia *American Journal of Veterinary Research* 30: 2099-2104

McGuire T C, Henson J B, and Quist S E 1969b Viral-induced hemolysis in equine infectious anemia *American Journal of Veterinary Research* 30: 2091-2097

McGuire T C, Crawford T B, and Henson J B 1974a Prevalence of antibodies to herpesvirus types 1 and 2, arteritis and infectious anemia viral antigens in equine serum *American Journal of Veterinary Research* 35: 181-185

McGuire T C, Poppie M J, and Banks K L 1974b Combined (B- and T-Lymphocyte) immunodeficiency: a fatal genetic disease of Arabian foals *Journal of the American*

Veterinary Medical Association 164: 70-76

McGuire T C, Crawford T B, Hallowell A L, and Macomber L E 1977 Failure of colostral immunoglobulin transfer as an explanation for most infections and deaths of neonatal foals *Journal of the American Veterinary Medical Association* 170: 1302-1304

McGuirk S M and Muir W W 1985 Diagnosis and treatment of cardiac arrhythmias *Veterinary Clinics of North America: Equine Practice* 1: 353-370

McIlwraith C W and James L F 1982 Limb deformities of foals associated with ingestion of locoweed by mares *Journal of the American Veterinary Medical Association* 181: 255

McIlwraith C W, Foerner J J, and Davis D M 1991 Osteochondritis dissecans of the tarsocrural joint: results of arthroscopic surgery *Equine Veterinary Journal* 23: 155-62

McKelvey W A C and Owen R 1979 Acquired torticollis in eleven horses *Journal of the American Veterinary Medical Association* 175: 295-297

McLaughlin B G and Doige C E 1981 Congenital musculoskeletal system lesions and hyperplastic goiter in foals *Canadian Veterinary Journal* 22: 130-3

McLaughlin B G, Doige C E, Fretz P B, and Pharr J M 1981 Carpal bone lesions associated with angular limb deformities in foals *Journal of the American Veterinary Medical Association* 178: 224

McLaughlin S A, Brightman A H, Helper L C, Manning J P, and Tomes J E 1983 Pathogenic bacteria and fungi associated with extraocular disease in the horse *Journal of the American Veterinary Medical Association* 182: 241-242

McLean J G 1973 Equine paralytic myoglobinuria ("azoturia"): a review *Australian Veterinary Journal* 49: 41-43

McMullan W C 1982 The skin: structure and diseases In Mannsmann R A, McAllister E S, and Pratt P W (eds) *Equine Medicine and Surgery, 3rd edition*, Santa Barbara, American Veterinary Publications

McPherson E A and Thomson J R 1983 Chronic obstructive pulmonary disease in the horse I. Nature of the disease *Equine Veterinary Journal* 15: 203-206

McPherson E A, Lawson G H K, Murphy J R, Nicholson J M, Fraser J A, Breeze, R G, Pirie H M 1978 Chronic obstructive pulmonary disease (COPD): identification of affected horses *Equine Veterinary Journal* 10(1): 47-53

McPherson E A, Lawson G H K, Murphy J R, Nicholson J M, Breeze R G, and Pirie H M 1979 Chronic obstructive pulmonary disease (COPD): Factors influencing the occurrence *Equine Veterinary Journal* 11: 167-171

Meagher D M, Pool R R, and O'Brien T R 1973 Osteochondritis of the shoulder joint in the horse. *Proceedings of the American Association of Equine Practitioners* 247-256.

Meagher D M, Pool R P, and O'Brien T R 1975 Osteochondrosis of the shoulder joint in horses *Proceedings Annual Convention American Association Equine Practitioners*

Meagher D M, Wheat J D, Hughes J P, Stabenfeldt G H, Harris B A 1977 Granulosa cell tumors in mares -A review of 78 cases *Proceedings Annual Convention American Association Equine Practitioners*

Medeiros L O, Martins L F, Ferri S, and Barcelos S R 1971 Effect of age on erythrogram values of thoroughbred horses from 1 to 12 months of age *Zentralblatte Veterinar Medizin* 18: 395-400

Mehlfeld R, Loeffler K, and Brehm H 1984 Der Einfluss der Bewegung auf die Bildung von Synovialgruben *Deutsch Tierärztliche Wochenschrift* 91: 360-4

Mehrle F 1926 Beitrag zum physiologie der Sehnen und Bänder am Unterfuss des Pferdes *Münchener Tierärztliche Wochenschrift* 77: 345-8

Mellor P S 1973 Studies on *Onchocerca cervicalis*, Railliet and Henry 1910: I. *Onchocerca cervicalis* in British horses Journal Helminthology 47: 97-118

Mellor P S and McCaig J 1974 The probable cause of "sweet itch" in England *Veterinary Record* 95: 411-15

Mendoza L and Alfaro A A 1986 Equine pythiosis in Costa Rica: Report of 39 cases *Mycopathologia* 94: 123-129

Meredith D, Elser A H, Wolf B, Soma L R, Donawick W J, and Lazary S 1986 Equine leukocyte antigens: relationships with sarcoid tumors and laminitis in two breeds *Immunogen* 23(4): 221-225

Merillat L A 1917 *Fistula of the withers and poll-evil* Chicago American Veterinary Publications

Merkt H, Klug E, Bohm K H, Weiss R 1974 Erfahrungen uber Klebsiellen als Genitalinfektionserreger beim Pferd *Berliner Munchener Tierarztliche Wochenschrift* 87: 405-409

Merritt A M 1983 Diabetes mellitus. In *Current Therapy Equine Medicine* Philadelphia, W.B. Saunders

Merritt A M, Merkal R S, Skye D, Selway S 1975 A case of avian tuberculosis in the intestinal tract of a horse *American Journal Digestive Disease* 20(6): 598

Merritt A M, Cimprich R E, and Beech J 1976 Granulomatous enteritis in nine horses *American Veterinary Medical Association* 169: 603

Merritt A M, Robbins J, and Brewer B 1982 Is salmonella infection a cause of the acute gastric dilatation/ileus syndrome in horses? *Equine Colic Research Symposium* Athens, Georgia

Meschter C L, Maylin G A, and Krook L 1984 Vascular pathology in phenylbutazone intoxicated horses *Cornell Veterinarian* 74: 282-297

Messer N T and Knight A P 1982 Pemphigus foliaceus in a horse *Journal of the American Veterinary Medical Association* 180: 938-940

Messow C 1952-3 Die Lebertumoren unserer Haustiere *Wissenschaft Zeitschrift Humboldt-Univ, Berlin* 2: 121-52

Mey G J W van der, Kleyn E F, and Watering C C 1967 Een onderzoek naar de erfalljke aanleg voor podotrochlitis *Tijdschrift Dieergeneesk* 92: 1261

Meyer E E, Morris PO G, Elcock L H, and Weil J 1986 Hindlimb hyperesthesia associated with rabies in two horses *Journal of the American Veterinary Medical Association* 188(6): 623-633

Meyer H 1984 The pathogenesis of disturbances of the alimentary tract of horses in the light of newer knowledge of digestive physiology *Proceedings Horse Nutrition Symposium*, Uppsala

Meyer H 1990 Beitrage zum Wasser- und Mineralstoffhaushault des Pferdes *Fort Tierphysiologie Tierernährung* 21: 1-102

Meyer H, Coenen M, and Gurer C 1985 Investigations on saliva production and chewing effects in horses fed various feeds *Proceedings 9th Equine Nutrition Physiology Symposium*

Meyer O 1948 Gefassberstungen bei der Stute *Deutsch Tierärztliche Wochenschrift* 55: 8-9

Meyer O 1949 Kritik und Vorschlag zum Abschluss des problems der Sehnenstelzfussbehandlung *Deutsch Tierärztliche Wochenschrift* 56: 261-3

Meyers K M, Menard M, and Wardrop K J 1987 Equine hemostasis: description, evaluation, and alteration *Vet Clinics of North America: Equine Practice* 3: 485-505

Meyling H A 1955 Das periphere Nervennetz und sin Zusammenhang mit den ortho- und parasympathetischen Nervenfasern *Acta Neurovegetativa* (Suppl) VI 35-63

Meyling H A and TerBorg N 1957 The conducting system of the heart in hoofed animals *Cornell Veterinarian* 47: 419

M'Fadyean J 1918 Tuberculosis in the horse caused by the bacilli of the avian type *Journal of Comparative Pathology Therapeutics* 31: 225-56

Michna S W 1970 Leptospirosis *Veterinary Record* 86: 484-96

Miers K C and Ley W B 1980 *Corynebacterium pseudotuberculosis* in the horse: study of 117 cases and consideration of etiopathogenesis *Journal of the American Veterinary Medical Association* 177: 250-52

Migulin V, Medvedev V, Mustel E, and Parygin V 1983 *Basic Theory of Oscillations* Moscow, Mir

Millar J W 1959 A clinical case of convulsive syndrome in a new-born foal *Austrialian Veterinary Journal* 35: 489-492

Miller C L and Todhunter R 1987 Acetabular osteochondrosis in a foal *Cornell Veterinarian* 77: 75-83

Miller L M, Reed S M, Gallina A M and Palmer G H 1985 Ataxia and weakness associated with fourth ventricle vascular anomalies in two horses *Journal of the American Veterinary Medical Association* 186: 601-603

Miller P J and Holmes J R 1985 Observations on seven cases of mitral insufficiency in the horse *Equine Veterinary Journal* 17: 181-90

Miller P J, Rose R J, Hoffman K, and Taylor G I 1987 Idioventricular tachycardia in a horse *Australian Veterinary Journal* 64: 55-57

Miller R I and Campbell R S F 1982a Clinical observations on equine phycomycosis *Australian Veterinary Journal* 58: 221-226

Miller R I and Campbell R S F 1982b Immunological studies on equine phycomycosis *Australian Veterinary Journal* 58: 227-231

Miller R I and Campbell R S F 1982c A survey of granulomatous and neoplastic diseases of equine skin in north Queensland *Australian Veterinary Journal* 59: 33-37

Miller R I and Campbell R S F 1983 Haematology of horses with phycomycosis *Australian Veterinary Journal* 60: 28-29

Miller R I and Campbell R S F 1984 The comparative pathology of equine cutaneous phycomycosis *Veterinary Pathology* 21: 325-332

Miller T R and Whitley R D 1987 Uveitis in horses *Modern Veterinary Practice* 68(6): 351-357

Miller T R, Gaskin J M, Whitley R D, and Wittcoff M L 1990 Herpetic keratitis in a horse *Equine Veterinary Journal* 10 (supplement): 15-17

Miller W C 1901/02 Comminuted fracture of the os suffraginus in a race horse *American Veterinary Revue* 24: 756-7

Millichamp N J, Carter G K, and Dziezyc J 1990 Idiopathic corneal oedema in a horse *Equine Veterinary Journal* 10 (supplement): 12-14

Milne E M, Doxey D L, and Gilmour J S 1990a Analysis of peritoneal fluid as a diagnostic aid in grass sickness (equine dysautonomia) *Veterinary Record* 127: 162-165

Milne E M, Doxey D L, and Gilmour J S 1990b Serum lipids and lipoproteins in equine colic and grass sickness *Research in Veterinary Science* 48: 170-174

Milne J C 1986 Malignant melanomas causing Horner's syndrome in a horse *Equine Veterinary Journal* 18: 74-75

Mirck M H 1977 *Strongyloides westeri* ihle. 1947 (Nematoda: Strongyloididae). I. Parasitologische aspecten van de natuurlijkke infectie *Tidjschift Diergeneesk* 102: 1039-43

Misdorp W 1967 Tumours in large domestic animals in the Netherlands *Journal of Comparative Pathology* 77: 211-217

Misdorp W and Nauta-van Gelder H L 1968 "Granular-cell myoblastoma" in the horse. A report of 4 cases *Pathologica Veterinaria (Veterinary Pathology)* 5: 385-394

Mishra P C and Leach D H 1983 Electron microscopic study of the veins of the dermal lamellae of the equine hoof wall *Equine Veterinary Journal* 15: 14-21

Mitchell W M 1930a Some aspects of osteoarthritis of the vertebral column *Veterinary Record* 10: 89-93

Mitchell W M 1930b Some further observations on pathological changes found in horses affected with "shivering" and their significance *Veterinary Record* 10: 535-37

Mitchell W M 1935 The problem of "Rheumatic Disease" (osteoarthritic and allied conditions) in the horse *Veterinary Record* 15: 1501-07

Mitchell W M 1937 "Rheumatic Disease" in the horse (osteoarthritis and allied conditions) *Journal of Comparative Pathology* 50: 282-86

Miura N, Senba H, Ogawa H, Sasaki N, Oishi H, Ohashi F, Takeuchi A, and Usui K 1987 A case of equine thrombasthenia *Japanese Journal of Veterinary Science* 49: 155-158

Modes E 1939 Zur Vorkommen echter Synovial gruben bei Mensche, Wiederkauern und Pferd *Virchows Archiv pathologishe Anatomie* 303: 603-10

Moens Y and Kombe A H 1988 Molluscum contagiosum in a horse *Equine Vet J* 20: 143-145

Mohamed F H A, Abu Samra M T, Ibrahim K E E, and Idris S O 1989 Cutaneous habronemiasis in horses and domestic donkeys (*Equus asinus asinus*) *Egyptian Veterinary Journal* 42: 535-538

Mohammed H O, Hill T, and Lowe J 1991 Risk factors associated with injuries in thoroughbred horses *Equine Veterinary Journal* 23: 445-48

Moll H D, Slone D E, Humburg J M, and Jagar J E 1987 Traumatic tarsal luxation repaired without internal fixation in three horses and three ponies *Journal of the American Veterinary Medical Association* 190: 297-300

Möller H, Frick H 1921 Vol 2 *Lehrbuch der Speziellen CHirurgie für Tierärzte* 6 Ed Stuttgart, Enke

Mollmann L H 1932 Zur Pathologie der sympathischen Bauch- Ganglien des Pferdes—Ganglien coeliacum plus mesentericum enterius—zugleich ein Beitrag zur pathogenese der Kolik *Zeitschrift Veterinarkiv* 44: 273-88

Monlux W S 1952 Primary pulmonary neoplasms in domestic animals *Southwest Veterinarian* 6: 17-20

Monlux W S and Luedke A J 1973 Brain and spinal cord lesions in horses inoculated with Venezuelan equine encephalomyelitis virus (epidemic American and Trinidad strains) *American Journal of Veterinary Research* 34: 465-473

Montali R J, Strandberg J D, and Squire R A 1970 Spinal ataxia in zebras *Laboratory Investigation* 23: 302-6

Montali R J, Bush M, Sauer R M, Gray C M, and Xanten W A Jr 1974a A histochemical and ultrastructural study of intimal bodies of horse arterioles *Veterinary Pathology* 11: 68

Montali R J, Bush M, Sauer R M, Gray C W and Xanten W A Jr 1974b Spinal ataxia in zebras. Comparison with the Wobbler syndrome of horses *Veterinary Pathology* 11: 68-78

Montané M and Morot Ch 1892 Epitheliome cylindrique due cheval avec transformation vibratile *Revue Veterinaire* 17: 185-89

Montgomerie R F and Rowlands W T 1937 Lamb dysentery in a foal *Veterinary Record* 49: 398

Montpelier D, Elser A H, Wolf B, Soma L R, Donawick W J, and Lazary S 1986 Equine leukocyte antigens: relationships with sarcoid tumors and laminitis in two breeds *Immunogen* 23(3): 221-225

Montpelier J, Deiuzeide R, and Badens P 1939 Greffe d'une tumeur schwannienne chez le mulet *Bulletin of the Academy of Veterinarians France* 12: 91

Monzon C M and Villavicencio V I 1990 Serum proteins in guinea-pigs and horses infected with *Trypanosoma evansi* (Steel, 1885) *Veterinary Parasitology* 36: 295-301

Moon F C 1987 *Chaotic Vibrations* New York, Wiley

Moore B O and Bryans J T 1969a Type specific antigenicity of group C streptococci from disease of the horse In Bryans J T and Gerber H *Proceedings 2nd International Conference Equine infectious Diseases* Basel, Karger 231-238

Moore B O and Bryans J T 1969b Antigenic classification of group C animal streptocci *Journal of the American Veterinary Medical Association* 155(2): 416-421

Moore C P 1984 Large animal ophthalmology *Veterinary Clinics of North America, Large Animal Practice* 6: 433-676

Moore C P, Sarazan R D, Whitley R D, and Jackson W F 1983 Equine ocular parasites: A review *Equine Veterinary Journal* 2 (supplement): 76-85

Moore J N, Garner H E, and Coffman J R 1981 Haematological changes during development of acute laminitis hypertension *Equine Veterinary Journal* 13: 240-242

Moore J N, Allen D, and Clark E S 1991a Pathophysiology of acute laminitis *Equine Practice* 13: 29-32

Moore J N, Dreesen D W, and Traldi A 1991b Evaluation of weather parameters and colonic distension, displacement and volvulus in broodmares *4th Equine Colic Research Symposium* Athens, Georgia

Moorthy A R S and Spradbrow P B 1978 Adenoviral infections of Arab foals with respiratory disease *Zentralblatte Veterinar Medizin* 25: 469-477

Moorthy A R S and Spradbrow P B 1985 The isolation of organisms resembling rickettsiae from respiratory tracts of horses *Zentralblatte Veterinar Medizin* 32: 46-54

Moraillon R 1985 Reanimation medicale et pathologie digestive des l'espece equine. *Recueil Médecine Vétérinaire* 161: 249-55

Morgan J P 1967 Necrosis of the third tarsal bone of the horse *Journal of the American Veterinary Medical Association* 151: 1334

Morgan J P, Carlson W D, and Adams O R 1962 Hereditary multiple exostosis in the horse *Journal of the American Veterinary Medical Association* 140: 1320-22

Morgan M H 1962 *The Art of Horsemanship by Xenophon* London, J.A. Allen

Morgan S E, Johnson B, Brewer B, and Walker J 1990 Sorghum cystitis ataxia syndrome in horses *Veterinary Human Toxicology* 32: 582

Morgan S J and Van Houten D S 1990 The ultrastructure of *Strongylus vulgaris*-mediated equine chronic mesenteric arteritis *Veterinary Research Communications* 14: 41-46

Morgan S J, Stromberg P C, Storts R W, Sowa B A, and Lay J C 1991 Histology and morphometry of *Strongylus vulgaris*-mediated equine mesenteric arteritis *Journal of Comparative Pathology* 104: 89-99

Mori T, Ishida T, Washizu T, Yamagami T, Umeda M, Sugiyama M, and Motoyoshi S 1991 Acute myelomonocytic leukemia in a horse *Veterinary Pathology* 28: 344-346

Morris Animal Foundation 1991, *Morris Animal Foundation Report*, Denver.

Morris C F, Robertson J L, Mann P C, Clark S, and Divers T J 1987 A hemolytic-uremic like syndrome in two horses *Journal of the American Veterinary Medical Association* 191: 1453-1454

Morris D D 1987 Cutaneous vasculitis in horses: 19 cases (1978-1985) *Journal of the American Veterinary Medical*

Association 191: 460-464

Morris D D 1988 Recognition and management of disseminated intravascular coagulation in horses *Veterinary Clinics of North America: Equine Practice* 4: 115-143

Morris D D and Beech J 1983 Disseminated intravascular coagulation in six horses *Journal of the American Veterinary Medical Association* 183: 1067-1072

Morris D D and Moore J N 1991 Tumor necrosis factor activity in derum from neonatal foals with presumed septicemia *Journal of the American Veterinary Medical Association* 199: 1584-1589

Morris D D and Whitlock R H 1983 Relapsing idiopathic thrombocytopenia in a horse *Equine Veterinary Journal* 15: 73-75

Morris D D, Miller W M Jr, Goldschmidt M H, and Trenka-Benthin S 1983 Chronic necrotizing vasculitis in a horse *Journal of the American Veterinary Medical Association* 183: 579-582

Morris D D, Aclund H M, and Hodge T G 1985 Pleural effusion secondary to metastasis of an ovarian adenocarcinoma in a horse *Journal of the American Veterinary Medical Association* 187: 272-274

Morris D D, Messick J, Whitlock R H, Palmer J, Ward M V, Feldman, B F 1988 Effect of equine ehrlichial colitis on the hemostatic system in ponies *American Journal of Veterinary Research* 49: 1030-1036

Morrison W I and Wright N G 1977 Viruses associated with renal disease of man and animals *Progress Medical Virology* 23: 22-50

Morrow A N, Baker K P, and Quinn P J 1987 Skin lesions of sweet itch and the distribution of dermal mast cells in the horse *Journal of Veterinary Medicine* 34: 347-355

Morter R L, Williams R D, Bolte H, Freeman M J 1969 Equine leptospirosis *Journal of the American Veterinary Medical Association* 155: 436-442

Mosier D A, Engelman R W, Confer A W, and McCarroll G D 1983 Bilateral multiple congenital ocular defects in Quarterhorse foals *Equine Veterinary Journal* 2 (supplement): 18-20

Mosselman M M and Hebriant 1899/90 Saturnism in horses *American Veterinary Revue* 23: 278

Moulton J E 1978 *Tumors in Domestic Animals*, Berkeley, University of California Press

Moyer W 1979 Disease of the equine heel *Proceedings Annual Conference American Association of Equine Practitioners*

Moyer W and Anderson J P 1975 Sheared heels *Journal of the American Veterinary Medical Association* 166: 53

Moyer W and Redden R R 1989 Chronic and severe laminitis: a critique of therapy with heart bar shoes and hoof wall resection *Equine Veterinary Journal* 21: 317-318

Mullaney T P and Brown C M 1988 Iron toxicity in neonatal foals *Equine Veterinary Journal* 20: 119-24

Mullenax C H 1957 A dietary cause of hair loss in Bahamian livestock *Journal of the American Veterinary Medical Association* 131: 302

Muller H 1991 Papillomatosen des Rindes und ihre Beziehungen zum equinen Sarkoid *Tierarztliche Praxis* 19: 39-43

Mumford J A 1985 Preparing for equine arteritis *Equine Vet Journal* 17: 6-11

Mumford J A and Rossdale P D 1980 Virus and its relationship to the "poor performance" syndrome *Equine Veterinary Journal* 12: 3-9

Munday B L, Monkhouse I M and Gallagher R T 1985 Intoxication of horses by lolitrem B in ryegrass seed cleanings *Australian Veterinary Journal* 62: 207

Munger R J 1983 Equine onchocercal keratoconjunctivitis *Equine Veterinary Journal* 2 (supplement): 65-70

Munger R J 1984 Equine ophthalmic emergencies *Veterinary Clinics of North America, Large Animal Practice* 6: 467-487

Munier 1890 Ruptur der hinteren Hohlvene während einer Geburt beim Pferde *Wochenschrift Tierheilkunde* 34: 338-9

Murphy F A, Bauer S P, Harrison A K and Winn W C 1973 Comparative pathogenesis of rabies and rabies-like viruses. Viral infection and transit from inoculation site to the central nervous system *Laboratory Investigation* 28: 361-376

Murphy J R, Breeze R G, and McPherson E A 1978 Myxoma of the equine respiratory tract *Modern Veterinary Practice* 59: 529-532

Murray D R, Ladds P W, and Campbell R S F 1978a Granulomatous and neoplastic diseases of the skin of horses *Australian Veterinary Journal* 54: 338-341

Murray D R, Ladds P W, Johnson, R H, and Pott B W 1978b Metastatic phycomycosis in a horse *Journal of the American Veterinary Medical Association* 172: 834-836

Murray M J, Grodinsky C, Anderson C W, Radue P F, and Schmidt G R 1989 Gastric ulcers in horses, a comparison of endoscopic findings in horses with and without clinical symptoms *Equine Veterinary Journal* (Suppl)7: 68-72

Murray M J et al. 1990 The prevalence of gastric lesions in foals without signs of gastric disease. An endoscopic survey *Equine Veterinary Journal* 22: 6-8

Musselman E E and LoGuidice R J 1984 Hypoplastic left ventricular syndrome in a foal *Journal of the American Veterinary Medical Association* 185: 542-543

Muybridge E 1957 *Animals in Motion*. New York, Dover

Muylle E 1974 Hypercalcemia and mineralization of non-osseous tissues in horses due to vitamin-D toxicity. *Zentrablatt Veterinäre Medicin* 21A: 638-43

Muylle E, De Roose P, Oyaert W, and Van Den Hende C 1974 An interventricular septal defect and a tricuspid valve insufficiency in a trotter mare *Equine Veterinary Journal* 6: 174-176

Muylle E, Vandenhende C, Oyaert W, Thoonen H, and Vlaeminck K 1981 Delayed monensin sodium toxicity in horses *Equine Veterinary Journal* 13: 107-108

Myers D D, Simon J, and Case M T 1964 Rhinosporidiosis in a horse *Journal of the American Veterinary Medical Association* 145

Naglic R, Herceg M, Hajsig D, Bambir S 1982 Bacteria in

equine pneumonia *Veterinarski Archiv* 52: 107-113

Nakamura R, Matsuhashi A, Yamashita N, and Yamamoto T 1956 Studies on "Kasen" of horses in Hokkaido III. Research on the actual state of the disease *Japanese Journal of Veterinary Research* 4: 81-90

Nappert G 1992 Atresia coli in foals *Equine Veterinary Data* 13: 261

Nation P N and Klavano G G 1986 Osteopetrosis in two foals *Canadian Veterinary Journal* 27: 74-7

Naughton G K, Mahaffey M, and Bystryn J C 1986 Antibodies to surface antigens of pigmented cells in animals with vitiligo *Proceedings of the Society for Experimental Biology and Medicine* 181: 423-426

Naylor J M, Kronfeld D S, and Acland H 1980 Hyperlipemia in horses: effects of undernutrition and disease *American Journal of Veterinary Research* 41: 899-905

Nemeth F 1974 Prognose, Therapie, und Pathogenese der Gleichbeinlahmheit *Tierärztliche Praxis* 2: 287-98

Nes M, Lomo O M, and Bjerkas I 1982 Hereditary lethal arthrogryposis ("muscle contracture") in horses *Nordiska Veterinärmedicin* 34: 425-30

Neufeld F and Schnitzer R 1928 *Pneumokokken Handbuch der Pathogenen Mikroorganismen* 3rd ed. Fisher, Jena

Neufeld J L 1973 Lymphosarcoma in the horse: a review *Canadian Veterinary Journal* 14: 129-135

Neumann-Kleinpaul K and Tabbert B 1936 Ätiologie und Pathologie der Recurrenslahmung des Pferdes *Archiv Tierheilkunde* 70: 413-25

Newberne J W, Robinson V B, and Bowen N E 1958 Histologic aspects of *Klosiella equi* in the kidney of a zebra *American Journal of Veterinary Research* 19: 304-307

Newsholme S J, Schneider D J, and Reid C 1985 A suspected lipofuscin storage disease of sheep associated with ingestion of the plant Trachyandra divaricata (Jacq.) Kunth) *Onderstepoort Journal of Veterinary Research* 52(2) 87-92

Ng B K Y and Vanselow B 1978 Outbreak of surra in horses and the pathogenesis of the anaemia *Kajian Veterinar Malayasia* 10: 88-98

Nicholas F W 1987 *Veterinary Genetics* Oxford, Clarendon Press

Nichols J M, Clayton H M, Pirie H M, and Duncan J L 1978 A pathological study of the lungs of foals infected expereimentally with *Parascarus equorum Journal of Comparative Pathology* 8: 261-74

Nickel R 1938 Über den Bau der Hufrorchen und seine Bedeutung für den Mechanismus des Pferdeshufes *Deutsch Tierärztliche Wochenschrift* 46: 449-552

Nickel R 1939 *Deutsch Tierärztliche Wochenschrift* 33: 521-24

Nickel R 1941 Anatomische bemerkungen zur hufrehe und zu den durchstromversuchen am huf *Deutsch Tierärztliche Wochenschrift* 49: 110-11

Nickel R 1949 Anordnung des Zwischenhorns in trachte und Eckstrebe der Hufplatte *Deutsch Tierärztliche Wochenschrift* 5/6 34-6

Nickel R, Schummer A, Seiferle E 1960 Vol 2 *Lehrbuch der Anatomie der Haustiere* Berlin, Parey.

Nickels F A, Grant B D, and Lincoln S D 1976 Villonodular synovitis of the equine metacarpophalangeal joint *Journal of the American Veterinary Medical Association* 168: 1043

Nighbert J D 1900/01 Spasms of the masseters, with complications *American Veterinary Revue* 24: 35-7

Niilo L and Chambers G A 1982 Hemorrhagic enterotoxemia caused by *Clostridium perfringens* type C in a foal *Canadian Veterinary Journal* 23: 299-301

Nilsson F 1947 Hästens goniter *Svensk Veterinärtidsskrift* 52: 1

Nilsson G, Dalin G, Drevemo S, Fredricson I, Jonsson K, and Olsson S E 1973 Lameness and pathological changes in the distal joints and the phalanges of the standardbred horse *Acta Veterinaria Scandia* (Suppl)44: 83

Nilsson S A 1982 Laminitis in cattle in comparison with equine laminitis *Acta Veterinaria Scandia* 53: 1-4

Nimmo-Wilkie J S, Yager J A, Nation D W, Clark E G, Townsend H G G, and Baird J D 1985 Chronic eosinophlic ermatitis: a manifestation of a multisystemic, eosinophilic, epitheliotropic disease in five horses *Veterinary Pathology* 22: 297-305

Nixon A J, Stashak T S, Ingram J T, Norrdin R W, and Park R D 1984 Cervical intervertebral disk protrusion in a horse *Veterinary Surgery* 13: 154-58

Noden D M and Lahunta de A 1985 *The Embryology of the Domestic Animals* Baltimore Williams & Wilkins

Noirjean P 1945 L'hydroarthrose du grasset chez le poulain de la race des Franches-Montagne *Schweizer Archiv Tierheilkunde* 87: 163,211

Nomina Anatomica Veterinaria 1983, 3rd Edition, Ithaca, New York International Committee

Norberg I 1967 Contracture *Personal communication*

Norval J and McPherson E A 1983 Dermatitis in the horse caused by acarus farinae *Veterinary Record* 112(16): 385-386

Norwood G L 1978 The bucked-shin complex in Thoroughbreds *Proceedings Annual Conference American Association of Equine Practitioners*

Numans S R and Watering C C van der 1973 Navicular disease Podotrochlitis chronica aseptica. *Equine Veterinary Journal* 5: 1

Nyack B, Morgan J P, Pool R, Meagher D 1981 Osteochondrosis of the shoulder joint of the horse *Cornell Veterinarian* 71: 149

Nyland T G, Blythe L L, Pool R R, Helhrey M G, and O'Brien T R 1980 Metrizimide myelography in the horse: clinical, radiographic, and pathologic changes *American Journal of Veterinary Research* 41(2): 204-211

Nyman G, Lindberg R, Weckner D, Bjork M, Kvart C, Persson S G B, Gustaffson H, and Hedenstierna G 1991 Pulmonary gas exchange correlated to clinical signs and lung pathology in horses with chronic bronchiolitis *Equine Veterinary Journal* 23: 253-260

Nyrop K A, DeBowes R M, Cox J H, and Goffman J R 1984 Rupture of the urinary bladder in two postparturient mares *Compendium Continuing Education* 6(9): 510-513

Obara J and Nakajima H 1961 Kinetics of iron metabolism in equine infectious anemia *Japanese Journal of Veterinary Science* 23: 247-252

Obel A-L 1955 Studies on grass disease. The morphological picture with special reference to the vegetative nervous system *Journal of Comparative Pathology* 65: 334-346

Obel A-L 1969 Vol I Die pulmonale hyperthropische Osteoarthropathie In Dobberstein J, Pallaske G, and Stünzi H (Eds) *Joest's Handbuch der SPeziellen Pathologischen Anatomie der Haustiere* 3rd Ed Berlin, Parey

Obel N 1948 *Studies on the histopathology of acute laminitis* Uppsala, Almqvist and Wiksells

O'Callaghan M W, Pascoe J R, Tyler W S, and Mason D K 1987 Exercise-induced pulmonary haemorrhage in the horse: I-VII *Equine Veterinary Journal* 19: 384-434

Ochoa R and Kern S R 1980 The effects of *Clostridium perfringens* Type A enterotoxin in Shetland ponies-clinical, morphologic and clinicopathologic changes *Veterinary Pathology* 17: 738-747

O'Connor G R 1981 The initiation of inflammation in uveitis *Transactions of the Ophthalmologic Society UK* 101(2): 297-300

Odberg F O 1978 A study of the hearing ability of horses *Equine Veterinary Journal* 10: 82-4

O'Dea J C 1969 Comments on vaccination against strangles *Journal of the American Veterinary Medical Association* 155: 427-431

Ogbourne C P 1978 *Pathogenesis of cyathostome (Trichonema) infection of the horse* Bucks, England, Commonwealth Agricultural Bureaux

Ogilvie T H, Rosendal S, Blackwell T E, Rostkowski C M, Julian R J, and Ruhnke L 1983 *Mycoplasma felis* as a cause of pleuritis in horses *Journal of the American Veterinary Medical Association* 182: 1374-1376

Oguri N and Tsutsumi Y 1972 Studies on lodging of the equine unfertilized ova in Fallopian tubes *Research Bulletin, Hokkaido University* 6: 32-43

Oikawa M, Yoshihara T, and Kaneko M 1989 Pathomorphological aspects of extremely small thymuses occurring spontaneously in thoroughbred foals *Japanese Journal of Veterinary Science* 51: 437-40

Oikawa M, Yoshihara T, Kaneko M, and Yoshikawa T 1990 Morphology of equine allantochorion at the tip of the pregnant horn *Journal of Comparative Pathology* 103: 343-49

Oikawa M, Kamada M, Yoshihara T, Kaneko M, and Yoshikawa T 1991 Clinico-pathological analysis of foal disease from 237 autopsy cases *Kitasato Archives Experimental Medicine* 64: 149-56

Oikawa M, Kaneko M, and Yoshikawa T 1992 Villous hypoplasia of the small intestine in neonatal foals *Journal of Veterinary Medicine* A 39: 121-29

Okumura M, Fujinaga T, Yamshita K, Tsunoda N, and Mizuno S 1991 Isolation, characterization, and quantitative analysis of ceruloplasmin from horses *American Journal of Veterinary Research* 52: 1979-1985

Oladosu L A and Olufemi B E 1992 Haematology of experimental babesiosis and ehrlichiosis in steroid immunosuppressed horses *Journal of Veterinary Medicine* 39: 345-352

Olander H J 1967 The migration of *Hypoderma lineatum* in the brain of a horse *Pathologica Veterinaria (Veterinary Pathology)* 4: 477-483

Olitsky P K, Traum J, and Schoening H W 1926 Comparative studies on vesicular stomatitis and foot-and-mouth disease *Journal of the American Veterinary Medical Association* 70: 147-167

Ono H, Satoh H, Miyake M, and Fujimoto Y 1969 On the development of "ovarian adrenocortical cell nodules" in the horse *Bulletin Equine Research Institute* 6: 59-90

Onuma H and Ohnami Y 1975 Retention of the tubal eggs in mares *Journal Reproduction Fertility* (Suppl) 23: 507-11

O'Rourke K I, Besola M L, and McGuire T C 1991 Proviral sequences detected by polymerase chain reaction in peripheral blood cells of horses with equine infectious anemia lentivirus *Archives Virology* 117: 109-119

Osbaldiston G W and Griffith P R 1972 Serum iron levels in normal and anemic horses *Canadian Veterinary Journal* 13: 105-108

Osbaldiston G W, Coffman J R, and Kruckenberg S M 1970 Biochemical differentiation of equine anemias *Journal of the American Veterinary Medical Association* 157: 322-325

O'Shea J D 1968 A histological study of nonfollicular cysts in the ovulation fossa region of the equine ovary *Journal Morphology* 124: 313-20

Ostblum L, Lund C, and Melsen F 1982 Histological study of navicular bone disease *Equine Veterinary Journal* 14: 199

Ostertag 1899 Vol 3 Die Krankheiten der Zähne In *Bayer-Fröhner Handbuch der tierärtzlichen chirurgie und Geburtshilfe* Braumuller, Wien

Ottaway C W 1944 The anatomical closure of the foramen ovale in the equine and bovine heart. A comparative study with observations on the foetal and adult states *Veterinary Journal* 199: 111-18,130-34

Owen J M 1975 Abnormal flexion of the corono-pedal joint of "contracted tendons" in unweaned foals *Equine Veterinary Journal* 7: 40-5

Owen L N 1958 Hair loss and other toxic effects of *Leucaenia glauca* ("Jumbey") *Veterinary Record* 70: 454-456

Owen R R 1975 Post stress diarrhoea in the horse *Veterinary Record* 96: 267-70

Owen R R, Moore J N, Hopkins J B, and Arthur D 1977 Dystrophic myodegeneration in adult horses *Journal of the American Veterinary Medical Association* 171: 343-49

Owens W R, Miller R I, Haynes P F, and Snider T G 1985 Phycomycosis caused by *Basidiobolus haptosporus* in two horses *Journal of the American Veterinary Medical Association* 186: 703-705

Oxspring G E 1935 The radiology of navicular disease with observations on its pathology *Veterinary Record* 15: 1433-47

Ozawa Y 1965 Experimental transmission of African horse-sickness by means of mosquitoes *American Journal of Veterinary Research* 26: 754
Pablo L S, Purohit R C, Teer P A, Newton J C, and Hammond L S 1983 Disseminated intravascular coagulation in experimental intestinal strangulation obstruction in ponies *American Journal of Veterinary Research* 44: 2115-2122
Pader J from Liautard A 1901/02 Filariosis of the suspensory ligament of the fetlock in horses *American Veterinary Revue* 25: 257-66
Pallaske G 1960 *Pathologische Histologie* Jena, Fischer
Palmer A C 1965 *Introduction to Animal Neurology* Oxford, Blackwell Publications
Palmer A C and Hickman J 1960 Ataxia in a horse due to angioma of the spinal cord *Veterinary Record* 72: 611-613
Palmer A C and Rossdale P D 1975 Neuropathy of the convulsive foal syndrome *Journal Reproduction Fertility* 23: 691-694
Palmer A C and Rossdale P D 1976 Neuropathological changes associated with the neonatal maladjustment syndrome in the Thoroughbred foal *Research Veterinary Science* 20: 267-275
Palmer A C, Blakemore W F, Cook W R, Platt H, and Whitwell K E 1973 Cerebellar hypoplasia and degeneration in the young Arab horse: clinical and neuorpathological features *Veterinary Record* 93: 62-66
Palmer A C, Leadon D P, Rossdale P D and Jeffcott L B 1984 Intracranial haemorrhage in pre-viable, premature and full term foals *Equine Veterinary Journal* 16: 383-389
Palomba E, Martone F, Meduri A, Vaccaro A, and Damiani N 1976 Biochemical studies on equine infectious anaemia *Folia Veterinaria Latina* 6: 275-288
Panciera R J 1972 Theiler's Disease In Catcott E J and Smithcors J E (Eds) *Equine Medicine Surgery* 2nd Ed Santa Barbara, American Veterinary Publications
Pandolfi F and Roperto F 1983 Seminoma with multiple metastases in a zebra *Equus zebra* X mare *(Equus caballus) Equine Veterinary Journal* 15: 70-72
Pankowski R L and Fubini S L 1987 Urinary bladder rupture in a two-year-old horse: Sequel to a surgically repaired neonatal injury *Journal of the American Veterinary Medical Association* 191: 560-562
Panovko Y G and Gubanova I 1965 *Stability and oscillations of elastic systems* New York, Consultants Bureau
Papa F O, Alvarenga M A, Lopes M D, and Campos Filho E P 1990 Infertility of autoimmune origin in a stallion *Equine Veterinary Journal* 22: 145-146
Parks A H, Doran R E, White N A, Allen D, and Baxter G M 1989 Ileal impaction in the horse: 75 cases *Cornell Veterinarian* 79: 83-91
Parry B W 1984 Resting blood pressure values in various equine clinical cases *Equine Veterinary Science* 4: 49-56
Parry B W 1987 Use of clinical pathology in evaluation of horse with colic *Veterinary Clinics of North America: Equine Practice* 3: 529-542
Pascoe J R, Ferraro G L, Cannon J H, Arthur R M, and Wheat J D 1981a Exercise-induced pulmonary haemorrhage in racing Thoroughbreds: a preliminary study *American Journal of Veterinary Research* 42: 703-707
Pascoe J R, Ellenburg T V, Culbertson M R, and Meagher D M 1981b Torsion of the spermatic cord in a horse *Journal of the American Veterinary Medical Association* 178: 242-245
Pascoe R R 1973 The nature and treatment of skin conditions observed in horses in Queensland *Australian Veterinary Journal* 49(1): 335-40
Pascoe R R 1976 Studies on the prevalence of ringworm among horses in racing and breeding stables *Australian Veterinary Journal* 52: 419-421
Pascoe R R 1979 The epidemiology of ringworm in racehorses caused by *Trichophyton equinum* var *autotrophicum Australian Veterinary Journal* 55: 403-407
Pascoe R R 1981a Clinical survey of tumours and tumour-like lesions in horses in south east Queensland *Equine Veterinary Journal* 13: 235-239
Pascoe R R 1981b *Equine Dermatoses* Sydney, University of Sydney
Pascoe R R 1984 Infectious skin diseases of horses *Veterinary Clinics North America: Large Animal Practice* 6: 27-46
Pascoe R R and Bagust T J 1975 Coital exanthema in stallions *Journal Reproduction Fertility* 23: 147-150 (supplement)
Pascoe R R and Connole M D 1974 Dermatomycosis due to *Microsporum gypseum* in horses *Australian Veterinary Journal* 50: 380-383
Pascoe R R and Summers P M 1981 Clinical survey of tumours and tumour-like lesions in south east Queensland *Equine Veterinary Journal* 13: 235-239
Pascoe R R, Spradbrow P B, and Bagust T J 1969 An equine genital infection resembling coital exanthema associated with a virus *Australian Veterinary Journal* 45: 166-170
Pass D A and Bolton J R 1982 Chronic eosinophilic gastroenteritis in the horse *Veterinary Pathology* 19: 486-96
Pass D A, Bolton J R, and Mills J N 1984 Basophilic enterocolitis in a horse *Veterinary Pathology* 21: 362-64
Paterson P Y, Ley H L Jr, Wiseman C L Jr, Pond W L, Smadel J E, Diercks F H, Heterington H D G, Sneath P H A, Witherington D H and Lancaster W E 1952 Japanese encephalitis in Malaya I. Isolation of virus and serologic evidence of human and equine infections *American Journal of Hygiene* 56: 320-330
Pauli B 1973 Koronärsklerose beim Pferd *Schweizer Archiv Tierheilkunde* 115: 517-26
Pauli B and Alroy J 1972 Veränderungen an Herzkranzgefassen bei Pferdefoten und wenige tage alten Saugfohlen *Schweizer Archiv Tierheilkunde* 114: 83-8
Pauli B, Gerber M, and Chuit P 1971 Dunndarminfarkte beim Pferd. II. Pathologie und Pathogenese *Schweizer Archiv Tierheilkunde* 113: 686-96
Pauli B, Gerber H, and Schatzmann U 1972 "Farmer's lung" beim Pferd *Pathologica et Microbiologica* 38: 200-14
Pearson E G 1991 Liver failure attributable to pyrrolizidine

alkaloid toxicosis and associated with inspiratory dyspnoea in ponies: Three cases (1982-1988) *Journal of the American Veterinary Medical Association* 198: 1651-1654

Peck A L (trans) 1979 *Aristotle Historia Animalum*. Books I-III. Cambridge, Loeb Classical Library, Harvard University Press

Pecquet Goad M E 1984 Pulmonary pythiosis in a horse *Veterinary Pathology* 21: 261-262

Peet R L, McDermott J, Williams J M, and Maclean A A 1981 Fungal myocarditis and nephritis in a horse *Australian Veterinary Journal* 57: 439-440

Peiffer R L Jr 1979 Keratomycosis in the horse *Equine Practice* 1: 32-37

Pemberton D H and Caple I W 1980 Australian stringhalt in horses *Veterinary Annual* 20: 167-71

Pepin G A and Austwick P K C 1968 II. Skin disease, mycological origin *Veterinary Record* 2/24/68: 208-224

Perce R B and Shideler R K 1976 Septic thrombosis in a foal *Veterinary Medicine/Small Animal Clinician* August: 1103-1107

Percivall W 1834 *Hippopathology. A systematic treatise on the disorders and lamenesses of the horse* London, Longman

Perdrizet J A and Scott D W 1987 Cellulitis and subcutaneous abscesses caused by *Rhodococcus equi* infection in a foal *Journal of the American Veterinary Medical Association* 190: 1559-1561

Peremans K, Verschooten F, DeMoor A, and Desmet P 1991 Laminitis in the pony: conservative treatment vs dorsal hoof wall resection *Equine Veterinary Journal* 23: 243-246

Perley H S 1899/1900 Extrauterine pregnancy *American Veterinary Revue* 23: 116-7

Perry B D 1988 Potomac horse fever *Veterinary Annual* 28: 108-13

Perryman 1988 Animal Genetics 19:

Perryman L E and Crawford T B 1979 Diagnosis and management of immune system failures of foals *Proceedings American Association Equine Practitioners* 25: 235-245

Perryman L E and McGuire T C 1980 Evaluation for immune system failures in horses and ponies *Journal of the American Veterinary Medical Association* 176: 1374-1377

Perryman L E and Torbeck R L 1980 Combined immunodeficiency of Arabian horses: confirmation of autosomal recessive mode of inheritance *Journal of the American Veterinary Medical Association* 176: 1250-1251

Perryman L E, Wyatt C R, and Magnuson N S 1984 Biochemical and functional characterization of lymphocytes from a horse with lymphosarcoma and IgM deficiency *Comparative Immunology Microbiology Infectious Disease* 7: 53-62

Peters 1935 Beitrag auf Kniescheibengelenkenentzundung bei Fohlen *Berliner Tierärztliche Wochenschrift* 51: 720-22

Peters 1938 Orthopädie an den Extremitäten der Fohlen *Deutsche Tierärztliche Wochenschrift* 46: 337,357

Peterson D E 1984 Equine testicular tumors *Equine Veterinary Science* 4: 25-27

Petersson H and Ryden G 1982 Avulsion fractures of the caudoproximal extremity of the first phalanx *Equine Veterinary Journal* 14: 333-35

Petrick S W, Roos C J, and Van Niekerk J 1978 Persistent right aortic arch in a horse *Journal South African Veterinary Association* 49: 355-358

Pettersson H 1970 Arbeitgemeinschaft fur Osteosynthesefragen *Svensk Vet Tidn* 22: 171-176

Pfaff G 1976 The incidence of epistaxis in racehorses in South Africa *Journal South African Veterinary Association* 47: 215-218

Pfeiffer C C 1935 Die habituelle laterale Dislokation der Kniescheibe bei Fohlen *Münchener Tierärztliche Wochenschrift* 86: 169-170

Pfeiffer C J, Spurlock S, and Ball M 1988 Ultrastructural aspects of equine pemphigus foliaceus-like dermatitis. Report of cases *Journal Submicroscopic Cytology Pathology* 20: 453-461

Physick-Sheard P W, Maxie M G, Palmer N C, and Gaul C 1985 Atrial septal defect of the persistent ostium primum type with hypoplastic right ventricle in a Welsh pony foal *Canadian Journal of Comparative Medicine* 49: 429-433

Picard L No Date *Origines de l'Ecole de Cavallerie et de ses traditions Equestre* Saumur, France, S. Milon et Fils

Pickar J G, Spier S J, Snyder J R, Carlsen R C 1991 Altered ionic permeability in skeletal muscle from horses with hyperkalemic periodic paralysis *American Journal of Physiology* 260: C926-C933

Pickett B W and Voss J L 1975 Abnormalities of mating behaviour in domestic stallions *Journal Reproduction Fertility, Suppl* 23: 129-134

Pierce K R, Joyce J R, England R B, and Jones L P 1972 Acute hemorrhagic anemia caused by wild onion poisoning in horses *Journal of the American Veterinary Medical Association* 160: 323-27

Pinkovsky DD and Butler JF 1978 Black flies (Diptera): simuliidae of Florida. I. Geographic and seasonal distribution *Flor Entom* 61(4): 257-267

Pinsent P J N 1989 Grass sickness of horses (grass disease; equine dysautonomia) *Veterinary Annual* 29: 169-74

Piot-Bey J B 1912 Mediate contusion causes bursting of the caecum *American Veterinary Revue* 41: 479

Platt H 1973 Septicaemia in the foal. A review of 61 cases *British Veterinary Journal* 129: 221-229

Platt H 1974 Causes of mortality in the young foal *Veterinary Annual* 15: 153-155

Platt H 1975 Haemorrhagic nasal polyps of the horse *Journal Pathology* 115: 51-55

Platt H 1982 Sudden and unexpected deaths in horses: a review of 69 cases *British Veterinary Journal* 138: 417-19

Platt H 1983 Caecal rupture in parturient mares *Journal of Comparative Pathology* 93: 343-46

Platt H 1986 Chronic inflammation and lymphoproliferative lesions of the equine small intestine *Journal of Comparative Pathology* 96: 671-84

Platt H 1987a Vascular malformation and angiomatous

lesions in horses: a review of 10 cases *Equine Veterinary Journal* 19: 500-4

Platt H 1987b Alimentary lymphomas in the horse *Journal of Comparative Pathology* 97: 1-10

Platt H and Whitwell K E 1971 Clinical and pathological observations on generalized steatitis in foals *Journal of Comparative Pathology* 81: 499-506

Platt H, Atherton J G, and Simpson D J 1978 The experimental infection of ponies with contagious equine metritis *Equine Veterinary Journal* 10: 153-59

Platt H, Singh H, and Whitwell K E 1980a Two cases of pancreatic adenocarcinoma in horses *Equine Veterinary Journal* 12: 118-26

Platt H, Singh H, and Whitwell K E 1980b Pathological observations on an outbreak of paralysis in broodmares *Equine Veterinary Journal* 12: 118-126

Platt H, Barnett K C, Barry D R, and Bell A S W 1983 Degenerative lesions of the optic nerve in Equidae *Equine Veterinary Journal* 2 (supplement): 91-97

Pohlenz J, Eckert J and Minder H P 1981 Zentralnervose storungen beim Pferde, versucht durch nematoden der gattung *Micronema* (Rhabditida) *Berliner Münchener Tierärtzliche Wochenschrift* 94: 216-220

Pohlenz J D, Schulze D, and Eckert J 1965 Spinale Nematodiasis beim Pferd, verursacht durch *Strongylus vulgaris Deutsche Tierärztliche Wochenschrift* 72: 510-11

Poland J 1978 Mycoplasms of the respiratory tract of horses and their significance in upper respiratory tract disease In Bryans J T and Gerber H (eds) *Equine Infectious Diseases IV*, Princeton, Vet Publications

Pollitt C C 1990a Clinical anatomy and physiology of the normal equine foot *Vet Conf Education* Massey University

Pollitt C C 1990b An autoradiographic study of equine hoof growth *Equine Veterinary Journal* 22: 366-368

Pollitt C C 1992 The role of arteriovenous anastomoses in the pathophysiology of equine laminitis *Proceedings of the American Society of Equity Practice* 37: 711-719

Pollitt C C and Molyneux G S 1987 An electron microscopic study of the laminar dermal microcirculation of the equine foot. I. Scanning electron microscopy. II. Ultrastructural innervation of the arteriovenous anastomoses (AVAs) *Proceedings 4th Australia New Zealand Microcirculation Symposium*

Pollitt C C and Molyneux G S 1990 A scanning electron microscopic study of the dermal microcirculation of the equine foot *Equine Veterinary Journal* 22: 79-87

Pomorski Z, Pinkiewicz E, and Grzebula S 1984 Proba wykazania wspoludzialu procesow autoagresyjnch w patogneezie okreswego zapelenia oczu u koni (Experimental demonstration of the participation of autoimmune processes in the pathogenesis of equine periodic ophthalmia) *Polskie Archiwum Weterynaryjne* 24: 155-164 (Polish)

Poncet P A, Montavon S, Gaillard C, Barrelet F, Straub R, and Gerber H A preliminary report on the possible genetic basis of laryngeal hemiplegia *Equine Veterinary Journal* 21: 137-138

Pool 1928 Grass sickness in horses *Veterinary Record* 8: 23

Popp E 1940 Ein Beitrag zur Kenntnis des juvenilen und des gravid gewese Uterus des Pferdes *Dissertation* Leipzig

Poppie M J and McGuire T C 1977 Combined immuno-defiency in foals of Arabian breeding: evaluation of mode of inheritance and estimation of prevalence of affected foals and carrier mares and stallions *Journal of the American Veterinary Medical Association* 170: 31-33

Posnett E S, Fehrsen J, De Waal D T, and Ambrosio R E 1991 Detection of *Babesia equi* in infected horses and carrier animals using a DNA probe *Veterinary Parasitology* 39: 19-32

Potel 1968 Vol 3 Die Zirbel In Dobberstein J, Pallaske G, and Stünzi H (Eds) *Joest's Handbuch der Speziellen Pathologischen Anatomie der Haustiere* 3rd Ed Berlin, Parey

Potratz Hanns A *Das Pferd in der Fruhzeit.*

Powell C A 1898/99 Untitled *American Veterinary Revue* 22: 679

Powell D G 1975 Equine infectious respiratory disease *Veterinary Record* 96: 30-34

Powell D G 1991 Viral respiratory disease of the horse *Veterinary Clinics North America: Equine Practice* 7: 27-52

Powell D G, Burrows R, and Goodridge D 1974 Respiratory viral infections among Thoroughbred horses in training during 1972 *Equine Veterinary Journal* 6: 19-24

Power H T, Watrous B J, Lahunta de A 1983 Facial and vestibulocochlear nerve disease in six horses *Journal of the American Veterinary Medical Association* 183: 1076-1080

Poynter D 1960 The arterial lesions produced by *Strongylus vulgaris* and their relationship to the migratory route of the parasite in its host *Research Veterinary Science* 1: 205-217

Prades M, Grant B D, Turner T A, Nixon A J, and Brown M P 1989 Injuries to the cranial cruciate ligament and its associated structures *Equine Veterinary Journal* 21: 354-7

Prasse K W, Lundvall R L, and Cheville N F 1975 Generalized mastocytosis in a foal, resembling urticaria pigmentosa of man *Journal of the American Veterinary Medical Association* 166: 68-70

Prasse K W, George L W, and Whitlock R H 1981 Idiopathic hypersegmentation of neutrophils in a horse *Journal of the American Veterinary Medical Association* 178: 303-305

Prasse K W, Allen D, Moore J N, and Duncan A 1990 Evaluation of coagulation and fibrinolysis during the prodromal stages of carbohydrate-induced acute laminitis in horses *American Journal of Veterinary Research* 51: 1950-1955

Prater P E, Patton C S, and Held J P 1989 Pleural effusion resulting from malignant hepatoblastoma in a horse *Journal of the American Veterinary Medical Association* 194: 383-385

Pratt G W and O'Connor J T 1976 Force plate studies of equine biomechanics *American Journal of Veterinary Research* 37: 1251-55

Prawochenski R 1936 A new lethal factor in the horse *Journal Heredity* 27: 411-14

Prescott J F 1987 Epidemiology of *Rhodococcus equi* infection in horses *Veterinary Microbiology* 14: 211-214

Prescott J F 1991 *Rhodococcus equi*: an animal and human pathogen *Clinical Microbiology Reviews* January: 20-34

Prescott J F, Travers M, and Yager-Johnson J A 1984 Epidemiological survey of *Corynebacterium equi* infection on five Ontario horse farms *Canadian Journal of Comparative Medicine* 48: 10-13

Preuss F and Eggers H 1951 Zur Radialislahmung des Pferdes *Tierärztliche Umschau* 6: 430-35

Preuss F and Henschel E 1969 Über die reitende Patella des Pferdes *Berliner Münchener Tierärztliche Wochenschrift* 82: 409-13

Preuss F, Budras K D, and Traeder W 1972 Arcus inguinalis und tendo praepubicus des Pferdes und deren vergleichend anatomische Bedeutung *Acta Anatomica* 82: 47-74

Prichard J T and Voss J L 1967 Fetal ankylosis associated with hybrid sudan grass pasture *Journal of the American Veterinary Medical Association* 150: 871

Prickett M E 1967 The pathology of the equine placenta and its effects on the fetus *Proceedings Annual Conference American Association of Equine Practitioners*

Prickett M E 1969 The pathology of disease caused by equine herpesvirus-1 In Bryans J T and Gerber H *Proceedings of the 2nd International Conference on Equine Infectious Diseases*, Karger, Basel 24-33

Prickett M E, Reeves J T, and Zent W W 1973 Tetralogy of Fallot in a Thoroughbred foal *Journal of the American Veterinary Medical Association* 162: 552-555

Priester W A, Glass G G, and Waggoner N S 1970 Congenital defects in domestic animals. General considerations *American Journal of Veterinary Research* 31: 1871-79

Prussian Army 1903 *Statistiches Jahrbuch Deutsche Reich. XIV Kriegwessen* Berlin, Puttkamer und Muhlbrecht

Pulley L T and Shively J N 1974 *Veterinary Pathology* 11: 203

Pulos W L and Hutt F B 1969 Lethal dominant white in horses *Journal of Heredity* 60(2): 59-63

Pulst H 1964 Listeriosis in a foal (in German) *Mh Vet Med* 19: 742-744

Purohit R C, Hammond L S, Slone D E, and Ganjam V K 1976 Evaluation of vasoactive drugs in equine hypertension and laminitis 21: 152-156

Putnam M R, Bransby D I, Schumacher J, Boosinger T R, and Bush L 1991 Effects of the fungal endophyte *Acremonium coenophialum* in fescue on pregnant mares and foal viability *American Journal of Veterinary Research* 52: 2071-74

Quinn P J, Baker K P, Morrow A N 1983 Sweet itch: response of clinically normal and affected horses to intradermal challenge with extracts of biting insects *Equine Veterinary Journal* 15: 266-72

Rabalais F C and Votava C L 1974 Cutaneous distribution of microfilariae of *Onchocerca cervicalis* in horses *American Journal of Veterinary Research* 35: 1369-1370

Radin M J, Eubank M C, and Weiser M G 1986 Electronic measurement of erythrocyte volume and volume heterogeneity in horses during erythrocyte regeneration associated with experimental anemias *Veterinary Pathology* 23: 656-660

Ragland W L and Spencer G R 1969 Attempts to relate bovine papilloma virus to the cause of equine sarcoid: Equidae inoculated intradermally with bovine papilloma virus *American Journal of Veterinary Research* 30: 743-752

Ragland W L, Keown G H, and Gorman J R 1966 An epizootic of equine sarcoid *Nature* 210: 1399

Ragland W L, Keown G H, and Spencer G R 1970 Equine sarcoid *Equine Veterinary Journal* 2: 2-11

Rahaley R S and Mueller R E 1983 Molluscum contagiosum in a horse *Veterinary Pathology* 20: 247-250

Rahaley R S, Gordon B J, Leipold H W, and Peter J E 1983 Sertoli cell tumour in a horse *Equine Veterinary Journal* 15: 68-70

Rajasekhar M and Keshavamurthy B S 1976 Acute cystitis due to *Pseudomonas aeruginosa* in a race-horse *Veterinary Record* 99: 214

Raker C W 1976 Diseases of the pharynx *Modern Veterinary Practice* 57: 396-400, 471-473

Ramadan R O 1975 Primary ocular melanoma in a young horse *Equine Veterinary Journal* 7: 49-50

Ramsay G, Rothwell L W, Gibson K T, Moore J D, and Rose R J 1987 Polycystic kidneys in an adult horse *Equine Veterinary Journal* 19: 243-244

Rantanen N W 1986 Diseases of the kidneys *Veterinary Clinics of North America: Equine Practice* 2: 89-103

Raphael C F 1982 Brain abscess in three horses *Journal of the American Veterinary Medical Association* 180: 874-877

Raphael C F and Beech J 1982 Pleuritis secondary to pneumonia or lung abscessation in 90 horses *Journal of the American Veterinary Medical Association* 181: 808-810

Raphael C F and Soma L R 1982 Exercise-induced pulmonary hemorrhage in Thoroughbreds after racing and breeding *American Journal of Veterinary Research* 43: 1123-1127

Rappeport J M and Nathan D G 1982 Acquired aplastic anemias: pathophysiology and treatment *Advance in Internal Medicine* 27: 547-590

Rasbech N O 1975 Ejaculatory disorders of the stallion *Journal Reproduction Fertility, Suppl* 23: 123-128

Rathor S S 1967 *Clinical aspects of the functional disorders of the equine and bovine femoro-patellar articulation with some remarks on its biomechanics* Utrecht, Drukkerij Hoeijenkos

Rawlings A and Bisgard G E 1975 Renal clearance and excretion of endogenous substances in the small pony *American Journal of Veterinary Research* 36: 45-48

Raymond 1899/90 Paralysis of the tail and sphincters in a mare *American Veterinary Revue* 23: 126-7

Read W K 1983 Renal medullary crest necrosis associated

with phenylbutazone therapy in horses *Veterinary Pathology* 20: 662-669

Rebar A, Fessler J F, Erb R 1979 Testicular teratoma in a horse: a case report and endocrinologic study *Journal of Equine Medicine and Surgery* 3: 361-6

Rebhun W C 1979 Diagnosis and treatment of equine uveitis *Journal of the American Veterinary Medical Association* 175: 803

Rebhun W C 1981 Bacterial ulcers of the equine cornea *Equine Practice* 3(1): 41-49

Rebhun W C 1983 Equine retinal lesions and retinal detachments *Equine Veterinary Journal* 2 (supplement): 86-90

Rebhun W C, Tennant B C, Dill S G, and King J M 1984 Vitamin K_3-induced renal toxicosis in the horse *Journal of the American Veterinary Medical Association* 184: 1237-1239

Rebhun W C, Shin S J, King J M, Baum K H, and Patten V 1985 Malignant edema in horses *Journal of the American Veterinary Medical Association* 187: 732-36

Redden R F 1989 Complicated laminitis: 311-319

Reed S M, Hegreberg G A, Bayly W M, Brown C M, Paradis M R, and Clemmons R M 1988 Progressive myotonia in foals resembling human dystrophia myotonica *Muscle & Nerve* II: 291-296

Reef V B 1983 *Clostridium perfringens* cellulitis and immune-mediated hemolytic anemia in a horse *Journal of the American Veterinary Medical Association* 182: 251-254

Reef V B 1985 Cardiovascular disease in the equine neonate *Veterinary Clinics of North America: Equine Practice* 1: 117-29

Reef V B 1987 Mitral valvular insuffiency associated with ruptured chordae tendineae in three foals *Journal Americal Veterinary Medical Association* 191: 329-331

Reef V B, Levitan C W, Spencer P A 1988 Factors affecting prognosis and conversion in equine atrial fibrillation *Journal of Veterinary Internal Medicine* 2: 1-6

Reef V B, Boy M G, Reid C F, and Elser A 1991 Comparison between diagnostic ultrasonography and radiography in the evaluation of horses and cattle with thoracic disease: 56 cases (1984-1985) *Journal of the American Veterinary Medical Association* 198: 2112-2118

Reeks H C 1911 Twist or displacement of the pelvic flexure in the horse *Journal of Comparative Pathology Therapeutics* 24: 306-27

Reid C H 1965 Habronemiasis and corynebacterium "chest" abscess in California horses" *VM SAC* 60: 233-242

Reif J S 1979 Epidemiology of equine infectious respiratory disease *Veterinary Clinics North America: Large Animal Practice* 1: 3-15

Rejno S and Strömberg B 1978 Osteochondrosis in horses *Acta Radiologica* (Suppl) 358, 153

Renaut J 1881 Recherche sur quelques points particular d'histologie des nerfs *Archiv Physiologie(Paris)* 8: 180-191

Reynolds D J and Nicholl T K 1978 Tetralogy of Fallot and cranial mesenteric arteritis in a foal *Equine Veterinary Journal* 10: 185-187

Rezabek G 1992 Unpublished observations.

Rezabek G and Rooney J R 1992 Unpublished observations.

Richardson D W 1985 Urogenital problems in the neonatal foal *Veterinary Clinics of North America: Equine Practice* 1: 179-187

Richardson D W 1991 Chronic proliferative (villonodular) synovitis In *Equine Medicine and Surgery, 4th Ed,* Goleta, California, Equine Medicine and Surgery American Veterinary Publications

Richardson D W and Kohn C W 1983 Uroperitoneum in the foal *Journal of the American Veterinary Medical Association* 182: 267-271

Richardson D W, Colahan P T 1991 Chronic proliferative (villonodular) synovitis In *Equine Medicine and Surgery* 4th Ed Goleta, California Equine Medicine and Surgery American Veterinary Publications

Richter H 1923 Physiologische Bedeutung und Erklarung des Luftsackes (Divertix tubae auditivae Eustachii) bei Equiden und verwaandten tierarten (Tapieren, Rhinocern, Hyradoiden) und bei Babirussa *Schweizer Archiv Tierheilkunde* 65: 61-74

Richters 1928 Experimentelle Untersuchungen über die histologische Veranderungen an den Beugesehnen des Pferdes durch perforiendes Brennen *Zeitschrift Veterinärkunde* 40: 321-28

Ricketts S W, Rossdale P D, and Samuel C A 1978 Endometrial biopsy studies of mares with contagious equine metritis *Equine Veterinary Journal* 10: 160-66

Rider J R 1932 Diverticula of the small intestine *Veterinary Record* 12: 1202-06

Ridge W 1891 Abscess of the guttural pouches *American Veterinary Revue* 15: 382-86

Riek R F 1953 Studies on allergic dermatitis ("Queensland itch") of the horse. I. Description, distribution, symptoms and pathology *Australian Veterinary Journal* 29: 177-187

Riemann H P, Smith A T, Stormont C, et al. 1975 Equine toxoplasmosis: a survey for antibodies to Toxoplasma gondii in horses *American Journal of Veterinary Research* 36(2): 1797-1800

Riemersma D J and Schamhardt H C 1985 In vitro mechanical properties of equine tendons in relation to cross-sectional area and collagen content *Research Veterinary Science* 39: 263-70

Ries J-N 1903 Guttaromycose chez le cheval *Recueil Médecine Vétérinaire* 80: 225-29

Ries J-N 1913 Note sur une myopathie progressive des poulains *Recueil Médecine Vétérinaire* 90: 634-36

Rigg D L, Ramey D W, and Reinerston E L 1985 Tracheal compression secondary to abscessation of cranial lymph nodes in a horse *Journal of the American Veterinary Medical Association* 186: 283-284

Riis R C 1981 Equine ophthalmology: Horse, ass, zebra In Gelatt K N (ed) *Textbook of Veterinary Opthalmology*, Philadelphia, Lea and Febiger

Riis R C and Rebhun W C 1990 Proliferative optic neuropathy in a horse caused by a granular cell tumour *Equine Veterinary Journal* 10 (supplement): 69-72

Riis R C and Smith J C 1975 Clinical investigation (1975) cited in Startup F G and Tatum S J (1990)

Riis R C, Scherlie P H Jr, and Rebhun W C 1990 Intraocular medulloepithelioma in a horse *Equine Veterinary Journal* 10 (supplement): 66-68

Rijkenhuizen A B, Nemeth F, Dik K J, and Goedegebuure S A 1989a The arterial supply of the navicular bone in adult horses with navicular disease *Equine Veterinary Journal* 21: 418-424

Rijkenhuizen A B, Nemeth F, Dik K J, Goedegebuure S A and Van Den Brom W E 1989b The effect of unilateral resection of segments of both palmar digital arteries on the navicular bone in ponies: An experimental study *Equine Veterinary Journal* 21: 413-417

Rimaila-Parnanen E 1976 Neuritis of the cauda equina in a horse *Nordsk Vet Med* 28: 464-467

Rimpau W 1947 Leptospirosis in the horse (periodic ophthalmia) *Tierartz. Umschr.* 2: 177-182

Ringen L 1966 Response of erythrocytes to *Leptospira pomona* hemolysins during infection *American Journal of Veterinary Research* 27: 1629-1632

Ris M 1924 Untersuchungen über Erkrankungen des Arteriellen Gefässsystems des Pferdes *Schweizer Archiv Tierheilkunde* 66: 1-14,35-47

Ristic M and Sibinovic S 1964 Equine babesiosis: diagnosis by a precipitation in gel and by a one-step fluorescent antibody-inhibition test *American Journal of Veterinary Research* 25: 1519-1526

Ritzenthaler M 1924 L'anaphylaxie du cheval *Archiv International Physiologie* 24: 54-72

Riviere J E, Traver D S, and Coppoc G L 1982 Gentamicin toxic nephropathy in horses with disseminated bacterial infection *Journal of the American Veterinary Medical Association* 180: 648-651

Roberts E D, Samartin C, Payan J and Mackenzie R B 1970 Neuropathologic changes in 15 horses with naturally occurring Venezuelan equine encephalomyelitis *American Journal of Veterinary Research* 31: 1223-1229

Roberts E D, Ochoa R, and Haynes P F 1980 Correlation of dermal-epidermal laminar lesions of equine hoof with various disease conditions *Veterinary Pathology* 17: 656-666

Roberts E J 1968 *Proceedings Annual Conference American Association of Equine Practitioners*

Roberts M C 1977 A case of primary lymphoid leukaemia in a horse *Equine Veterinary Journal* 9: 216-219

Roberts M C 1979 Ascending urinary tract infection in ponies *Australian Veterinary Journal* 55: 191-193

Roberts M C 1982 Development of a drug-induced impaction colic model in the horse *Equine Colic Research Symposium*, Athens, Georgia

Roberts M C and Kelly W R 1982 Renal dysfunction in a case of purpura haemorrhagica in a horse *Veterinary Record* 110: 144-146

Roberts M C and Pinsent P J N 1975 Malabsorption in the horse associated with alimentary lymphosarcoma *Equine Veterinary Journal* 7(3): 166-172

Roberts M C and Seawright A A 1978 Mercury toxicosis studies in the horse *Australian Advances in Veterinary Science* 22-3

Roberts M C, Seawright A A, and Ng J C 1979 Chronic phenylmercuric acetate toxicity in a horse *Vet Hum Tox* 21(5): 321-327

Roberts M C, Seawright A A, and Norman P D 1982 Some effects of chronic mercuric chloride intoxication on renal function in a horse *Vet Hum Toxicol* 24: 415-420

Roberts S J 1969 Comments on equine leptospirosis *Journal of American Veterinary Medical Association* 155(2): 442-445

Roberts S J 1971 *Veterinary Obstetrics and Gynecology*, Ithaca, Cornell University Press

Robertson J 1991 Arytenoid Chondritis In Beech J (Ed) *Equine Respiratory Disease* Philadelphia, Lea and Febiger

Robertson J B 1910 *The Principles of Heredity Applied to the Racehorse* London, The Winning Post

Robertson J L 1993 Fibrinous pericarditis in a Percheron gelding (in preparation)

Robertson J T and Copelan R W 1990 Surgery of the upper respiratory tract in the racehorse *Veterinary Clinics of North America* 6(1): 197-222

Robertson W A N 1932 The hereditary character of sidebone *Veterinary Record* 12: 83-90

Robertson-Smith R G, Jeffcott J B, Friend S C B, and Badcoe I M 1986 *Australian Veterinary Journal* 62: 6-12

Robie S M, Smith S C, and O'Connor J T 1975a Equine serum lipids: serum lipoprotein profiles of Morgan and Thoroughbred horses *American Journal of Veterinary Research* 36: 1709-1713

Robie S M, Janson C H, Smith S C, and O'Connor J T 1975b Equine serum lipids: lipid composition and electrophoretic mobility of equine serum lipoprotein fractions *American Journal of Veterinary Research* 36(12): 1715-1717

Robin V and Charton A 1945 L'enevination du cheval pars les piques d'abeilles *Recueil Médecine Vétérinaire* 121: 289-98

Robinson J A, Marr C M, Reef V B, and Sweeney R W 1992 Idiopathic, aseptic, effusive, fibrinous, nonconstrictive pericarditis with tamponade in a Standardbred filly *Journal of the American Veterinary Medical Association* 201: 1593-1598

Robinson N E 1987 Exercise induced pulmonary haemorrhage (EIPH): could Leonardo have got it right? *Equine Veterinary Journal* 19: 370-371

Robinson N E 1990 Digital blood flow, arteriovenous anastomoses and laminitis *Equine Veterinary Journal* 22: 381-383

Robinson N E and Sorensen P R 1978 Pathophysiology of airway obstruction in horses: A review *American Review Respiratory Disease* 127 (Supplement): 16-25

Robinson N E, Dabney J M, Weidner W J, Jones G A, and Scott J B 1975a Vascular responses in the equine digit *American Journal of Veterinary Research* 36: 1249-1253

Robinson N E, Jones G A, Scott J B, and Dabney J M 1975b Effects of histamine and acetylcholine on equine digital lymph flow and composition *Proceedings Society*

for Experimental Biology and Medicine 149: 805-807
Robinson N E, Scott J B, Dabney J M, Jones G A 1976 Digital vascular responses and permeability in equine alimentary laminitis *American Journal of Veterinary Research* 37: 1171-6
Roby T O and Anthony D W 1963 Transmission of equine piroplasmosis by *Dermacentor nitens* Neumann *Journal of the American Veterinary Medical Association* 142: 768-769
Roderick L M, Kimball A, McLeod W M, and Frank E R 1948 A study of equine fistulous withers and poll evil *American Journal of Veterinary Research* 9: 5-10
Roeland 1910 Ossified cardiac auricles in a horse *American Veterinary Revue* 37: 539-40
Roesti W 1941 Ueber Drusenbildung am Schnervenkopf des Pferdes: Neuritis exsudativa nervi optici *Arch Wiss Prakt Tierheilk* 77: 81-103
Rohrback B W and Rooney J R 1980 Congenital esophageal ectasia in a thoroughbred foal *Journal of the American Veterinary Medical Association* 177: 65-7
Ronen N, Van Heerden J, and Van Amstel S R 1992 Clinical and biochemistry findings,and parathyroid hormone concentrations in three horses with secondary hyperparathyroidism *Journal South African Veterinary Association* 63: 134-136
Rooney J R 1963 Epiphyseal compression in young horses *Cornell Veterinarian* 53: 567
Rooney J R 1964 Gastric ulceration in foals *Veterinary Pathology* 1: 497-503
Rooney J R 1965 Volvulus, strangulation, and intussusception in the horse *Cornell Veterinarian* 55: 644-53
Rooney J R 1966 *Corynebacterium equi* infection in foals *Modern Veterinary Practice* 47: 43-5
Rooney J R 1967 Aortic ring rupture in stallions *Veterinary Pathology* 4: 268-74
Rooney J R 1968 Biomechanics of equine lameness *Cornell Veterinarian* (Suppl) 58: 49-58
Rooney J R 1969 *Biomechanics of Lameness in Horses* Baltimore, Williams and Wilkins
Rooney J R 1970 *Autopsy of the Horse* Baltimore, Williams and Wilkins
Rooney J R 1971 Rupture of the urinary bladder in the foal *Veterinary Pathology* 8: 445-51
Rooney J R 1973a Functional anatomy of the equine suspensory ligament *Modern Veterinary Practice* 54: 43-44
Rooney J R 1973b The primary site of damage in bowed tendon of the horse *Modern Veterinary Practice* 54: 58-59
Rooney J R 1973c Bog spavin and tibiotarsal joint lesions in the horse *Modern Veterinary Practice* 54: 45-56
Rooney J R 1974 Distal condylar fractures of the cannon bone in the horse *Modern Veterinary Practice* 55: 113
Rooney J R 1975 Osteochondrosis in the horse *Modern Veterinary Practice* 56: 41-3, 113-16
Rooney J R 1977 Sacroiliac arthrosis and "stifle lameness" *Modern Veterinary Practice* 58(2): 138-139
Rooney J R 1979a Ruptured aneurysm of the uterine artery *Modern Veterinary Practice* 60: 316-317
Rooney J R 1979b Cauda equina neuritis *Modern Veterinary Practice* 60: 228-230
Rooney J R 1981 An hypothesis on the pathogenesis of curb in horses *Canadian Veterinary Journal* 22: 300-01
Rooney J R 1982 The relationship of season of the year to lameness and breakdown in thoroughbred horses *Journal of Equine Veterinary Science* 2: 174-76
Rooney J R 1984 Arteriovenous anastomoses in the digit of the horse *Equine Veterinary Science* 4: 182-183
Rooney J R 1985 Vascular "rests" in the fibrocartilage of the navicular bone of the horse *Journal of Equine Veterinary Science* 5: 298-99
Rooney J R 1986 A model for horse movement *Journal of Equine Veterinary Science* 6: 30-34
Rooney J R 1989 Stability theory in equine biomechanics *Proceedings 7th Conference Racing Analysts and Veterinarians*
Rooney J R 1990a The jump behaviour of the humeroradial and tarsocrural joints of the horse *Journal of Equine Veterinary Science* 10: 311-14
Rooney J R 1990b An hypothesis for a type of lameness of the rearleg *Journal of Equine Veterinary Science* 10: 388-89
Rooney J R 1991a Stress relaxation of the equine forelimb in vitro *Journal of Equine Veterinary Science* 11: 75-6
Rooney J R 1991b A principle of least action and equine locomotion *Journal of Equine Veterinary Science* 11: 256-57
Rooney J R 1991c Postnatal contracture of young horses *Journal of Equine Veterinary Science* 11: 148-51
Rooney J R and Genovese R L 1981 A survey and analysis of bowed tendon in thoroughbred racehorses *Journal of Equine Veterinary Science* 1: 49-53
Rooney J R and Jeffcott L B 1968 Muscular hypertrophy of the ileum in a horse *Veterinary Record* 83: 217-19
Rooney J R and Prickett M E 1966 Foreleg splints in horses *Cornell Veterinarian* 56: 259
Rooney J R and Prickett M E 1967a Congenital lordosis of the horse *Cornell Veterinarian* 57: 417-28
Rooney J R and Prickett M E 1967b Shaker foal syndrome *Modern Veterinary Practice* 48: 44-45
Rooney J R and Turner L W 1985 The mechanics of pulling loads. *Journal of Equine Veterinary Science* 5:355-59
Rooney J R, Bryans J T, Prickett M E, and Zent W W 1966 Exhaustion shock in the horse *Cornell Veterinarian* 56: 220-35
Rooney J R, Prickett M E, and Crowe M W 1967 Aortic ring rupture in stallions *Path Vet* 4: 268-274
Rooney J R, Delaney F M, and Mayo J 1969 Sacroiliac luxation in horses *Equine Veterinary Journal* 1: 287-89
Rooney J R, Prickett M E, Delaney F M, Crowe M W 1970 Focal myelitis-encephalitis in horses *Cornell Veterinarian* 60: 494-501
Rooney J R, Raker C W, and Harmany K J 1971 Congenital lateral luxation of the patella in the horse *Cornell Veterinarian* 61: 670-73
Rose A L, Gardner C A, McConnell, and Bull L B 1957

Field and experimental investigation of "Walk-about" disease of horses (Kimberley horse disease) in Northern Australia: *Crotolaria* poisoning in horses. Part II. *Australian Veterinary Journal* 33: 49-62

Rose R J, Hartley W J, and Baker W 1981 Laryngeal paralysis in Arabian foals associated with oral haloxon administration *Equine Veterinary Journal* 13: 171-176

Rosen L 1986 The natural history of Japanese encephalitis virus *Annual Review of Microbiology* 40: 395-414

Ross M W and Martin B B 1992 Dorsomedial articular fractures of the proximal aspect of the third metacarpal bone in standardbred racehorses: Seven cases (1978-1990) *Journal of the American Veterinary Medical Association* 201: 332-35

Ross M W, Donawick W J, Sellars A F, and Lowe J E 1986 Normal motility of the cecum and right ventral colon in ponies *American Journal of Veterinary Research* 47: 1756-62

Ross P F, Rice L G, Reagor J C, Osweiler G D, Wilson T M, Nelson H A, Owens D L, Plattner R D, Harlin K A, Richard J L, Colvin B M, and Banton M I 1991 Fumonisin B_1 concentrations in feeds from 45 confirmed equine leukoencephalomalacia cases *Journal of Veterinary Diagnostic Investigation* 3: 238-241

Rossdale P D 1967 Respiratory distress in a newborn foal with failure to form lung lining film *Nature* 215: 1498-1499

Rossdale P D 1972a Modern concepts of neonatal disease in foals *Equine Veterinary Journal* 4(3): 117-128

Rossdale P D 1972b Differential diagnosis and treatment of equine neonatal disease *Veterinary Record* 91(224: 581-588

Rossdale P D 1979 Neonatal respiratory problems of foals *Veterinary Clinics North America: Large Animal Practice* 1: 205-217

Rossier Y, Sweeney C R, and Ziemer E L 1991 Broncho-alveolar lavage fluid cytologic findings in horses with pneumonia or pleuropneumonia *Journal of the American Veterinary Medical Association* 198: 1001-1004

Roth H and Christensen N O 1942 On parasitic gastritis in the horse due to *Trichostrongylus axei Skandinaviska Veterinär Tidsskrift* 32: 488-514

Round M C 1972 A study of the natural history of lungworm infection of Equidae Cambridge, *Dissertation*

Round M C 1976 Lungworm infection (*Dictyocaulus arnfeldi*) of horses and donkeys *Veterinary Record* 99: 393-395

Rous R C 1975 Mesenteric thrombosis *Journal of the South African Veterinary Association* 46: 79-80

Rubarth S 1943 Plotsliga dodsfall hos hast och derar samband med fokalinfectioner *Svensk Militarvetsallskap Kvarfalskrit* 30: 1

Rubarth S 1967 Leber In Dobberstein J, Pallaske G, and Stünzi H (Eds) *Joest's Handbuch der Speziellen pathologischen Anatomie der Haustiere* 3rd Ed Berlin, Parey

Rubarth S and Krook L 1968 Etiology and pathogenesis of so-called mucoid degeneration of the nasal conchae of the horse *Acta Veterinaria Scandinavia* 9: 253

Rubin H L and Woodard J C 1974 Equine infection with *Micronema deletrix Journal of the American Veterinary Medical Association* 165: 256-258

Rudolph W, Correa J, Zorita L, and Manley W 1975 Equine piroplasmosis: leukocytic response to *Babesia equi* (Laveran, 1901) infection in Chile *British Veterinary Journal* 131: 601-609

Rugh K S, Garner H E, Sprouse R F, and Hatfield D G 1987 Left ventricular hypertrophy in chronically hypertensive ponies *Laboratory Animal Science* 37: 335-338

Rumbaugh G E 1977 Disseminated septic meningitis in a mare *Journal of the American Veterinary Medical Association* 171: 452-454

Runnells R A and Benbrook E A 1941a Malignant melanomas of horses and mules *American Journal of Veterinary Research* 2: 340-344

Runnells R A and Benbrook E A 1941b Connective tissue tumors of horses and mules *American Journal of Veterinary Research* 2: 427-430

Runnells R A and Benbrook E A 1942 Epithelial tumors of horses *American Journal of Veterinary Research* 3: 176-179

Runnells R A and Benbrook E A 1944 Malignant lymphoid tumors in horses *Journal of the American Veterinary Medical Association* 104: 148-149

Ruoff W W, Baker D C, Morgan S J, and Abbitt B 1986 Type II diabetes mellitus in a horse *Equine Veterinary Journal* 18: 143-144

Ruppaner R, de G-Gelinas L, and Marcoux M 1972 Equine incoordination *Canadian Veterinary Journal* 13: 180-183

Russ J C 1989 Automatic methods for the measurement of curvature of lines, features, and feature alignment in images *Journal Computer-Assisted Microscopy* 1: 39-77

Rutkowski J A and Richardson D W 1989 A retrospective study of 100 pelvic fractures in horses *Equine Veterinary Journal* 21: 256-59

Ryan A F and Ramey J W 1945 *Australian Veterinary Journal* 21: 146

Ryan M J and Wand D S 1981 Cryptococcus as a cause of neonatal pneumonia and abortion in two horses *Veterinary Pathology* 18: 270-72

Ryshkov V P 1944 Water metabolism and elimination by horses fasting and on normal diets *Veterinary Bulletin* 12: 26

Sabnis S G, Gunson D E, and Antonovych T T 1984 Some unusual features of mesangioproliferative glomerulonephritis in horses *Veterinary Pathology* 21: 574-581

Sack W O 1991 *Rooney's Guide to the Dissection of the Horse* Ithaca, Veterinary Textbooks

Sainsbury D W B 1981 Ventilation and environment in relation to equine respiratory disease *Equine Veterinary Journal* 13: 167-170

Salama S A 1984 Epidemiological and immunological studies on South African horsesickness and trials of production of inactivated vaccine *United States Agricultural Research Program Public Law 480, Cairo*: 205

Salinovich O, Payne S L, Montelaro R C, Hussain K A, Issel C J, Schnorr K L 1986 Rapid emergence of novel antigenic and genetic variants of equine infectious anemia virus during persistent infection *Journal of Virology* 57: 71 80

Salis-Schindler E von 1967 Bestehen Anhaltspunkte für eine erbliche Disposition zur Strahlbeinlahmheit des Pferdes Zurich, *Semesterarbeit*, ETH

Salonen A 1955 Hippologica Accadica *Annales Acadamie Science Fennicae B*, 100: 1-318

Salsbury D L 1970 Pine tar irritation in a horse *VM SAC* 65(1): 60-61

Samuelson D A, Andressen T L, Gwin R M 1984 Conjunctival fungal flora in horses, cattle, dogs, and cats *Journal of American Veterinary Medical Association* 184(10): 1240-1241

Sandersleben, J von and Schlotke B 1977 Die Muskeldystrophie (Weissmuskelkrankheit) bei Fohlen, eine offensichlich im Zunehmen begriffene Erkrankung *Deutsch Tierärztliche Wochenschrift* 84: 105-7

Sandgren B 1988 Bony fragments in the tarsocrural and metacarpo-or metatarsophalangeal joints in the standardbred horse—a radiological survey *Equine Veterinary Journal* (Suppl) 6: 66-9

Sanford J, Ewbank, R, Molony, V, Tavernor, W D, and Uvarov O 1986 Guidelines for the recognition and assessment of pain in animals *Veterinary Record* 118: 334-338

Santschi E M and Foreman J H 1989 Equine bacterial meningitis—Part I. Key facts *Compendium of Continuing Education for Veterinarians* 11: 479-483

Sartin E A and Hodge T G 1982 Congenital dermal hemangioendothelioma in two foals *Veterinary Pathology* 19: 569-571

Sarton G 1927 *Introduction to the History of Science* Vol 1 Washington, Carnegie Institution of Washington

Saunders L Z 1953 Cerebrovascular siderosis in horses *American Medical Association Archives Pathology* 56: 637-42

Saunders L Z and Rubin L F 1975 *Ophthalmic Pathology of Animals: An Atlas and Reference Book*, Basel, Karger

Saunders L Z, Bistner S I, and Rubin L F 1972 Proliferative optic neuropathy in horses *Veterinary Pathology* 9: 368-378

Saxegaard S and Svenkerud R 1974 Pasteurella haemolytica associated with pneumonia in a foal *Acta Vet Scand* 15(3): 439-441

Saxegaard F, Teige J, Fjellheim P 1971 Equine bronchopneumonia caused by Bordetella bronchiseptica: a case report *Acta Vet Scand* 12(1): 114-115

Saxer E 1974 Die serolgische Diagnose der infektiosen Anamie der Einhufer (AIE) *Schweiz Arch Tierheilk* 116: 679-692

Schalm O W 1981 Lymphosarcoma in the horse *Equine Practice* 3(2): 23-27

Schalm O W, Knight H D, and Osburn B I 1974 Idiopathic gammopathy and plasmacytosis in a horse *California Veterinarian* 28(2): 13-20

Schaper W 1939 Über die Erblikchkeit des Kehlkopfpfeifens beim Pferd *Deutsche Tierärztliche Wochenschrift* 47: 385-8

Schäper W and Weischer F 1938 Entstehung und Bekampfung des Hufkrebses im Lichte Konstitutionsforschung *Tierärztliche Rundschau* 44: 216-22

Schatzmann U and Gerber H 1972 Etiology of chronic lung disease in the horse (in German) *Zentralbl Vetmed A* 19(2): 89-101

Schatzmann U, De Weck A L, Gerber H, Lazary S, Straub, R, and Pauli B 1973 Active and passive cutaneous anaphylaxis in the horse following immunization with Benzylpeniciloyl-BovineGammaGlobulin(BPO2O-BGG) *Research Veterinary Science* 15: 347-52

Schebitz H 1968 Degenerative arthritis of the shoulder joint following asaeptic necrosis of the humeral head in foals *Proceedings Annual Conference American Association of Equine Practitioners*

Schebitz H and Harwigk H 1950 Myositis sacosporidica beim Pferde *Tierartz umsch* 5: 351-353

Schebitz H, Dämmrich K, and Waibl H 1975 Intra-artikuläre Absprengungsfrakturen im Articulus talocruralis beim Pferd *Berlin München Tierärztliche Wochenschrift* 88: 309-17

Scheunert A and Illing G 1906 Ein Beitrag zur Kenntnis der Grösse der Speichelsekretion und ihrer Abhangigheit von der physikalischen Beschaffenheit der Nahrungsmittel *Zablonski Physiologie* 19: 853-56

Scheunert A and Trautmann A 1976 Lehrbuch für Veterinär Physiologie Berlin Parey

Schifferli A 1908 Die aseptischen Beugesehneneveranderungen des Pferdes unter besonderer Berucksichtigung der histologischen Vorgange *Schweizer Archiv Tierheilkunde* 59: 1-29; 63-89

Schlotthauer C 1931 The incidence and types of disease of the thyroid gland of adult horses *Journal of the American Veterinary Medical Association* 78: 211

Schmall L M, Muir W W, and Robertson J T 1990 Haematological, serum electrolyte and blood gas effects of small volume hypertonic saline in experimentally induced haemorrhagic shock *Equine Veterinary Journal* 22: 278-283

Schmidt G M 1985 Onchocerca cervicalis in horses: dermal histopathology *Acta Trop* 42(1): 55-61

Schmidt G M, Kerhbiel J D, Coley S C, Leid R W 1982 Equine onchocerciasis: histopathologic study *American Journal of Veterinary Research* 43(8): 1371-1375

Schmidt G M, Coley S C, and Leid R W 1985 *Onchocerca cervicalis* in horses: dermal histopathology *Acta Tropica* 42: 55-61

Schmidt G R, Dueland R, and Vaughan J T 1975 Osteochondrosis dissecans of the equine shoulder joint *Veterinary Medicine Small Animal Clinician* 70: 542

Schmidt J 1937 Die Oesophaguserkrankung des Pferdes *Berliner Tierärztliche Wochenschrift* 1: 1-5

Schneider J E and Leipold H W 1978 Recessive lethal white in two foals *Journal of Equine Medicine and Surgery* 2(11): 479-482

Schneider R K, Milne D W, and Kohn C W 1982 Acquired inguinal hernia in the horse: A review of 27 cases *Journal of the American Veterinary Medical Association* 180: 317-320

Schoeb T R and Panciera R J 1979 Pathology of blister beetle poisoning in horses *Veterinary Pathology* 16: 18-31

Schofield F W 1933 Enzootic hypertrophic cirrhosis of the horse caused by the feeding of alsike clover *Annual Report, Ontario Veterinary College*

Schonbauer M and Schonbauer-Langle A 1983 Seminome beim Pferd Eine Retrospektivuntersuchung *Zentralblatte Veterinar Medizin A* 30: 189-198

Schoon H-A and Deegen E 1983 Histopathologie der chronisch obstruktiven Bronchitis bei klinisch manifest erkrankten Pferden *Tierärztliche Praxis* 11: 213-21

Schotman A J H and Wagenaar G 1969 Hyperlipemia in ponies *Zentralblatte Veterinar Medizin* 16: 1-7

Schott H C, Major M D, Grant B D, and Bayly W M 1990 Melanoma as a cause of spinal cord compression in two horses *Journal of the American Veterinary Medical Association* 196: 1820-1822

Schougaard H, Ronne J F, and Phillipson J 1990 A radiographic survey of tibiotarsal osteochondrosis in a selected population of trotting horses in Denmark and its possible genetic significance *Equine Veterinary Journal* 22: 288-90

Schroeder W G 1969 Suggestions for handling horses exposed to rabies *Journal of the American Veterinary Medical Association* 155: 1842-1843

Schulte F 1950 Idiopathische Muskularishypertrophie des Huft-und Leerdarmes sowie Divertikelbildung beim Pferd. *Monatshrift Veterinär Medicin* 5: 63-4

Schulte F 1970 Vol 5 In Dobberstein J, Pallaske G, and Stünzi H (Eds) *Joest's Handbuch der Speziellen Pathologischen Anatomie der Haustiere* 3rd Ed Berlin, Parey

Schultze A E, Sonea I, and Bell T G 1988 Primary malignant pulmonary neoplasia in two horses *Journal of the American Veterinary Medical Association* 193: 477-480

Schulz W 1914/15 Untersuchungen über die sogenannten Synovialgruben, Fossa nudatae, beim Pferd *Archiv Tierheilkunde* 41: 245-71

Schumacher J, Wilson R C, Spano J S, Hammond L S, McGuire J, Duran S H, Kemppainen R J, and Hughes F E 1991 Effect of diet on gentamicin-induced nephrotoxicosis in horses *American Journal of Veterinary Research* 52: 1274-1278

Schummer A 1949 Zirkulationsfordernde einrichtungen am Zehnenendorgan des Pferdes *Deutsche Tierärztliche Wochenschrift* 56: 36-8

Schummer A 1951 Zirkulationsfordernde einrichtungen am Zehnenendorgan des Pferdes *Gegenbauers Morph Jb* 91: 586-649

Schummer A 1953 Morphologische Untersuchungen über die Funktionszustandedes Ileums *Tierärztliche Umschau* 8: 244-47

Schurmann E 1933 Pathologische Organbefunde beim sogenannten Hoppegartner Husten *Berliner Tierärtzliche Wochenschrift* 49: 161-4

Schuster E 1941 Über deb Funktionellen Bau des Hufknorpels *Dissertation*, Hannover

Schwarte L H 1938 Moldy corn poisoning in horses *Journal of the American Veterinary Medical Association* 92: 152-158

Schwarte L H, Biester H E and Murray C 1937 A disease of horses caused by feeding moldy corn *Journal of the American Veterinary Medical Association* 90: 76-85

Schwartz L W, Knight H D, Whittig L D, Malloy R L, Abraham J L, and Tyler N K 1981 Silicate pneumoconiosis and pulmonary fibrosis in horses from the Monterey-Carmel Peninsula *Chest* 80: 82S-85S

Schwink K 1987 Factors influencing morbidity and outcome of equine ocular squamous cell carcinoma *Equine Veterinary Journal* 19: 198-200

Scott A M and Jeffcott L B 1978 Haemolytic disease of the newborn foal *Veterinary Record* 103: 71-74

Scott D W 1983 Pemphigus in domestic animals *Clinics in Dermatology* 1: 141-152

Scott D W 1985 Sterile nodular panniculitis in a horse *Equine Practice* 7: 30-35

Scott D W 1989 Lymphoid nodules in skin biopsies from dogs, cats and horses with nonneoplastic dermatoses *Cornell Veterinarian* 79: 267-272

Scott D W Veterinary dermatohistopathology: What's new and exciting

Scott D W and Manning T O 1980 Equine folliculitis and furunculosis *Equine Practice* 2: 11-32

Scott D W and White K K 1983 Demodicosis associated with systemic glucocorticoid therapy in two horses (Demodex folliculorum var. equi) *Equine Practice* 5(4): 31-35

Scott D W, Wolfe M J, Smith C A, and Lewis R M 1980 The comparative pathology of non-viral bullous skin diseases in domestic animals *Veterinary Pathology* 17: 257-281

Scott D W, Manning T O, Smith C A, and Lewis R M 1982 Pemphigus and pemphigoid in dogs, cats, and horses *Journal of the American Veterinary Medical Association* 180: 353-360

Scott E A, Duncan J R and McCormack J E 1974 Cryptococcus involving the postorbital area and frontal sinus in a horse *Journal of the American Veterinary Medical Association* 165: 626-627

Scott E A, Kneller S K, and Witherspoon D M 1975 Closure of ductus ateriosus determined by cardiac catheterization and angiography in newborn foals *American Journal of Veterinary Research* 36: 1021-1023

Scott E A, Chaffee A, Eyster G E, and Kneller S K 1978 Interruption of aortic arch in two foals *Journal of the American Veterinary Medical Association* 172: 347-50

Scott E A, McDole M, and Shires M H 1979 A review of third phalanx fractures in the horse. Sixty-four cases *Journal of the American Veterinary Medical Association* 174: 1337

Seanor J W, Byars T D, and Boutcher J K 1984 Renal disease associated with colic in horses *Modern Veterinary*

Practice: A26-A29

Seiler R J, Omar S, and Jackson A R B 1981 Meningoencephalitis in naturally occurring *Trypanosoma evansi* infection (surra) of horses *Veterinary Pathology* 18: 120-122

Sellers A F and Lowe J E 1986 Review of large intestinal motility and mechanisms of impaction in the horse *Equine Veterinary Journal* 18: 261-63

Sellers A F, Lowe, J E, and Rendano V T 1984 Equine colonic motility: Interactions among wall motion, propulsion, and fluid flow *American Journal of Veterinary Reserch* 45: 357-360

Selye H 1950 *Stress* Montreal, Acta

Sentsui H and Kono Y 1988 Studies on viral-induced anemia in horses infected with equine infectious anemia virus *Japanese Journal of Veterinary Science* 50: 303-311

Severin G A 1974 Common eye problems in the horse-examination and treatment *American Association of Equine Practice* 2: 20-23

Shad-del F, Nakata G, and Navai S 1970 Transmission of African horsesickness by means of mosquito bites and replication of the virus in *Aedes aegypti Archives Institute Razi* 22: 113

Shaw D D, Gunson D E, and Evans L 1987 Nasal amyloidosis in four horses *Veterinary Pathology* 24: 183-5

Shaw D P and Roth J E 1986 Testicular teratocarcinoma in a horse *Veterinary Pathology* 23: 327-328

Shaw J G 1966 Ear mange in horses *New Zealand Veterinary Journal* 14: 127

Sheahan B J, Atkins G J, Russell R J, and O'Connor J P 1980 Histiolymphocytic lymphosarcoma in the subcutis of two horses *Veterinary Pathology* 17: 123-133

Sherman J, Thorsen J, Barnum D A, Mitchell W R, and Ingram D G 1977 Infectious causes of equine respiratory disease on Ontario Standardbred racetracks *Journal Clinical Microbiology* 5: 285-289

Shively J N, Moe K K, and Dellers R W 1974 Fine structure of spontaneous *Pneumocytis carinii* pulmonary infection in foals *Cornell Veterinarian* 64: 72-88

Shively M A, Banks K L, Greenlee A, and Klevjer-Anderson P 1982 Antigenic stimulation of T lymphocytes in chronic nononcogenic retrovirus infection: equine infectious anemia *Infection and Immunity* 36(1): 38-46

Shull R M 1981 Biochemical changes in equine erythrocytes during experimental regenerative anemia *Cornell Veterinarian* 71: 280-287

Shupe J L 1972 Hereditary Multiple Exostosis In Catcott E J and Smithcors J E (Eds) *Equine Medicine Surgery* 2nd Ed Santa Barbara American Veterinary Publications

Shupe J L and Olson A E 1971 Clinical aspects of fluorosis in horses *Journal of the American Veterinary Medical Association* 158: 167-74

Shupe J L, Olson A E, Sharma R P, and Kampen K R van 1970 Multiple exostosis in horses *Modern Veterinary Practice* 34-6

Siedamgrotsky 1891 Einiges über Sehnenkrankungen der Pferde *Wissenshaftliche Praktike Tierheilkunde* 17: 173-209

Siedamgrotsky 1900 Vol 4 Krankheiten der Sehnen, Sehnenscheiden, und Schleimbeutel. In *Bayer-Fröhner Handbuch der tierärztlichen chirurgie und Geburtshilfe* Vienna Braumuller

Silbersiepe E, Berge E, Muller 1986 *Lehrbuch der speziellen Chirurgie* 16th Ed Stuttgart Enke

Silva-Curiel J M A da, Murphy C J, Jang S S, and Bellhorn R W 1990 Nutritionally variant streptococci associated with corneal ulcers in horses: 35 cases (1982-1988) *Journal of the American Veterinary Medical Association* 197: 626

Silver I A, Brown P N, Goodship A E, Lanyon L E, Mc-Cullagh K G 1983 A clinical and experimental study of tendon injury, healing, and treatment in the horse *Equine Veterinary Journal* (Suppl) 1: 1-43

Simmons H A, Cox J E, Edwards G B, Neal P A, and Urquhart K A 1985 Paraphimosis in seven debilitated horses *Veterinary Record* 116: 126-127

Simmons T R, Gaughan E M, Ducharme N G, Dill S G, King J S, and Anderson W I 1990 Treatment of right dorsal ulcerative colitis in a horse *Journal of the American Veterinary Medical Association* 196: 455-58

Simpson C F and Buergelt C D 1981 Congealed amniotic fluid in the alveoli of lungs of aborted foals *Equine Veterinary Journal* 13: 109-111

Simpson C F and Mayhew I G 1980 Evidence for *Sarcocytis* as the etiologic agent of equine protozoal myeloencephalitis *Journal of Protozoology* 27: 288-292

Simpson G G 1951 *Horses* New York, Oxford University Press

Simpson J G 1966 A case of chromoblastomycosis in a horse *Veterinary Medicine/Small Animal Clinician* 61: 1207-1209

Sippel W L 1942 Equine degenerative arthritis Thesis, Cornell University

Sippel W L, Cooperrider D E, Gainer, J H, Allen, R W, Mouw J E B, and Teigland M B 1962 Equine piroplasmosis in the United States *Journal of the American Veterinary Medical Association* 141: 694-698

Sippel W L, Keahey E E, and Bullard T L 1968 *Corynebacterium* infection in foals: Etiology, pathogenesis, and laboratory diagnosis *Journal of the American Veterinary Medical Association* 153: 1610-1613

Sisson S 1914 Some mechanical factors in digestion *American Veterinary Revue* 45: 408-22,513-26

Sisson S and Grossman J D 1953 *The Anatomy of Domestic Animals* 4th Ed Philadelphia, Saunders

Sjolte I P 1944 Polyneuritis equi *Maanedskrift Dyrlaeger* 56: 357-413

Skoda K 1911 Über die Bedeutung der Tubendivertikel (Luftsacke) bei den Equiden *Anatomische Hefte* 42: 503-604

Slatter D H 1981 *Fundamentals of Veterinary Ophthalmology*, Philadelphia, Saunders

Slatter D H and Huxtable C R 1983 Retinal degeneration and granulomatous optic neuritis in a horse *Equine Veterinary Journal* 2 (supplement): 98-100

Slauson D O and Cooper B J 1990 *Mechanisms of Disease* 2nd Ed Baltimore, Williams and Wilkins

Slipjer E J 1946 Over de wervelkolom van onze huisdieren *Tidjschr Diergeensk* 71: 677-687

Sloan J A 1898/99 A case of rupture of the flexor metatarsi *American Veterinary Revue* 22: 767-7

Slocombe R F and Slauson D O 1988 Invasive pulmonary aspergillosis of horses: An association with acute enteritis *Veterinary Pathology* 25: 277-281

Slocombe R F, Huntington P J, Friend S C E, Jeffcott L B, Luff A R, and Finkelstein D K 1992 Pathological aspects of Australian stringhalt *Equine Veterinary Journal* 24: 174-83

Slone D E, Humburg J M, Jagar J E, and Powers R D 1982 Noniatrogenic rectal tears in three horses *Journal of the American Veterinary Medical Association* 180: 750-751

Slone D E, Purhoit R C, and Ganjam V K 1981 Effects of dexamethasone and triamcinolone that may predispose to laminitis in horses *Proceedings of the American Association of Equine Practitioners* 27: 469-71

Smetzer D L, Smith C R, and Senta T 1969 Second-degree atrioventricular block in the horse *American Journal of Veterinary Research* 30: 933-946

Smith B P 1977 Pleuritis and pleural effusion in the horse: A study of 37 cases *Journal of the American Veterinary Medical Association* 170: 208-211

Smith B P 1979 Disease of the pleura *Veterinary Clinics North America: Large Animal Practice* 1: 197-204

Smith B P and Robinson R C 1981 Studies of an outbreak of *Corynebacterium equi* pneumonia in foals *Equine Veterinary Journal* 13: 223-228

Smith B P, Reina-Guerra M, Hardy A J, and Habasha F 1979 Equine salmonellosis: experimental production of four syndromes *American Journal of Veterinary Research* 40: 1072-77

Smith F 1886 The pathology of navicular disease *Veterinary Journal* 23: 73

Smith F 1917 *A Manual of Veterinary Physiology* 4th Ed London, Bailliere, Tindall & Cox

Smith F 1976 *The Early History of Veterinary Literature and its British Development* 4 Vols London, J A Allen

Smith H A and Frankson M C 1961 Rhinosporidiosis in a Texas horse *Southwest Veterinarian* 15: 22

Smith H M S 1978 Diagnosis and control of idiopathic thrombocytopenia in a horse *Journal of Equine Medicine and Surgery* 2: 257-267

Smith J A 1973 The occurrence of larvae of *Strongylus edentatus* in the testicles of stallions *Veterinary Record* 104: 604-606

Smith J E and Agar N S 1976 Studies on erythrocyte metabolism following acute blood loss in the horse *Equine Veterinary Journal* 8: 34-37

Smith J E and Cipriano J E 1987 Inflammation-induced changes in serum iron analytes and ceruloplasmin of Shetland ponies *Veterinary Pathology* 24: 354-356

Smith P J, Samuelson D A, and Brooks D A 1988 Aqueous drainage paths in the equine eye: scanning electron microscopy of corrosion cast *Journal Morphology* 198: 33-40

Smith R, Hunt R, Jones T, *Veterinary Pathology* 1983 Philadelphia, Lea and Febiger

Smyth G B 1979 Testicular teratoma in an equine cryptorchid *Equine Veterinary Journal* 11: 21-23

Snow D H, Douglas T A, Thompson H, Parkins J J, and Holmes P H 1981 Phenylbutazone toxicosis in equidae: A biochemical and pathophysiologic study *American Journal of Veterinary Research* 42: 1754-1759

Snyder S P, England J J, and McChesney A E 1978 Cryptosporidiosis in immunodeficient Arabian foals *Veterinary Pathology* 15: 12-17

Snyder J R, Olander H J, Pascoe J R, Holland M, and Kupershock C J 1988 Morphologic alterations observed during experimental ischemia of the equine large colon *American Journal of Veterinary Research* 49: 801-809

Snyder J R, Pascoe J R, Olander H J, Spier S J, Meagher D M, and Bleifer D R 1989a Strangulating volvulus of the ascending colon in horses *Journal of the American Veterinary Medical Association* 195: 757-64

Snyder J R, Tyler W S, Pascoe J R, Olander H J, and Bleifer D R 1989b Microvascular circulation of the ascending colon in the horse *American Journal of Veterinary Research* 50: 2075-83

Sockett D C, Traub-Dargatz J, and Weiser M G 1987 Immune-mediated hemolytic anemia and thrombocytopenia in a foal *Journal of the American Veterinary Medical Association* 190: 308-310

Sojka J E and Colahan P T 1991 In *Equine Medicine and Surgery 4th Ed* Goleta, California, American Veterinary Publications

Solleysel S de 1711 *The Compleat Horseman or Perfect Farrier* London

Solomons B 1984 Equine cutis hyperelastica *Equine Veterinary Journal* 16: 541-542

Sonnenberg E 1912 Ruckenmarkskrankungen unserer Haustiere und Vorbemerkungen hierzu *Archiv Wissenshaftliche Praktische Tierheilkunde* 39: 141-68

Sorensen D K 1972 Hemorrhagic diseases In Catcott E J and Smithcors J F (eds) *Equine Medicine and Surgery* Wheaton, Illinois, American Veterinary Publications

Soulsby E J L 1965 *Textbook of Veterinary Clinical Parasitology*, Oxford, Blackwell Scientific Publications

Soulsby E J L 1968 Helminths, arthropods and protozoa of domesticated animals In *Sixth Edition of Monnig's Veterinary Helminthology and Entomology*, London, Balliere, Tindall and Cassell

Sparks 1968, unpublished

Specht T E, Breuhaus B A, Manning T O, Miller R T, and Cochrane R B 1991 Skin pustules and nodules caused by *Actinomyces viscosus* in a horse *Journal of the American Veterinary Medical Association* 198: 457-459

Speirs V C and Wrigley R 1979 A case of bilateral hip dysplasia in a foal *Equine Veterinary Journal* 11: 202-4

Speirs V C, Veenendaal J C van, Harrison I W, Smyth G B, Anderson G A, Wilson D V, and Gilbo B 1982 Pulmonary haemorrhage in standardbred horses after racing *Australian Veterinary Journal* 59: 38-40

Spier S J 1992 In Robinson N E (Ed) *Current Therapy in Equine Medicine* Philadelphia, Saunders

Spier S J, Carlson G P, Holliday T A, Cardinet G H III, and Pickar J G 1990 Hyperkalemic periodic paralysis in horses *Journal of the American Veterinary Medical Association* 197: 1009-1016

Spier S J, Carlson G P, Harrold D, Bowling A, Byrns G, and Bernoco D 1993 Genetic study of hyperkalemic periodic paralysis in horses *Journal of the American Veterinary Medical Association* 202: 933-937

Splitter G A, Incefy G S, Dardenne M, Iwata T, McGuire T C 1979 Arabian horses with severe combined immunodeficiency-evaluation of functional thymic hormones *Developmental and Comparative Immunology* 3: 359-363

Splitter G A, Perryman L E, Magnuson N S, and McGuire T C 1980 Combined immunodeficiency of horses: a review *Developmental Comparative Immunology* 4: 21-32

Sponseller M L 1967 Equine cerebellar hypoplasia and degeneration *Proceedings American Association Equine Practitioners* 13: 123-126

Sponseller M L, Binn L N, Wooding W L, Yager R H 1965 Field strains of Western encephalitis virus in ponies: Virologic, clinical and pathologic observations *American Journal of Veterinary Research* 27: 1591-1598

Sporri H and Wittke G 1956 In *Scheunert and Trautmann Lehrbuch der Veterinär Physiologie* Berlin, Parey

Sprinkle F P, Swerczek T W, and Crowe M W 1984 Meckel's diverticulum in the horse *Journal of Equine Veterinary Science* 4: 175-76

Sprinkle F P, Swerczek T W, and Crowe M W 1985 Gastrocnemius rupture and hemorrhage in foals *Equine Practice* 7: 10-17

Sprouse R F, Garner H E, and Green E M 1987 Plasma endotoxin levels in horses subjected to carbohydrate induced laminitis *Equine Veterinary Journal* 19: 25-28

Spurlock G H and Gabel A A 1983 Apical fractures of the proximal sesamoid bones in 109 standardbred horses *Journal of the American Veterinary Medical Association* 183: 76

Stachak T S 1991 *Equine Wound Management*, Philadelphia, Lea and Febiger

Stadler P, Van de Berg S S, and Tustin R C 1987 Cervical intervertebral disk prolapse in a horse *Journal South African Veterinary Association* 59: 31-2

Staempfli H R, Townsend H G G, and Prescott J F 1991 Prognostic features and clinical presentation of acute idiopathic enterocolitis in horses *Canadian Veterinary Journal* 32: 232-237

Stanek Ch and Hantak E 1986 Bilateral atavistic polydactyly in a colt and its dam *Equine Veterinary Journal* 18: 76-9

Stanek V C, Mayr B, Graninger W, and Hofmann R 1984 Immunkomplexe im peripheren Blut bei gesunden und an Hufrehe erkrankten Pferden *Berliner Munchener Tierarztliche Wochenschrift* 97: 25-28

Stanley O and Hillidge J 1982 Alopecia associated with hypothyroidism in a horse *Equine Veterinary Journal* 14: 165-167

Stannard A A 1972 Some important dermatoses in the horse *Modern Veterinary Practice* August: 31-36

Stannard A A 1976 Equine dermatology *Proceedings American Association Equine Practitioners*

Stannard A A and Cello R M 1975 *Onchocerca cervicalis* infection in horses from the western United States *American Journal of Veterinary Research* 36: 1029-1031

Stannard A A and Pulley T 1978 Tumours of the skin and soft tissues In Moulton J E (ed) 1978 *Tumors in Domestic Animals*, Berkeley, University of California Press

Startup F G and Tatum S J 1990 Bibliography of equine ophthalmology 1818 to 1989: an update In Equine ophthalmology *Equine Veterinary Journal* (Suppl 10) September

Stashak T S 1987 *Adam's Lameness in Horses* 4th Ed Philadelphia, Lea and Febiger

Stavrou D 1967 Zur zerebrospinalen Nematodiasis der Equiden *Berliner und Meunchener tierartzliche Wochenschrift* 80: 471-474

Stecher R M 1962 Anatomical variations of the spine of the horse *Journal Mammology* 43: 205-19

Stecher R M and Goss L J 1961 *Journal of the American Veterinary Medical Association* 138: 248

Steck W 1969 Investigations on the epidemiology of equine infectious anemia In Bryans J T and Gerber H (eds) *Proceedings 2nd International Conference Equine Infectious Diseases* Basel, Karger 172-177

Steck W and Roost E 1949 Zur Pathogenese der chronischen Bronchiolitis beim Pferde *Schweizer Archiv Tierheilkunde* 91: 427-36

Steckel R R, Adams S B, Long G G, and Rebar A H 1982 Antemortem diagnosis and treatment of cryptococcal meningitis in a horse *Journal of the American Veterinary Medical Association* 180: 1085-1089

Stede M, Preuss F, and Stede G 1977 Angewandt-Anatomische Grundlagen zur Gleichbein-fraktur des Pferdes *Berlin München Tierärztliche Wochenschrift* 90: 212-15

Steenhaut M 1988 La chirurgie des coliques due cheval. Une etude retrospective *Pratique Vétérinaire Equine* 20: 59-66

Stein C D and Mott L O 1942 Studies on congenital transmission of equine infectious anemia *Veterinary Medicine* 37: 370-377

Stein C D, Lucker J T, Osteen O L, and Gochenour W S 1939 Studies on the possible role of endoparasites in the transmission of infectious anemia *Journal of the American Veterinary Medical Association* 95: 536-541

Stein C D, Osteen O L, Mott L O, and Shahan M S 1944 Action of chemical and physical agents on the virus of equine infectious anemia *American Journal of Veterinary Research* 5: 291-302

Stein C D, Mott L O, and Gates D W 1955 Some observations on carriers of equine infectious anemia *Journal of the American Veterinary Medical Association* 126: 277-287

Stenius P L 1941 Equine liver and brain disease in Finland in 1934 *Skandinavisk Veterinärtidskrift* 31: 192

Steven D H, Jeffcott L B, Mallon K A, Ricketts S W,

Rossdale P D, Samuel C A 1979 Ultrastructural studies of the equine uterus and placenta following parturition *Journal Reproduction Fertility* (Suppl) 27: 579-86

Stewart J and McCallum J W 1944 The anhydraemia of oxalate poisoning in horses *Veterinary Record* 56: 77

Stewart R H 1987 Central nervous system trauma *Veterinary Clinics of North America: Equine Practice* 3: 371-377

Stewart S 1903/04 Verminous bronchopneumonia in the ass *American Veterinary Revue* 27: 1174-77

Stick J A 1980 Teratoma and cyst formation of the equine cryptorchid testicle *Journal of the American Veterinary Medical Association* 176: 211-214

Stick J A 1981 Surgical management of genital habronemiasis in a horse *Veterinary Medicine/Small Animal Clinician* 76: 410-414

Stickle R L and Fessler J F 1978 Retrospective study of 350 cases of equine cryptorchidism *Journal of the American Veterinary Medical Association* 172: 343-346

Stiers M, Newman L, and Duncan R 1993 Personal communication

Stoker J J 1950 *Nonlinear Vibrations in Mechanical and Electrical Systems* New York, Interscience

Stone W M, Stewart T B and Parkham J C 1970 *Micronema deletrix* Anderson and Bemrick, 1965, in the central nervous system of a pony *Journal of Parasitology* 56: 986-987

Stormont C 1975 Neonatal isoerythrolysis in domestic animals: a comparative review *Advances in Veterinary Science Comparative Medicine* 19: 23-45

Stornetta D 1988 Etude comparative de la frequence d'apparition de la maladie naviculaire (podotrocholose) dans la descendance de deux etalons de la race franches-montagnes. *Dissertation*, Berne

Stoss A O 1923 Anatomie und Kinematik der Gelenke der Pferde extremitäten *Zeitschrift Anatomie Entwicklgeschicte* 69: 5-31

Strafuss A C, Smith J E, Dennis S M, and Anthony, H D 1973 Sarcoid in horses *Veterinary Medicine/Small Animal Clinician* 68: 1246-1247

Straunard R 1939 Les efforts de tendons *Annales Médecine Vétérinaire* 84: 49-67,119-30,159-79

Strömberg B 1976 Osteochondritis dissecans of the stifle joint in the horse. A clinical, radiographic, and pathologic study *Journal American Veterinary Radiology Society* 17: 117

Strömberg B 1979 A review of the salient features of osteochondrosis in the horse *Equine Veterinary Journal* 11: 211

Strömberg B and Rejno S 1976 Osteochondrosis in the horse *Acta Radiologica* 1-15

Stuart B P, Martin B R, Williams L P, and Von Byern H 1973 Salmonella-induced meningoencephalitis in a foal *Journal of the American Veterinary Medical Association* 162: 211-213

Studdert M J 1978 Primary, severe, combined immunodeficiency disease of Arabian foals *Australian Veterinary Journal* 54: 411-417

Stunzi H and Pohlenz J 1974 Zur Pathologie den Neuritis caudae equinae beim Pferd *Schweizer Archiv Tierheilkunde* 116: 533-41

Sugawa Y 1953 Histo-pathological studies on the horses artificially infected with the virus of Japanese B encephalitis *Norin Suisansho Kachiku Eisei Shikenjo kenkyu hokoku* 27: 1-16

Sundberg J P, Burnstein T, Page E H, Kirkham W W, and Robinson F R 1977 Neoplasms of equidae *Journal of the American Veterinary Medical Association* 170: 150-152

Supperer R 1953 Filariosen der Pferde in Österreich *Wiener Tierärztliche Monatschrift* 40: 194-220

Sutherland R J, Cambridge H, and Bolton J R 1989 Functional and morphological studies on blood platelets in a thrombasthenic horse *Australian Veterinary Journal* 66: 366-370

Svalastoga E, Reimann I, and Nielson K 1983 Changes of the fibrocartilage in navicular disease *Nordiska Veterinärmedicin* 35: 372-78

Svenkerud R R 1948 Listerellainfeksjoner, spesielt med henblikk pa deres forekomst hos hesten *Norsk Veterinaer-Tiddsskrift* 9: 321-340

Svinhufvud A Ch 1978 *A Late Middle English Treatise on Horses* Stockholm, Acta Universitatis Stockholmiensis XLVII

Swanstrom O G, Rising J L, and Carlton W W 1969 Spinal Nematodosis in a horse *Journal of the American Veterinary Medical Association* 155: 748-753

Sweeney C R 1988 Bacterial infections of the equine lung *Proceedings American College Veterinary Internal Medicine* 6: 31-32

Sweeney C R and Beech J 1983 Retrobulbar melanoma in a horse *Equine Veterinary Journal* 2 (supplement): 117-122

Sweeney C R, Divers T J, and Benson C E 1985 Anaerobic bacteria in 21 horses with pleuropneumonia *Journal of the American Veterinary Medical Association* 187: 721-724

Sweeney C R, Whitlock R H, Meirs D A, Whitehead S C, and Barningham S O 1987 Complications associated with *Streptococcus equi* infection on a horse farm *Journal of the American Veterinary Medical Association* 191: 1446-1448

Sweeney C R, Soma L R, Maxson A D, Thompson J, and Holcombe S J 1990 Effects of furosemide on the racing times of Thoroughbreds *American Journal of Veterinary Research* 51: 772-78

Sweeney C R, Holcombe S J, Barningham S C, and Beech J 1991 Aerobic and anaerobic bacterial isolates from horses with pneumonia or pleuropneumonia and antimicrobial susceptibility patterns of the aerobes *Journal of the American Veterinary Medical Association* 198: 839-842

Sweeney R W, Saik J, and Lichtensteiger C 1986 Chronic granulomatous bowel disease in three sibling horses *Journal of the American Veterinary Medical Association* 188: 1192-94

Sweeney R W, MacDonald M, Hall J, Divers T J, Sweeney C R 1988 Kinetics of gentamicin elimination in two horses with acute renal failure *Equine Veterinarian* 20:

182-184

Swerczek T W 1977 Multifocal hepatic necrosis and hepatitis in foals caused by *Bacillius piliformis* (Tyzzer's disease) *Veterinary Annual* 17: 130-32

Swerczek T W 1980 Toxicoinfectious botulism in foals and adult horses *Journal of the American Veterinary Medical Association* 176: 217-220

Swerczek T W and Crowe M W 1983 Hepatotoxicosis in neonatal foals (letter) *Journal of the American Veterinary Medical Association* 183: 388

Swerczek T W, Crowe M W, Prickett M E, and Bryans J T 1973 Focal bacterial hepatitis in foals *Modern Veterinary Practice* 54: 66-7

Szakall J 1899 Beiträge zur Anatomie und Funktion des oberes Gleichbeinbandes beim Pferde *Zeitschrift Tiermedicin* 3: 334-38

Szeleky G 1930 Ligamentum intersesamoideum des Pferdes *Dissertation*, Budapest

Tadmor A, Fischel R, and Shem Tov A 1983 A condition resembling hypoplastic left heart syndrome in a foal *Equine Veterinary Journal* 15: 175-177

Taira T, Fujinaga T, Okumura M, Yamashita K, Tsunoda N, Mizuno S 1992a Equine haptoglobin: isolation, characterization, and the effects of ageing, delivery and inflammation on its serum concentration *Journal of Veterinary Medical Science* 54: 435-442

Taira T, Fujinaga T, Tamura K, Izumi M, Itoh H, Tsunoda N, Yamashita K, Okumura M, and Mizuno S 1992b Isolation and characterization of $alpha_1$-acid glycoprotein from horses, and its evaluation as an acute-phase reactive protein in horses *American Journal of Veterinary Research* 53: 961-965;

Tajima M 1953 Neuro-histopathological studies on epidemic equine encephalomyelitis (Japanese equine encephalitis) *Veterinary Research Japan* 1: 64

Takatori K 1981 Fungal flora of equine skin with and without dermatophytosis *Nippon Juishikai Zasshi* 34: 580-584

Tasker J B 1967 Fluid and electrolyte studies in the horse. III. Intake and output of water, sodium and potassium in normal horses. IV. The effects of fasting and thirsting. V. The effects of diarrhea *Cornell Veterinarian* 57: 649-667

Tasker J B, Whiteman C E, and Martin B R 1966 *Journal of the American Veterinary Medical Association* 149: 393-99

Tasler G R W and Hartley W J 1981 Foal abortion associated with *Mycobacterium terrae* infection *Veterinary Pathology* 18: 122-25

Taylor F G R 1990 Clinicopathologic diagnosis in the adult horse *Veterinary Annual* 30: 155-61

Taylor H W, Vandevelde M, and Firth E C 1977 Ischemic myelopathy caused by fibrocartilaginous emboli in a horse *Veterinary Pathology* 14: 479

Taylor W M, Bryant J E, Anderson J B, and Willers K H 1969 Equine piroplasmosis in the United States- a review *Journal of the American Veterinary Medical Association* 155: 915-919

Teeter S 1969 Experimental production of laminitis *Personal communication*

Tennant B, Dill S G, Glickman L T, Mirro E J, King J M 1981 Acute hemolytic anemia, methemoglobinemia, and Heinz body formation associated with ingestion of red maple leaves by horses *Journal of the American Veterinary Medical Association* 179: 143-50

Tennant B, Bettleheim P, and Kaneko J J 1982 Paradoxic hypercalcemia and hypophosphatemia associated with chronic renal failure in horses *Journal of the American Veterinary Medical Association* 180: 630-634

Tennant B D, Wheat J D, and Meagher D M 1972 *Proceedings Annual Conference American Association Equine Practitioners*

Tenter A M and Friedhoff K T 1986 Serodiagnosis of experimental and natural *Babesia equi* and *B. caballi* infections *Veterinary Parasitology* 20: 49-61

Theilen G H and Fowler M E 1962 Lymphosarcoma (lymphocytic leukemia) in the horse *Journal of the American Veterinary Medical Association* 140: 923-930

Theiler A 1919 Acute liver atrophy and parenchymatous hepatitis in horses *Report Director Veterinary Research* South Africa

Thein P 1981 Infection of the central nervous system of horses with equine herpesvirus serotype 1 *Journal South African Veterinary Association* 52: 239-241

Thein P and Mayr A 1974 Untersuchungen über die Bedeutung von Reovirus-Infektion für respiatorische Erkrankungen beim Pferd *Zablonski Veterinärmedicin B* 21: 219-233

Thein P and Bohm D 1976 Atiologie und Klink einer virusbedingten Keratokonjunktivitis beim Fohlen *Zentralblatte Veterinarmedizin* 23 B: 507-519

Thein P and Hartl G 1976 Isolierun eines Reovirus aus einem respiratorisch erkrankten Pferd *Zablonski Veterinarmedicin B* 23: 698-701

Thesing B 1950 Beitrag zur Aetiologie und Therapie des Stelzfusses beim Pferd *Tierärztliche Umschau* 5: 322-4

Thieke A 1911 Die Hippomanes des Pferdes *Anatomischer Anzeiger* 38: 454-86

Thompson D B, Studdert M J, Beilharz R G, and Littlejohns I R 1975 Inheritance of a lethal immunodeficiency disease of Arabian foals *Australian Veterinary Journal* 51(3): 109-113

Thompson J M T and Stewart H B 1986 *Nonlinear Dynamics and Chaos* New York, John Wiley

Thompson K N 1986 The influence of high planes of nutrition upon skeletal development in the growing equine *Dissertation* Lexington, University of Kentucky

Thompson K N 1989 Calcium deficiency and condylar fractures of the cannon bone *Personal communication*

Thompson K N and Rooney J R 1992 The dynamics of the standing horse *Unpublished observations*

Thompson K N, Rooney J R, and Petrites-Murphy M B 1991 Considerations on the pathogenesis of navicular disease *Journal of Equine Veterinary Science* 11: 4-8

Thompson K N, Cheung T, and Rooney J R 1992 Soft-spring behaviour of equine extensor tendon Unpublished observations

Thomsett L R 1984 Noninfectious skin diseases of horses *Veterinary Clinics of North America: Large Animal Practice* 6: 59-78

Thomson G R, Mumford J A, Campbell J, Griffiths L, and Clapham P 1976 Serological detection of equid herpesvirus 1 infections of the respiratory tract *Equine Veterinary Journal* 8: 58-65

Thomson G W, McCready R, Sanford E and Gagnon A 1979 Case report: An outbreak of herpesvirus myeloencephalitis in vaccinated horses *Canadian Veterinary Journal* 20: 22-25

Thomson J R, McPherson E A, Lawson G H K, Wooding P, and Brown R 1983 A study on the possible role of chymotrypsin in the aetiology of equine chronic obstructive pulmonary disease (COPD) *Veterinary Immunology Immunopathology* 4: 387-395

Thorp F Jr and Graham R 1932 An urticaria-like syndrome accompanied by multiple eosinophilic granulomas of the skin *North American Veterinarian* 13: 19-22

Threlfall W R, Carleton C L, Robertson J, Rosol T, and Gabel A 1990 Recurrent torsion of the spermatic cord and scrotal testis in a stallion *Journal of the American Veterinary Medical Association* 196: 1641-1643

Thurman J D, Johnson B J, and Lichtenfels J R 1984 Dirofilariasis with arteriosclerosis in a horse *Journal of the American Veterinary Medical Association* 185: 532-533

Timoney P J 1971 Adenovirus precipitating antibodies in the sera of some domestic animal species in Ireland *British Veterinary Journal* 127: 567-571

Timoney J F and Eggers D 1985 Serum bactericidal responses to *Streptococcus equi* of horses following infection or vaccination *Equine Veterinary Journal* 17: 306-310

Timoney J F, Donnelly W C, Clements C, and Fenlon M 1974 Letter: Louping ill infection in the horse *Veterinary Record* 95(23): 540

Timoney P J, Donnelly W J C, Clements L O, and Fenlon M 1976 Encephalitis caused by louping ill virus in a group of horses in Ireland *Equine Veterinary Journal* 8: 113-117

Timoney P J, McArdle J F and Byrne M J 1983 Abortion and meningitis in a Thoroughbred mare associated with *Klebsiella pneumoniae*, type 1 Equine Veterinary Journal 15: 64-65

Timoney P J, McCollum W H, Murphy T W, and Roberts A W 1987a The carrier state in equine arteritis virus infection in the stallion with special emphasis on the venereal mode of virus transmission *Journal Reproduction Fertility* (Suppl) 35: 95-102

Timoney P J, McCollum W H, and Roberts A W, McDonald M J 1987b Status of equine viral arteritis in Kentucky for 1986 *Vet Rec* 120(12): 282

Timoney P J, McCollum W H, Roberts A W, and McDonald M J 1987c Status of equine viral arteritis in Kentucky, 1985 *Journal of the American Veterinary Medical Association* 191: 36-39

Torres C M, De Salles J F, and Jansen G 1944 Neurite no mal de cadersas *Rev Brasil Biol* 4: 319-322

Tóth J 1989 Ein Beitrag zu den Insertionsdesmopathien des Strahlbeins *Pferdeheilkunde* 5: 111-14

Townsend H G G, Leach D H, Doige C E, Kirkaldy J and Willis W H 1986 Relationship between spinal biomechanics and pathologic changes in the equine thoracolumbar spine *Equine Veterinary Journal* 18: 107-12

Traub J L, Rantanen N, Reed S, and Schecter L 1982 Cholelithiasis in four horses *Journal of the American Veterinary Medical Association* 181: 59-62

Traub-Dagartz J L 1991 Bacterial pneumonia *Veterinary Clinics North America: Equine Practice* 7: 53-61

Traub-Dargatz J L, Salman M D, and Voss J L 1991 Medical problems of adult horses, as ranked by equine practitioners *Journal of the American Veterinary Medical Association* 198: 1745-1747

Trautmann A 1924 Beitrage zur pathologischen Anatomie der Innersekretorishen Organe der Haustiere *Zeitschrift Infektionskrankheiten Haustiere* 27: 20-9

Trautmann A, Fiebiger J 1952 Habel R E and Biberstein E L (Eds) *Histology of the Domestic Animals* Ithaca, Comstock Publishing

Traver D S, Moore J N, Thornburg L P, Johnson J H and Coffman J R 1977 Epidural melanoma causing posterior paresis in a horse *Journal of the American Veterinary Medical Association* 170: 1400-1403

Trenfeld K, Spradbrow P B, and Vanselow B 1985 Sequences of papillomavirus DNA in equine sarcoids *Equine Veterinary Journal* 17(6): 449-452

Trigo F J, Miller R A, and Torbeck R L 1984 Metastatic equine seminoma: report of two cases *Veterinary Pathology* 21: 259-260

Trommershausen-Smith A 1980 Aspects of genetics and disease in the horse *Journal Animal Science* 51: 1087-95

Trommershausen-Smith A, Stormont C, and Suzuki Y 1975 Allo antibodies: their role in equine neonatal isoerythrolysis *Proceedings International Symposium on Equine Hematology* 349-355

Trotter G W, McIlwraith C W, Norrdin R W, and Turner A S 1982 Degenerative joint disease with osteochondrosis of the proximal interphalangeal joint in young horses *Journal of the American Veterinary Medical Association* 180: 1312-18

Trotter G W, Miller D, Parks A, and Arden W 1986 Type II renal tubular acidosis in a mare *Journal of the American Veterinary Medical Association* 188: 1050-1051

Trout D R, Hornof W J, Linford R L, O'Brien T R 1990 Scintigraphic evaluation of digital circulation during the developmental and acute phases of equine laminitis *Equine Veterinary Journal* 22: 416-421

Trueta J and Trias A 1961 The vascular contribution to osteogenesis. IV. The effect of pressure upon the epiphyseal cartilage of the rabbit *Journal Bone Joint Surgery* 43B: 800

Tulamo R M, Bramlage L R, and Gabel A A 1983 Fractures of the central and third tarsal bones in the horse *Journal of the American Veterinary Medical Association* 82: 1234

Tulleners E P, Harrison I W, and Raker C W 1988 Management of arytenoid chondropathy and failed laryngoplasty in horses: 75 cases (1979-85). *Journal of the American Veterinary Medical Association* 192: 670-75

Tumova B 1980 Equine influenza—a segment in influenza virus ecology *Comparative Immunology Microbiology Infectious Disease* 3: 45-59

Turk J R, Brown C M, and Johnson G C 1981 Diffuse alveolar damage with fibrosing alveolitis in a horse *Veterinary Pathology* 18: 560-561

Turner A S 1982 In Mansmann R A and McAllister G S (Eds) *Equine Medicine and Surgery* 3rd Ed Wheaton, American Veterinary Publications

Turrentine M A, Sculley P W, Green E M, and Johnson G S 1986 Prekallikrein deficiency in a family of miniature horses *American Journal of Veterinary Research* 47: 2464-2467

Turtinen L W 1983 Studies on the antigenic and genetic variations between the two subtypes of equine herpesvirus-1 *Dissertation, University of Kentucky*

Uberreiter O 1937 Zungengrundzysten bim Pferde *Berliner Tierärztliche Wochenschrift* 28: 434-36

Uberreiter O 1968 Zungengrundzysten aussgehend von Resten des Ductus thyroglossus beim Pferd *Wiener Tierärztliche Monatschrift* 55: 175-77

Ubertini T R and King J M 1972 A case of pneumonia in a foal morphologically similar to bovine proliferative pneumonia (atypical interstitial pneumonia) *Cornell Veterinarian* 62: 532-539

Ueda Y 1990 Aniridia in a Thoroughbred horse *Equine Veterinary Journal* 10 (supplement): 29

Ueno H and Ishihara T 1957 Studies on the summer mange ("Kasen" disease) of the horse in Japan. II. Histopathological findings on the affected skin. III. Skin sensitivity tests with insect allergens. *Bulletin of the National Institute of Animal Health* 32: 200-231

Ugorski L, Kaminski J, and Strojna S 1959 Pryspadek listeriozy u koni *Medycyna weterynaryjna* 15: 153-156

Uhlinger C 1991a Investigations into the incidence of field colic *4th Equine Colic Research Symposium* Athens, Georgia

Uhlinger C 1991b Clinical and epidemiologic features of an epizootic of equine leukoencephalomalacia *Journal of the American Veterinary Medical Association* 198: 126-128

U S Communicable Diseases Center Bulletin, 1983 Atlanta

Updike S J 1984 Functional anatomy of the equine tarsocrural ligaments *American Journal of Veterinary Research* 5: 867-74

Uphoff C S and Lyncoln J A 1987 A primary pulmonary tumor in a horse *Equine Practice* 9: 19-20

Uppal P K, Yadav M P, Singh B K, and Prasad S 1989 Equine coital exanthema (EHV-3 virus) infection in India *Journal of Veterinary Medicine B* 36: 786-788

Usry J L 1989 Simulating digesta movement through the gastrointestinal tract of the growing pig *Dissertation* Lexington, University of Kentucky

Vaala W E, Clark E S, and Orsini J A 1988 Omphalophlebitis and osteomyelitis associated with *Klebsiella* septicemia in a premature foal *Journal of the American Veterinary Medical Association* 193: 1273-1277

Valentine B and Cooper B 1993, Personal communication

Valentine B A and Weinstock D 1986 Metastatic testicular embryonal carcinoma in a horse *Veterinary Pathology* 23: 92-96

Valladares J F Equine biliary fever in Madras: 88-94

Valpotic I, Kastelan M, Rudolf M, Gerencer M, Jukic B, Basic I 1989 T and B lymphocytes in horses persistently infected with equine infectious anaemia virus *Veterinary Research Communications* 57-65

Van Amstel S R, Ross M, and Van Den Bergh S S 1984 Maduromycosis (*Madurella mycetomatis*) in a horse *Journal South African Veterinary Association* 55: 81-83

Van Andel A C J, Gruys E, Kroneman J, and Veerkamp J 1988 Amyloid in the horse: a report of nine cases *Equine Veterinary Journal* 20: 277-85

Vandeplassche M, Simoens P, Bouters R, De Vos N, and Verschooten F 1984 Aetiology and pathogenesis of congenital torticollis and head scoliosis in the equine foetus *Equine Veterinary Journal* 16: 419-424

Van Der Linde-Sipman J S, Goedege Boore S A, and Kroneman J 1979 Interventricular septal defect in a horse *Veterinary Quarterly* 1: 189

Van Der Linde-Sipman J S, Kroneman J, Meulenaar H, Vos J H 1985 Necrosis and rupture of the aorta and pulmonary trunk in four horses *Veterinary Pathology* 22: 51-53

Van der Luer R J T and Kroneman J 1982a Biliary atresia in a foal *Equine Veterinary Journal* 14: 91-3

Van der Luer R J T and Kroneman J 1982b Three cases of cholelithiasis and biliary fibrosis in the horse *Equine Veterinary Journal* 14: 251-52

Van der Molen E J 1979 Een onderzoek naar de bacteriele oorzaken van de neonatale motaliteit bij het veulen (Studies on the bacterial causes of neonatal mortality in foals. Report on post-mortem findings) *Tijdschrift Diergeneeskunde* 104: 165-177 (Dutch)

Van Kampen K R 1970 Sudan grass and sorghum poisoning of horses: A possible lathyrogenic disease *Journal of the American Veterinary Medical Association* 156: 629-630

Van Mol K A C and Fransen J L A 1986 Renal carcinoma in a horse *Veterinary Record* 119: 238-239

Van Nie C J 1968 Anomalous origin of the coronary arteries in animals *Veterinary Pathology* 5: 313-26

Van Niekerk C H and Gerneke W H 1966 Persistence and parthenogenetic cleavage of tubal ova in the mare *Onderstepoort Journal of Veterinary Research* 31: 195-232

Van Rensburg I B J, Stadler P, and Soley J 1989 Bronchiolo-alveolar adenocarcinoma in a horse *Journal South African Veterinary Association* 60: 212-214

Vanselow B A, Abetz I, and Jackson A R B 1988 BCG emulsion immunotherapy of equine sarcoid *Equine Veterinary Journal* 20: 444-447

Van Veenendaal J C and Moffat R E 1980 Soft tissue masses in the fetlock joint of horses *Australian Veterinary Journal* 56: 533

Vaughn L C 1961 Fractures of the navicular bone *Veterinary Record* 73: 95

Velling A J 1926 Luxation des Kreuz-Darmbeingelenkes beim Pferde *Monadskrift Dyrlaeger* 38: 49-70

Verhaar W M 1965 Operatieve fractuurbehandeling bij grote huisdieren *Dissertation* Utrecht

Verney F A 1911 Dunsickness *Journal of Comparative Pathology Therapeutics* 24: 226-29

Verschooten F 1989 Radiographic measurements from the lateromedial projection of the equine foot with navicular disease. *Research Veterinary Science* 46: 15-21

Verschooten F and Picavet T-M 1988 Desmitis of the fetlock annular ligament of the horse *Veterinary Annual* 28: 198-201

Vestre W A, Turner T A, and Carlton W W 1982 Proliferative optic neuropathy in a horse *Journal of the American Veterinary Medical Association* 181: 490-491

Vethy A 1901/02 *Filaria papilosa* in the anterior chamber of the eye *American Veterinary Revue* 25: 680

Vetterling J M and Thompson D E 1972 *Klosiella equi* Baumann, 1946 (Sporozoa: Eucoccidia: Adeleina) from equids *Journal Parasitology* 58: 589-594

Viidik A 1966 Biomechanics and functional adaptation of tendons and joint ligaments In Evans F G (Ed) *Studies on the Anatomy and Function of Bones and Joints* Berlin, Springer-Verlag

Virchow H 1916 Der Senkrucken des Pferdes *Berliner Kliniker Wochenschrift* 53: 888-90

Vitums A and Bayly W M 1982 Pulmonary atresia with dextroposition of the aorta and ventricular septal defect in three Arabian foals *Veterinary Pathology* 19: 160-168

Vogelsang E G and Narvaez P 1956 Notas de la practica. *Setaria equina* (Abilgaard, 1789) en las meningeas de un equino *Revista de medicina veterinaria y parasitologia* 15: 61-62

Vogt 1906 Sattelzwang *Deutscher Tierärztliche Wochenschrift* 14: 557-8

Volckart W and Loeffler K 1971 Atrioventikulare Herzblockbildungen be einem Pferde mit Lymphosarkomen in der Milz *Deutsche Tierärztliche Wochenschrift* 78(16): 446-449

Volkmann 1936 Die Ursachen der Verknocherung der Hufknorpel *Tierärztliche Rundschau* 380-84

Vonderfecht S L, Bowling A T, and Cohen M 1983 Congenital intestinal aganglionosis in white foals *Veterinary Pathology* 20: 65-70

Vos J H, Gaag I, van der Dijk J E, and Wouda W 1986 Lobular capillary haemangiomas in young horses *Journal of Comparative Pathology* 96: 637-44

Voss J L 1969 Transmission of equine sarcoid *American Journal of Veterinary Research* 30: 183

Voss J L and Pickett B W 1975 Diagnosis and treatment of haemospermia in the stallion *Journal Reproduction Fertility, Suppl* 23: 151-154

Vrins A and Feldman B F 1893 Lupus erythematosus-like syndrome in a horse *Equine Practice* 5(6): 18-25

Wada R, Imagawa H, Kamoda M, Fukunaga Y, and Kumanomido T 1984 Pathological studies on foals experimentally infected with equine rotavirus *Bulletin Equine Research Institute* 21: 72-80

Wahl A M 1963 *Mechanical Springs* New York, McGraw-Hill

Walde I 1983a Some observations on congenital cataracts in the horse *Equine Veterinary Journal* 2 (supplement): 27-28

Walde I 1983b Band opacities *Equine Veterinary Journal* 2 (supplement): 32

Waldvogel A, Wild P, and Wegmann C 1983 Membrano-proliferative glomerulonephritis in a horse *Veterinary Pathology* 20: 500-503

Walker D 1975 Defining the equine sarcoid *Veterinary Record* 96: 494

Walter P 1958 Die vegetative-nervose Peripherie und ihre Darstellunsmöglichkeit nach untersuchungen an Materiel von Haustieren *Zentralblatt Veterinärmedicin* 5: 692-741

Walthall J C and McKenzie 1976 Osteodystrophia fibrosa in horses at pasture in Queensland *Australian Veterinary Journal* 52: 11-16

Walton T E and Johnson K M 1972 Epizootiology of Venezuelan equine encephalomyelitis in the Americas *Journal of the American Veterinary Medical Association* 161: 1509-1515

Walton T E, Alvarez O Jr, Buckwalter R M and Johnson K M 1973 Experimental infection of horses with enzootic and epizootic strains of Venezuelan equine encephalomyelitis virus *Journal of Infectious Diseases* 128: 271-282

Wang Y J, Gu P W, and Liu P S 1982 Japanese B encephalitis virus infection of horses during the first epidemic season following entry into an infected area *Chain Medical Journal of England* 95(1): 63-66

Warner A E and Mayhew I G 1982 Equine anhidrosis: a survey of affected horses in Florida *Journal of the American Veterinary Medical Association* 180: 627-29

Warner A and Mayhew I G 1983 Equine anhidrosis: A review of pathophysiologic mechanisms *Veterinary Research Communications* 6: 249-264

Watson E D, Mair T S, and Sweeney C R 1990 Immunoreactive prostaglandin production by equine monocytes and alveolar macrophages and concentrations of PGE2 and PGF in bronchoalveolar lavage fluid *Research Veterinary Science* 49: 88-91

Watson T D G, Burns L, Love S, Packard C J, and Shepherd J 1992a Plasma lipids, lipoproteins and post-heparin lipases in ponies with hyperlipaemia *Equine Veterinary Journal* 24: 341-346

Watson T D G, Murphy D, and Love S 1992b Equine hyperlipaemia in the United Kingdom: clinical features and blood biochemistry of 18 cases *Veterinary Record* 131: 48-51

Watters J W, Lebel J L, and Park R D 1978 Morphometric analysis of radiographic changes in the distal phalanges of quarterhorse with lower leg lameness *American Journal of Veterinary Radiology Society* 19: 60-4

Weaver A D 1969 Fracture of the equine pedal bone *Equine Veterinary Journal* 1: 283-86

Webb J 1882 Abscess in the pelvic cavity *Veterinary Journal* 13: 205-6

Webbon P M 1973 Equine tendon stress injuries *Equine Veterinary Journal* 5: 58

Webbon P M 1978a A postmortem study of equine digital flexor tendons *Equine Veterinary Journal* 9: 61-7

Webbon P M 1978b A histological study of macroscopically normal equine digital flexor tendons *Equine Veterinary Journal* 10: 253-59

Webster R G and Yuanji G 1991 New influenza virus in horses *Nature* 351: 527

Webster's Third New International Dictionary 1964 Springfield, Massachusetts, Merriam

Weinmann J P and Sicher H 1955 *Bone and Bones* 2nd Ed Saint Louis, Mosby

Weirup M 1977 Equine intestinal clostridiosis *Acta Veterinaria Scandinavia* (Suppl) 62: 1-182

Weirup M 1983 Intestinal clostridiosis *Current Therapy Equine Practice*. Philadelphia, Saunders

Welch R D, Watkins J P, Taylor T S, Cohen N D, and Carter G K 1992 Disseminated intravascular coagulation associated with colic in 23 horses (1984-1989) *Journal of Veterinary Internal Medicine* 6: 29-35

Weldon A D, Zhang C, Antczak D F, and Rebhun W C 1992 Selective IgM deficiency and abnormal B-cell response in a foal *Journal of the American Veterinary Medical Association* 201: 1396-1398

Wensing T H, Schotman A J H, and Kroneman J 1973 Various new clinical chemical data in the blood of normal ponies and ponies affected with hyperlipaemia (hyperlipoproteinaemia) *Tijdschrift Diergeneesk* 98: 673-680

Wentink C H 1978 Biomechanics of the hind limb of the horse and the dog *Dissertation*, Utrecht

Werner L L, Gross T L, and Hillidge C J 1984 Acute necrotizing vasculitis and thrombocytopenia in a horse *Journal of the American Veterinary Medical Association* 185: 87-90

West H J, Kelly D F, and Ritchie H E 1987 Renal carcinomatosis in a horse *Equine Veterinary Journal* 19: 548-551

Westhues M 1937 Über das Wesen und die Behandlung des Hufkrebses *Berliner Tierärztliche Wochenschrift* 28: 436-40

Westhues M 1938 Über das Wesen, die Diagnostik, und die Therapie der Podotrochlitis chronica des Pferds *Berliner Münchener Tierärztliche Wochenschrift* 51: 781,791

Wetzel R and Enigk K 1938 Zur Biologie von Dictyocaulus arnfeldi, dem Lungenwurm der Einhufer *Arch Wiss Prakt Teirheilk* 73: 91-114

Wetzel R and Kersten W 1956 Die Leberphase der Entwicklung von *Strongylus edentatus* *Wiener Tierärztliche Monatschrift* 43: 664-73

Weyers H 1954 Uber das erste Auftreten der Oldenberger Fohlenataxie in Hessen *Tierärztliche Umschau* 9: 283-284

Wheat J D 1962 New aspects on the pathology of tendon injury *Proceedings Annual Conference American Association Equine Practitioners*

Wheeler C A and Collier L L 1990 Bilateral colobomas involving the optic discs in a Quarterhorse *Equine Veterinary Journal* 10 (supplement): 39-41

Whitcomb R W, Schneyer A L, Roser J F, and Hughes J P 1991 Circulating antagonist of luteinizing hormone in association with infertility in stallions *Endocrinology* 128: 2497-2502

White L Jr 1978 *Medieval Religion and Technology* Berkeley, University California Press

White N A 1981 Intestinal infarction associated with mesenteric vascular thrombotic disease in the horse *Journal of the American Veterinary Medical Association* 178: 259-262

White N A 1987 Epizootology, risk factors, and prognostic factors in colic *Current Therapy Equine Medicine* Philadelphia, Saunders

White N A, Moore J N, and Douglas M 1983 SEM study of *Strongylus vulgaris* larva-induced arteritis in the pony *Equine Veterinary Journal* 15: 349-353

White N A, Cowgill L M, and Brown J 1986 Epizootology and risk factors in equine colic at university hospitals *Newsletter #1 American Association Equine Practitioners*

White N A, Tyler D E, Blackwell R B, and Allen D 1987 Hemorrhagic fibrinonecrotic duodenitis-proximal jejunitis in horses: 20 cases (1977-1984) *Journal of the American Veterinary Medical Association* 190: 311-15

White N A, Lessard P, Tinker M K, Thatcher C D, Pelzer K D, Davis B 1991 Colic risk assessment: initial report on a prospective study *4th Equine Colic Research Symposium* Athens, Georgia

White R A S, Gerring E L, Jackson P G G, and Noakes D E 1984 Persistent vaginal haemorrhage in five mares caused by varicose veins of the vaginal wall *Veterinary Record* 115: 263-264

White S 1991 Chronic active hepatitis *Equine Veterinary Data* 12: 147-48

Whitley R D and Gelatt K N 1981 Ocular manifestations of systemic disease. Part II. Horse In Gelatt K N (ed) *Textbook of Veterinary Ophthalmology*, Philadelphia, Lea and Febiger

Whitley R D and Moore C P 1984 Microbiology of the equine eye in health and disease *Veterinary Clinics North America: Large Animal Practice* 6: 451-466

Whitley R D, Burgess E C, and Moore C P 1983 Microbial isolates of the normal equine eye *Equine Veterinary Journal* 2 (supplement): 138-140

Whitley R D, McLaughlin S A, Gilger B C, Lindley D M 1991 The treatment of keratoconjunctivitis sicca *Veterinary Medicine* 86(11): 1076-1093

Whitwell K E 1976 Four cases of Tyzzer's disease in foals in England *Equine Veterinary Journal* 8: 118

Whitwell K E 1988 In Powell D E (Ed) *Equine Infectious Diseases V* Lexington, Kentucky Universities Press

Whitwell K E and Jeffcott L B 1975 Morphological studies on the foetal membranes of the normal singleton foal at term *Research Veterinary Science* 19: 44-55

Whitwell K E, Harris P, and Farrington P G 1988 Atypical myoglobinuria: an acute myopathy in grazing horses *Equine Veterinary Journal* 20: 357-63

Wilcke J R, Crissman M V, and Pleasant R S 1993 Investigation into the role of microvascular endothelium in the pathogenesis of laminitis *Personal communication*

Wilkie B N 1982 Respiratory tract immune response to microbial pathogens *Journal of the American Veterinary Medical Association* 181: 1074-1079

Wilkie J S N, Yager J A, Nation P N, Clark E G, Townsend H G G, and Baird J D 1985 Chronic eosinophilic dermatitis: A manifestation of a multisystemic, eosinophilic, epitheliotropic disease in five horses *Veterinary Pathology* 22: 297-305

Wilkinson J E, Smith C A, Castleman W L, and Lewis R M 1985 Fibrillary deposits in glomerulonephritis in a horse *Veterinary Pathology* 22: 647-649

Williams I F, Heaton A, and McCullugh K G 1980 Cell morphology and collagen types of equine tendon scar *Research Veterinary Science* 28: 302-310

Williams I F, Heaton A, and McCullagh K G 1982 Connective tissue composition of the equine sarcoid *Equine Veterinary Journal* 14: 305-10

Williams R D 1973 Equine uveitis: a model for the study of immunologically mediated tissue injury (Dissertation) *Dissertation Abstracts International* 33 B: 4578-4579

Williams R D, Morter R C, Freeman M J, Lavignette AM 1971 Experimental chronic uveitis ophthalmic signs following equine leptospirosis *Investigative Ophthalmology* 12: 948-953

Williams W L 1891/92 A clinical study of odontomas *American Veterinary Revue* 15: 1-17,64-74

Williams W L 1897/98 Extreme luxation of the patellae in a foal *American Veterinary Revue* 21: 444-52

Williams W L 1899/90 Notes on odontomes *American Veterinary Revue* 23: 82-94

Williams W L 1905/6 Rupture of the prepubian tendon in the pregnant mare *American Veterinary Revue* 29: 360-9

Williams W L, Fisher C W, and Udall D H 1906 The spavin group of lamenesses *Proceedings 42nd Annual Conference American Veterinary Medical Association*

Willis R A and Rudduck H B 1943 Testicular teratomas in horses *Journal Pathology Bacteriology* 55: 165-171

Willoughby R A and McDonell W N 1979 Pulmonary function testing in horses *Veterinary Clinics North America: Large Animal Practice* 1: 171-196

Willoughby R A, MacDonald A E, McSherry B J, and Brown G 1972 Lead and zinc poisoning and the interaction between lead and zinc in the foal *Canadian Journal of Comparative Medicine* 36: 348-59

Wilmes H 1938 Kehlkopfkrebs beim Pferde *Zeitschrift Infektious Krankheiten Haustiere* 52: 328-30

Wilmes H and Schneider 1933 Eigneartige Kehlkopfmissbildung beim Pferd (Hypoplasia der Epiglottis) *Berliner Tierärztliche Wochenschrift* 49: 133-34

Wilson B J, Maronpot R R, and Hildebrandt P K 1973 Equine leukoencephalomalacia *Journal of the American Veterinary Medical Association* 163: 1293-95

Wilson B J, Garst J E, Linnabary R D, and Channel R B 1977 Perilla ketone: a potent lung toxin from the mint plant, *Perilla frutescens*, Britton *Science* 197: 573-574

Wilson J H 1989 Serial gastric endoscopy of foals in a research herd *Equine Veterinary Journal* (Suppl) 7: 138

Wilson M, Morrison H A, Palmer N C, Finley G, Dreumel A A van 1976 Myodegeneration and suspected selenium/vitamin E deficiency in horses *Journal of the American Veterinary Medical Association* 169: 213-217

Wilson R B and Haffner J C 1987 Right atrioventricular atresia and ventricular septal defect in a foal *Cornell Veterinarian* 77: 187-191

Wilson T M, Ross P F, Rice L G, Osweiler G D, Nelson H A, Owens D L, Plattner R D, Reggiardo C, Noon T H, and Pickrell J W 1990 Fumonisin B_1 levels associated with an epizootic of equine leukoencephalomalacia *Journal of Veterinary Diagnostic Investigation* 2: 213-216

Wimberley H C, Andrews E J, and Haschek W M 1977 Diaphragmatic hernia in the horse: a review of the literature and an analysis of six additional cases *Journal of the American Veterinary Medical Association* 170: 1404-1407

Wimberly H C, Antonovych T T, and Lewis R M 1981 Focal glomerulosclerosis-like disease with nephrotic syndrome in a horse *Veterinary Pathology* 18: 692-694

Winder N C and von Fellenberg R 1987 Chronic small airway disease in horses slaughtered in Switzerland *Schweizer Archiv Tierheilkunde* 129: 585-593

Winder N C and von Fellenberg R 1988 Chronic small airway disease in the horse: Immunohistochemical evaluation of lungs with mild, moderate and severe lesions *Veterinary Record* 122: 181-183

Winder N C, Ehrenspreger F, Hermann M, Howald B, and von Fellenberg R 1988 Interstitial pneumonia in the horse: Two unusual cases *Equine Veterinary Journal* 20: 298-301

Winder N C, Gruenig G, Hermann M, Howald B, and von Fellenberg R 1989 Comparison of respiratory secretion cytology and pulmonary histology in horses *Journal of Veterinary Medicine A* 36: 32-38

Winder N C, Grünig G, Hermann M, and von Fellenberg R 1990 Fibrin/ fibrinogen in lungs and respiratory secretions of horses with chronic pulmonary disease *American Journal of Veterinary Research* 51: 945-949

Wingate D L 1992 Autonomic dysfunction and the gut. In Bannister R and Mathias C J (Eds) *Autonomic Failure* New York, Oxford

Winqvist G 1945 A topographical and etiological study of cases of fibrinous and ulcerative endocarditis in some of our domestic animals *Skandinavisk Veterinärtidskrift* 35

Wintzer H-J 1986 *Equine Diseases* Berlin, Springer-Verlag

Wintzer H-J and Dämmrich K 1971 Untersuchungen zur Pathogenese der sogenannten Strahlbeinlahmheit des Pferdes *Berliner Münchener Tierärztliche Wochenschrift* 84: 221-225

Wintzer H-J and Glasnap H von 1973 Über eine localae Myopathie bei Trabbenpferden *Berliner Münchener Tierärztliche Wochenschrift* 86: 221-225

Wirstad H F 1948 En förlopig meddelse om den patologiste hoftleddsluxasjon hos Dolehest *Festskrift Prof Per Tuff*,

Oslo

Wirstad H F 1962 Fractures of the proximal sesamoid bones in the horse *Nordiska Veterinärmedicin* 14: 33

Wirstad H F 1963 Fractures of the proximal sesamoid bones in the horse *Veterinary Record* 75: 509-13

Wirth D and Pommer A 1931 Akropachie beim Pferde *Archiv Tierheilkunde* 63: 230-8

Wirth K 1985 Statistiche Auswertung der Pferdsektionen in Institut für Pathologie der tierärtzlichen Hochschule Hannover zwischen 1933-1983. *Dissertation*, Hannover

Wirth W W and Blaton F S 1970 A review of the Culicoides nigrigenus group, with two new species *Entomological News* 81(6): 141-151

Wiseman A, Petrie L, and Murray M 1974 Diarrheoa in the horse as a result of alimentary lymphosarcoma *Veterinary Record* 95(20): 454-457

Wisner E R, O'Brien T R, Pool R R, Pascoe J R, Koblik P, Hornoff W J, and Poulos P W 1991 Osteomyelitis of the axial border of the proximal sesamoid bones in seven horses *Equine Veterinary Journal* 23: 383-89

Witmer R 1953 The diagnosis, aetiology, and therapy of periodic ophthalmia in the horse *Schweiz Arch Tierheilk* 95: 419-427

Wolkoff K 1924 Über Altersveränderungen der Arterien bei Tieren *Virchows Archiv* 252: 208-28

Wong P L, Nickel L S, Bowling A T, and Steffey E P 1986 Clinical survey of antibodies against red blood cells in horses after homologous blood transfusion *American Journal of Veterinary Research* 47: 2566-2571

Woo S L-Y, Ritter M A, Amiel D, Sanders T M, Gomez M A 1970 The biomechanical and biochemical properties of swine tendons—long term effects of exercise on the digital extensors *Connective Tissue Research* 7: 177-83

Woo S L-Y, Ritter D A, Sanders T M, Gomez M A, Kuei S C, Garfin S R, and Akeson W H 1980 The biomechanical and biochemical properties of swine tendons—long term effects of exercise on the digital extensors. *Connective Tissue Research* 7: 177-183

Wood R N and Davis G R 1950 The correlation of periodic ophthalmia with leptospira agglutinins in horses *American Journal of Ophthalmology* 33: 961-965

Woods A C and Chesney A M 1930 The transmission of periodic ophthalmia by means of a filterable agent *Journal Experimental Medicine* 52: 637-47

Woods G L, Garcia M C, and Kenney R M 1980 Variations in testicular size of Standardbred stallions *Proceedings of the American Association of Equine Practitioners* 26: 117-121

Woods P R, Helman R G, Schmitz, G G 1993 Granulomatous enteritis and cutaneous arteritis in a horse *Journal of the American Veterinary Medical Association* 203(11): 1 1573-1575

Wright J A and Giles C J 1986 Diffuse carcinomatosis involving the meninges of a horse *Equine Veterinary Journal* 18: 147-150

Wright J A and Hodson N P 1988 Pathological changes in the brain in equine grass sickness *Journal of Comparative Pathology* 98: 247-252

Wright J A, Fordyce P, and Edington N 1987 Neuritis of the cauda equina in the horse *Journal of Comparative Pathology* 97: 667-675

Wyburn R S and Goulden B E 1974 Fractures of the equine carpus: a report of 57 cases *New Zealand Veterinary Journal* 22: 133-42

Wyman M, Rings M D, Tarr M J, and Alden C L 1977 Immunotherapy in equine sarcoid: a report of two cases *Journal of the American Veterinary Medical Association* 171: 449-451

Yager J A 1987 The pathogenesis of *Rhodococcus equi* pneumonia in foals *Veterinary Microbiology* 14: 225-232

Yager J A and Scott D W 1985 In Jubb, K, Kennedy P C, and Palmer N (Eds) *Pathology of Domestic Animals* 3rd Ed Orlando, Academic Press

Yamashita K, Fujinaga T, Okumura M, Takiguchi M, Tsunoda N, and Mizuno S 1991 Serum C-reactive protein (CRP) in horses: the effect of ageing sex, delivery and inflammations on its concentrations *Journal of Veterinary Medical Science* 53: 1019-1024

Yenne K, Dreesen D W, Moore J N, and Embertson R M 1991 A retrospective study of colonic disorders in central Kentucky (1975-1990) *4th Equine Colic Research Symposium* Athens, Georgia

Yilma T, Perryman L E, and McGuire T C 1982 Deficiency of interferon-gamma but not interferon-beta in Arabian foals with severe combined immunodeficiency *Journal Immunology* 129: 931-933

Yoeli M, Roden A T, and Abbott J D 1948 Smears from subcutaneous nodules of a mule showing microfilaria from *Onchocerca* sp. *Transactions of the Royal Society of Tropical Medicine and Hygiene* 41: 444

Yong-ji W, Pei-wei G and Pei-sheng L 1982 Japanese B encephalitis virus infection of horses during the first epidemic season following entry into an infected area *Chinese Medical Journal* 95: 63-66

Yoshihara T, Kanemaru T, Hasegawa M, Tomoika Y, Kaneko M, Kiryu K, Wada R, and Watanabe O 1985 *Micronema deletrix* infection in the central nervous system of a horse *Bulletin Equine Research Institute* 22: 30-37

Young S, Brown W W, and Klinger B 1970a Nigropallidal encephalomalacia in horses fed Russian knapweed *American Journal of Veterinary Research* 31: 1393-1404

Young S, Brown W W, and Klinger B 1970b Nigropallidal encephalomalacia in horses caused by ingestion of weeds of the genus *Centaurea Journal of the American Veterinary Medical Association* 157: 1602-1605

Yovich J V, Hilbert B J, and McGill C A 1982 Fractures of the distal phalanx in horses *Australian Veterinary Journal* 59: 180-82

Yovich J V, McIlwraith C W, and Stashak T S 1985a Osteochondritis dissecans of the sagittal ridge of the third metacarpal and metatarsal bones in horses *Journal of the American Veterinary Medical Association* 186: 1186-91

Yovich J V, Stashak T S, and Bertone A L 1985b Incarceration of small intestine through rents in the gastrosplenic ligament in the horse *Veterinary Surgery* 14:

303-6

Yovich J V, McIlwraith C W, and Stashak T S 1986 Osteochondrosis dissecans am sagittalen Rollkamm von McIII und MtIII beim Pferd *Pferdeheilkunde* 2: 109-13,115-6

Zakrzewski A 1970 Vol 5 Mund u. Rachenhöhle mit Speicheldrusen In Dobberstein J, Pallaske G, and Stünzi H (Eds) *Joest's Handbuch der Speziellen Pathologische Anatomie der Haustiere* 3rd Ed Berlin, Parey

Zeller R, Hertsch B, and Samy M T 1978 Vorkommen und Klinische Beurteilung der Osteochondrosis dissecans (OCD) im talocruralgelenk beim Pferd *Deutsche Tierärztliche Wochenschrift* 85: 223-26

Zenker W 1992 Hufprobleme bei Lipizzanern und ein Behandlungsversuch mit Biotin *Dissertation* (in progress), Zurich

Zeskov B 1959 A study of the discontinuity of the fibula in the horse *American Journal of Veterinary Research* 30: 852

Zhang J, Ricketts S W, and Tanner S J 1990 Antisperm antibodies in the semen of a stallion following testicular trauma *Equine Veterinary Journal* 22: 138-141

Zicker S C, Marty G D, Carlson G P, Madigan J E, Smith J M, Goetzman B W 1990 Bilateral renal dysplasia with nephron hypoplasia in a foal *Journal of the American Veterinary Medical Association* 196: 2001-2005

Zicker S C, Spensley M S, Rogers Q R, and Willits N H 1991 Concentrations of amino acids in the plasma of neonatal foals with septicemia *American Journal of Veterinary Research* 152: 1010-1013

Ziegler M 1969 Muskeln, Sehnen, Schleimbeutel In Dobberstein J, Pallaske G, and Stünzi H (Eds) *Joest's Handbuch der Speziellen pathologishcen Anatomie der Haustiere* 3rd Ed Berlin, Parey

Ziemer E L, Parker H R, Carlson G P, and Smith B P 1987a Clinical features and treatment of renal tubular acidosis in two horses *Journal of the American Veterinary Medical Association* 190: 295-296

Ziemer E L, Whitlock R H, Palmer J E, and Spencer P A 1987b Clinical and hematologic variable in ponies with experimentally induced equine ehrlichial colitis (Potomac horse fever) *American Journal of Veterinary Research* 48: 63-67

Zietzschmann O and Krölling O 1955 *Lehrbuch der Entwicklungsgeschichte der Haustiere* Berlin, Parey

Zietzschmann O, Ackerknecht E, and Grau H 1943 *Ellenberger-Baum Handbuch der Vergleichenden Anatomie der Haustiere, 18th Edition*, Berlin, Springer

Zitnik W 1945 Über die Verdauungsleukocytose beim Pferd Cited *Veterinary Bulletin* 15: 272

Zschokke E 1892 Untersuchungen über das Verhaltniss der Knochenbildung *Anatomical Institut Orell Fussli*, Zurich

Zschokke E 1898 Über degenerationsformen der Stammesmuskulatur *Schweizer Archiv Tierheilkunde* 40: 97-113

Zschokke E 1900 Vol 4 Die Krankheiten der Knochen In *Bayer-Fröhner Handbuch der tierärztlicher chirurgie und Geburtshilfe* Vienna, Braumuller

Zuill W L 1894 Typhoid fever; or, contagious influenza in the horse *American Veterinary Revue* 17: 1-13, 91-101, 193-202

Index

ISBN 0-8138-2334-X

9 780813 823348 90000>